Medical Radiology

Diagnostic Imaging

Series Editors

Hans-Ulrich Kauczor
Paul M. Parizel
Wilfred C. G. Peh

The book series *Medical Radiology - Diagnostic Imaging* provides accurate and up-to-date overviews about the latest advances in the rapidly evolving field of diagnostic imaging and interventional radiology. Each volume is conceived as a practical and clinically useful reference book and is developed under the direction of an experienced editor, who is a world-renowned specialist in the field. Book chapters are written by expert authors in the field and are richly illustrated with high quality figures, tables and graphs. Editors and authors are committed to provide detailed and coherent information in a readily accessible and easy-to-understand format, directly applicable to daily practice.

Medical Radiology - Diagnostic Imaging covers all organ systems and addresses all modern imaging techniques and image-guided treatment modalities, as well as hot topics in management, workflow, and quality and safety issues in radiology and imaging. The judicious choice of relevant topics, the careful selection of expert editors and authors, and the emphasis on providing practically useful information, contribute to the wide appeal and ongoing success of the series. The series is indexed in Scopus.

Michael Fuchsjäger
Elizabeth Morris · Thomas Helbich
Editors

Breast Imaging

Diagnosis and Intervention

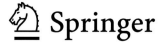

Editors
Michael Fuchsjäger
Department of Radiology
Medical University of Graz
Graz, Austria

Thomas Helbich
Department of Biomedical Imaging and
Image-guided Therapy
Medical University of Vienna
Vienna, Austria

Elizabeth Morris
Department of Radiology
University of California, Davis (UCD)
School of Medicine
Sacramento, CA
USA

ISSN 0942-5373 ISSN 2197-4187 (electronic)
Medical Radiology
ISSN 2731-4677 ISSN 2731-4685 (electronic)
Diagnostic Imaging
ISBN 978-3-030-94920-4 ISBN 978-3-030-94918-1 (eBook)
https://doi.org/10.1007/978-3-030-94918-1

© Springer Nature Switzerland AG 2022
This work is subject to copyright. All rights are reserved by the Publisher, whether the whole or part of the material is concerned, specifically the rights of translation, reprinting, reuse of illustrations, recitation, broadcasting, reproduction on microfilms or in any other physical way, and transmission or information storage and retrieval, electronic adaptation, computer software, or by similar or dissimilar methodology now known or hereafter developed.
The use of general descriptive names, registered names, trademarks, service marks, etc. in this publication does not imply, even in the absence of a specific statement, that such names are exempt from the relevant protective laws and regulations and therefore free for general use.
The publisher, the authors and the editors are safe to assume that the advice and information in this book are believed to be true and accurate at the date of publication. Neither the publisher nor the authors or the editors give a warranty, expressed or implied, with respect to the material contained herein or for any errors or omissions that may have been made. The publisher remains neutral with regard to jurisdictional claims in published maps and institutional affiliations.

This Springer imprint is published by the registered company Springer Nature Switzerland AG
The registered company address is: Gewerbestrasse 11, 6330 Cham, Switzerland

To my parents Edith and Norbert, to my wife Nina and to my children Sophie, Maximilian, Livia, Alexander, Johannes and Laia, for their love and support; without you this wouldn't have been possible.

– Michael Fuchsjäger

To my children who are my greatest joy...

– EAM

To my parents, Ilse and Rudolf, who inspired me and helped me live my dreams.

To my wife, Angelika, who supports me endlessly and makes life rich in love.

To my children, Matthaeus Elisa, Julian Augustus, and Klara Paulina, who make everything worthwhile.

– Thomas Helbich

Preface

The book you are about to read is important, not only because breast cancer remains a major health problem globally—in Europe and in the USA every year 576,000 and 264,000 women are diagnosed with breast cancer, respectively—but also as it contains the most up-to-date information on breast imaging, screening, diagnosis, intervention and therapy. Advances in screening, diagnosis and therapeutics happen at an accelerated pace. In order to keep up we need to have an open mind, and a nimble ability to adapt rapidly, a skill that is fortunately innate to radiologists.

Through the imaging options available for women these days, not just mammography but also digital breast tomosynthesis, ultrasound, and breast MRI, the radiologist could improve the rate of successful treatments within cancer patients significantly, with an outcome not just for the lives of women but also for their families and society in general.

By focusing on personal screening as an additional testing to the mammogram, we radiologists strive to lower the risk of each woman with breast cancer. Radiology sets new measures in this field, introducing quality standards, reporting standards and now the implementation of artificial intelligence into the workflow and interpretations of mammograms. We no longer remain hidden behind our results; we have become the face of the breast care expert, doing biopsy procedures, discussing results and managing options with and for our patients.

And we love being so close to our patients, being engaged in the whole diagnostic and therapeutic journey from detection at screening through diagnostic imaging, image-guided biopsy, staging, minimally invasive treatment, treatment monitoring and follow-up.

We are the gatekeepers in medicine who help start the process getting our patients to be good or at least better in the end. As a multi-discipline matter we spend a large amount of time talking and consulting with colleagues from Surgery, Gynaecology, Oncology, Pathology as well as Family Medicine, to take care of patients in the best possible way.

All of this makes Breast Imaging the probably most exciting subspecialty and brings us even closer to our patients, involving us into the whole diagnostic and therapeutic journey. We are not just doctors, we are also advisers, carers and guides through a sometimes-difficult pathway which challenges us to find the best outcome for each woman.

By reading this book you will come to an even better understanding of the multiple roles of the breast imager and the numerous aspects of breast imaging from screening to minimally invasive therapy, including AI. Almost everything you need to know on breast imaging and breast intervention can be found in this book. All imaging techniques are brilliantly described from intermediate to expert knowledge. Furthermore, there is a focus on breast interventions with all guidance methods as well as image-guided minimally invasive therapy, a step into the future. Burning topics like breast density, the practical value of artificial intelligence or the most challenging histopathologies with high-risk lesions and DCIS are given special attention.

The highest standard, our maximum effort, the closest working together, the best findings, all come together for the one purpose we all serve, the well-being of the women who come to us for help. They are our focus and they are the reason this book is in your hands, to improve the rate of successful outcome within our breast cancer patients.

Graz, Austria   Michael Fuchsjäger
Sacramento, CA, USA   Elizabeth Morris
Vienna, Austria   Thomas Helbich

Contents

Mammography and Digital Breast Tomosynthesis: Technique 1
Ioannis Sechopoulos

Contrast-Enhanced Mammography 25
Anand Narayan and Maxine Jochelson

Mammography Screening 43
Carin Meltzer and Per Skaane

Stereotactic Guided Breast Interventions 69
Daniela Bernardi and Vincenzo Sabatino

How to Use Breast Ultrasound 95
Boris Brkljačić, Gordana Ivanac, Michael Fuchsjäger,
and Gabriel Adelsmayr

Breast Ultrasound: Advanced Techniques 113
Andy Evans

Automated Breast Ultrasound 127
Ritse M. Mann

Ultrasound-Guided Interventions 143
Eva Maria Fallenberg

Breast MRI: Techniques and Indications 165
Francesco Sardanelli, Luca A. Carbonaro, Simone Schiaffino,
and Rubina M. Trimboli

Abbreviated Breast MRI: Short and Sweet? 215
Michelle Zhang, Victoria L. Mango, and Elizabeth Morris

Breast MRI: Multiparametric and Advanced Techniques 231
Maria Adele Marino, Daly Avendano, Thomas Helbich, and Katja
Pinker

MRI-Guided Breast Interventions 259
Karim Rebeiz and Elizabeth Morris

Imaging the Axilla 271
Fleur Kilburn-Toppin

Imaging of Ductal Carcinoma In Situ (DCIS) 287
Paola Clauser, Marianna Fanizza, and Pascal A. T. Baltzer

Cystic and Complex Cystic and Solid Lesions 303
Panagiotis Kapetas and Thomas Helbich

High-Risk Lesions of the Breast: Diagnosis and Management...... 337
Maria Adele Marino, Katja Pinker, and Thomas Helbich

Minimal Invasive Therapy 359
Gabriel Adelsmayr, Gisela Sponner, and Michael Fuchsjäger

Post-therapy Evaluation (Including Breast Implants)............. 375
Silvia Pérez Rodrigo and Julia Camps-Herrero

Impact and Assessment of Breast Density 419
Georg J. Wengert, Katja Pinker, and Thomas Helbich

Artificial Intelligence in Breast Imaging....................... 435
Xin Wang, Nikita Moriakov, Yuan Gao, Tianyu Zhang,
Luyi Han, and Ritse M. Mann

Mammography and Digital Breast Tomosynthesis: Technique

Ioannis Sechopoulos

Contents

1	**Introduction**	2
2	**Basics of X-Ray-Based Breast Imaging**	2
	2.1 Breast Lesions	3
	2.2 Digital Mammography	4
	2.3 Digital Breast Tomosynthesis	4
	2.4 Mammographic Views	6
3	**Imaging Systems**	6
	3.1 X-Ray Source	7
	3.2 Compression Paddle	8
	3.3 Anti-scatter Grid	8
	3.4 Digital Detector	9
4	**Breast Compression**	10
5	**Clinical Performance of Digital Breast Tomosynthesis**	11
	5.1 Lesion Visibility	11
	5.2 Detection	11
	5.3 Diagnosis	13
6	**Population Screening with Digital Breast Tomosynthesis**	13
7	**Radiation Dose**	15
	7.1 Basics of Breast Dosimetry	15
	7.2 Meaning of Breast Dose Estimates	16
	7.3 Mammography vs. Tomosynthesis Dose	16
	7.4 Radiation Dose vs. Clinical Performance	18
	7.5 Total Breast Dose During a Screening Examination	18
	References	19

I. Sechopoulos (✉)
Department of Medical Imaging, Radboud University
Medical Center, Nijmegen, The Netherlands

Dutch Expert Centre for Screening (LRCB),
Nijmegen, The Netherlands

Technical Medical Centre, University of Twente,
Enschede, The Netherlands
e-mail: ioannis.sechopoulos@radboudumc.nl

© Springer Nature Switzerland AG 2022
M. Fuchsjäger et al. (eds.), *Breast Imaging*, Medical Radiology Diagnostic Imaging,
https://doi.org/10.1007/978-3-030-94918-1_1

Abstract

The introduction of mammography as a radiographic imaging modality optimized for breast imaging revolutionized breast cancer care. Throughout the decades, conventional, screen-film-based mammography has given way to digital mammography, resulting in many benefits, including a streamlined workflow and improved performance in certain subgroups of patients. More importantly, the introduction of digital technology in mammographic imaging resulted in the development of even more advanced technologies, such as digital breast tomosynthesis. Tomosynthesis, with its ability to result in pseudo-tomographic imaging of the breast with a system that has the same footprint and workflow as mammography, has had an important impact in the breast imaging clinic.

In this chapter, the basic concepts of X-ray-based breast imaging, common for both mammography and tomosynthesis, are reviewed. The major components of these imaging systems are described, and the resulting and potential clinical and screening performance of these modalities is discussed. Finally, considering their widespread use in asymptomatic women during screening, the dosimetry aspects of X-ray-based breast imaging are explained.

1 Introduction

Even after years of research and development of more advanced imaging techniques, some of them involving acquisition of functional, multiparametric, and/or dynamic data, mammography is still the most common modality used for breast cancer imaging. Its relatively high performance, ease of use, affordability, few requirements for installation, and speed of acquisition and interpretation have made it, and its newly developed offspring, digital breast tomosynthesis, the main workhorse of breast imaging.

Mammography is based on the principles of standard radiography, but modified and optimized to image the breast. Due to specific clinical and physical requirements, breast imaging, especially for detection of features that suggest the presence of cancer, necessitated the development of a separate system. The end result is a device that can acquire an image of the breast in a couple of seconds, with the ability to depict both very fine calcifications and very subtle masses and spiculations at the same time. These different suspicious features, which can be the result of malignancy, require very different imaging capabilities, a problem that has been solved by the optimization of a radiography system for this specific clinical application.

Due to its benefits, mammography is not only used in clinics and hospitals for diagnosis of breast disease in (mostly) women presenting with symptoms, but more importantly, for screening for breast cancer in asymptomatic women. Mammographic screening for breast cancer has become common practice throughout the industrialized world, with some countries even implementing population-based screening programs. As part of these programs, all women of a certain age group are invited to undergo mammographic imaging for detection of suspicious findings that may indicate the presence of breast cancer. This widespread use of mammography can only be performed due to its aforementioned advantages, such as noninvasiveness, affordability, ease and speed of use, and high detection performance.

In this chapter, the basics of mammography and digital breast tomosynthesis, their capabilities and limitations, clinical use, and other characteristics, such as radiation dose, are discussed.

2 Basics of X-Ray-Based Breast Imaging

Mammography is an X-ray-based transmission imaging technique. This means that the mammographic image is formed by transmitting a field of X-rays through the breast and detecting the X-rays that exit it. The resulting mammogram shows the differences in how the different breast tissues attenuate the X-rays traveling through them (Fig. 1). At the macroscopic scale, in terms

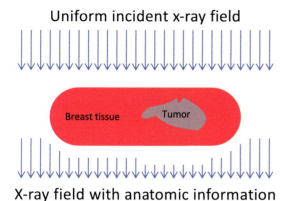

Fig. 1 Diagram of the acquisition of a mammogram. An incident X-ray field, as uniform as possible, is emitted towards the breast. The tissue attenuates the field, with each type of tissue attenuating the field differently. The differences in the intensity of the X-ray field that exit the other side of the breast reflect the differences in attenuation of the tissues contained inside the breast. The detector captures the X-rays and the resulting image is related to the amount of X-ray energy arriving at the detector. In this diagram, the length of the arrows representing the X-rays corresponds to the number of X-rays at each location

of absorption of X-rays, the breast can be assumed to be composed of largely three different tissues: skin, adipose, and fibroglandular tissue. Adipose tissue attenuates X-rays less than fibroglandular tissue (Hammerstein et al. 1979). Therefore, a dense area of the breast, composed mainly of fibroglandular tissue, appears brighter in a mammogram than a more fatty area.[1] Meanwhile, malignant tissue attenuates X-rays at a very similar rate to that of fibroglandular tissue (Hammerstein et al. 1979; Johns and Yaffe 1987). This means that a malignant lesion can appear with the same brightness in a mammogram as normal fibroglandular tissue. Therefore, detection of lesions depends on their irregular shape being visible against an adipose background. If a lesion is completely surrounded or superimposed by fibroglandular tissue, then it might not be visible. This is why the sensitivity of mammography is substantially reduced with increasing breast density (Wanders et al. 2017).

2.1 Breast Lesions

The main types of suspicious features that mammography aims to depict in the detection and diagnosis of breast cancer are the following:

- Masses: In general, dense areas, usually with low contrast, of round, oval, or irregular shape, well-defined or ill-defined margins which could include spiculations (thin, low contrast, fiber-like structures) radiating outwards. Irregular shape, ill-defined margins, presence of spiculations, and other features are markers of malignancy.
- Architectural distortions: Distortions in the normal parenchymal pattern of the breast, with no associated visible mass. These include radiating spiculations, which are fine fiber-like tissues of low contrast.
- Microcalcifications: Specks (usually high contrast) that could be as small as 100 μm in size, usually grouped in clusters. Their size and shape, and more importantly the shape and distribution of the cluster, are determinants of the probability of malignancy present.
- Asymmetries: Fibroglandular tissue patterns tend to be symmetric between the left and right breasts. Deviations from this, i.e., presence of asymmetry, can be markers of malignant development.

Although other signs of pathologic processes exist, these are the main features of breast cancer in mammograms, and, importantly, the ones that define the capabilities that a mammography system must possess. As can be seen, soft-tissue lesions (masses and architectural distortions, especially) require high contrast, while depiction of calcifications requires very high spatial resolution. Mammography systems are optimized to

---

[1] Dense areas appear brighter in the already processed "for presentation" mammogram. In the original raw "for processing" mammogram, dense areas appear darker. The image is inverted during the image processing that every digital mammogram undergoes.

deliver these two demanding capabilities in the same image, a challenging feat.

2.2 Digital Mammography

Until the turn of the century, mammography was performed using screen-film. However, the development of digital detectors allowed for the introduction of digital mammography. The benefits of digital over screen-film mammography are numerous, the most important being the following:

- Linear response with high dynamic range: Digital detectors cannot be under- or overexposed (until saturated), in terms of resulting contrast. Whereas films had a narrow exposure range in which an image had adequate contrast, changes in the overall exposure in digital mammography will only affect the level of noise, but not the contrast between tissues. This reduces the number of retakes.
- Lower dose: Especially in more recent generation of digital mammography, the dose required per acquisition has been substantially reduced (Hendrick et al. 2010; Bouwman et al. 2015).
- Easy transmission and archiving: Of course, a digital signal is much easier to transmit and archive than a film.
- Improved workflow: Images can be checked immediately after acquisition at the acquisition workstation, resulting in a faster check of the need for a retake.
- Production of a digital image: This might be the most important advantage, since it allows for easy post-processing of the image to optimize its display, and, perhaps even more importantly, for more advanced imaging methods, such as contrast-enhanced spectral mammography and digital breast tomosynthesis.

Of course, screen-film mammography is cheaper and was the established technology, so there was a significant cost in upgrading to digital mammography. Finally, the spatial resolution of screen-film mammography is superior to that of digital mammography.

Even though the DMIST trial showed only a detection performance improvement with digital mammography over screen-film for specific subgroups of the general population it did not show an overall detection performance improvement with digital mammography over screen-film (Pisano et al. 2005). However, the other benefits of digital mammography beyond clinical performance, as listed above, have resulted in screen-film mammography being completely phased out in the developed world.

2.3 Digital Breast Tomosynthesis

Digital mammography, however, is not without limitations. Chief among them is its 2D nature, which results in the need to represent the 3D breast tissue distribution information onto a single 2D plane. This results in tissue superposition, where two features of the breast that are actually separated in the vertical direction coincide in the mammographic image. If one of these features is a malignant lesion, it could be rendered undetectable due to it being superimposed by the other, resulting in a loss of sensitivity. In addition, if both of these tissues are normal, they could project in such a way that they appear to be something suspicious, resulting in a loss of specificity. Therefore, the ability to represent the breast in its true 3D form, or at least in a form that approximates it, held great promise in improving clinical performance.

With the introduction of digital detectors for breast imaging, Niklason et al. introduced in 1997 the first practical study on digital breast tomosynthesis (Niklason et al. 1997). One of the major advantages of digital breast tomosynthesis, also called *limited-angle tomography*, is its similarity to mammography. As can be seen in Fig. 2, in its simplest implementation, breast tomosynthesis involves the acquisition of several mammography-like images, *projections*, while the X-ray source rotates around the compressed breast. By acquiring a number of such projections over a certain angular range, enough information about the

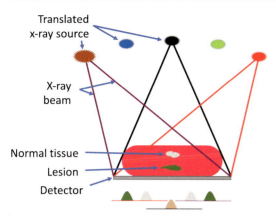

Fig. 2 Diagram of the acquisition of a digital breast tomosynthesis image. The breast is positioned in the same manner as for mammography. The X-ray source rotates over a limited angle around the breast, acquiring several low-dose mammography-like images at each preset acquisition angle. Depending on the vertical location of the features inside the breast, these shift differently in their location in each projection. This provides enough information to the reconstruction algorithm to generate a pseudo-3D image of the breast volume

relative position of the different tissues in the breast is obtained that a *pseudo*-3D image of the breast can be reconstructed.

As a result of the reconstruction process, the imaged breast is represented as a stack of slices parallel to the detector entrance (and therefore to the breast support table). It is important to note that tomosynthesis is not a true 3D modality, given that the limited angle covered during projection acquisition does not allow for a full recovery of the vertical (direction perpendicular to the detector surface) distribution of tissue. Rather, the tissues that are actually located above and below the currently viewed tomosynthesis slice are preferentially blurred out from the image, but not necessarily completely removed.

The visibility of these out-of-plane structures depends on their contrast and on the angular range of the acquisition (Sechopoulos and Ghetti 2009). A large or very bright signal, e.g., a large calcification, might be visible in many or all tomosynthesis slices, while a small or faint mass might be well constrained to only appearing in a few slices, even if beyond the ones that it actually occupies (Fig. 3). Therefore, strictly speaking the reconstructed tomosynthesis slices do not have a

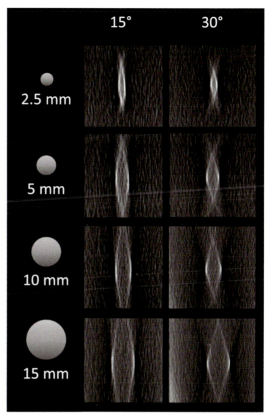

Fig. 3 Simulated digital breast tomosynthesis images of a circular disk of various sizes for two different total angular ranges, shown from the side. The size of the disk affects over how many slices, beyond the ones it actually occupies, the signal can still be seen. As can be seen, therefore, being a pseudo-3D modality, the effective vertical resolution in DBT is size and contrast dependent. (Image courtesy of Dr. John Boone, from Nosratieh et al., "Comprehensive assessment of the slice sensitivity profiles in breast tomosynthesis and breast CT," *Medical Physics*. 39(12), 7254–7261 (2012). © American Association of Physicists in Medicine)

specific thickness, since what is depicted in them depends on the nature of the signal. As done by Niklason et al. in their original paper, most tomosynthesis systems today still reconstruct one slice every 1 mm in the vertical direction. This does not mean that the slices are 1 mm thick, but rather that they are separated by 1 mm.

Even though tomosynthesis results in a limited vertical spatial resolution, its ability to partially suppress the effect of tissue superposition is enough to have an important impact on the sensitivity and specificity for breast cancer detection, compared to standard digital mammography, as will be discussed in Sects. 5 and 6.

After the advent of tomosynthesis, which was at first introduced in the clinic as an adjunct to mammography, the vendors introduced the concept of the *synthetic mammogram*. The intent of this image was to generate a mammogram-like 2D image from the tomosynthesis data that would replace and avoid the acquisition of a real mammogram. For this, computer algorithms were developed that would summarize the information in the reconstructed tomosynthesis stack of slices into one 2D image, with the aim of replicating, as closely as possible, what a mammogram of that same breast would look like (Gur et al. 2012). Although initial attempts of generating these synthetic mammograms resulted in a loss of performance compared to the use of real digital mammograms, even when used together with the tomosynthesis stacks, subsequent generations of synthetic mammograms have been shown to result in equivalent performance as digital mammograms, again, when in combination with the tomosynthesis stacks (Gur et al. 2012; Skaane et al. 2014).

Synthetic mammogram-generating algorithms have continued to evolve, including even introducing a rotating synthetic for easier visibility of feature depth (Tani et al. 2014). However, although it is still not recommended to be used without the corresponding tomosynthesis stack for detection, early comparisons of the performance of synthetic mammograms compared to digital mammography and tomosynthesis stack have been performed, yielding disparate results (Murphy et al. 2018; Rodriguez-Ruiz et al. 2018c). In addition, currently it is thought that the synthetic mammogram should not attempt to replicate a mammogram as closely as possible, but rather should attempt to summarize the interesting features found in the tomosynthesis stack onto one 2D image. This is an important change in the thinking behind the synthetic mammogram. Given the original intent of the synthetic mammogram, its generation involved the attempting to replicate the projection of the 3D tissue information onto one plane. The newer role of the synthetic requires the analysis of the 3D image content from a diagnostic point of view, similar to that of a computer-aided detection or diagnosis algorithm.

2.4 Mammographic Views

For both mammographic and breast tomosynthesis acquisitions the breast is positioned, and compressed, in specific orientations. There are a number of possible views, some for imaging the whole breast (or as much tissue as possible), while others, such as spot or magnification views, involve special equipment and are aimed at imaging only a specific portion of the breast. In the former set are included the two most common views, which are the ones used for screening: the craniocaudal (CC) and the mediolateral oblique (MLO) views.

The CC view is acquired with the breast compression paddle and the breast support table horizontal (parallel to the floor), with the breast laid on the latter. For compression, the breast is compressed downward by the paddle until the appropriate level of compression is achieved. The MLO view involves rotating the mammography gantry to approximately 45°, positioning the support table on the lateral side of the patient, below the axilla, and compressing from the medial side. In the MLO view the pectoralis muscle should be included in the field of view. There are various guidelines that determine what is an appropriate positioning for these and the other mammographic views (e.g., Kopans 2007; European Commission 2006).

3 Imaging Systems

To acquire mammography (and digital breast tomosynthesis) images, mammography systems are adaptations of radiography systems optimized for the requirements of breast imaging. The main components of a (digital) mammography/tomosynthesis system are the X-ray source, the compression paddle, the breast support table, the anti-scatter grid, and the (digital) detector (Fig. 4). Of course, there are many other

Mammography and Digital Breast Tomosynthesis: Technique

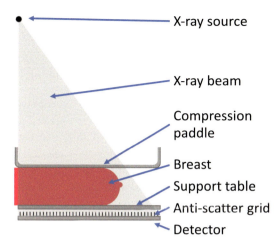

Fig. 4 Diagram showing the main components of a (digital) mammography/tomosynthesis system: X-ray source, compression paddle, breast support table, anti-scatter grid, and (digital) detector

components that make the acquisition of an image possible, but these, in addition to the acquisition workstation, form the main components of the image acquisition chain.

3.1 X-Ray Source

Although some alternative X-ray sources are being investigated, especially for digital breast tomosynthesis (Qian et al. 2012), currently all mammography systems use a traditional X-ray tube as the source of X-rays. X-ray tubes do not emit X-rays of a single energy, but rather a spectrum of X-rays, which include a range of X-ray energies, with a varying number of X-rays at each energy. The energy range of these X-rays and the number of X-rays at each energy level are important determinants in the trade-off among the resulting image contrast, image noise, and dose to the breast.

To obtain the high contrast required for breast imaging, the mammographic X-ray tube uses lower tube voltages than those used in any other radiographic application. For mammography, voltages between 25 and 32 kV are the most commonly used, while for tomosynthesis higher voltages, up to ~38 kV, may be used (Feng and Sechopoulos 2012). Using such low tube volt-

ages has the benefit of increasing tissue contrast, but results in the need for higher tube currents and/or exposure times; in mammography and tomosynthesis, exposures at anywhere between ~60 and ~200 mAs are commonplace, while general radiography values are typically below 10 mAs.

In addition to using lower voltages, mammographic X-ray tubes have traditionally used anodes of materials other than tungsten, the commonly used material in radiographic X-ray tubes. Tubes with anodes made of molybdenum and rhodium were common. However, current state-of-the-art mammography systems mostly use tungsten-anode X-ray tubes.

To further optimize the shape of the X-ray spectrum used to acquire the images, additional filtration is added to mammographic X-ray tubes. These filters are intended to preferentially absorb X-rays of specific energy ranges, for different purposes. In the first place, one fundamental requirement is to remove the X-rays of very low energy from the beam. These X-rays, if allowed to reach the breast, would all be absorbed in the first few mm of tissue, increasing the dose to the breast without providing any additional information to the resulting image. Depending on the X-ray tube anode, filtration is also used to absorb the higher energy X-rays emitted by the X-ray source. Allowing too many of these X-rays in the beam would, due to their high energy, reduce the contrast in the image. However, a balance needs to be achieved, since more X-rays being detected result in a lower image noise.

The motion of the X-ray source during digital breast tomosynthesis projection acquisition varies across commercial systems. In most tomosynthesis systems, the X-ray tube continues to rotate during acquisition of each projection. This decreases acquisition time and simplifies the motion mechanism, but introduces a loss of spatial resolution (Zhou et al. 2007). Currently one tomosynthesis vendor uses a stop-and-shoot method, in which the X-ray tube stops completely at each projection acquisition position before performing the projection acquisition. This has the benefit of avoiding the loss of spatial resolution due to the effective increase in the size of the

3.2 Compression Paddle

During acquisition of a mammographic or breast tomosynthesis image, the breast is mechanically compressed against the breast support table by a compression paddle. Compression paddles are composed of different types of transparent plastic, a few mm thick. They can be of different sizes, some being as large as the active detector area (usually 24 cm × 30 cm), while others are specific for diagnostic spot views, and therefore could be as small as 7.5 cm in diameter.

Compression paddles are designed to remain relatively horizontal and therefore parallel to the breast support, while some incorporate a flexible attachment to their holder, therefore tilting upwards towards the posterior of the breast as compression force is increased (Mawdsley et al. 2009; Tyson et al. 2009). Although this adjustment to the natural breast anatomy is proposed to result in decreased pain, in a study of 288 women undergoing screening no difference in perceived pain was detected, while the flexible paddle resulted in a reduction in the amount of fibroglandular tissue in the posterior section of the breast and a reduction in contrast (Broeders et al. 2015).

Other innovations aiming at reducing discomfort or pain and/or increasing tissue coverage have been introduced by several manufacturers, such as curved compression paddles, breast cushioning pads, and positioning sheets. In general, there have been few independent studies on the effectiveness of these devices in reducing discomfort or improving image quality, and the studies that have been performed report equivocal results (Timmers et al. 2015; Markle et al. 2004). Another option aimed at reducing patient discomfort is giving the women the option of performing the breast compression themselves (Kornguth et al. 1993; Balleyguier et al. 2018). This alternative has yielded very promising results, with no loss of image quality and with the women expressing a willingness to repeat the experience. The more recent study included a quantitative comparison on compression level, breast thickness, and average glandular dose between technologist compression and self-compression (Balleyguier et al. 2018). Perhaps surprisingly, the women applied a higher final compression force to themselves than that used by the technologist, resulting in statistically, though probably not clinically, significant reductions in compressed breast thickness and dose (Balleyguier et al. 2018).

3.3 Anti-scatter Grid

The most important component to the imaging chain in the breast support table, aside from the detector itself, is the anti-scatter grid. The inclusion of the signal from scattered X-rays in the image results in a reduction of contrast. To reduce this effect, a grid is located between the breast support and the detector entrance surface that preferentially absorbs scattered X-rays while transmitting through non-scattered (also called *primary*) X-rays. To accomplish this, anti-scatter grids consist of a series of very fine walls, called *septa*, closely spaced, that are either parallel to each other or focused so that they are parallel to the expected incident primary X-rays. Since scattered X-rays tend to travel at other, larger, angles, these are more probable to encounter one of these septa. Since the septa are composed of highly attenuating material, these X-rays are absorbed, while the primary X-rays that traverse the grid parallel to the septa continue straight through (Fig. 5).

Of course, since the septa has some thickness to them, they are not perfect in transmitting all primary X-rays. Therefore, in a high-spatial-resolution application like mammography, the shadows of the septa would be visible if this is not accounted for. To avoid this, the anti-scatter grid is moved during acquisition of the mammogram, so as to blur out the shadow of the septa. This, unfortunately, results in an added complexity to the system, since a motion system needs to be added within the detector housing to perform

Mammography and Digital Breast Tomosynthesis: Technique

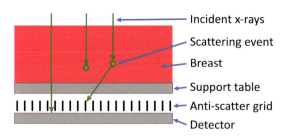

Fig. 5 Diagram showing how an anti-scatter grid works. X-rays that are incident on the breast may travel straight through (leftmost X-ray), be absorbed in the breast (center X-ray), or scatter in the breast (rightmost X-ray). The X-rays that do not undergo any interaction with the breast tissue travel through the anti-scatter grid parallel to the septa, so most of them are transmitted through. The X-rays that undergo a scattering event change direction, and are therefore more likely to be absorbed by the septa of the grid

this movement. In general, inadequate motion of the anti-scatter grid is the main source of artifacts when any grid-related problem arises in the images.

Two types of anti-scatter grid are common in mammography systems: linear and cellular. Linear grids have septa in one direction, and therefore need to be separated, for structural reasons, with a solid material, which is commonly carbon fiber. Cellular grids are composed of septa in both perpendicular directions, so they result in improved scatter rejection. The honeycomb-like structure of the septa eliminates the need for a solid material in between, so the space simply consists of the ambient air. Due to these factors, cellular grids result in a somewhat better contrast improvement compared to linear grids (Rezentes et al. 1999). However, cellular grids require a more complex motion path to blur out the septa shadow, and therefore are more prone to malfunctioning.

Given the varying incident angle of primary X-rays due to the rotating X-ray source, in general the anti-scatter grid is not used during acquisition of tomosynthesis projections. This results in the signal from the scattered X-rays being included in the acquired projections, which has been found to reduce contrast and signal-to-noise ratio (Liu et al. 2006; Wu et al. 2009). The digital breast tomosynthesis systems from one commercial vendor do use the anti-scatter grid during tomosynthesis, however.

Recently, one manufacturer has, for breast thicknesses up to 69 mm, replaced the use of the anti-scatter grid with a software-based post-acquisition correction for the effects of X-ray scatter (Fieselmann et al. 2013; Monserrat et al. 2018; Abdi et al. 2018). Removal of the anti-scatter grid avoids its (unwanted) attenuation of the primary X-rays. After evaluation of screening outcomes of over 70,000 patients, Abdi et al. found an equivalent performance with the software-based solution but with a reduction in the dose of 13–36%, depending on breast thickness.

3.4 Digital Detector

Currently two main types of digital detectors are used in commercial digital mammography/digital breast tomosynthesis systems, the indirect and the direct detectors.

Indirect detectors, only used by one system vendor, involve a two-stage detection process, in which the incident X-rays are first absorbed in a crystal layer that, upon absorption of each X-ray, emits light. This light is the one that is then actually detected and quantified by the digital detector, resulting in a digital signal that corresponds with the amount of X-ray energy arriving at the detector. This two-stage behavior is similar to that used in screen-film.

Direct detectors rely on a detection layer in which the incident and absorbed X-rays directly result in an electrical charge, which is then quantified by the electronics of the detector.

Both types of detectors result in digital images composed of ~2400–3500 pixels × 3000–4500 pixels, depending on their pixel size, to cover the current standard full field size of ~24 cm × 30 cm. Although previous-generation digital mammography systems included detectors of the order of 24 cm × 20 cm, the current larger area detectors minimize the number of tiled acquisitions that were needed to fully image a larger compressed breast. For tomosynthesis, it is also common, to decrease acquisition time, for the pixels to be *binned* (combined) during readout by 2 × 2 pixels. This results in pixels in tomosynthesis projections being double the size of those in mammography images, with a consequent loss of spatial resolution (Zhou et al. 2007). Newer and upcoming digital breast tomosynthesis systems do not perform this pixel binning, and count with newer electronics that still allows them to have fast image acquisitions.

During tomosynthesis acquisition, some imaging systems also rotate the detector with the X-ray source, while in others the detector remains stationary. To date, there do not seem to be any reports on if there is any benefit to either approach.

4 Breast Compression

There are many reasons why the breast is compressed during acquisition:

- Dose reduction: The thinner the breast, the lower the dose needed to acquire an adequate image.
- X-ray scatter reduction: Breast thickness is the largest factor in the amount of X-ray scatter generated in the breast, which reduces image contrast. Therefore, a thinner breast is important to reduce this effect.
- Tissue immobilization: To minimize the possibility of motion blur in the images, especially important for sharp depiction of calcifications, it is important to achieve good breast compression.
- Tissue coverage increase: During breast compression, additional posterior tissue is brought into the field of view.
- Exposure time reduction: A thinner breast, resulting in the need for lower exposure, allows for a faster acquisition, reducing the chances for tissue motion.
- Thickness equalization: Constant breast thickness results in a more consistent signal throughout the image, decreasing the requirements of dynamic range and post-processing.
- Geometric distortion reduction: Features farther away from the detector are magnified differently from those close to the detector, seeming larger even if of the same size. Breast compression minimizes this effect.

For all these reasons, adequate breast compression is important, allowing for the acquisition of adequate images at the lowest dose possible. Unfortunately, there are too many factors involved in determining what is an "appropriate" compression for each breast, with perhaps some of them unknown (e.g., overall breast density). Therefore, it is impossible to prospectively give appropriate, breast-specific guidelines of what level of compression should be achieved per acquisition. In some screening protocols, a minimum compression force is set, but these are general, not evidence based (Waade et al. 2017a, b), and probably result in many cases in over-compression of the breast (Agasthya et al. 2017; Lau et al. 2017).

It is obvious that not achieving an appropriate compression level, and therefore under-compressing the breast, can affect clinical performance due to increased tissue superposition, in addition to increase in dose, scatter, risk of motion blur, etc., resulting in a loss in sensitivity and a need for repeated acquisitions. However, it has also been found that over-compression may also affect clinical performance, resulting in lower sensitivity during screening (Holland et al. 2017b). Therefore, avoiding over-compression not only is important to not subject the woman to unnecessary pain or discomfort beyond what is truly necessary, but might also be important to optimize screening performance. The mechanisms involved as to why over-compressing might lead to a loss of detectability of some lesions is not yet understood.

In an effort to optimize the level of compression used for each patient, it has also been suggested that compression pressure as opposed to compression force should be the metric of choice to determine and set compression level. Pressure is defined as the amount of force divided by the area over which it is applied. Therefore, the same amount of compression force applied on a smaller breast results in a higher compression pressure. Some reports show that monitoring and setting

Mammography and Digital Breast Tomosynthesis: Technique

pressure level result in a more consistent level of compression compared to using force (de Groot et al. 2013).

5 Clinical Performance of Digital Breast Tomosynthesis

There have been a large number of studies comparing digital breast tomosynthesis compared to digital mammography both for detection and for diagnosis. These have included side-by-side comparative studies; multi-reader multi-case receiver operating characteristic retrospective interpretation studies; retrospective evaluation of performance in both the screening and diagnostic setting; and prospective population screening studies, among others. In addition, some review articles have already comprehensively evaluated the available literature (Baker and Lo 2011; Gilbert et al. 2016; Houssami and Skaane 2013; Vedantham et al. 2015; Hodgson et al. 2016; Yun et al. 2017). Here we will discuss some of the findings of these studies, although a comprehensive review of all such literature is beyond the scope of this chapter.

5.1 Lesion Visibility

Some early studies before and upon introduction of digital breast tomosynthesis to the clinical realm compared the depiction of lesions between this modality and that in mammography. In one of the earliest such studies, Poplack et al. compared the conspicuity of recalled lesions with breast tomosynthesis to that of diagnostic screen-film mammography (Poplack et al. 2007), finding that the former yielded superior lesion conspicuity more often than the latter. However, calcifications were judged better visualized with mammography in 8 out of the 14 available lesions.

Andersson et al. compared the visibility of 40 cancers in single-view tomosynthesis to single- and two-view digital mammography (Andersson et al. 2008). Interestingly, all lesions were chosen due to their subtlety or non-visibility in digital mammography, and the tomosynthesis view acquired was the one that depicted the lesion in mammography the least. Even in these conditions, breast tomosynthesis showed an improvement in visibility for 22 cancers vs. one-view mammography and 11 cancers vs. two-view mammography. The authors reported equal calcification detectability, with the distribution of the clusters well depicted but the morphology of the individual calcifications not as well visualized in tomosynthesis.

In a second study from the same group, Lång et al. (2014) investigated the visibility and the reasons behind discrepant interpretations of a subset of lesions from a previously performed observer study (Svahn et al. 2012). Breast tomosynthesis again depicted the lesions more clearly, with only 1 lesion out of 26 being assessed as more clearly visible in mammography. Lång et al. also performed a very interesting evaluation of these discrepant lesions, using the opinions of three expert radiologists to evaluate why the discrepant lesions were missed by each modality. The reason for each false negative was deemed to be as either due to a lack of visibility (is the lesion visible?), a lack in the radiographic visibility of lesion characteristics (does the lesion look malignant?), or an interpretative error by the reader (did the radiologist decide incorrectly?). All lesions were visible in tomosynthesis, and in only one case were its features not suggestive enough of malignancy to be recalled. In other words, the information to (correctly) detect the lesion was there in the vast majority of cases. This was not the case for digital mammography, for which the vast majority of lesions were deemed not visible or their features of malignancy not being sufficiently clear. These findings suggest a potential radical change in the conduct and performance of screening for breast cancer.

5.2 Detection

In the same study by Poplack et al. referred above, the addition of digital breast tomosynthesis to the digital mammography screening exam would have reduced the recall rate by approximately 40% (Poplack et al. 2007). However, the acquisition of tomosynthesis images was not performed during the same compression event as that of the mammographic image. Therefore, the effect of repositioning on the ability to resolve a substantial number of overlapping tissue-mimicking lesions is unknown.

Various multi-reader multi-case observer studies compared the detection performance of digital breast tomosynthesis to mammography (Rafferty et al. 2013, 2014; Gur et al. 2009; Clauser et al. 2016; Gennaro et al. 2010; Spangler et al. 2011; Wallis et al. 2012; Rodriguez-Ruiz et al. 2018b). In general, breast tomosynthesis, especially with two views, outperformed mammography for all types of lesions. The use of single-view tomosynthesis resulted in different conclusions, ranging from no benefit over two-view mammography to a substantial benefit. In one study, the increase in performance of single-view tomosynthesis was half of that of two-view tomosynthesis (Rafferty et al. 2014). Two studies specifically compared the performance in detecting calcifications, failing to detect a difference in the overall calcification detection (Clauser et al. 2016; Spangler et al. 2011), even though Spangler et al. did detect an increased sensitivity for calcification detection with mammography. These studies were important due to the early studies that showed a decrease in conspicuity of calcifications with tomosynthesis.

Retrospective studies on the impact of screening with digital breast tomosynthesis have reported, in general, an important decrease in the recall rate, and mostly an increase in the cancer detection rate (Destounis et al. 2014; Lourenco et al. 2015; Friedewald et al. 2014; Rose et al. 2013; McCarthy et al. 2014; Greenberg et al. 2014; Durand et al. 2015; Sharpe et al. 2016; Powell et al. 2017). It should be noted that, as is standard in the USA, the recall rate before introduction of breast tomosynthesis was in the vicinity of 10% for all studies. In addition, standard screening practice in the USA is the single reading of exams.

In Europe, meanwhile, investigators have performed large prospective screening trials to estimate the potential impact of breast tomosynthesis on screening performance (Skaane et al. 2013; Bernardi et al. 2016; Ciatto et al. 2013; Zackrisson et al. 2018; Romero Martin et al. 2018; Gilbert et al. 2015; Lång et al. 2016). Given some major differences in the way that screening is performed in these European programs compared to the institutional screening performed in the USA, the impact of this new modality was expected to be different. These trials show an important increase in the cancer detection rate, in the order of 30–40%, while the effect of tomosynthesis on recall rate seems to depend on the baseline (mammography) recall rate. Specifically, the effect of using breast tomosynthesis for screening is to tend to homogenize the recall rate, with higher baseline values decreasing, while low recall rates increasing, resulting in a recall rate approaching 3.5–5.0%.

All these observational studies and, especially, the prospective screening trials were performed with different tomosynthesis systems, and with a variability of acquisition and reading strategies. The use of two- and single-view tomosynthesis, tomosynthesis as an adjunct or a replacement of mammography, single-reading tomosynthesis while double-reading mammography, or single or double reading of both are all parameters that have been varied in these studies. In any case, overall it does appear that tomosynthesis increases the sensitivity of screening, with the aforementioned impact on recall rate. The use of single-view tomosynthesis, single-reading tomosynthesis, and/or tomosynthesis as a replacement of mammography seems to be feasible, but, given the variety in characteristics of the systems evaluated and the methods used, it is challenging to provide a single conclusion for what implementation is possible.

Of course, an actual outcome benefit from the introduction of tomosynthesis into screening would be a reduction in interval cancers and, eventually, mortality. Given its relatively new introduction, any impact that screening with breast tomosynthesis has on mortality would be impossible to evaluate for many more years to come. Several studies have compared the interval cancer rates after standard mammographic screening compared to after screening with digital breast tomosynthesis, the majority of them in the context of the large prospective screening trials performed in Europe. For the most part, interval cancer rates have not been detected to be lower after tomosynthesis screening, or have been marginally lower with no statistical significance (McDonald et al. 2016; Bahl et al. 2017; Houssami et al. 2018; Hovda et al. 2019; Skaane et al. 2018; Bernardi et al. 2020; Conant et al. 2020). It should be noted, however, that these studies have not been powered for this endpoint, and therefore the numbers of interval cancers involved up to now have been low. New larger trials, like the TOSYMA trial in Germany and TMIST in North America, may provide a more definitive answer as to the impact of tomosynthesis screening on interval cancers.

5.3 Diagnosis

The impact of digital breast tomosynthesis in the diagnostic setting has also been evaluated. Brandt et al. compared, using a multi-reader multi-case observer study design, the diagnostic performance of two-view breast tomosynthesis to multiple-view diagnostic mammography for non-calcified lesions (Brandt et al. 2013). The average number of mammographic views acquired for the included cases was three. Tomosynthesis, even with the lower number of views acquired, achieved similar performance as that of diagnostic mammography.

Zuley et al. performed a similar study, comparing two-view breast tomosynthesis to multiple-view diagnostic mammography, again for the diagnosis of noncalcified lesions (Zuley et al. 2013). Zuley et al. did find an increase in performance, with a significant increase in the area under the ROC curve for tomosynthesis compared to that obtained for diagnostic mammography.

In a recent study, Bahl et al. performed a retrospective evaluation of the performance of breast tomosynthesis for the diagnosis of clinical concerns, excluding screening recall cases (Bahl et al. 2019). For these types of cases it was also found that tomosynthesis could outperform mammography, with an equivalent cancer detection rate, and a slightly decreased abnormal interpretation rate. A comparison of the number of views acquired per modality was not provided, however.

Of course, if breast tomosynthesis is used for screening, there would be no benefit in acquiring these images again during workup due to abnormal findings at screening. Therefore, it is expected that the diagnostic workup of screen-detected lesions, especially noncalcified ones, could involve only the use of ultrasound, to discard the presence of cysts.

6 Population Screening with Digital Breast Tomosynthesis

As mentioned previously, population screening with digital breast tomosynthesis has not yet been widely implemented. Even though the observational trials in the USA and the large prospective screening trials in Europe have shown important benefits with this modality, one of the major concerns of transitioning to tomosynthesis for population screening is the increase in reading time with this modality. Therefore, there has been an intense interest in reducing the effort in reading digital breast tomosynthesis exams for the detection of suspicious lesions at screening. It is possible that a combination of time-saving strategies could be the final solution to make breast tomosynthesis feasible for widespread screening. These strategies could include both the reduction of time spent in reviewing each case and reducing the number of cases needing human reading. A number of alternative strategies are being investigated to determine which one, or a combination thereof, could result in tomosynthesis screening requiring similar resources to mammography screening.

In the first place, given the ability of DBT to reduce tissue superposition, the acquisition of only the MLO view for screening could be feasible. The Malmö Tomosynthesis Breast Screening Trial was performed using single-view tomosynthesis (Lång et al. 2016; Zackrisson et al. 2018), resulting in an important increase in cancer detection rate. As mentioned above, since the baseline recall rate with mammography was low, tomosynthesis did result in an increase in the recall rate. Rodriguez-Ruiz et al. 2018c evaluated and compared the detection performance of single-view DBT to three other combinations of DBT and DM views, and found the former non-inferior to all other strategies (Rodriguez-Ruiz et al. 2018b, c). Single-view DBT resulted in a 25% reading time increase compared to two-view DM, considerably less than the doubling in reading time due to two-view DBT (Skaane et al. 2013). It should be noted that both of these studies were performed with a wide-angle tomosynthesis system, so the generalization of these findings with a tomosynthesis device that covers a narrower angular range remains to be investigated.

Although screening mammography in Europe is mainly performed with double reading (with either consensus or arbitration), the possibility of single-reading breast tomosynthesis images for screening has been investigated. Houssami et al. showed that single-reading tomosynthesis screening during the STORM trial would still result in a 41.5% increase in cancer detection rate (from 5.3 to 7.5 cancers per 1000 women screened) with a reduction in the recall rate of 26.5%, from 4.9% to 3.6% (Houssami et al. 2014). In another large prospective screening trial, Romero Martin et al. also showed substantial improvement in performance with single-reading tomosynthesis, with a 21.3% increase in cancer detection rate (4.7 to 5.7 per 1000) and an almost halving of the recall rate from 5.0% to 2.5%, a 42.0% reduction (Romero Martin et al. 2018).

Due to the limited vertical resolution of DBT, the usual DBT slices separated by 1 mm, resulting in dozens of slices to be read per view, could be reduced without compromising performance by combining the information into thicker (~8 mm) slabs. This was first proposed by Diekmann et al., proposing an advanced method to combine the slices into thicker slabs that is a good compromise between maximizing the visibility of masses and calcifications (Diekmann

et al. 2009). This method was evaluated in a retrospective observer study by Agasthya et al. who showed a significant reduction in interpretation time of about 28% with a nonsignificant increase in performance with the 8 mm slabs (Agasthya et al. 2016). Dustler et al. evaluated the quality of depiction of lesions in 2 mm thick slabs, finding no loss in image quality, while interpretation of such images was found to be 20% faster (Dustler et al. 2013). In another study from the same group, combining slices to 10 mm thick slabs was found to hamper lesion detectability, however (Petersson et al. 2016).

In a fraction of *simple* cases, it could be possible that the review of only the synthetic mammography image obtained from the tomosynthesis acquisition information could be enough to discard the case as normal, substantially reducing the reading time. For *difficult* cases, in which the presence of dense glandular tissue results in the potential for false positives or negatives, then the entire tomosynthesis stack would need to be reviewed. The optional review of the stack should not affect the specificity of interpretation, since before recalling based on a synthetic mammography finding, the radiologist would review the stack. To estimate the fraction of *difficult* cases due to tissue masking that would need full stack review, a previous study on quantification of the masking effect could be used (Holland et al. 2017a). Using a very conservative threshold for full tomosynthesis stack review in which 90% of interval cancers are included, about 40% of cases could be defined as *easy*, and therefore possible to only review the synthetic image. In a study evaluating the visibility of cancers in synthetic 2D images alone, Murphy et al. found that all cancers visible in the tomosynthesis stacks were visible in the synthetic mammograms, including all cancers that were not visible in the digital mammography images (Murphy et al. 2018). The review of the synthetic mammogram only for a certain number of cases is an exciting and promising strategy, but one that needs further study before it can be used. Since the creation of the synthetic mammogram is purely based on software algorithms, it is expected that the quality of these images will continue to evolve as manufacturers improve their algorithms further.

Finally, using artificial intelligence (AI), we should be able to avoid the human interpretation of a substantial portion of screening cases, resulting in a substantial reduction in the case volume to be read. The introduction of deep learning algorithms for computer-aided detection (CAD) has increased CAD performance in mammography to levels equivalent to an average breast radiologist (Rodriguez-Ruiz et al. 2019). Recently, breast tomosynthesis CAD algorithms, also based on AI, have become commercially available, and have shown to result in both an improvement in performance and a substantial reduction in reading time (Conant et al. 2019). Now that these computer algorithms are as good as humans in interpreting digital mammography and breast tomosynthesis images, they could be used as a first reader to triage between the cases that need to be human-read and those that do not. With such a computer-based triaging system, half of the screening cases could be automatically labeled normal, and hence not human-read, with only a 7% of cancer cases being incorrectly included in that category (Rodriguez-Ruiz et al. 2018a). It should be noted that human reading results in ~25% of cancer cases being interpreted as normal (National Evaluation Team for Breast cancer screening in the Netherlands (NETB) 2016). The possibilities to improve performance and/or reduce reading time with AI in screening with tomosynthesis are varied and numerous. Although a full review of this topic is beyond the scope of this chapter, several recent review articles on this fast-evolving topic are available (Sechopoulos et al. 2020; Sechopoulos and Mann 2020; Geras et al. 2019). Of course, double reading of two-view digital breast tomosynthesis examinations (including digital mammography images) for screening would most probably yield the highest performance, as opposed to incorporating any or a combination of the abovementioned strategies. However, in many screening programs, implementation of screening tomosynthesis with this *standard* strategy is not feasible, due to the important increase in radiologist reading time needed. Therefore, it must be realized that the potential of these strategies should be investigated, and eventually they should be implemented, if by doing so a substantial portion of the benefit of tomosynthesis screening is maintained while the increase in reading time is manageable. To achieve this, additional studies on the generalizability of these methods for the different types of tomosynthesis systems and the possible combination of various of these strategies should be undertaken.

7 Radiation Dose

Mammography and digital breast tomosynthesis are low-dose X-ray imaging examinations. However, their use for screening of the general population results in there being an intense interest in the characterization and optimization of the dose involved in these modalities. These are, after all, by far the most commonly performed screening tests on asymptomatic people that use ionizing radiation. Therefore, not only should the level of radiation dose be well understood and minimized, but also its meaning and the current limitations of our methodology and knowledge also need to be communicated.

7.1 Basics of Breast Dosimetry

The metric that quantifies the radiation dose to the breast is the average glandular dose (AGD). The dose is qualified as being the "glandular dose" because, as opposed to the dose to all of the breast tissue, only the dose to the fibroglandular tissues in the breast is of interest. This is because these are the ones most at risk to develop breast cancer. The term "average" is used to reflect that the dose is the average of the dose to all the glandular tissue in the breast. Since breast imaging uses relatively low-energy X-rays, there is a very large variation in the dose deposited throughout the breast during a single acquisition. The dose at the top surface of the compressed breast, closest to the X-ray source, can be an order of magnitude higher than that at the bottom of the breast, closest to the detector (Sechopoulos et al. 2010). The current models that translate organ dose to risk are based on the average dose to the entire organ, so any large differences in dose within an organ are not taken into account.

The average glandular dose in the breast, just like any other organ dose, cannot be measured, only estimated. This is done by measuring the intensity and characteristics of the X-rays that the breast is exposed to, and then converting this value to an AGD using specific conversion coefficients. These conversion coefficients to obtain AGD were obtained by assuming a simplified model of the breast, in which all the fibroglandular and adipose tissues are perfectly mixed and are spread evenly throughout the breast (Dance 1990; Dance et al. 2000, 2009, 2011).

7.2 Meaning of Breast Dose Estimates

This means that even when we estimate the dose resulting from a mammographic or breast tomosynthesis acquisition, we are not estimating *that patient's breast dose*. Even if we take into account the exposure technique used for that acquisition, we only consider the number and type of X-rays to which we exposed that breast. The dose we calculated estimated on those factors is the dose to a *model breast*, which does not represent that patient's breast characteristics. This model breast could be of the correct thickness, since conversion coefficients are available for different thicknesses of breast. In addition, perhaps some consideration of the density (fraction of glandular tissue) of the breast could be taken into account, since conversion coefficients for different densities are also available. However, the true structure of the fibroglandular tissue inside the breast, i.e., where it is located, is not considered in the current dose estimations. Assuming that the fibroglandular tissue is spread out evenly throughout the whole breast makes our dose estimates not *patient specific* but model estimates. It has been found that using these model dose estimates can overestimate the dose to the actual patient breast by up to a factor of 2 and, on average, overestimates the dose by 30% (Sechopoulos et al. 2012; Hernandez et al. 2015).

Other patient-specific factors, such as the thickness of the skin of that specific breast, and the mammographic view (CC, MLO, etc.), are also not taken into account. As can be expected, the thicker the breast skin, the lower the AGD (Huang et al. 2008), while the dose in the MLO view, for the same acquisition technique, is lower than that in the CC view (Sechopoulos et al. 2007). However, conversion coefficients are not available for different skin thicknesses nor different mammographic views.

Therefore, it must be remembered that our current breast dose methods and estimates are not aimed at estimating the AGD to each specific patient for each specific view acquired. Even if the breast density of the patient is considered, as in some commercial breast dosimetry products, the resulting AGD is not *patient specific*. Rather, these estimates aim to obtain a relative estimate of the dose, useful for controlling the constancy of the behavior of the systems, the appropriateness of their use, and the optimization of techniques and technologies.

7.3 Mammography vs. Tomosynthesis Dose

During the introduction of digital breast tomosynthesis, especially for screening of asymptomatic women, one major concern was how does the dose from tomosynthesis compared to that from mammography. Furthermore, if tomosynthesis were used as an adjunct to rather than a replacement of mammography, would the total dose be doubled, or more?

Early phantom-based characterization and comparison of the dose from mammography and tomosynthesis using the first commercial digital breast tomosynthesis system were performed by Feng and Sechopoulos (2012). Using simple phantoms that represented a range of breast thicknesses and densities, the authors found that the dose ratio between that from breast tomosynthesis to that from mammography varied considerably. For the traditional "standard" breast, i.e., 5 cm thick and 50% density, the dose from the two modalities was essentially equal, with only an 8% increase with breast tomosynthesis. For a more clinically relevant standard breast, now considered to be about 6 cm thick and ~15% dense, tomosynthesis resulted in almost a doubling of the dose of that of mammography.

In a review paper, Svahn et al. collected all the comparisons of the dose between mammography and tomosynthesis provided in the early clinical performance comparisons between the two modalities (Svahn et al. 2015). Of course, the dose comparison varied greatly, depending on the system used, and, presumably, depending on the characteristics of the breast. However, as expected, the greatest variation in how the dose from mammography compares to that of tomosynthesis depended on how the two modalities would be implemented, that is, if tomosynthesis were used as an adjunct to mammography, and if tomosynthesis would involve the acquisition of one or two views. As a result of this variability, the dose from a tomosynthesis exam could be as low as a third of that of a standard two-view mammographic exam (if single-view tomosynthesis replaces mammography), to resulting in more than doubling of the dose (if two-view tomosynthesis is used in combination with mammography).

Once digital breast tomosynthesis was introduced to normal clinical practice, then more extensive patient-based dose data became available and could be compared, especially on a patient-by-patient basis. In a comprehensive study, Bouwman et al. compared the dose between both modalities for thousands of women imaged with systems of various vendors (Bouwman et al. 2015). Again, the ratios between the modalities varied depending on the breast characteristics, and, especially, depending on the system vendor. Figure 6 shows the resulting AGD values for both modalities with one system, based on the acquisitions of 2500 women. As can be seen, the dose from breast tomosynthesis is less variable for a given compressed breast thickness than that from digital mammography. In addition,

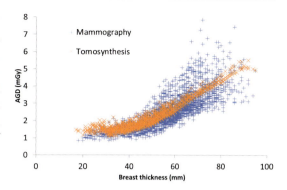

Fig. 6 Comparison of the average glandular dose (AGD) resulting from mammography (DM) and digital breast tomosynthesis (DBT) with one system, based on the acquisitions of 2500 women. The dose from DBT is less variable for a given compressed breast thickness than that from DM. The former tends to be higher than the latter for thin breasts, while for thicker breasts there is a smaller difference, and for many thick breasts DBT results in a lower dose. (Adapted from Bouwman et al. "Average Glandular Dose in Digital Mammography and Digital Breast Tomosynthesis: Comparison of Phantom and Patient Data." *Physics in Medicine and Biology* 60(20): 7893–7907. © Institute of Physics and Engineering in Medicine. Reproduced by permission of IOP Publishing. All rights reserved)

for thin breasts the dose from tomosynthesis is mostly higher than that from mammography, while for thicker breasts there is a smaller difference, and for many thick breasts tomosynthesis results in a lower dose. For the latter, the tomosynthesis dose distribution is well within the range of dose values resulting from mammography. Overall, with this system, the dose from digital breast tomosynthesis is 8% higher, on average, than that from digital mammography. For other systems, Bouwman et al. found varying differences overall for the dose from tomosynthesis compared to that from mammography.

Overall, the dosimetric consequences of moving from mammography to tomosynthesis imaging will be settled, in the big picture, not due to any dose penalty or savings due to physics- or technical-based optimization work on either modality, but by the clinical decision of how many views of each modality will be involved in one complete breast examination. This is because acquiring a single view as opposed to two, and/or replacing the mammographic acquisition with the computation of a synthetic mammogram, introduces much larger savings in dose than those that can be achieved by optimization of the acquisition technique or the technology involved in the imaging systems.

7.4 Radiation Dose vs. Clinical Performance

Even if, as mentioned above, the dose during X-ray-based breast imaging is of particular interest due to its use for screening, the main focus of concern and interest should still be the optimization of clinical performance.

The amount of radiation used for acquisition of a mammogram or a breast tomosynthesis image has a direct consequence on the level of noise in the image. Lesion detectability, especially of calcifications, is limited by image noise (Burgess et al. 2001). Therefore, it is important that the appropriate levels of dose are used to obtain an adequate, diagnostic, image. Compromising the clinical performance to save some fraction of the dose used, even for screening, should not be considered.

Furthermore, as discussed above, the choice of modality or combination of modalities has a much larger impact on the total dose of a breast exam than image acquisition technique selection. Implementing screening as one-view or two-view tomosynthesis, as a replacement or an adjunct to mammography, has, of course, the largest impact on the level of dose used for screening. The decision as to what modality or combination should be used for screening should be taken based on expected outcomes and other factors that determine feasibility: reading time, human and economic resources, etc.

As discussed in Sects. 5 and 6, digital breast tomosynthesis results in important increases in cancer detection rate, and, in some cases, in an important reduction in recall rate. Even if for widespread screening of the general (asymptomatic) population it is determined that the optimal implementation of tomosynthesis screening results in an increase in dose, then the benefit in outcomes should be considered above any increase in risk due to radiation.

According to the current model of risk based on exposure to ionizing radiation, a mammography-based screening program, even involving annual mammography between 40 and 55 years of age and biennially up to 74 years of age, would potentially result in 10.6 deaths due to radiation-induced breast cancers per 100,000 women (Yaffe and Mainprize 2011). This is in comparison to 2070 breast cancer deaths in that same cohort of women between 40 and 74 years old, of which 497 could be saved by breast cancer screening (Yaffe and Mainprize 2011). Clearly, any discussion on the appropriateness of breast cancer screening with mammography or breast tomosynthesis should not be based on appropriateness of the radiation doses involved, but on clinical, economic, and other factors.

Furthermore, it should be noted that the current model used to relate the dose to risk of cancer development, as also used by Yaffe and Mainprize for the calculations above, assumes that there is no *safe* level of radiation. This means that no matter how low the radiation dose, if enough people are exposed to it, some cancers, and therefore some deaths, will be induced. Especially at the diagnostic imaging dose levels there is a lack of consensus on the effects and risks of this level of radiation, and they might be nonexistent (American Association of Physicists in Medicine (AAPM) 2018). Therefore, as stated by this Position Statement of the AAPM, given the uncertainty in these risk models, the use and recommendations for use of these imaging modalities should be based on their clinical appropriateness, and should be used with the levels of radiation that are needed to achieve the required image quality.

7.5 Total Breast Dose During a Screening Examination

Let us consider a hypothetical scenario of a mammographic screening exam consisting of the usual two views (CC and MLO) of each of the two breasts. For this exercise, let us assume that both breasts are exactly the same size and density, and that all the fibroglandular tissue present in the imaged breast is exposed during both the CC and the MLO views. However, due to the MLO view compression resulting in the breast being a little thicker, the two views result in a slight difference in AGD; both left and right CC views each result in an AGD of 1.0 mGy while the left and right MLO views each result in an AGD of 1.2 mGy.

What is the total dose to the breasts for this screening exam?

It is tempting to answer that the total dose is simply the sum of the dose of the four acquisitions: 4.4 mGy. However, to obtain the correct answer, the definition of dose needs to be considered:

Dose = Energy deposited in tissue
/ Amount of tissue the energy is deposited in

The amount of tissue, in the case of breast imaging, as mentioned, is the mass of fibroglandular tissue.

If we first consider the dose to each individual breast only, e.g., the left breast only, then the total dose to the left breast from the acquisition of both views is 2.2 mGy. This is because whatever X-ray energy was deposited during the acquisition of each of the two views, it was in the same fibroglandular tissue, the one of the left breast. Now, when the right breast is imaged, it also results in a total dose due to acquisition of both views of 2.2 mGy. However, the X-ray energy deposition that resulted in this other dose was deposited in different fibroglandular tissue, that present in the right breast. Therefore, when calculating the total dose to both breasts, we do not only have double the energy deposition, but also have double the amount of tissue it is deposited on. As a result, the total breast dose due to this bilateral two-view screening examination is the average of the total dose received by each breast due to the two views. Since each breast was exposed to an AGD of 2.2 mGy, the total AGD to the breasts from this exam was also 2.2 mGy.

In short, when the dose from multiple views of the same breast is being calculated, the individual dose values are added. However, when the total dose to both breasts is being calculated, then the total dose received by each breast is averaged together.

References

Abdi AJ, Fieselmann A, Pfaff H, Mertelmeier T, Larsen LB (2018) Comparison of screening performance metrics and patient dose of two mammographic image acquisition modes in the Danish National Breast Cancer Screening Programme. Eur J Radiol 105(August):188–194. https://doi.org/10.1016/j.ejrad.2018.06.010

Agasthya GA, D'Orsi CJ, Holbrook A, Ho C, Piraner M, Newell M, Gilliland L, Sechopoulos I (2016) Reduction in digital breast tomosynthesis interpretation time by slabbing of the reconstructed slices. In: European Congress of Radiology, Vienna, Austria

Agasthya GA, D'Orsi E, Kim Y-J, Handa P, Ho CP, D'Orsi CJ, Sechopoulos I (2017) Can breast compression be reduced in digital mammography and breast tomosynthesis? Am J Roentgenol 209(5):W322–W332. https://doi.org/10.2214/AJR.16.17615

American Association of Physicists in Medicine (AAPM) (2018) AAPM position statement on radiation risks from medical imaging procedures. https://www.aapm.org/org/policies/details.asp?id=439&type=PP

Andersson I, Ikeda D, Zackrisson S, Ruschin M, Svahn T, Timberg P, Tingberg A (2008) Breast tomosynthesis and digital mammography: a comparison of breast cancer visibility and BIRADS classification in a population of cancers with subtle mammographic findings. Eur Radiol 18(12):2817–2825

Bahl M, Gaffney S, McCarthy AM, Lowry KP, Dang PA, Lehman CD (2017) Breast cancer characteristics associated with 2D digital mammography versus digital breast tomosynthesis for screening-detected and interval cancers. Radiology 287(1):49–57. https://doi.org/10.1148/radiol.2017171148

Bahl M, Mercaldo S, Vijapura CA, McCarthy AM, Lehman CD (2019) Comparison of performance metrics with digital 2D versus tomosynthesis mammography in the diagnostic setting. Eur Radiol 29(2):477–484. https://doi.org/10.1007/s00330-018-5596-7

Baker JA, Lo JY (2011) Breast tomosynthesis: state-of-the-art and review of the literature. Acad Radiol 18(10):1298–1310. https://doi.org/10.1016/j.acra.2011.06.011

Balleyguier C, Cousin M, Dunant A, Attard M, Delaloge S, Arfi-Rouche J (2018) Patient-assisted compression helps for image quality reduction dose and improves patient experience in mammography. Eur J Cancer 103(November):137–142. https://doi.org/10.1016/j.ejca.2018.08.009

Bernardi D, Macaskill P, Pellegrini M, Valentini M, Fantò C, Ostillio L, Tuttobene P, Luparia A, Houssami N (2016) Breast cancer screening with tomosynthesis (3D mammography) with acquired or synthetic 2D mammography compared with 2D mammography alone (STORM-2): a population-based prospective study. Lancet Oncol 17(8):1105–1113. https://doi.org/10.1016/S1470-2045(16)30101-2

Bernardi D, Gentilini MA, De Nisi M, Pellegrini M, Fantò C, Valentini M, Sabatino V, Luparia A, Houssami N (2020) Effect of implementing digital breast tomosynthesis (DBT) instead of mammography on population screening outcomes including interval cancer rates: results of the Trento DBT pilot evaluation. Breast 50(April):135–140. https://doi.org/10.1016/j.breast.2019.09.012

Bouwman RW, van Engen RE, Young KC, den Heeten GJ, Broeders MJ, Schopphoven S, Jeukens CR, Veldkamp WJ, Dance DR (2015) Average glandular dose in digital mammography and digital breast tomosynthesis: comparison of phantom and patient data. Phys Med Biol 60(20):7893–7907. https://doi.org/10.1088/0031-9155/60/20/7893

Brandt KR, Craig DA, Hoskins TL, Henrichsen TL, Bendel EC, Brandt SR, Mandrekar J (2013) Can digital breast tomosynthesis replace conventional diagnostic mammography views for screening recalls without calcifications? A comparison study in a simulated clinical setting. Am J Roentgenol 200(2):291–298. https://doi.org/10.2214/ajr.12.8881

Broeders MJM, ten Voorde M, Veldkamp WJH, van Engen RE, van Landsveld-Verhoeven C, 't Jong-Gunneman MNL, de Win J, Greve K D-d, Paap E, den Heeten GJ (2015) Comparison of a flexible versus a rigid breast compression paddle: pain experience, projected breast area, radiation dose and technical image quality. Eur Radiol 25(3):821–829. https://doi.org/10.1007/s00330-014-3422-4

Burgess AE, Jacobson FL, Judy PF (2001) Human observer detection experiments with mammograms and power-law noise. Med Phys 28(4):419–437

Ciatto S, Houssami N, Bernardi D, Caumo F, Pellegrini M, Brunelli S, Tuttobene P et al (2013) Integration of 3D digital mammography with tomosynthesis for population breast-cancer screening (STORM): a prospective comparison study. Lancet Oncol 14(7):583–589. https://doi.org/10.1016/S1470-2045(13)70134-7

Clauser P, Nagl G, Helbich TH, Pinker-Domenig K, Weber M, Kapetas P, Bernathova M, Baltzer PAT (2016) Diagnostic performance of digital breast tomosynthesis with a wide scan angle compared to full-field digital mammography for the detection and characterization of microcalcifications. Eur J Radiol 85(12):2161–2168. https://doi.org/10.1016/j.ejrad.2016.10.004

Conant EF, Toledano AY, Periaswamy S, Fotin SV, Go J, Boatsman JE, Hoffmeister JW (2019) Improving accuracy and efficiency with concurrent use of artificial intelligence for digital breast tomosynthesis. Radiol Artif Intell 1(4):e180096. https://doi.org/10.1148/ryai.2019180096

Conant EF, Zuckerman SP, McDonald ES, Weinstein SP, Korhonen KE, Birnbaum JA, Tobey JD, Schnall MD, Hubbard RA (2020) Five consecutive years of screening with digital breast tomosynthesis: outcomes by screening year and round. Radiology 295(2):285–293. https://doi.org/10.1148/radiol.2020191751

Dance DR (1990) Monte Carlo calculation of conversion factors for the estimation of mean glandular breast dose. Phys Med Biol 35(9):1211–1219

Dance DR, Skinner CL, Young KC, Beckett JR, Kotre CJ (2000) Additional factors for the estimation of mean glandular breast dose using the UK mammography dosimetry protocol. Phys Med Biol 45(11):3225–3240

Dance DR, Young KC, van Engen RE (2009) Further factors for the estimation of mean glandular dose using the United Kingdom, European and IAEA breast dosimetry protocols. Phys Med Biol 54(14):4361–4372

Dance DR, Young KC, van Engen RE (2011) Estimation of mean glandular dose for breast tomosynthesis: factors for use with the UK, European and IAEA breast dosimetry protocols. Phys Med Biol 56(2):453

de Groot JE, Broeders MJM, Branderhorst W, den Heeten GJ, Grimbergen CA (2013) A novel approach to mammographic breast compression: improved standardization and reduced discomfort by controlling pressure instead of force. Med Phys 40(8):081901. https://doi.org/10.1118/1.4812418

Destounis S, Morgan R, Arieno A (2014) Initial experience with combination digital breast tomosynthesis plus full field digital mammography or full field digital mammography alone in the screening environment. J Clin Imaging Sci 4(1):9. https://doi.org/10.4103/2156-7514.127838

Diekmann F, Meyer H, Diekmann S, Puong S, Muller S, Bick U, Rogalla P (2009) Thick slices from tomosynthesis data sets: phantom study for the evaluation of different algorithms. J Digit Imaging 22(5):519–526

Durand MA, Haas BM, Yao X, Geisel JL, Raghu M, Hooley RJ, Horvath LJ, Philpotts LE (2015) Early clinical experience with digital breast tomosynthesis for screening mammography. Radiology 274(1):85–92. https://doi.org/10.1148/radiol.14131319

Dustler M, Andersson M, Förnvik D, Timberg P, Tingberg A (2013) A study of the feasibility of using slabbing to reduce tomosynthesis review time. Proc SPIE 8673:86731L

European Commission (2006) European guidelines for quality assurance in breast cancer screening and diagnosis, 4th edn. European Communities, Brussels, Belgium

Feng SSJ, Sechopoulos I (2012) Clinical digital breast tomosynthesis system: dosimetric characterization. Radiology 263(1):35–42. https://doi.org/10.1148/radiol.11111789

Fieselmann A, Fischer D, Hilal G, Dennerlein F, Mertelmeier T, Uhlenbrock D (2013) Full field digital mammography with grid-less acquisition and software-based scatter correction: investigation of dose saving and image quality. In: Nishikawa RM, Whiting BR (eds) Proceedings of SPIE, Lake Buena Vista (Orlando Area), Florida, USA, p 86685Y. https://doi.org/10.1117/12.2007490

Friedewald SM, Rafferty EA, Rose SL, Durand MA, Plecha DM, Greenberg JS, Hayes MK et al (2014) Breast cancer screening using tomosynthesis in combination with digital mammography. JAMA 311(24):2499. https://doi.org/10.1001/jama.2014.6095

Gennaro G, Toledano A, di Maggio C, Baldan E, Bezzon E, La Grassa M, Pescarini L et al (2010) Digital breast tomosynthesis versus digital mammography: a clinical performance study. Eur Radiol 20(7):1545–1553. https://doi.org/10.1007/s00330-009-1699-5

Geras KJ, Mann RM, Moy L (2019) Artificial intelligence for mammography and digital breast tomosynthesis: current concepts and future perspectives. Radiology 293(2):246–259. https://doi.org/10.1148/radiol.2019182627

Gilbert F, Lorraine Tucker M, Gillan PW, Julie Cooke K, Duncan M, Michell H, Dobson YL, Purushothaman H (2015) The TOMMY trial: a comparison of TOMosynthesis with digital MammographY in the UK NHS Breast Screening Programme. Health Technol Assess 19(4). https://doi.org/10.3310/hta19040

Gilbert FJ, Tucker L, Young KC (2016) Digital breast tomosynthesis (DBT): a review of the evidence for use as a screening tool. Clin Radiol 71(2):141–150. https://doi.org/10.1016/j.crad.2015.11.008

Greenberg JS, Javitt MC, Katzen J, Michael S, Holland AE (2014) Clinical performance metrics of 3D digital breast tomosynthesis compared with 2D digital mammography for breast cancer screening in community practice. Am J Roentgenol 203(3):687–693. https://doi.org/10.2214/AJR.14.12642

Gur D, Abrams GS, Chough DM, Ganott MA, Hakim CM, Perrin RL, Rathfon GY, Sumkin JH, Zuley ML, Bandos AI (2009) Digital breast tomosynthesis: observer performance study. Am J Roentgenol 193(2):586–591. https://doi.org/10.2214/ajr.08.2031

Gur D, Zuley ML, Anello MI, Rathfon GY, Chough DM, Ganott MA, Hakim CM, Wallace L, Amy L, Bandos AI (2012) Dose reduction in digital breast tomosynthesis (DBT) screening using synthetically reconstructed projection images: an observer performance study. Acad Radiol 19(2):166–171. https://doi.org/10.1016/j.acra.2011.10.003

Hammerstein GR, Miller DW, White DR, Masterson ME, Woodard HQ, Laughlin JS (1979) Absorbed radiation dose in mammography. Radiology 130(2):485–491

Hendrick RE, Pisano ED, Averbukh A, Moran C, Berns EA, Yaffe MJ, Herman B, Acharyya S, Gatsonis C (2010) Comparison of acquisition parameters and breast dose in digital mammography and screen-film mammography in the American College of Radiology Imaging Network digital mammographic imaging screening trial. Am J Roentgenol 194(2):362–369. https://doi.org/10.2214/ajr.08.2114

Hernandez AM, Seibert AJ, Boone JM (2015) Breast dose in mammography is about 30% lower when realistic heterogeneous glandular distributions are considered. Med Phys 42(11):6337–6348. https://doi.org/10.1118/1.4931966

Hodgson R, Heywang-Köbrunner SH, Harvey SC, Edwards M, Shaikh J, Arber M, Glanville J (2016) Systematic review of 3D mammography for breast cancer screening. Breast 27(Suppl C):52–61. https://doi.org/10.1016/j.breast.2016.01.002

Holland K, van Gils CH, Mann RM, Karssemeijer N (2017a) Quantification of masking risk in screening mammography with volumetric breast density maps. Breast Cancer Res Treat 162(3):541–548. https://doi.org/10.1007/s10549-017-4137-4

Holland K, Sechopoulos I, Mann RM, den Heeten GJ, van Gils CH, Karssemeijer N (2017b) Influence of breast compression pressure on the performance of population-based mammography screening. Breast Cancer Res 19(1):126. https://doi.org/10.1186/s13058-017-0917-3

Houssami N, Skaane P (2013) Overview of the evidence on digital breast tomosynthesis in breast cancer detection. Breast 22(2):101–108. https://doi.org/10.1016/j.breast.2013.01.017

Houssami N, Macaskill P, Bernardi D, Caumo F, Pellegrini M, Brunelli S, Tuttobene P et al (2014) Breast screening using 2D-mammography or integrating digital breast tomosynthesis (3D-mammography) for single-reading or double-reading – evidence to guide future screening strategies. Eur J Cancer 50(10):1799–1807. https://doi.org/10.1016/j.ejca.2014.03.017

Houssami N, Bernardi D, Caumo F, Brunelli S, Fantò C, Valentini M, Romanucci G, Gentilini MA, Zorzi M, Macaskill P (2018) Interval breast cancers in the 'screening with tomosynthesis or standard mammography' (STORM) population-based trial. Breast 38(April):150–153. https://doi.org/10.1016/j.breast.2018.01.002

Hovda T, Holen ÅS, Lång K, Albertsen JL, Bjørndal H, Brandal SHB, Sahlberg KK, Skaane P, Suhrke P, Hofvind S (2019) Interval and consecutive round breast cancer after digital breast tomosynthesis and synthetic 2D mammography versus standard 2D digital mammography in BreastScreen Norway. Radiology 294(2):256–264. https://doi.org/10.1148/radiol.2019191337

Huang S-Y, Boone JM, Yang K, Kwan ALC, Packard NJ (2008) The effect of skin thickness determined using breast CT on mammographic dosimetry. Med Phys 35(4):1199–1206

Johns PC, Yaffe MJ (1987) X-ray characterisation of normal and neoplastic breast tissues. Phys Med Biol 32(6):675–695

Kopans DB (2007) Breast imaging, 3rd edn. Lippincott Williams & Wilkins, Baltimore, MD

Kornguth PJ, Rimer BK, Conaway MR, Sullivan DC, Catoe KE, Stout AL, Brackett JS (1993) Impact of patient-controlled compression on the mammography experience. Radiology 186(1):99–102. https://doi.org/10.1148/radiology.186.1.8416595

Lång K, Andersson I, Zackrisson S (2014) Breast cancer detection in digital breast tomosynthesis and digital mammography-a side-by-side review of discrepant cases. Br J Radiol 87(1040):20140080. https://doi.org/10.1259/bjr.20140080

Lång K, Andersson I, Rosso A, Tingberg A, Timberg P, Zackrisson S (2016) Performance of one-view breast tomosynthesis as a stand-alone breast cancer screening modality: results from the Malmö breast tomosynthesis screening trial, a population-based study. Eur Radiol 26(1):184–190. https://doi.org/10.1007/s00330-015-3803-3

Lau S, Aziz YFA, Ng KH (2017) Mammographic compression in Asian women. PLoS One 12(4):e0175781. https://doi.org/10.1371/journal.pone.0175781

Liu B, Tao W, Moore RH, Kopans DB (2006) Monte Carlo simulation of X-ray scatter based on patient model from digital breast tomosynthesis. Proc SPIE 6142:61421N

Lourenco AP, Barry-Brooks M, Baird GL, Tuttle A, Mainiero MB (2015) Changes in recall type and patient treatment following implementation of screening digital breast tomosynthesis. Radiology 274(2):337–342. https://doi.org/10.1148/radiol.14140317

Markle L, Roux S, Sayre JW (2004) Reduction of discomfort during mammography utilizing a radiolucent cushioning pad. Breast J 10(4):345–349. https://doi.org/10.1111/j.1075-122X.2004.21352.x

Mawdsley GE, Tyson AH, Peressotti CL, Jong RA, Taffc MJ (2009) Accurate estimation of compressed breast thickness in mammography. Med Phys 36(2):577–586

McCarthy AM, Kontos D, Synnestvedt M, Tan KS, Heitjan DF, Schnall M, Conant EF (2014) Screening outcomes following implementation of digital breast tomosynthesis in a general-population screening program. J Natl Cancer Inst 106(11):dju316. https://doi.org/10.1093/jnci/dju316

McDonald ES, Oustimov A, Weinstein SP, Synnestvedt MB, Schnall M, Conant EF (2016) Effectiveness of digital breast tomosynthesis compared with digital mammography: outcomes analysis from 3 years of breast cancer screening. JAMA Oncol 2(6):737–743. https://doi.org/10.1001/jamaoncol.2015.5536

Monserrat T, Prieto E, Barbés B, Pina L, Elizalde A, Fernández B (2018) Impact on dose and image quality of a software-based scatter correction in mammography. Acta Radiol 59(6):649–656. https://doi.org/10.1177/0284185117730100

Murphy MC, Coffey L, O'Neill AC, Quinn C, Prichard R, McNally S (2018) Can the synthetic C view images be used in isolation for diagnosing breast malignancy without reviewing the entire digital breast tomosynthesis data set? Ir J Med Sci. https://doi.org/10.1007/s11845-018-1748-7

National Evaluation Team for Breast cancer screening in the Netherlands (NETB) (2016) NETB monitor 2014 - nation-wide breast cancer screening in the Netherlands, results 1990–2014. Erasmus MC and Radboudumc, Rotterdam

Niklason LT, Christian BT, Niklason LE, Kopans DB, Castleberry DE, Opsahl-Ong BH, Landberg CE et al (1997) Digital tomosynthesis in breast imaging. Radiology 205(2):399–406

Petersson H, Dustler M, Tingberg A, Timberg P (2016) Evaluation of the possibility to use thick slabs of reconstructed outer breast tomosynthesis slice images. In: Abbey CK, Kupinski MA (eds) Proceedings of SPIE, San Diego, California, United States, p 97871. https://doi.org/10.1117/12.2216688

Pisano ED, Gatsonis C, Hendrick E, Yaffe M, Baum JK, Acharyya S, Conant EF et al (2005) Diagnostic performance of digital versus film mammography for breast-cancer screening. N Engl J Med 353(September):1–11

Poplack SP, Tosteson TD, Kogel CA, Nagy HM (2007) Digital breast tomosynthesis: initial experience in 98 women with abnormal digital screening mammography. Am J Roentgenol 189(3):616–623. https://doi.org/10.2214/ajr.07.2231

Powell JL, Hawley JR, Lipari AM, Yildiz VO, Selnur Erdal B, Carkaci S (2017) Impact of the addition of digital breast tomosynthesis (DBT) to standard 2D digital screening mammography on the rates of patient recall, cancer detection, and recommendations for short-term follow-up. Acad Radiol 24(3):302–307. https://doi.org/10.1016/j.acra.2016.10.001

Qian X, Tucker A, Gidcumb E, Shan J, Yang G, Calderon-Colon X, Sultana S et al (2012) High resolution stationary digital breast tomosynthesis using distributed carbon nanotube X-ray source array. Med Phys 39(4):2090–2099

Rafferty EA, Park JM, Philpotts LE, Poplack SP, Sumkin JH, Halpern EF, Niklason LT (2013) Assessing radiologist performance using combined digital mammography and breast tomosynthesis compared with digital mammography alone: results of a multicenter, multireader trial. Radiology 266(1):104–113. https://doi.org/10.1148/radiol.12120674

Rafferty EA, Park JM, Philpotts LE, Poplack SP, Sumkin JH, Halpern EF, Niklason LT (2014) Diagnostic accuracy and recall rates for digital mammography and digital mammography combined with one-view and two-view tomosynthesis: results of an enriched reader study. Am J Roentgenol 202(2):273–281. https://doi.org/10.2214/AJR.13.11240

Rezentes PS, de Almeida A, Barnes GT (1999) Mammography grid performance. Radiology 210(1):227–232

Rodriguez-Ruiz A, Gubern-Mérida A, Gennaro G, Chevalier M, Zackrisson S, Andersson I, Sechopoulos I, Mann R (2018a) Can the breast cancer screening case-load be reduced by deep-learning based identification of normal cases? An international multi-centre retrospective analysis. In: European Congress of Radiology, Vienna, Austria

Rodriguez-Ruiz A, Gubern-Merida A, Imhof-Tas M, Lardenoije S, Wanders A, Andersson I, Zackrisson S et al (2018b) One-view digital breast tomosynthesis as a stand-alone modality for breast cancer detection: do we need more? Eur Radiol 28(5):1938–1948

Rodriguez-Ruiz A, Lardenoije S, Wanders AJT, Sechopoulos I, Mann RM (2018c) Comparison of breast cancer detection and depiction between planar and rotating synthetic mammography generated from breast tomosynthesis. Eur J Radiol 108(November):78–83. https://doi.org/10.1016/j.ejrad.2018.09.022

Rodriguez-Ruiz A, Lång K, Gubern-Merida A, Broeders MJM, Gennaro G, Clauser P, Helbich TH et al (2019) Stand-alone artificial intelligence for breast cancer detection in mammography: comparison with 101 radiologists. J Natl Cancer Inst 111(9):916–922. https://doi.org/10.1093/jnci/djy222

Romero Martin S, Raya Povedano JL, Cara Garcia M, Santos Romero AL, Pedrosa Garriguet M, Alvarez Benito M (2018) Prospective study aiming to compare 2D mammography and tomosynthesis + synthesized mammography in terms of cancer detection and recall. From double reading of 2D mammography to single reading of tomosynthesis. Eur Radiol. https://doi.org/10.1007/s00330-017-5219-8

Rose SL, Tidwell AL, Bujnoch LJ, Kushwaha AC, Nordmann AS, Sexton R (2013) Implementation of breast tomosynthesis in a routine screening practice: an observational study. Am J Roentgenol 200(6):1401–1408. https://doi.org/10.2214/AJR.12.9672

Sechopoulos I, Ghetti C (2009) Optimization of the acquisition geometry in digital tomosynthesis of the breast. Med Phys 36(4):1199–1207. https://doi.org/10.1118/1.3090889

Sechopoulos I, Mann RM (2020) Stand-alone artificial intelligence - the future of breast cancer screening? Breast 49(February):254–260. https://doi.org/10.1016/j.breast.2019.12.014

Sechopoulos I, Suryanarayanan S, Vedantham S, D'Orsi C, Karellas A (2007) Computation of the glandular radiation dose in digital tomosynthesis of the breast. Med Phys 34(1):221–232. https://doi.org/10.1118/1.2400836

Sechopoulos I, Feng SSJ, D'Orsi CJ (2010) Dosimetric characterization of a dedicated breast computed tomography clinical prototype. Med Phys 37(8):4110–4120. https://doi.org/10.1118/1.3457331

Sechopoulos I, Bliznakova K, Qin X, Fei B, Feng SSJ (2012) Characterization of the homogeneous tissue mixture approximation in breast imaging dosimetry. Med Phys 39(8):5050–5059. https://doi.org/10.1118/1.4737025

Sechopoulos I, Teuwen J, Mann R (2020) Artificial intelligence for breast cancer detection in mammography and digital breast tomosynthesis: state of the art. Semin Cancer Biol. https://doi.org/10.1016/j.semcancer.2020.06.002

Sharpe RE, Venkataraman S, Phillips J, Dialani V, Fein-Zachary VJ, Prakash S, Slanetz PJ, Mehta TS (2016) Increased cancer detection rate and variations in the recall rate resulting from implementation of 3D digital breast tomosynthesis into a population-based screening program. Radiology 278(3):698–706. https://doi.org/10.1148/radiol.2015142036

Skaane P, Bandos AI, Gullien R, Eben EB, Ekseth U, Haakenaasen U, Izadi M et al (2013) Prospective trial comparing full-field digital mammography (FFDM) versus combined FFDM and tomosynthesis in a population-based screening programme using independent double reading with arbitration. Eur Radiol 23(8):2061–2071. https://doi.org/10.1007/s00330-013-2820-3

Skaane P, Bandos AI, Eben EB, Jebsen IN, Krager M, Haakenaasen U, Ekseth U, Izadi M, Hofvind S, Gullien R (2014) Two-view digital breast tomosynthesis screening with synthetically reconstructed projection images: comparison with digital breast tomosynthesis with full-field digital mammographic images. Radiology 271(3):655–663. https://doi.org/10.1148/radiol.13131391

Skaane P, Sebuødegård S, Bandos AI, Gur D, Østerås BH, Gullien R, Hofvind S (2018) Performance of breast cancer screening using digital breast tomosynthesis: results from the prospective population-based Oslo tomosynthesis screening trial. Breast Cancer Res Treat 169(3):489–496. https://doi.org/10.1007/s10549-018-4705-2

Spangler ML, Zuley ML, Sumkin JH, Abrams G, Ganott MA, Hakim C, Perrin R, Chough DM, Shah R, Gur D (2011) Detection and classification of calcifications on digital breast tomosynthesis and 2D digital mammography: a comparison. Am J Roentgenol 196(2):320–324. https://doi.org/10.2214/ajr.10.4656

Svahn TM, Chakraborty DP, Ikeda D, Zackrisson S, Do Y, Mattsson S, Andersson I (2012) Breast tomosynthesis and digital mammography: a comparison of diagnostic accuracy. Br J Radiol 85(1019):e1074–e1082. https://doi.org/10.1259/bjr/53282892

Svahn TM, Houssami N, Sechopoulos I, Mattsson S (2015) Review of radiation dose estimates in digital breast tomosynthesis relative to those in two-view full-field digital mammography. Breast 24(2):93–99. https://doi.org/10.1016/j.breast.2014.12.002

Tani H, Uchiyama N, Machida M, Kikuchi M, Arai Y, Otsuka K, Jerebko A, Fieselmann A, Mertelmeier T (2014) Assessing radiologist performance and microcalcifications visualization using combined 3D rotating mammogram (RM) and digital breast tomosynthesis (DBT). In: Fujita H, Hara T, Muramatsu C (eds) International workshop on digital mammography. Springer International Publishing, Cham, pp 142–149

Timmers J, ten Voorde M, van Engen RE, van Landsveld-Verhoeven C, Pijnappel R, Greve K D-d, den Heeten GJ, Broeders MJM (2015) Mammography with and without radiolucent positioning sheets: comparison of projected breast area, pain experience, radiation dose and technical image quality. Eur J Radiol 84(10):1903–1909. https://doi.org/10.1016/j.ejrad.2015.07.005

Tyson AH, Mawdsley GE, Yaffe MJ (2009) Measurement of compressed breast thickness by optical stereoscopic photogrammetry. Med Phys 36(2):569–576

Vedantham S, Karellas A, Vijayaraghavan GR, Kopans DB (2015) Digital breast tomosynthesis: state of the art. Radiology 277(3):663–684. https://doi.org/10.1148/radiol.2015141303

Waade GG, Moshina N, Sebuødegård S, Hogg P, Hofvind S (2017a) Compression forces used in the Norwegian breast cancer screening program. Br J

Radiol 90(1071):20160770. https://doi.org/10.1259/bjr.20160770

Waade GG, Sanderud A, Hofvind S (2017b) Compression force and radiation dose in the Norwegian breast cancer screening program. Eur J Radiol 88(March):41–46. https://doi.org/10.1016/j.ejrad.2016.12.025

Wallis MG, Moa E, Zanca F, Leifland K, Danielsson M (2012) Two-view and single-view tomosynthesis versus full-field digital mammography: high-resolution X-ray imaging observer study. Radiology 262(3):788–796. https://doi.org/10.1148/radiol.11103514

Wanders JOP, Holland K, Veldhuis WB, Mann RM, Pijnappel RM, Peeters PHM, van Gils CH, Karssemeijer N (2017) Volumetric breast density affects performance of digital screening mammography. Breast Cancer Res Treat 162(1):95–103. https://doi.org/10.1007/s10549-016-4090-7

Wu G, Mainprize JG, Boone JM, Yaffe MJ (2009) Evaluation of scatter effects on image quality for breast tomosynthesis. Med Phys 36(10):4425–4432

Yaffe MJ, Mainprize JG (2011) Risk of radiation-induced breast cancer from mammographic screening. Radiology 258(1):98–105. https://doi.org/10.1148/radiol.10100655

Yun SJ, Ryu C-W, Rhee SJ, Ryu JK, Ji Young O (2017) Benefit of adding digital breast tomosynthesis to digital mammography for breast cancer screening focused on cancer characteristics: a meta-analysis. Breast Cancer Res Treat 164(3):557–569. https://doi.org/10.1007/s10549-017-4298-1

Zackrisson S, Lång K, Rosso A, Johnson K, Dustler M, Förnvik D, Förnvik H et al (2018) One-view breast tomosynthesis versus two-view mammography in the Malmö breast tomosynthesis screening trial (MBTST): a prospective, population-based, diagnostic accuracy study. Lancet Oncol 19(11):1493–1503. https://doi.org/10.1016/S1470-2045(18)30521-7

Zhou J, Zhao B, Zhao W (2007) A computer simulation platform for the optimization of a breast tomosynthesis system. Med Phys 34(3):1098–1109. https://doi.org/10.1118/1.2558160

Zuley ML, Bandos AI, Ganott MA, Sumkin JH, Kelly AE, Catullo VJ, Rathfon GY, Lu AH, Gur D (2013) Digital breast tomosynthesis versus supplemental diagnostic mammographic views for evaluation of noncalcified breast lesions. Radiology 266(1):89–95. https://doi.org/10.1148/radiol.12120552

Contrast-Enhanced Mammography

Anand Narayan and Maxine Jochelson

Contents

1   **Background**.. 26

2   **Techniques**... 26
    2.1   Temporal Technique.. 27
    2.2   Dual-Energy Technique................................... 27

3   **Clinical Studies**... 28
    3.1   Comparisons of CEDM with Digital Mammography.... 29
    3.2   Comparisons of CEDM with MRI.................. 29
    3.3   Comparisons of CEDM with Ultrasound........ 32

4   **Current and Potential Indications for Contrast-Enhanced Mammography**.. 34

5   **Risks**.. 38
    5.1   Iodinated Contrast... 38
    5.2   Renal Toxicity.. 38
    5.3   Radiation Dose.. 38

6   **Conclusions**... 39

  References... 39

A. Narayan (✉)
Department of Radiology, University of Wisconsin - Madison, Madison, WI, USA
e-mail: anarayan@uwhealth.org

M. Jochelson
Department of Radiology, Memorial Sloan Kettering Cancer Center, New York, NY, USA
e-mail: jochelsm@mskcc.org

Abstract

Screening mammography is known to decrease breast cancer mortality. It is relatively inexpensive and available to large populations of women. However, sensitivity is reduced in women with dense breast tissue. Consequently, other imaging techniques are used to improve upon the performance of digital mammography both for screening and to better evaluate the breast once cancer is diagnosed. Ultrasound and contrast-enhanced breast MRI are two of

---

© Springer Nature Switzerland AG 2022
M. Fuchsjäger et al. (eds.), *Breast Imaging*, Medical Radiology Diagnostic Imaging,
https://doi.org/10.1007/978-3-030-94918-1_2

the most commonly used examinations for supplemental imaging. Using contrast to enhance tumor vascularity, MRI provides significant improvements in sensitivity but MRI is limited by lack of widespread availability and high costs. Contrast-enhanced digital mammography (CEDM) is an emerging technology that utilizes the MRI concept of imaging enhancing neovascularity on an adapted digital mammography platform to improve the sensitivity and specificity of mammography alone. The purpose of this book chapter is to review the current status of CEDM.

1 Background

In randomized control trials, screening mammography has consistently been associated with reduction in breast cancer mortality (Siu 2016). Mammography is relatively inexpensive and broadly available to large populations of women. The overall sensitivity of mammography is 70–85%, but for women with dense breasts who are at increased risk for developing breast cancer (Boyd et al. 2007), it is reduced to 30–50% (Carney et al. 2003). Consequently, a wide variety of additional imaging techniques have been developed to supplement screening mammography as well as to evaluate the breast once cancer has been diagnosed.

Screening breast ultrasound and breast MRI are two such imaging techniques. Screening breast ultrasound is a purely anatomic method for evaluating for mammographically occult breast cancer. Multiple investigators have demonstrated that ultrasound detects an approximately 4 additional cancers per 1000 women (Berg 2016). Nevertheless, while ultrasound is theoretically less costly and widely accessible, it is limited by a large number of false-positive findings (Hooley et al. 2012). The ACRIN 6666 trial, a large multi-center study, randomized 2809 women with elevated cancer risk and dense breasts to three yearly independent rounds of screening mammography and ultrasound in a randomized order (Berg et al.

2012). Supplemental ultrasound yielded an additional cancer detection rate of 3.7 per 1000 women per year screened. However, among the substantial number of biopsies prompted by screening ultrasound (5.0%), only 7.4% were found to have cancer. After three rounds of both screenings, 612 women chose to undergo an MRI. Sixteen of these women had breast cancer that had not been detected on either mammography or screening ultrasound; for 9 of these 16 women, breast cancer could not be seen on subsequent targeted ultrasound.

Studies including the EVA trial also demonstrated that MRI has significant additional value over and above mammographic and ultrasound screening, making a strong statement that physiologic imaging improves cancer detection over purely anatomic imaging (Kuhl et al. 2010). By utilizing contrast to enhance tumor vascularity, contrast-enhanced breast MRI screening significantly improves sensitivity of mammography, detecting up to 97% of all breast cancers. However, MRI is expensive with limited availability for large numbers of women (Saslow et al. 2007). Additionally, women who are claustrophobic, have metallic implants, or are allergic to gadolinium cannot undergo MRI.

Contrast-enhanced digital mammography (CEDM) is an emerging technology that utilizes the MRI concept of imaging enhancing neovascularity to detect early breast cancers on an adapted digital mammography platform (Jochelson 2014). The purpose of this book chapter is to review the current status of CEDM.

2 Techniques

The two techniques that have been utilized for performing contrast-enhanced mammography are temporal (dynamic post-contrast imaging) and dual-energy contrast mammography. Initially, the temporal technique was used but at this time dual-energy contrast mammography is the standard technique.

2.1 Temporal Technique

The temporal or dynamic post-contrast technique relies on similar principles as dynamic post-contrast-enhanced breast MRI. After a unilateral single-view pre-contrast mammogram, iodinated contrast is administered. Sequential post-contrast mammograms are then acquired for 5–7 min.

The pre-contrast mammogram is subtracted from post-contrast mammograms to remove background non-enhancing parenchyma to produce subtraction images. Post-contrast-enhanced mammograms at multiple time points can be used to produce dynamic curves to evaluate kinetics (initial and delayed phases) with the purpose of using kinetics to determine which enhancing lesions are most likely to be malignant.

Initial results were reported by Diekmann et al. and were somewhat promising. The technique resulted in an improvement in sensitivity from 35% to 59% (Diekmann et al. 2011). However, the acquisition of multiple post-contrast mammograms over 5–7 min was frequently plagued by motion artifact. Additionally, only one view of one breast was imaged for each contrast injection, limiting sensitivity and the ability to localize tumors. And while the idea of using kinetic analysis seemed promising, kinetic information using this technique was different from that of MRI, limiting its specificity. As a result, the temporal technique has been abandoned.

2.2 Dual-Energy Technique

In this now standard technique, CEDM utilizes characteristics of the X-ray spectrum to provide an iodine image. Incoming X-ray photons interact with electrons in K-shells. Photons with sufficient energy cause electrons from the K-shell to be ejected, causing vacancies in the K-shell. Vacancies can be filled by electrons from other shells, generating characteristic X-rays in the process. Each substance has its own unique K-shell binding energy known as the k-edge. CEDM utilizes the k-edge of iodine to depict enhancing lesions.

The dual-energy technique involves acquisition of both low- and high-energy images nearly simultaneously. Low-energy images are obtained by utilizing X-ray photons with energy levels slightly below the k-edge of iodine (33.2 keV), similar to the energies utilized in conventional full-field digital mammography but insufficiently high to cause electrons from the K-shell to be ejected and produce characteristic X-rays. High-energy images are obtained by utilizing X-ray photons with energy levels above the k-edge of iodine (approximately 45–49 keV) with sufficient energy levels to be absorbed by K-shell electrons and produce characteristic X-rays. High-energy images are subtracted from low-energy images to subtract background parenchyma yielding only contrast-enhancing lesions.

CEDM is performed using intravenous iodinated contrast material. Peripheral access is obtained with a 20 G needle in an antecubital or other large vein when possible, and contrast is injected via a power injector at 3.0 mL/s followed by a saline bolus. The total amount of contrast is based on the patient's weight (1.5 mL/kg with a maximum dose of 150 mL). After completion of the injection, the patient is positioned for her mammogram. The breast is placed under standard compression. The first exposure occurs approximately 2 min and 45 s after injection. For each perceived exposure both low- and high-energy images are obtained with standard mammographic views: low-energy images are acquired using the routine filter while high-energy images are acquired using a copper filter. Post-processing yields what is essentially a subtraction image, i.e., generated to eliminate normal-background parenchyma. Low-energy and subtraction images are sent to a picture archiving and communication system for review (Fig. 1). The total examination time is approximately 8–9 min.

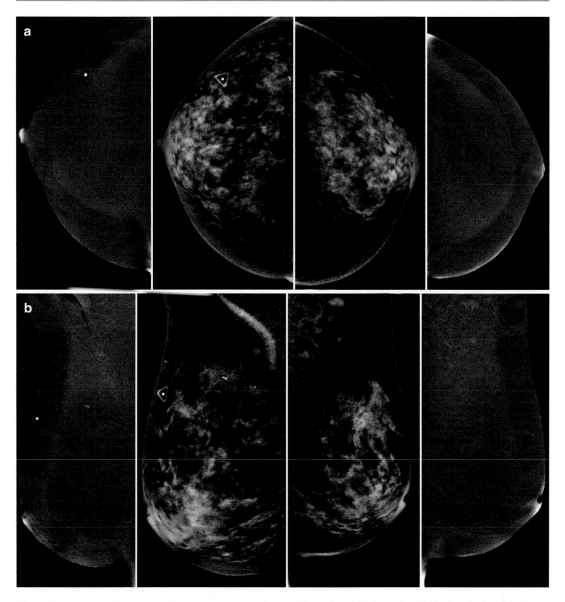

Fig. 1 Standard set of contrast-enhanced mammography images in a 68-year-old woman who presented for evaluation of a palpable finding in her right breast but whose workup was negative for underlying suspicious abnormality. Craniocaudal (**a**) and mediolateral oblique (**b**) views with marker denoting palpable finding in the right breast with post-processing images (outer panels) demonstrating the marker in the right breast but no suspicious enhancement

3 Clinical Studies

Lewin et al. conducted an initial feasibility study using a standard mammography unit (not designed as a dual-energy unit) to perform dual-energy mammography after intravenous contrast administration (Lewin et al. 2003). They evaluated 26 patients, 13 of whom had invasive cancers. Eleven of these tumors enhanced strongly, 1 enhanced moderately, and 1 enhanced weakly.

Dromain et al. demonstrated the feasibility of unilateral CEDM using a filter adapted for CEDM (Dromain et al. 2012). Jochelson et al. demonstrated that it was feasible to perform bilateral CEDM after a single contrast injection in 52 patients with known breast carcinoma (Jochelson et al. 2013).

3.1 Comparisons of CEDM with Digital Mammography

Studies comparing CEDM with digital mammography have universally found that CEDM consistently demonstrates statistically significant improvements in sensitivity compared with digital mammography alone (Luczyńska et al. 2014, 2016; Lalji et al. 2016; Mori et al. 2017; Fallenberg et al. 2014b; Cheung et al. 2014; Lobbes et al. 2014; Dromain et al. 2011, 2012) with sensitivities ranging from 86% to 100%. Additionally, these improvements in sensitivity persist even in the setting of combining digital mammography with ultrasound. Dromain et al. studied 110 women undergoing both mammography and ultrasound and found that the addition of CEDM was associated with statistically significant improvements in AUC (0.87 vs. 0.83, $p = 0.045$) (Dromain et al. 2012). Moreover, CEDM is especially sensitive for women with dense breasts. Fallenberg et al. studied 118 patients with histologically proven breast cancers of whom 56% had heterogeneously dense or extremely dense breast tissue. Sensitivity improved from 71.6% to 93.3% with CEDM (Fallenberg et al. 2014b). Similarly, Cheung et al. studied 89 women with heterogeneously dense or extremely dense breast tissue who had benign and malignant lesions in whom sensitivity improved from 71.5% to 92.7% while specificity increased from 51.8% to 67.9% (Cheung et al. 2014).

Tennant et al. studied women presenting at a clinic for breast symptoms undergoing contrast-enhanced mammography (Tennant et al. 2016). One hundred CEDM examinations with histopathology (73 malignant, 27 benign) were evaluated. Compared with low-energy digital images, CEDM was associated with improved sensitivity (94.5% vs. 84.4%, $p = 0.023$) and specificity (80.7% vs. 63.0%, $p = 0.014$) (Fig. 2).

Specificity of CEDM is superior to that of mammography (Fallenberg et al. 2014a, b).

Overall, eight studies (Lalji et al. 2016; Mori et al. 2017; Luczyńska et al. 2014; Fallenberg et al. 2017; Cheung et al. 2014; Lobbes et al. 2014; Dromain et al. 2012; Diekmann et al. 2011) have demonstrated statistically significant improvements in specificity when compared with digital mammography while two (Luczyńska et al. 2016; Dromain et al. 2011) have found no statistically significant improvements in specificity. Lobbes et al. reported results on 116 women referred for CEDM to evaluate abnormalities detected during breast cancer screening (Lobbes et al. 2014). One hundred thirteen of these women underwent CEDM. Sensitivity increased from 96.9% (these women were referred for abnormal imaging) to 100%. Specificity increased from 42.0% to 87.7%. Mori et al. evaluated accuracy of CEDM compared with conventional digital mammography in 143 breasts in 72 women in whom 90% of the breasts were dense (Mori et al. 2017). Sensitivity was 90.9% and specificity 94.1%.

To evaluate the utility of CEDM in assessing patients with microcalcifications, Cheung et al. studied 94 lesions in 87 women who underwent CEDM prior to undergoing stereotactic biopsy for microcalcifications without an underlying mass (Cheung et al. 2016). Of the 27 malignant lesions, 8 contained invasive components on core biopsy, all of which (8/8, 100%) demonstrated enhancement. Of the 19 patients with ductal carcinoma in situ (DCIS), 16/19 (84.2%) demonstrated enhancement. Of the 35 benign lesions, only 8.6% (3/35) demonstrated enhancement. With a negative predictive value of 95.1%, the results suggest that CEDM can be used to risk stratify microcalcifications without evidence of underlying mass, but the absence of enhancement should not preclude biopsy of suspicious calcifications (Fig. 3).

3.2 Comparisons of CEDM with MRI

Studies evaluating CEDM have demonstrated sensitivities ranging from 72% to 96%, comparable to contrast-enhanced breast MRI (Fallenberg et al. 2017; Chou et al. 2015; Wang et al. 2016;

Jochelson et al. 2013; Łuczyńska et al. 2015). Several studies have directly compared CEDM and MRI (Fig. 4). In a multi-reader study, Fallenberg et al. reported comparable diagnostic AUC for CEDM and MRI (0.84 vs. 0.85, respectively) in 178 women with either invasive ductal carcinoma or ductal carcinoma in situ (Fallenberg et al. 2017). Chou et al. studied 185 patients with benign and malignant lesions and found no statistically significant differences in AUC for CEDM and MRI (0.88 vs. 0.90, respectively) (Chou et al. 2015). Wang et al. studied 68 patients with pathologically proven malignant and benign lesions who underwent breast MRI and CEDM and found that CEDM was associated with higher sensitivities (95.8% vs. 93.8%) but lower specificities (65.5% vs. 82.8%) (Wang et al. 2016). On the other hand, in a study of 52 women with known breast cancer, Jochelson et al. prospectively compared breast cancer detection by mammography, MRI, and CEDM in 52 women with known carcinoma. Sensitivity for detecting the index cancer was 96% for CEDM and MRI, significantly better than mammography (81%). They found lower sensitivities for CEDM compared to MRI when evaluating for additional cancers beyond the index lesions but significantly higher specificities (Jochelson et al. 2013). Luczynska et al. studied 102 patients with benign and malignant lesions and found comparable sensitivities and AUC (0.83 vs. 0.84, respectively) (Łuczyńska et al. 2015).

Investigators have demonstrated that CEDM is very accurate in determining the actual cancer size. Luczynska et al. demonstrated that CEDM provided estimates of lesion size which were

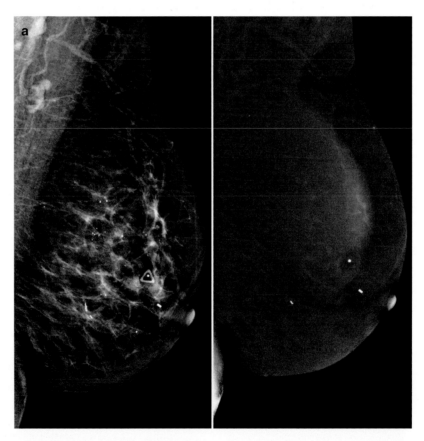

Fig. 2 Standard and CEDM mediolateral oblique (**a**) and craniocaudal images (**b**) of a patient with a palpable left breast finding with no suspicious underlying findings on CEDM. On ultrasound, the patient was found to have a possible hypoechoic lesion (**c**), biopsied yielding dense stromal fibrosis

Fig. 2 (continued)

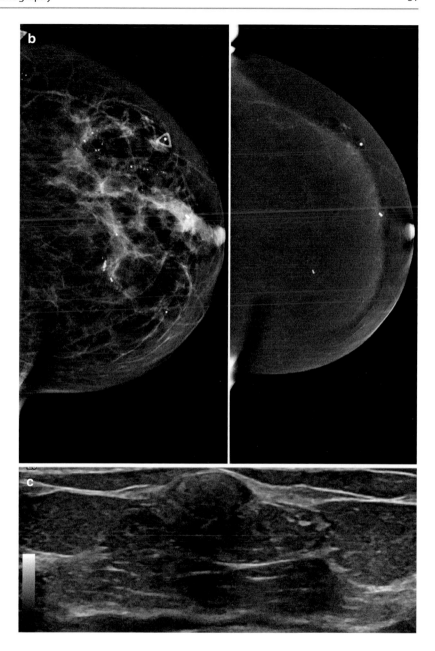

comparable to contrast-enhanced MRI (Łuczyńska et al. 2015). Lobbes et al. also found good correlation between CEDM and pathology and CEDM and MRI in 58 breast cancers evaluated by both exams (Lobbes et al. 2015). Mean differences between histopathology and CEDM were smaller (0.03 mm) compared with mean differences between histopathology and MRI (2.12 mm); however for the large majority of cases (84.5%), no size discrepancies were observed comparing CEDM with MRI. Similarly, Fallenberg et al. found no significant differences between lesion size measurement on MRI and CESM (27.7 vs. 31.6 mm, respectively, $p = 0.938$) compared with histopathology in 80 women with newly diagnosed breast cancer (Fallenberg et al. 2014a).

Increased background parenchymal enhancement (BPE) on breast MRI has been linked to

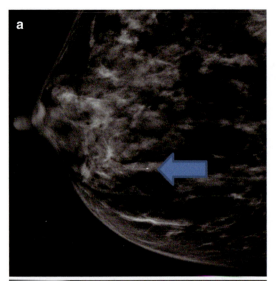

Fig. 3 Patient with suspicious microcalcifications in the inner right breast (**a**) without suspicious enhancement on CEDM (**b**), biopsied yielding intermediate-grade ductal carcinoma in situ with marked necrosis

study found substantial agreement between CEDM and MRI among the four categories of BPE: minimal, mild, moderate, and marked. Clinical characteristics' associations with increased or decreased BPE were similar for CEDM and MRI. On the other hand, Li et al. found that CEDM was associated with significantly decreased BPE compared with breast MRI in 48 women in a population weighted towards women with breast cancer (Li et al. 2017). Neither study was designed to determine if BPE on CEDM was associated with increased breast cancer risk; this is an ongoing investigation.

On the whole, patients prefer CEDM to MRI. Hobbs et al. surveyed 49 patients who underwent both MRI and CEDM and found that patients preferred the experience of CEDM (Hobbs et al. 2015). The most commonly cited reasons were faster procedure times, greater patient comfort, and decreased noise levels. In a survey of 38 patients undergoing both breast MRI and CEDM, Phillips et al. found that if CEDM and MRI had comparable sensitivities, the patients would prefer CEDM (Phillips et al. 2017).

Patel et al. used standard Medicare prices in 2015 to evaluate the costs associated with contrast-enhanced mammography compared with contrast-enhanced MRI (Patel et al. 2017). One CEDM examination costs $196.01 compared with $775.10 for one MRI examination (including the costs of contrast agents and computer-aided detection). They also used median equipment prices and maintenance costs to compare CEDM with MRI and found that equipment costs were approximately half for CEDM compared with MRI ($635,000 vs. $1,355,000).

3.3 Comparisons of CEDM with Ultrasound

Luczynska et al. compared CEDM and US in 116 symptomatic patients (Luczyńska et al. 2016). The sensitivity of CEDM was statistically significantly higher than US (100% vs. 92%, $p < 0.01$). CEDM accuracy was statistically significantly

increased breast cancer risk (Fig. 5) (Dontchos et al. 2015). Sogani et al. evaluated 287 women who underwent both CEDM and MRI within 30 days of each other (Sogani et al. 2017). This

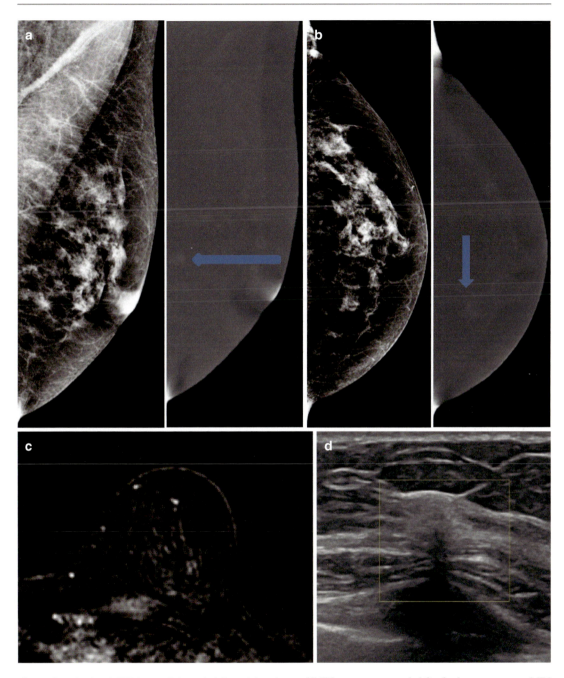

Fig. 4 Standard and CEDM mediolateral oblique (**a**) and craniocaudal (**b**) images of the left breast in a 61-year-old female presenting for high-risk screening for a history of lobular carcinoma in situ. CEDM demonstrated enhancement that was considered suspicious (denoted by arrow) and MRI was recommended for further assessment. MRI was negative (**c**). The patient returned 6 months later for ultrasound which demonstrated irregular mass corresponding to CEDM finding (**d**), biopsied yielding invasive lobular carcinoma

higher than US (78% vs. 70%, $p = 0.03$). AUC for both CEDM and US was 0.83. Klang et al. evaluated the utility of performing ultrasound after CEDM examinations (Klang et al. 2018). Among 87 biopsied lesions (37 malignant, 50 benign), CEDM findings given BI-RADS 0, 4, or 5 were

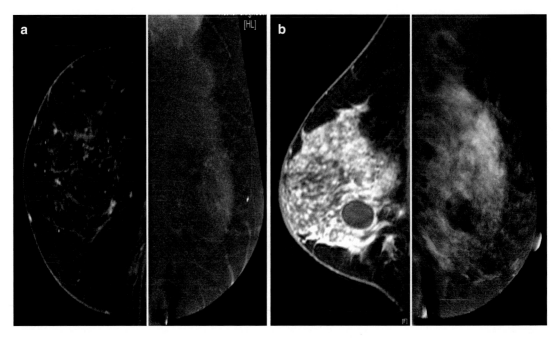

Fig. 5 Corresponding CEDM and MRI examples of mild (**a**) and marked background parenchymal enhancement (**b**)

associated with malignancy ($p < 0.0001$); however ultrasound findings given BI-RADS 0, 4, or 5 were not associated with malignancy ($p = 0.985$). Specificity of CESM was 40% (95% CI 26.4–54.8), significantly higher than US: 8% (95% CI 2.2–19.2).

4 Current and Potential Indications for Contrast-Enhanced Mammography

Many of the indications for breast MRI represent potential indications for CEDM, including of course CEDM for patients with contraindications to breast MRI. At this time, CEDM is mostly performed for additional evaluation of patients with abnormal screening mammograms and/or symptoms of breast cancer (Dromain et al. 2011; Lobbes et al. 2014) or for preoperative staging of known breast cancer (Fallenberg et al. 2014b; Jochelson et al. 2013; Lee-Felker et al. 2017). Occasionally CEDM can be used for problem-solving.

Increasing numbers of women are receiving neoadjuvant chemotherapy (NAC) for breast cancer (Fig. 6). Contrast-enhanced breast MRI is known to be the best imaging method to assess the response to chemotherapy (Martincich et al. 2004) but there has been an increasing interest in the ability of CEDM to accurately assess tumor response. Iotti et al. have reported results on 46 prospectively evaluated women who underwent both MRI and CEDM at baseline, halfway through treatment and at the end of treatment. Both MRI and CEDM underestimated residual tumor size: CEDM by 4.1 mm and MRI by 7.5 mm (Iotti et al. 2017). Of interest, CEDM was more likely to predict pathologic complete response than MRI. Travieso-Aja et al. retrospectively studied 204 breast cancers in 158 patients who underwent CEDM prior to surgery (Travieso-Aja et al. 2018). Mean tumor size at pathology was 20.7 mm while tumor size measured by CEDM was 23.6 mm (2.9 mm overestimation). Similarly, El-Said studied 21 patients with stage II and III breast cancer undergoing NAC and found that CEDM had an overall sensitivity of 40% and a specificity of 91%

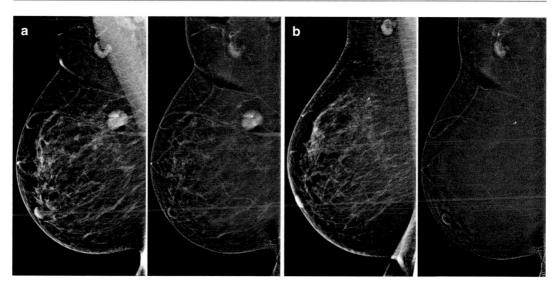

Fig. 6 (**a**) Pre- and (**b**) post-neoadjuvant chemotherapy standard and CEDM mediolateral oblique images in a 30-year-old female with ER/PR/HER2-positive invasive ductal carcinoma. No suspicious enhancement was found on CEDM post-neoadjuvant chemotherapy. Patient subsequently underwent mastectomy revealing no residual tumor. (Source: Bhavika Patel, MD, Mayo Clinic, Phoenix, AZ)

with 100% sensitivity for detecting complete response (El-Said et al. 2017). Barra et al. compared the size of residual malignancy on surgical pathology with the size of residual malignancy on CEDM and MRI in 33 women post-NAC (Barra et al. 2018). They found that CEDM measurements were comparable to MRI and had good correlation and agreement with surgical pathology measurements. Patel et al. studied 65 patients who underwent CEDM and MRI before and after neoadjuvant chemotherapy (Patel et al. 2018). Mean tumor size measured by CEDM or MRI was equivalent to the mean tumor size measured on surgical pathology within 1 cm. Additional studies are ongoing to clarify the potential benefits of using CEDM in patients after NAC.

Another potential indication for CEDM is screening for women at increased risk for breast cancer (Figs. 7 and 8) including post-lumpectomy patients, patients with a family history of breast cancer, patients with a history of high-risk lesions such as atypical ductal hyperplasia or lobular neoplasia, and women with dense breasts. Sung et al. evaluated the performance of CEDM in 904 women undergoing screening CEDM for a variety of indications (intermediate or high risk, personal history of breast cancer, high-risk lesion) (Sung et al. 2019). They found that CEDM had a cancer detection rate of 15.5 of 1000. The sensitivity of CEDM was 87.5%, compared with 50.0% for digital mammography ($p = 0.03$). The specificity of CEDM was 93.7%, compared with 97.1% for digital mammography ($p < 0.001$). Sorin et al. evaluated the performance of CEDM in a retrospective cohort of 611 women with intermediate breast cancer risk and/or dense breast tissue (Sorin et al. 2018). In 21 malignancies, CEDM demonstrated statistically significant improvements in sensitivity (90.5% vs. 52.4%, $p = 0.008$) compared with digital mammography. Specificity was higher in patients undergoing digital mammography compared with patients undergoing CEDM (90.5% vs. 76.1%, $p < 0.001$). The incremental cancer detection rate of CEDM was 13.1/1000 women (95% CI, 6.1–20.1). Jochelson et al. performed a prospective trial comparing CEDM with MRI in 307 women at increased risk for breast cancer (Jochelson et al. 2017). Too few cancers were found to be able to assess sensitivity, but both

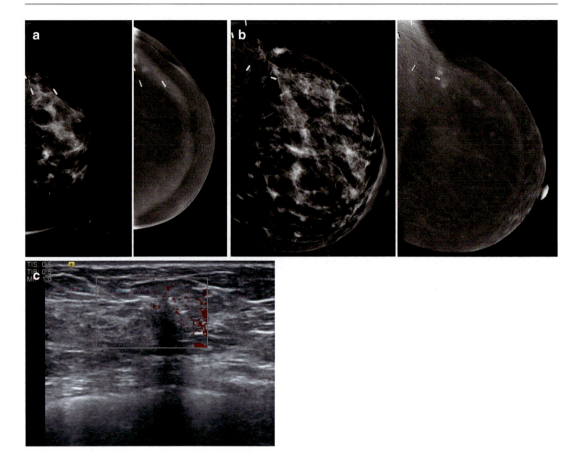

Fig. 7 CEDM in a 40-year-old patient 1 year post-lumpectomy with clear margins and radiation therapy, with corresponding ultrasound images of the lumpectomy site. Standard and CEDM craniocaudal (**a**) and mediolateral oblique (**b**) images with CEDM demonstrated suspicious enhancement within the lumpectomy bed. Ultrasound correlate (**c**) was biopsied yielding recurrent invasive ductal carcinoma

CEDM and MRI found the two mammographically occult invasive lobular cancers. No differences were found in specificity comparing CEDM to MRI (94.7% vs. 94.1%). Another clinical trial is underway to compare CEDM with screening ultrasound. Preliminary results in 126 women with five cancers were presented by Sung et al. at the Radiological Society of North America annual meeting in 2016 (Sung et al. 2016). Only two of the five cancers were detected on ultrasound while all five were seen on CEDM. Preliminary results of 1197 screening CEDM examinations in women, 27% of whom had a family history of breast cancer in a first-degree relative and 39% of whom had a personal history of breast cancer, were presented by Sung et al. at the Radiological Society of North America annual meeting in 2017 (Sung et al. 2017). Twenty-two cancers were detected for a PPV3 of 31% with a cancer detection rate of 18/1000.

There are preliminary efforts to integrate CEDM with tomosynthesis. There remain some technical difficulties in performing tomosynthesis after contrast. Chou et al. evaluated CEDM and contrast-enhanced tomosynthesis versus MRI. They found no statistically significant differences in AUC between contrast-enhanced tomosynthesis and MRI (0.89 vs. 0.90, respectively, $p = 0.891$), and between contrast-enhanced

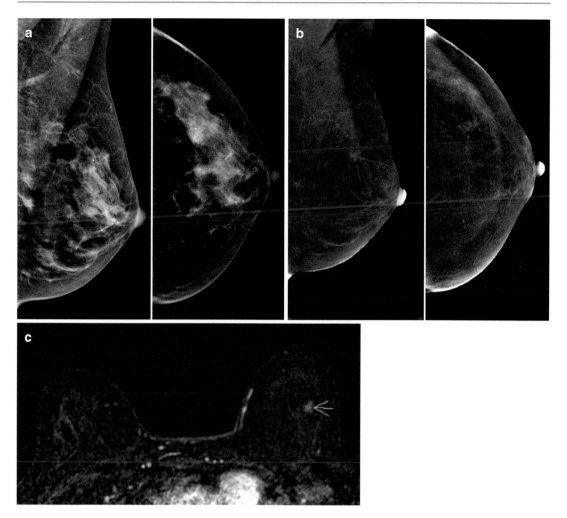

Fig. 8 CEDM in a 52-year-old patient with a childhood history of mantle radiation for Hodgkin's lymphoma. The patient presented for high-risk screening. Standard mediolateral oblique and craniocaudal images (**a**) did not reveal suspicious findings. Mediolateral oblique and craniocaudal CEDM images of the left breast (**b**) demonstrating suspicious enhancement, seen on the corresponding bilateral breast MRI (**c**). Ultrasound was negative. The enhancement was biopsied under MRI guidance and confirmed to be ductal carcinoma in situ

tomosynthesis and CEDM (0.89 vs. 0.88, respectively, $p = 0.717$) (Chou et al. 2015). Huang et al. studied 21 adult women with suspicious breast lesions (BI-RADS 4 or 5) prior to biopsy to compare CEDM with contrast-enhanced tomosynthesis (Huang et al. 2019). Using a 5-point scale (−2 to +2) comparing CEDM or contrast-enhanced tomosynthesis, they found that contrast-enhanced tomosynthesis depicted lesion margins better. Contrast-enhanced tomosynthesis with a synthetic 2D CEDM image delivered a 35.7% decreased radiation dose compared with CEDM + DBT.

Efforts are underway to adapt BI-RADS language to contrast-enhanced mammography, drawing from BI-RADS 5 terminology for mammography as well as BI-RADS for contrast-enhanced MRI without including kinetics.

5 Risks

Despite all of its advantages, CEDM has its own unique set of risks:

5.1 Iodinated Contrast

The utilization of iodinated contrast is associated with certain risks, the most common of which involves iodine allergies (Cochran et al. 2001; Hunt et al. 2009). Zanardo et al. identified 84 articles with 14,012 patients in a systematic review of CEDM protocols and adverse reactions (Zanardo et al. 2019). Among all these patients, only one severe-nonfatal adverse reaction event was reported. Overall adverse reaction rates were comparable to previously reported reaction rates from CT scans. Reactions to iodinated contrast occur in less than 1% of all patients but are higher in patients with prior allergic reactions (Mortelé et al. 2005). Therefore prior to CEDM it is critical to determine if the patient is an appropriate candidate for contrast. Patients with histories of allergies to intravenous contrast should be asked about the nature and severity of their contrast reaction. Severe contrast reactions (respiratory difficulty, throat swelling, etc.) to iodinated contrast material represent an absolute contraindication to CEDM and these patients should obtain supplemental screening with contrast-enhanced breast MRI or screening ultrasound. Patients with a history of minor contrast reaction could theoretically be pretreated with corticosteroids and antihistamines prior to CEDM or alternatively obtain supplemental screening with other modalities such as ultrasound or contrast-enhanced breast MRI. At our institution, patients with any history of contrast reaction do not undergo CEDM because there are other options. Additionally, it is critical that all members of the team performing CEDM are familiar with the guidelines for treating contrast reactions (ACR Committee 2017).

5.2 Renal Toxicity

A second less common risk is that of renal toxicity. Potential CEDM patients should be screened in the same fashion as for computerized tomography patients. Glomerular filtration rates obtained within 12 weeks of CEDM are required for high-risk patients, defined at our institution as patients over 70 years of age, or those who have a history of diabetes, hypertension, prior renal transplantation, etc. Again, since there are other available imaging options, any patient with low GFR (under 45) should not undergo CEDM.

5.3 Radiation Dose

CEDM uses both low- and high-energy images with standard 2D mammographic projections, thereby increasing radiation doses. James et al. found that CEDM increases the average glandular dose by approximately 0.9 mGy compared with 2D examinations and 0.5 mGy compared with 3D examinations (James et al. 2017). Although these doses are higher than standard 2D and 3D mammographic examinations, Jeukens et al. found that the average glandular doses were within the dose limits of 3 mGy set by the Mammography Quality Standards Act (Jeukens et al. 2014).

Since CEDM has been used primarily in the diagnostic setting, patients have frequently already had routine mammograms. In the screening setting, it was originally uncertain as to whether, as with tomosynthesis, a separate mammogram would be necessary in addition to the routine CEDM. Francescone et al. studied 88 women undergoing CEDM and found no statistically significant differences in technical parameters or imaging findings when comparing low-energy images with conventional full-field digital mammography images (Francescone et al. 2014). Similarly, Lalji et al. studied 147 cases with both low-energy images and conventional full-field digital mammography images and found no statistically significant differences in image quality (Lalji et al. 2015). Finally, Fallenberg et al. studied 118 patients undergoing CEDM and found that CEDM without additional conventional full-field digital mammogram had comparable sensitivity and improved size assessment with only a 6.2% increase in average glandular dose (Fallenberg et al. 2014b). They concluded that conventional full-field digital mammography can be avoided resulting in potential radiation dose savings of up to 61%, particularly in patients with dense breasts.

6 Conclusions

CEDM is a promising emerging tool in breast imaging which utilizes the enhancement of neovascularity of breast cancers for improved cancer detection, similar to contrast-enhanced breast MRI. Initial studies have suggested that CEDM has comparable sensitivity to contrast-enhanced breast MRI with lower costs, preferred by patients and potentially more available. Potential indications include diagnostic workup after abnormal screening or clinical symptoms, screening of women at increased risk for breast cancer including some women with dense breasts, assessment of response to neoadjuvant chemotherapy, and evaluation of the extent of disease in patients with known breast cancer. Ongoing studies will help to define the role of this emerging technology in both screening and diagnostic imaging settings.

References

ACR Committee on Drugs and Contrast Media (2017) ACR manual on contrast media, Version 10.3
Barra FR, Sobrinho AB, Barra RR, Magalhães MT, Aguiar LR, de Albuquerque GFL, Costa RP, Farage L, Pratesi R (2018) Contrast-enhanced mammography (CEM) for detecting residual disease after neoadjuvant chemotherapy: a comparison with breast magnetic resonance imaging (MRI). Biomed Res Int 2018:8531916
Berg WA (2016) Current status of supplemental screening in dense breasts. J Clin Oncol 34(16):1840–1843

Berg WA, Zhang Z, Lehrer D, Jong RA, Pisano ED, Barr RG, Böhm-Vélez M, Mahoney MC, Evans WP III, Larsen LH, Morton MJ, Mendelson EB, Farria DM, Cormack JB, Marques HS, Adams A, Yeh NM, Gabrielli G, ACRIN 6666 Investigators (2012) Detection of breast cancer with addition of annual screening ultrasound or a single screening MRI to mammography in women with elevated breast cancer risk. JAMA 307(13):1394–1404
Boyd NF, Guo H, Martin LJ, Sun L, Stone J, Fishell E, Jong RA, Hislop G, Chiarelli A, Minkin S, Yaffe MJ (2007) Mammographic density and the risk and detection of breast cancer. N Engl J Med 356(3):227–236
Carney PA, Miglioretti DL, Yankaskas BC, Kerlikowske K, Rosenberg R, Rutter CM, Geller BM, Abraham LA, Taplin SH, Dignan M, Cutter G, Ballard-Barbash R (2003) Individual and combined effects of age, breast density, and hormone replacement therapy use on the accuracy of screening mammography. Ann Intern Med 138(3):168–175
Cheung YC, Lin YC, Wan YL, Yeow KM, Huang PC, Lo YF, Tsai HP, Ueng SH, Chang CJ (2014) Diagnostic performance of dual-energy contrast-enhanced subtracted mammography in dense breasts compared to mammography alone: interobserver blind-reading analysis. Eur Radiol 10:2394–2403
Cheung YC, Juan YH, Lin YC, Lo YF, Tsai HP, Ueng SH, Chen SC (2016) Dual-energy contrast-enhanced spectral mammography: enhancement analysis on BI-RADS 4 non-mass microcalcifications in screened women. PLoS One 11(9):e0162740
Chou CP, Lewin JM, Chiang CL, Hung BH, Yang TL, Huang JS, Liao JB, Pan HB (2015) Clinical evaluation of contrast-enhanced digital mammography and contrast enhanced tomosynthesis—comparison to contrast-enhanced breast MRI. Eur J Radiol 84(12):2501–2508
Cochran ST, Bomyea K, Sayre JW (2001) Trends in adverse events after IV administration of contrast media. AJR Am J Roentgenol 176(6):1385–1388
Diekmann F, Freyer M, Diekmann S, Fallenberg EM, Fischer T, Bick U, Pöllinger A (2011) Evaluation of contrast-enhanced digital mammography. Eur J Radiol 78(1):112–121
Dontchos BN, Rahbar H, Partridge SC, Korde LA, Lam DL, Scheel JR, Peacock S, Lehman CD (2015) Are qualitative assessments of background parenchymal enhancement, amount of fibroglandular tissue on MR images, and mammographic density associated with breast cancer risk? Radiology 276(2):371–380
Dromain C, Thibault F, Muller S, Rimareix F, Delaloge S, Tardivon A, Balleyguier C (2011) Dual-energy contrast-enhanced digital mammography: initial clinical results. Eur Radiol 21(3):565–574
Dromain C, Thibault F, Diekmann F, Fallenberg EM, Jong RA, Koomen M, Hendrick RE, Tardivon A, Toledano A (2012) Dual-energy contrast-enhanced digital mammography: initial clinical results of a multireader, multicase study. Breast Cancer Res 14(3):R94

El-Said N et al (2017) Role of contrast enhanced spectral mammography in predicting pathological response of locally advanced breast cancer post neo-adjuvant chemotherapy. Egypt J Radiol Nucl Med 48(2):519–527

Fallenberg EM, Dromain C, Diekmann F, Engelken F, Krohn M, Singh JM, Ingold-Heppner B, Winzer KJ, Bick U, Renz DM (2014a) Contrast-enhanced spectral mammography versus MRI: initial results in the detection of breast cancer and assessment of tumour size. Eur Radiol 24(1):256–264

Fallenberg EM, Dromain C, Diekmann F, Renz DM, Amer H, Ingold-Heppner B, Neumann AU, Winzer KJ, Bick U, Hamm B, Engelken F (2014b) Contrast-enhanced spectral mammography: does mammography provide additional clinical benefits or can some radiation exposure be avoided? Breast Cancer Res Treat 146(2):371–381

Fallenberg EM, Schmitzberger FF, Amer H, Ingold-Heppner B, Balleyguier C, Diekmann F, Engelken F, Mann RM, Renz DM, Bick U, Hamm B, Dromain C (2017) Contrast-enhanced spectral mammography vs. mammography and MRI – clinical performance in a multi-reader evaluation. Eur Radiol 27(7):2752–2764

Francescone MA, Jochelson MS, Dershaw DD, Sung JS, Hughes MC, Zheng J, Moskowitz C, Morris EA (2014) Low energy mammogram obtained in contrast-enhanced digital mammography (CEDM) is comparable to routine full-field digital mammography (FFDM). Eur J Radiol 83(8):1350–1355

Hobbs MM, Taylor DB, Buzynski S, Peake RE (2015) Contrast-enhanced spectral mammography (CESM) and contrast enhanced MRI (CEMRI): patient preferences and tolerance. J Med Imaging Radiat Oncol 59(3):300–305

Hooley RJ, Greenberg KL, Stackhouse RM, Geisel JL, Butler RS, Philpotts LE (2012) Screening US in patients with mammographically dense breasts: initial experience with Connecticut Public Act 09-41. Radiology 265(1):59–69

Huang H, Scaduto DA, Liu C, Yang J, Zhu C, Rinaldi K, Eisenberg J, Liu J, Hoernig M, Wicklein J, Vogt S, Mertelmeier T, Fisher PR, Zhao W (2019) Comparison of contrast-enhanced digital mammography and contrast-enhanced digital breast tomosynthesis for lesion assessment. J Med Imaging (Bellingham) 6(3):031407

Hunt CH, Hartman RP, Hesley GK (2009) Frequency and severity of adverse effects of iodinated and gadolinium contrast materials: retrospective review of 456,930 doses. AJR Am J Roentgenol 193(4):1124–1127

Iotti V, Ravaioli S, Vacondio R, Coriani C, Caffarri S, Sghedoni R, Nitrosi A, Ragazzi M, Gasparini E, Masini C, Bisagni G, Falco G, Ferrari G, Braglia L, Del Prato A, Malavolti I, Ginocchi V, Pattacini P (2017) Contrast-enhanced spectral mammography in neoadjuvant chemotherapy monitoring: a comparison with breast magnetic resonance imaging. Breast Cancer Res 19(1):106

James JR, Pavlicek W, Hanson JA, Boltz TF, Patel BK (2017) Breast radiation dose with CESM compared with 2D FFDM and 3D tomosynthesis mammography. AJR Am J Roentgenol 208(2):362–372

Jeukens CR, Lalji UC, Meijer E, Bakija B, Theunissen R, Wildberger JE, Lobbes MB (2014) Radiation exposure of contrast-enhanced spectral mammography compared with full-field digital mammography. Invest Radiol 49(10):659–665

Jochelson M (2014) Contrast-enhanced digital mammography. Radiol Clin North Am 52(3):609–616

Jochelson MS, Dershaw DD, Sung JS, Heerdt AS, Thornton C, Moskowitz CS, Ferrara J, Morris EA (2013) Bilateral contrast-enhanced dual-energy digital mammography: feasibility and comparison with conventional digital mammography and MR imaging in women with known breast carcinoma. Radiology 266(3):743–751

Jochelson MS et al (2017) Comparison of screening CEDM and MRI for women at increased risk for breast cancer: a pilot study. Eur J Radiol 97:37–43

Klang E, Krosser A, Amitai MM, Sorin V, Halshtok Neiman O, Shalmon A, Gotlieb M, Sklair-Levy M (2018) Utility of routine use of breast ultrasound following contrast-enhanced spectral mammography. Clin Radiol 73(10):908.e11–908.e16. https://doi.org/10.1016/j.crad.2018.05.031

Kuhl C, Weigel S, Schrading S, Arand B, Bieling H, König R, Tombach B, Leutner C, Rieber-Brambs A, Nordhoff D, Heindel W, Reiser M, Schild HH (2010) Prospective multicenter cohort study to refine management recommendations for women at elevated familial risk of breast cancer: the EVA trial. J Clin Oncol 28(9):1450–1457

Lalji UC, Jeukens CR, Houben I, Nelemans PJ, van Engen RE, van Wylick E, Beets-Tan RG, Wildberger JE, Paulis LE, Lobbes MB (2015) Evaluation of low-energy contrast-enhanced spectral mammography images by comparing them to full-field digital mammography using EUREF image quality criteria. Eur Radiol 25(10):2813–2820

Lalji UC, Houben IP, Prevos R, Gommers S, van Goethem M, Vanwetswinkel S, Pijnappel R, Steeman R, Frotscher C, Mok W, Nelemans P, Smidt ML, Beets-Tan RG, Wildberger JE, Lobbes MB (2016) Contrast-enhanced spectral mammography in recalls from the Dutch breast cancer screening program: validation of results in a large multireader, multicase study. Eur Radiol 26(12):4371–4379

Lee-Felker SA, Tekchandani L, Thomas M, Gupta E, Andrews-Tang D, Roth A, Sayre J, Rahbar G (2017) Newly diagnosed breast cancer: comparison of contrast-enhanced spectral mammography and breast MR imaging in the evaluation of extent of disease. Radiology 285(2):389–400

Lewin JM, Isaacs PK, Vance V, Larke FJ (2003) Dual-energy contrast-enhanced digital subtraction mammography: feasibility. Radiology 229(1):261–268

Li L, Roth R, Germaine P, Ren S, Lee M, Hunter K, Tinney E, Liao L (2017) Contrast-enhanced spectral mammography (CESM) versus breast magnetic resonance imaging (MRI): a retrospective comparison in 66 breast lesions. Diagn Interv Imaging 98(2):113–123

Lobbes MB, Lalji U, Houwers J, Nijssen EC, Nelemans PJ, van Roozendaal L, Smidt ML, Heuts E, Wildberger JE (2014) Contrast-enhanced spectral mammography in patients referred from the breast cancer screening programme. Eur Radiol 24(7):1668–1676

Lobbes MB, Lalji UC, Nelemans PJ, Houben I, Smidt ML, Heuts E, de Vries B, Wildberger JE, Beets-Tan RG (2015) The quality of tumor size assessment by contrast-enhanced spectral mammography and the benefit of additional breast MRI. J Cancer 6(2):144–150

Luczyńska E, Heinze-Paluchowska S, Dyczek S, Blecharz P, Rys J, Reinfuss M (2014) Contrast-enhanced spectral mammography: comparison with conventional mammography and histopathology in 152 women. Korean J Radiol 15(6):689–696

Łuczyńska E, Heinze-Paluchowska S, Hendrick E, Dyczek S, Ryś J, Herman K, Blecharz P, Jakubowicz J (2015) Comparison between breast MRI and contrast-enhanced spectral mammography. Med Sci Monit 21:1358–1367

Luczyńska E, Heinze S, Adamczyk A, Rys J, Mitus JW, Hendrick E (2016) Comparison of the mammography, contrast-enhanced spectral mammography and ultrasonography in a group of 116 patients. Anticancer Res 36(8):4359–4366

Martincich L, Montemurro F, De Rosa G, Marra V, Ponzone R, Cirillo S, Gatti M, Biglia N, Sarotto I, Sismondi P, Regge D, Aglietta M (2004) Monitoring response to primary chemotherapy in breast cancer using dynamic contrast-enhanced magnetic resonance imaging. Breast Cancer Res Treat 83(1):67–76

Mori M, Akashi-Tanaka S, Suzuki S, Daniels MI, Watanabe C, Hirose M, Nakamura S (2017) Diagnostic accuracy of contrast-enhanced spectral mammography in comparison to conventional full-field digital mammography in a population of women with dense breasts. Breast Cancer 24(1):104–110

Mortelé KJ, Oliva MR, Ondategui S, Ros PR, Silverman SG (2005) Universal use of nonionic iodinated contrast medium for CT: evaluation of safety in a large urban teaching hospital. AJR Am J Roentgenol 184(1):31–34

Patel BK, Gray RJ, Pockaj BA (2017) Potential cost savings of contrast-enhanced digital mammography. AJR Am J Roentgenol 208(6):W231–W237

Patel BK, Hilal T, Covington M, Zhang N, Kosiorek HE, Lobbes M, Northfelt DW, Pockaj BA (2018) Contrast-enhanced spectral mammography is comparable to MRI in the assessment of residual breast cancer following neoadjuvant systemic therapy. Ann Surg Oncol 25(5):1350–1356

Phillips J, Miller MM, Mehta TS, Fein-Zachary V, Nathanson A, Hori W, Monahan-Earley R, Slanetz PJ (2017) Contrast-enhanced spectral mammography (CESM) versus MRI in the high-risk screening setting: patient preferences and attitudes. Clin Imaging 42:193–197

Saslow D, Boetes C, Burke W, Harms S, Leach MO, Lehman CD, Morris E, Pisano E, Schnall M, Sener S, Smith RA, Warner E, Yaffe M, Andrews KS, Russell CA, American Cancer Society Breast Cancer Advisory Group (2007) American Cancer Society guidelines for breast screening with MRI as an adjunct to mammography. CA Cancer J Clin 57(2):75–89

Siu AL, U.S. Preventive Services Task Force (2016) Screening for breast cancer: U.S. Preventive Services Task Force recommendation statement. Ann Intern Med 164(4):279–296

Sogani J, Morris EA, Kaplan JB, D'Alessio D, Goldman D, Moskowitz CS, Jochelson MS (2017) Comparison of background parenchymal enhancement at contrast-enhanced spectral mammography and breast MR imaging. Radiology 282(1):63–73

Sorin V, Yagil Y, Yosepovich A, Shalmon A, Gotlieb M, Neiman OH, Sklair-Levy M (2018) Contrast-enhanced spectral mammography in women with intermediate breast cancer risk and dense breasts. AJR Am J Roentgenol 11(5):W267–WW74

Sung J, Jochelson M, Lee C, Bernstein J, Reiner A, Morris E, Comstock C (2016) Comparison of contrast enhanced digital mammography and whole breast screening ultrasound for supplemental breast cancer screening. In: Abstract presented at the Radiological Society of North America 2016 Scientific Assembly and Annual Meeting, Chicago, IL, 27 November–2 December, 2016

Sung J, Lebron L, D'Alessio D, Keating D, Lee C, Morris EA, Jochelson MS (2017) Utility of contrast enhanced digital mammography for breast cancer screening. In: Abstract presented at the Radiological Society of North America 2017 Scientific Assembly and Annual Meeting, Chicago, IL, 26 November 26–1 December, 2017

Sung JS, Lebron L, Keating D, D'Alessio D, Comstock CE, Lee CH, Pike MC, Ayhan M, Moskowitz CS, Morris EA, Jochelson MS (2019) Performance of dual-energy contrast-enhanced digital mammography for screening women at increased risk of breast cancer. Radiology 293(1):81–88

Tennant SL, James JJ, Cornford EJ, Chen Y, Burrell HC, Hamilton LJ, Girio-Fragkoulakis C (2016) Contrast-enhanced spectral mammography improves diagnostic accuracy in the symptomatic setting. Clin Radiol 71(11):1148–1155

Travieso-Aja MDM, Naranjo-Santana P, Fernández-Ruiz C, Severino-Rondón W, Maldonado-Saluzzi D, Rodríguez Rodríguez M, Vega-Benítez V, Luzardo OP (2018) Factors affecting the precision of lesion sizing with contrast-enhanced spectral mammography. Clin Radiol 73(3):296–303

Wang Q, Li K, Wang L, Zhang J, Zhou Z, Feng Y (2016) Preclinical study of diagnostic performances of contrast-enhanced spectral mammography versus MRI for breast diseases in China. Springerplus 5(1):763

Zanardo M, Cozzi A, Trimboli RM, Labaj O, Monti CB, Schiaffino S, Carbonaro LA, Sardanelli F (2019) Technique, protocols and adverse reactions for contrast-enhanced spectral mammography (CESM): a systematic review. Insights Imaging 10(1):76

Mammography Screening

Carin Meltzer and Per Skaane

Contents

1	**Introduction**	44
2	**History of Mammography Screening**	44
3	**Scientific Basis for Current Screening: The Randomized Controlled Trials**	45
4	**Digital Mammography in Breast Cancer Screening**	47
5	**Recommendations for Organized Mammographic Screening**	47
6	**Guidelines and Quality Assurance of Screening Programs**	48
	6.1 Performance Indicators	49
	6.2 Quality of the Mammographic Report	49
	6.3 Single Versus Double Reading	51
7	**Mammographic Diagnosis of Early Preclinical Breast Cancer**	51
	7.1 Ductal Carcinoma In Situ (DCIS)	52
	7.2 Early Invasive Breast Cancer	53
8	**Personalized Screening for Women at Average Risk**	55
	8.1 Ultrasound as Supplemental Imaging	55
	8.2 Magnetic Resonance Imaging (MRI) as Supplemental Imaging	56
	8.3 Digital Breast Tomosynthesis (DBT) as Supplemental Screening (Chapter "Mammography and Digital Breast Tomosynthesis: Technique")	56
	8.4 Other Imaging Modalities as Supplemental Screening	59
9	**Screening for Women at Higher Risk**	60
10	**Adverse Effects of Mammography Screening**	60
	10.1 Radiation Exposure	60
	10.2 False Positives	61
	10.3 False Negatives and Interval Cancer	61
	10.4 Overdiagnosis	62
11	**The Future of Breast Cancer Screening**	62
	References	63

C. Meltzer (✉) · P. Skaane
Oslo University Hospital, Oslo, Norway
e-mail: camelt@ous-hf.no

© Springer Nature Switzerland AG 2022
M. Fuchsjäger et al. (eds.), *Breast Imaging*, Medical Radiology Diagnostic Imaging,
https://doi.org/10.1007/978-3-030-94918-1_3

Abstract

Breast cancer screening with mammography is a validated and effective method, with a mortality reduction among women attending the program in the range of 25–45%. European guidelines recommend biannual screening for women 50–69 years, but target groups vary somewhat among countries. American societies recommend annual screening, often from the age of 40. The goal of mammographic screening is to detect small node negative cancers, and according to guidelines, at least 50% of screen-detected cancers should be less than 15 mm. Detection of small invasive cancers is a difficult task and a great challenge. In order to have a high cancer detection rate and a low recall rate, independent double reading with consensus or arbitration is a common approach in Europe. Full-field digital mammography (FFDM) is the current standard examination for screening of women at average risk. Conventional mammography has two serious limitations: low specificity and sensitivity in women with dense breasts. Ongoing discussion is whether the current practice of FFDM for all women ("one-size-fits-all" concept) should be replaced by "personalized" screening also for women at average risk. Implementation of advanced techniques for population-based screening is, however, a great problem and challenge. Adjunct ultrasound has so far been most used. Other potential modalities for supplemental screening include MRI and digital breast tomosynthesis. Adverse effects of mammography screening (radiation exposure, false positives, false negatives, and overdiagnosis) should be kept as low as possible in order to optimize the balance between benefit and harms of breast cancer screening.

1 Introduction

Breast cancer is the most frequent cancer among women worldwide, with almost 1.7 million new cancers diagnosed in 2012 (Ferlay et al. 2015).

Women in Northern America, Northern and Western Europe, Australia, and New Zealand have the highest incidence of breast cancer, with an estimated age-standardized incidence of more than 80 per 100,000 and year. Approximately 12% of women in Northern America will develop breast cancer during their lifetime. The lowest incidence is seen in Africa and Asia, where mammographic screening is not available, and these cases are often diagnosed in a late stage with poor outcome (Ferlay et al. 2015).

The prognosis of breast cancer is greatly dependent on the stage at the time of diagnosis, and 5-year survival rates range from close to 100% for the earliest, localized types to about 25% for late stages with spread to other organs (Jemal et al. 2017). Despite an overall good prognosis, the high incidence makes breast cancer the most common cause of cancer deaths, leading to approximately 500,000 deaths worldwide each year (Ferlay et al. 2015). Early-stage breast cancer is often asymptomatic, and typical clinical symptoms as a palpable mass, skin changes, pain, nipple retraction, or discharge from nipple are often a sign of a more advanced stage. The high incidence and good prognosis for localized disease made way for the introduction of breast cancer screening programs, which is the most widespread screening program worldwide.

2 History of Mammography Screening

The potential of mammography, an X-ray examination of the breast, has been known for many decades. However, it took several decades before the image quality opened for breast cancer screening. The first radiographies of breast cancer were mastectomy specimens published in 1913 by the German surgeon Albert Salomon (Gold et al. 1990). Imaging technique and mammographic studies of the breast were presented in the USA by the radiologist Stafford L. Warren in the 1930s. However, it was not until late 1950s that the cooperation between the radiologist Gershon-Cohen and the pathologist Ingleby resulted in the first published study on mammography for breast disease (Gershon-Cohen and Ingleby 1958). Their second publication in 1961 showed that periodic mammography of women over 40 years of age might have the potential to reduce the mortality rate from breast cancer (Gershon-Cohen et al. 1961). Of much importance was the first breast-dedicated X-ray imaging equipment developed by the French radiologist Charles Gros and "Compagnie Générale de Radiologie" which was introduced to the market in 1966 (Gold et al. 1990).

The first randomized controlled trial (RCT) to prove the efficiency of mammographic screening was the Health Insurance Plan (HIP) study performed in the state of New York between 1963 and 1967. The study demonstrated a significant reduction in breast cancer mortality (Shapiro et al. 1971) in the group randomized to screening. Following the HIP study, the Breast Cancer Detection Demonstration Project (BCDDP), initiated in 1973, was designed to evaluate the usefulness of mammographic screening in women aged 35–74 years. This study showed that a large proportion of the detected cancers were small preclinical tumors, but the results of the BCDDP left some open questions since no control group was included (Baker 1982).

The promising results from the US pioneer studies initiated the interest in Europe for mammography screening. The earliest case-control study in Europe started in Florence in 1970 (Palli et al. 1986). This study was followed by two Dutch case-control studies, the DOM project in Utrecht in 1974 (Collette et al. 1984) and the Nijmegen project in 1975 (Verbeek et al. 1984), and thereafter by the Edinburgh trial in 1978 (Roberts et al. 1990). An important study for the further development was the so-called Sandviken study, a Swedish pilot project conducted by B. Lundgren in 1974 showing that single-view (MLO-view) mammography has the potential to be a simple and cost-efficient approach for breast cancer screening (Lundgren and Jakobsson 1976). The program "Europe Against Cancer" was launched in 1986 and aimed to introduce systematic screening for breast cancer for women

aged 50–69 years (De Waard et al. 1994; del Moral Aldaz et al. 1994). It became obvious that mammography might have a great potential in breast cancer screening, but the effect could only be proven in prospective randomized trials.

3 Scientific Basis for Current Screening: The Randomized Controlled Trials

The early randomized controlled trials (RCTs) were initiated in Europe and North America in the period between 1963 and 1982, and the results provided the scientific basis for the development of guidelines for mammographic screening. The RCTs are listed in Table 1.

Overall, the RCTs showed a mortality reduction of about 25% for women invited to the mammography screening (Smith 2003). It is important today to keep in mind that the RCTs were carried out with screen-film mammography (SFM), with a much lower image quality as compared with the digital technique, which is the current gold standard for mammography screening. Furthermore, differences in study design including randomization, target groups, screening interval, and imaging technique (one-view and two-view mammography) have contributed to diverging results and much debate.

RCTs involve a randomization where one group of women is offered screening and the control group not. Today most Western countries have implemented breast cancer screening programs, and it is therefore unrealistic to believe that such randomized trials will ever be carried out again, and it would be unethical to randomize a group to non-screening. Consequently, we still need to use the results from these early trials, based on the examinations with poor-quality SFM in our never-ending debate on the benefit of mammography screening.

Radiologists need to keep in mind the concept of randomized trials: One group is invited to intervention (mammography) and the other is not offered mammography (control group). However, some women in the intervention group

Table 1 The randomized controlled trials of breast cancer screening

Trial	Year of initiation	Screening age	Intervention	Intervention group	Control group	RR	RR (95% CI)
HIP[a]	1963	40–64	M + CE	31,000	31,000	0.78	0.61–1.00
Malmo[b]	1976	45–69	M	20,695	20,783	0.81	0.62–1.07
Two county[c]	1977	40–74	M	77,080	55,985	0.68	0.59–0.80
Edinburgh	1978	45–64	M + CE	28,628	26,026	0.78	0.62–1.02
Canadian[d]	1980	40–59	M + CE	44,925	44,910	1.02	0.84–2.21
Stockholm	1981	40–64	M	38,525	20,651	0.90	0.53–1.22
Gothenburg	1982	39–59	M	20,724	28,809	0.78	0.54–1.37

M mammography, *CE* clinical breast examination, *RR* relative risk, *CI* confidence interval
[a] Health Insurance Plan of Greater New York, USA
[b] Malmo mammographic screening trial (MMST) I and II
[c] Two-County (WE) trial: Ostergotaland and Kopparberg
[d] Canadian National Breast Screening Study (CNBSS) 1 (40–49 years) and 2 (50–59 years)

invited to screening will not attend to mammography (nonattenders) whereas some women in the control group will have mammography outside the trial (contamination). Evaluation of randomized trials does not consider these aspects when interpreting the results, and consequently, the benefit for women who actually undergo screening will therefore be underestimated. The International Agency for Research on Cancer (IARC) Working Group has estimated the mortality reduction for women attending the mammography screening program to be about 35% (Smith 2003). Several studies on European screening programs have reported even greater benefit with a mortality reduction of women undergoing mammographic screening in the range of 38–48% (Gabe et al. 2007; Hofvind et al. 2013; Broeders et al. 2012).

4 Digital Mammography in Breast Cancer Screening

At the end of the 1990s it became obvious that most or all radiologic imaging was going to be digital. Only mammography was still considered to be kept as a screen-film technology. The RCTs had shown that screen-film mammography (SFM) was an efficient technique to reduce mortality from breast cancer. But it was obvious that digital mammography would offer several potential benefits in organized mammographic screening: elimination of technical failure recalls; reduction of the glandular dose; a higher workflow; a simplified archival, retrieval, and transmission of images; and the potential for simpler implementation of computer-aided detection (CAD), telemammography, teleconsultations, and breast cancer screening program reorganizations. However, there were two main concerns regarding the implementation of full-field digital mammography (FFDM) in screening: soft-copy reading on monitors instead of hard copies on alternators, and the spatial resolution with respect to fine microcalcifications, which are often of most importance for early detection of subtle breast cancer. Again trials were necessary to show whether the new digital technology was

ready for implementation in breast imaging and especially in screening.

The two pioneer studies comparing SFM and FFDM in breast cancer screening were the US Colorado-Massachusetts (Co-Ma) study (Lewin et al. 2001) and the Oslo I trial (Skaane et al. 2003). The results of these two pioneer studies were promising, but somewhat disappointing since slightly lower cancer detection rates were found in both studies, although the difference was not statistically significant. A breakthrough came with the following Oslo II trial which showed a significantly higher cancer detection rate for FFDM (Skaane and Skjennald 2004). When the DMIST trial (Pisano ct al. 2005) was published the next year, demonstrating a significantly higher cancer detection rate for FFDM in younger women and in women with dense breast parenchyma, the decision for future mammography screening was obvious: It was going to be digital. Several studies comparing SFM and FFDM in breast cancer screening published during the following years mostly confirmed the results from the DMIST trial, although some studies showed divergent and somewhat conflicting results. Overall, the higher cancer detection rate for FFDM was close to statistically significant for women presenting with microcalcifications and dense breast parenchyma, but these higher detection rates were often achieved at the cost of a higher recall rate and consequently there was often no significant difference in the positive predictive values between the two techniques (Skaane 2009).

Full-field digital mammography is today's "gold standard" for breast cancer screening in women at average risk for developing cancer.

5 Recommendations for Organized Mammographic Screening

The European Parliament Resolution on Breast Cancer in the Enlarged European Union presented the following statement in 2006: "The resolutions call for every woman in Europe to have access to the same first-class early detection, diagnosis, treatment and aftercare, irrespective of where she lives, her social status, and her level of education. Women between the ages of 50 and 69 must have the right to attend high-quality mammography screening at two-year intervals in dedicated and certified centres paid for by health insurance schemes," though the statement remains yet to be implemented in several European countries. The recommended age span for screening is chosen according to the highest beneficial effects in terms of mortality reduction, but there are some national differences (Giordano et al. 2012).

The USA strongly recommends screening, but does not offer an organized population-based screening program. The US Preventive Services Task Force (USPSTF) recommends biennial screening mammography for women aged 50–74 years, a program intended to offer the best balance of benefit to harm, and that screening between the ages of 40 and 50 can be considered on an individual basis. The American College of Radiology (ACR) (Monticciolo et al. 2017) recommends annual screening starting at age 40 for women at average risk. The American Cancer Society recommends annual screening for women aged 45–54 years, and biannual or annual screening for women 55 years or older. ACR recommends that there is an opportunity for screening from age 40, and that screening continous as long as the overall health is good and that life expectancy is 10 years or longer. Breast cancer screening of women younger than 50 years is widely discussed, and the scientific evidence shows various results. A greater number of small, localized tumors are found, but the effect on mortality and balance against the potential harms of screening is still unclear.

The national screening program in Australia invites all women aged 50–74 to undergo free biannual mammograms, and screening is also available for women aged 40–49 and over 74 upon request (Lee and Peters 2013). New Zealand offers free, biannual mammograms for women aged 45–69 (Morrell et al. 2017), Canadian guidelines recommend screening for women aged 50–69 (Warner et al. 2012), and the Republic of Korea recommends biannual screening for women over 40 years (Lee et al. 2016). In other Asian and Latin American countries, there are considerable national differences of the screening programs.

6 Guidelines and Quality Assurance of Screening Programs

The ideal screening program enables early detection of a potential lethal disease, identified by an inexpensive, safe test with high sensitivity and specificity, where effective treatment is available. Wilson and Junger wrote the paper "Principles and practice of screening for disease" for the World Health Organization (WHO) in 1968, and despite being published 50 years ago, the ten criteria for screening are still considered as central in the planning, conduction, and evaluation of screening programs. The paper emphasizes that the target condition should be associated with important health problems, with an accepted and available method for detection, diagnosis, and treatment. Further, there should be an understanding of the natural history of the disease, and the cost should be balanced against the available resources for health care, with a continuous evaluation of case findings within the program.

A successful screening program requires quality in every step, including a complete registry of the defined target population, personal invitations to screening, adequate information about the pros and cons of participation, and follow-up of non-responders. The method and interval for screening must be well defined, with a management team responsible for implementation of the program. A quality assurance structure should be responsible for the quality of the examinations and radiological reports, and a health-care team responsible for the workup of abnormal index tests, as well as treatment and long-term follow-up of detected cancers. The program should also include guidelines on how to address incidental findings detected in screening. Continuous evaluation of all aspects of the program is important in order to assure a high quality, and to assess profits and harms.

Mammography Screening

Screening can be population based, where all women in the target group are personally invited to a high-volume, standardized examination, or personalized, where imaging technique and frequency are tailored according to individual factors such as family history, age, and breast density. There are numerous guidelines for screening of women at average risk, but the establishment of guidelines for screening of high-risk women, and suggestion for suitable imaging modalities for women with dense breast, is a challenge, which requires further research upon settlement.

6.1 Performance Indicators

The European Guidelines for Quality Assurance in Breast Cancer Screening and Diagnosis (Perry et al. 2008) from 2006 presented a comprehensive list of performance indicators for breast cancer screening including detection rates, follow-up of abnormal screening results, invasive diagnostics, and maximum time for diagnosis and treatment. Some of the indicators are listed in Table 2.

6.2 Quality of the Mammographic Report

A standard report should include the indication for examination, assessment of breast composition, important findings, comparison to previous studies, classification of assessment category, and management recommendations. Detection of discrete, early signs of malignancy requires optimal reading environment and a systematic reading strategy, and a standardized hanging protocol should be used for FFDM soft-copy reading, where the previous examination is used for comparison. Older images should also be accessible upon request.

The density of the breast parenchyma is of great importance for the expected diagnostic value of a mammogram, since both sensitivity and specificity are higher for fatty breasts than for dense breasts. For the referring physician, as well as for the women themselves, information about breast density is important. As to date 38 states in the USA have introduced a "Breast density notification law" (Freer 2015), saying that the referring physician must inform the women about their breast density at screening mammography so that, if desirable, further examination with supplemental imaging procedures might be initiated. This information and such recommendations are so far not implemented in the European population-based screening programs.

Current recommendations say that each report should include an estimate of the breast composition according to the BI-RADS criteria (Winkler et al. 2015) presented by the American College of Radiology. Density category A is given to almost entirely fatty breast, B in breasts with scattered areas of fibroglandular density, C represents heterogeneously dense breast, and D is extremely

Table 2 Performance indicators in breast cancer screening according to the European Guidelines for Quality Assurance in Breast Cancer Screening and Diagnosis

Performance indicator	Desired level
Participant rate	≥75%
Radiographically acceptable screening examination	≥97%
Recall rate	<5% for initial screening <3% for subsequent screening
Node-negative cancers	>75%
Percentage of invasive cancer ≤10 mm	≥30%
Percentage of invasive cancer ≤15 mm	≥50%
Detection rate of breast cancer in the first screening examination	≥3 times higher than the expected incidence in a non-screening population
Detection rate of breast cancer in subsequent screening examinations	≥1.5 higher than the expected incidence in a non-screening population
Rate of interval cancer	≤50% of the expected in a non-screening population

dense breast; imaging examples are presented in Fig. 1.

The breast parenchyma density has traditionally been estimated subjectively by the radiologist. However, radiologists' interobserver variability is a huge challenge regarding breast density classification (Sprague et al. 2016) and this fact causes problems not only for the individual women having a mammographic examination, but also with respect to the application of supplemental imaging techniques in women having density above a defined threshold (Bernardi et al. 2012; Ciatto et al. 2005b; Ekpo et al. 2016; Irshad et al. 2016; Lehman et al. 2002; Redondo et al. 2012; Winkler et al. 2015). Methods for automated breast density measurements have recently been developed, and the software calculates the proportion (volume or area) of dense tissue in the breast, based on a given pixel threshold in the mammogram (Østerås et al. 2016a, b). Both the volumetric and area-based automated methods have proven superior to the subjective BI-RADS estimate by the radiologist (Østerås et al. 2016a, b; Winkler et al. 2015; Alonzo-Proulx et al. 2015), and the method will probably be the reference standard for density assessment in the future.

The conclusion of a mammographic examination is often categorized according to the BI-RADS Final Assessment Categories 0–6, presented in Table 3. The assessment categories can be used in quality assurance of screening

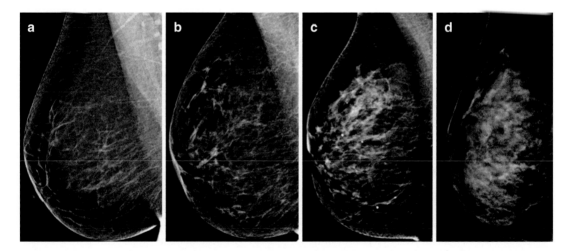

Fig. 1 Breast density according to BI-RADS atlas 5th edition. (**a**) Category A: almost entirely fatty breast. (**b**) Category B: scattered fibroglandular tissue. (**c**) Category C: heterogeneously dense breast. (**d**) Category D: extremely dense breast

Table 3 BI-RADS Final Assessment Categories

Category	Management	Likelihood of cancer
0—Need additional imaging or prior examinations	Recall for additional imaging and/or await prior examinations	n/a
1—Negative	Routine screening	~0%
2—Benign	Routine screening	~0%
3—Probably benign	Short-interval follow-up (6 months)	(>0% to ≤2%)
4—Suspicious	Tissue diagnosis	4a. Low suspicion for malignancy (>2% to ≤10%)
		4b. Moderate suspicion for malignancy (>10% to ≤50%)
		4c. High suspicion for malignancy (>50% to <95%)
5—Highly suggestive of malignancy	Tissue diagnosis	≥95%
6—Known biopsy-proven malignancy	Surgical excision	

programs, and for evaluation of the performance of the radiologists. The system is also designed to improve the communication between radiologists and clinicians. The BI-RADS category 3 ("short-term follow-up") is not used in several screening programs since it can expose women with low risk of cancer to considerable anxiety during the 6-month follow-up period. Some radiologists prefer therefore to categorize these "probably benign" lesions as BI-RADS 4 and consequently perform an immediate workup, or dismiss (category 2) with a calculated small risk of missing a malignancy which might present as interval cancer or next screening round cancer.

6.3 Single Versus Double Reading

Most European population-based screening programs recommend double reading of the mammograms by two independent radiologists. Interobserver variability is a huge challenge in mammography screening, and discordant interpretations have been reported in 23% of screening-detected cancers in a population-based screening program (Hofvind et al. 2009). Basically, double reading might be performed in a parallel or in a serial setup. Double reading in serial setup means that only images with a suspicious finding by the first reader are reread by the second radiologist, and only cases where both readers assess the examination as positive (suspicious) are referred to diagnostic workup. This approach results in a lower cancer detection rate but a higher specificity (lower recall rate). A parallel testing is where two readers independently read each examination, and the test is considered positive when at least one reader marks it as suspicious for malignancy. The most common approach is initial independent double reading by two radiologists, followed by a consensus or arbitration meeting for examinations with positive interpretations by one or both readers. The aim of independent double reading with consensus or arbitration is to achieve both high sensitivity and high specificity. Studies have shown an increased cancer detection rate of 10–12% using double reading, and implementation of consensus or arbitration significantly reduces the recall rate (Dinnes et al. 2001; Klompenhouwer et al. 2015; Ciatto et al. 2005a). However, the cost-effectiveness of double reading has been under discussion and one study found similar performance for single and double reading, and concluded that single reading might be a more cost-effective strategy (Posso et al. 2016).

Computer-aided detection (CAD) is designed to help the radiologists increase the cancer detection rate, and especially the detection of small early-stage cancers. The CAD system is beneficial when it shows (by marks for calcifications or densities) malignant lesions that are visible and actionable, but are overlooked by the radiologist, and when the radiologist recognizes and acts on the missed cancers identified by the CAD system. The intention was that CAD might replace the second reader without reducing the cancer detection rates. A large study concluded that single reading combined with CAD could be an alternative to double reading by two radiologists (Gilbert et al. 2008). CAD might even have a potential in mammography screening using independent double reading as shown in an experimental study (Skaane et al. 2007). However, a large retrospective study and a systematic review concluded that CAD did not improve screening performance and that scientific evidence is insufficient to determine whether double reading can be replaced by single reader and CAD (Lehman et al. 2015; Azavedo et al. 2012).

7 Mammographic Diagnosis of Early Preclinical Breast Cancer

The goal of mammographic screening should be to detect node-negative preclinical breast cancers. According to the European Guidelines, at least 50% of invasive screen-detected cancers should be less than 15 mm in size, and at least 30% should be less than 10 mm (Perry et al. 2008). Introduction of new imaging techniques including digital breast tomosynthesis, contrast-enhanced mammography, MRI, and advanced biopsy techniques such as vacuum-assisted biopsy has led to higher detection rates of cancers including ductal carcinoma in situ (DCIS). The detection of small, early-stage breast cancers at screening with mammography only remains a great challenge to the interpreting radiologists.

7.1 Ductal Carcinoma In Situ (DCIS)

DCIS often presents with "typical" microcalcifications in the more advanced cases. In the very early stage, however, the calcifications are often nonspecific and differentiation from benign microcalcifications may be difficult or impossible. It must also be borne in mind that areas of DCIS may not present with calcifications at all. The evaluation of the extent of DCIS may therefore occasionally be extremely difficult, but this is an important problem at the diagnostic workup of suspected DCIS. The great challenge for the radiologist in the reading session is not only the detection (perception) of small microcalcifications, but also the decision on which calcifications are suspicious and consequently need further diagnostic assessment (Fig. 2). It is also important to characterize calcifications that are

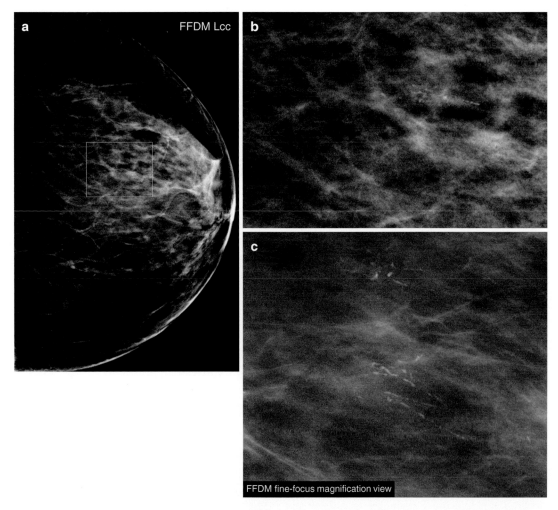

Fig. 2 (**a–c**) Screening mammography. Sixty-six-year-old asymptomatic woman. (**a**) The cluster of microcalcifications might easily be overlooked in the dense breast. (**b**) Zoomed image showing highly suspicious calcifications. (**c**) Fine-focus magnification view at diagnostic workup demonstrates "casting-type" calcifications consistent with high-grade (grade 3) DCIS, which was confirmed at histology

most likely benign, and thereby keep the unnecessary false-positive callbacks low. The mammographic findings of DCIS often reflect the breast anatomy, and calcifications' morphology and distribution may indicate the type and grade of DCIS.

Low-grade DCIS may often present with fine amorphous ("powdery") microcalcifications which are located anatomically within the terminal ductal lobular units (TDLUs). These mammographic features of low-grade DCIS may also be seen in a variety of benign conditions. The differential diagnosis of these microcalcifications is a challenge since the more common benign fibrocystic changes also originate in the TDLUs, with similar calcification pattern as DCIS (Tabár et al. 2008). The so-called casting (or linear branching) type calcifications are typically observed in high-grade DCIS (Fig. 2c). These casting-type calcifications may manifest as a fragmented casting type and a dotted casting type (Tabár et al. 2007). It is important in mammographic screening to diagnose cancers manifesting as casting-type calcifications at an early stage since these cancers have a much poorer prognosis than cancer of comparable size without such calcifications (Tabar et al. 2004). Unfortunately, calcifications are frequently rather nonspecific in the very early stages. In a large study it was found that "only" 50% of high-grade DCIS measuring less than 10 mm presented with casting-type calcifications, and that size is a major determinant of the mammographic features of DCIS (Evans et al. 2010).

Association between screen-detected DCIS and subsequent invasive cancers in mammography screening has been shown, and consequently the detection and treatment of DCIS are worthwhile in the prevention of future invasive breast cancers (Duffy et al. 2016).

7.2 Early Invasive Breast Cancer

The mammographic findings in invasive breast cancer are often divided into primary and secondary (indirect) signs. The most invasive cancers in a mammography screening program present with primary signs, and the BI-RADS atlas should be used for further characterization of suspicious findings (Fig. 3).

The secondary signs of invasive breast cancer include skin retraction, nipple retraction, and skin thickening ("peau d'orange"). History (previous biopsy or operation) is important in cases of skin or nipple retraction seen on screening mammograms. Skin edema is rarely diagnosed on screening mammograms since most women presenting with this finding will consult their physician and not attend the screening program. Differential diagnosis may rarely include enlarged axillary lymph nodes, thrombosis in the subclavian vein, or heart failure. Enlarged axillary lymph node(s) on screening mammography with normal findings within the breasts may include several differential diagnoses.

The mammographic findings in cases of invasive breast cancer rarely suggest a specific type of cancer, and in general a suspicious finding requires histologic examination. Invasive cancer may present as a circumscribed or spiculated mass, architectural distortion, asymmetric density, and/or calcifications, often in combination with densities. A single dilated duct is an extremely rare sign of cancer. An asymptomatic asymmetric density without suspicious mammographic features is in general a normal variation of the fibroglandular tissue. A developing asymmetric density, however, is suggestive of malignancy and requires further diagnostic workup. Comparison with previous mammograms is therefore of utmost importance in screening mammography interpretation.

The detection of early, subtle mammographic findings indicating early cancer requires optimal reading environment and a systematic search for abnormalities. Full-field digital mammography (FFDM) with soft-copy reading is today the gold standard for screening mammography. In the high-volume population-based European screening programs batch reading mode is the common procedure for interpretation of screening mammograms. Batch reading sessions might be a great challenge, and good hanging protocols including previous screening examinations are important. A systematic search for abnormalities

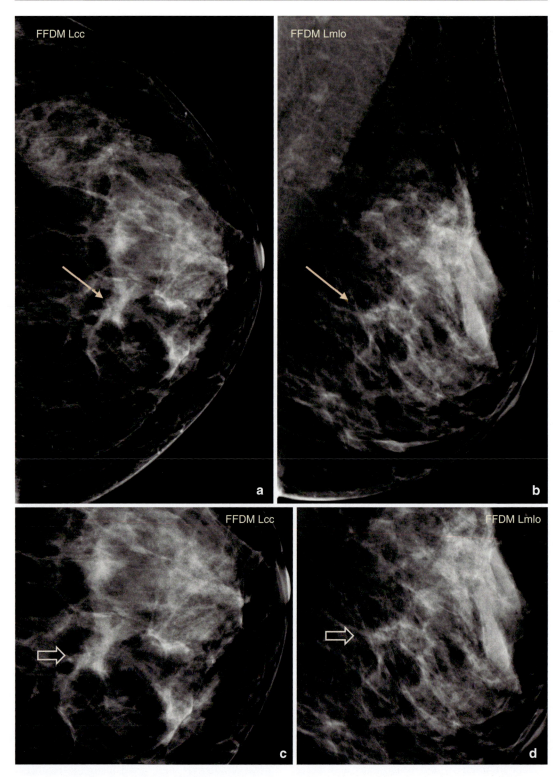

Fig. 3 (**a**–**d**) Sixty-six-year-old woman. Screening mammography, left breast. (**a**) CC mammogram and (**b**) MLO mammogram show a suspicious area (arrows), but a definite mass is difficult to identify. Zoomed images (**c** and **d**) demonstrate a spiculated mass, but the extension of the tumor is not possible to delineate. Histology revealed invasive ductal carcinoma, 18 mm

is important as otherwise subtle cancers may easily be missed. Interobserver variability is a great challenge as mentioned above, and more than 20% discordant interpretations of screen-detected cancers in population-based screening have been reported (Hofvind et al. 2009).

8 Personalized Screening for Women at Average Risk

Conventional mammography, SFM as well as FFDM, has two main inherent limitations: first, a low sensitivity, i.e., a low cancer detection rate in women with dense breast parenchyma due to a "masking effect." Tumors having a density similar to the surrounding parenchyma may easily be missed due to superimposed dense tissue. Second, summation of overlapping tissue may often simulate a tumor ("pseudotumor") causing unnecessary recalls and workup. Carney et al. (2003) found a sensitivity regarding cancer detection in mammographic screening of 87% among women with fatty breasts, decreasing to 62.9% for women with extremely dense breast, and even lower sensitivities have been reported. This means that subgroups of women are invited to breast cancer screening programs using a diagnostic test (mammography) having an unacceptable poor sensitivity, a fact that has led to the previously mentioned mandatory information of breast density, and possible need for supplemental screening for women attending mammographic screening in an increasing number of states in the USA (Freer 2015).

Since up to 50% of breasts examined in mammographic screening programs are BI-RADS category C or D, there is a need for a cost-effective and diagnostic sufficient alternative imaging for a great number of women. These mammography limitations together with the discussion in the last years on optimizing the balance between benefit and harms of breast cancer screening have initiated the focus on the so-called personalized screening. So far organized, population-based screening has been a "one-size-fits-all" approach: two-view mammography for all participants. In order to optimize benefit and

harms, the future screening might be "personalized" based on age, risk models including breast density, and medical history. A difficult topic in the discussion on personalized screening has been which supplemental imaging techniques and modalities should be used for the different categories of women. The most actual modalities to be implemented as adjunct to mammography have so far been ultrasound (US), MRI, and digital breast tomosynthesis (DBT).

8.1 Ultrasound as Supplemental Imaging

US has been the most used supplemental imaging modality for women with dense breast parenchyma. US may often miss tumors in fatty breasts, but in these women there is in general no indication for adjunct US examination, since mammography has a high sensitivity in this group. On the other hand, hypoechoic tumors in women with dense breast parenchyma having echogenic tissue are easily detected. Adjunct ultrasound is often of great value for detecting cancers in women with dense breast. In a retrospective study US detected more cancers than digital breast tomosynthesis in lesions surrounded by a small amount of fatty tissue (Garcia-Barquin et al. 2017).

Handheld ultrasound (HHUS) has several limitations as an adjunct method in breast cancer screening: Images are often not reproducible, documentation is limited, comparison with prior examinations is difficult, it is time consuming, double reading is not possible, and especially US as a stand-alone test has a very low specificity with many false-positive results. Nevertheless, cancer detection rate with ultrasound screening is comparable with mammography, but false positives are more common (Berg et al. 2016). In the prospective ASTOUND trial, women with mammography-negative dense breasts were offered adjunct screening with ultrasound or tomosynthesis (Tagliafico et al. 2016). US detected significantly more cancers than DBT. Only one country, Austria, has so far implemented supplemental ultrasound in organized high-volume screening (Oberaigner et al. 2011), offering handheld ultrasound to the approximately 45% of participating women with dense breast parenchyma (BI-RADS C or D). Evaluation of this program shows promising results with an increased cancer detection rate for women at average risk with dense as well as non-dense breasts, but with an increase in recall rate although the recalls were low (Buchberger et al. 2018; Geiger-Gritsch et al. 2018). The ultrasound examinations are carried out during the same visit and by the same radiologist as a "second line screening procedure," with a final BI-RADS category after both exams, and consequently the additional value of adjunct ultrasound per se is difficult to evaluate. The higher costs of combined screening with mammography and ultrasound would be a challenge in population-based screening. Austria uses single reading, and the physician-performed ultrasound is covered by social insurance.

Automated breast ultrasound (ABUS) (Chapter "Automated Breast Ultrasound") would overcome some of the limitations of HHUS in breast cancer screening. The examination is carried out by radiographers and consequently can be done in the screening unit after automatic breast density measurement (single-visit diagnosis). Addition of ABUS to screening mammography in women with dense breasts increased the cancer detection of clinically important cancers, but also increased the number of false-positive findings (Brem et al. 2015). Another study combining mammography with ABUS in women with dense breasts, however, showed significantly improved cancer detection without substantially affecting specificity (Giger et al. 2016).

8.2 Magnetic Resonance Imaging (MRI) as Supplemental Imaging

MRI has a very high sensitivity not only for invasive breast cancer but also for DCIS, with cancer detection rates significantly higher than mammography in women with dense breast parenchyma (Kuhl et al. 2007). The modality has been used for several years in women at high risk. A decade ago it was also suggested that "mammography is going to be replaced by MRI, not only in high-risk women but increasingly in those at average risk"(Hall 2008). Development of fast MRI techniques like "short first-pass MRI" (Fischer et al. 2012) and abbreviated breast magnetic resonance imaging ("ABB-MRI") (Chapter "Abbreviated Breast MRI: Short and Sweet?") (Kuhl et al. 2014) may open the door for implementing this modality even in breast cancer screening of women at average risk for developing cancer, either as adjunct or as single examination. Of importance is that MRI not only improves the detection of prognostically relevant invasive cancers but also has the potential to reduce the number of interval cancers (Bakker et al. 2019; Comstock et al. 2020; Kuhl et al. 2017).

Although ABB-MRI may solve some practical problems, the two main limitations of MRI implementation in organized high-volume (population-based) screening for women at average risk remain: cost and availability.

8.3 Digital Breast Tomosynthesis (DBT) as Supplemental Screening (Chapter "Mammography and Digital Breast Tomosynthesis: Technique")

The most promising supplemental screening technique to conventional mammography as of today is digital breast tomosynthesis (DBT or "3D mammography"), approved by the FDA in 2011 (Vedantham et al. 2015). DBT is based on a full-field digital mammography (FFDM) platform, and images are obtained in the same craniocaudal and mediolateral oblique projection as conventional mammography. The moving X-ray tube acquires multiple low-dose projections over a limited angular range, and the projection images are reconstructed to 1 mm section images. DBT, only a quasi-3D examination due to the limited angle of scanning, reduces the obscuring effect of superimposed breast tissue, thus improving the detection of lesions otherwise hidden by the dense parenchyma. Cancers are more conspicuous at DBT than at digital mammography, but cancers may occasionally be detected at only one of the two views (Korhonen et al. 2019). Furthermore, DBT can replace conventional supplemental views for evaluation of noncalcified lesions earlier needed to be recalled from screening, thus further reducing the number of false-positive interpretations and unnecessary recalls. Thus, the modality has a great potential for improving breast cancer screening (Vedantham et al. 2015); image example is presented in Fig. 4. Some prospective European trials and several retrospective US studies have confirmed that DBT has the potential to significantly improve the quality of breast cancer screening. All European trials except one have shown a significantly higher detection rate of invasive cancer but some conflicting results regarding recall rates (Ciatto et al. 2013; Skaane et al. 2013; Lang et al. 2016; Zackrisson et al. 2018). One study found as much as 90% more cancers using DBT but with similar recall rates in the two groups (Pattacini et al. 2018). The only prospective trial that did not demonstrate an increased cancer detection rate was the To-Be trial (Hofvind et al. 2019). All US studies have demonstrated a significant reduction in recall rates, but some conflicting results regarding cancer detection (Rafferty et al. 2016; Friedewald et al. 2014; McDonald et al. 2015). Different screening environments in Europe and the USA, with single reading vs. double reading and much higher recalls in the USA, might explain these differences. A recently published Australian study found a higher cancer detection rate and a higher recall rate using DBT in a prospective population-based screening trial (Houssami et al. 2019).

The first screening studies evaluating the implementation of tomosynthesis compared FFDM with FFDM plus DBT, i.e., the so-called combo mode. This "combo mode" means a doubling of the radiation dose which is not acceptable in population-based screening. The solution is synthesized 2D images ("syn2D"). Synthetic 2D images are created from the DBT dataset and need no extra radiation exposure. The diagnostic performance of syn2D plus DBT is comparable to FFDM plus DBT (Zuley et al. 2014; Aujero et al. 2017; Bernardi et al. 2016; Skaane et al. 2014; Caumo et al. 2018). An example of screening examination using synthesized 2D image in combination with DBT is presented in Fig. 5. Synthesized 2D images will eliminate the need for FFDM in breast cancer screening, and the next future mammography screening tends to be DBT with reconstructed syn2D.

DBT is increasingly used in breast cancer screening in the USA but has so far not been implemented in any population-based European screening program. The effect of DBT screening on subsequent interval cancer rates and stage of advanced cancers is still not known, and the potential for the so-called overdiagnosis when implementing new advanced technologies is a hot topic. Screening with DBT is associated with an increased proportion of smaller breast cancers with better prognosis compared with FFDM (Conant et al. 2019a, b; Johnson et al. 2019). Screening using DBT depicts more cancers in all density and age groups compared with digital mammography owing to the higher number of cancers presenting as either spiculated masses or architectural distortions (Østerås et al. 2019). Some studies have shown similar rates of interval cancers with FFDM (Bahl et al. 2018) but other studies found a decline in interval cancers (McDonald et al. 2016). Cost-effectiveness studies have shown that DBT screening might be cost effective in the USA (Lee et al. 2015; Kalra et al. 2016), but such studies in European screening programs with much lower recall rates might demonstrate that DBT is not cost effective at lower willingness-to-pay thresholds (Sankatsing et al. 2020) and further European studies need to be carried out. A matter of concern is the longer reading time for DBT. The Australian study

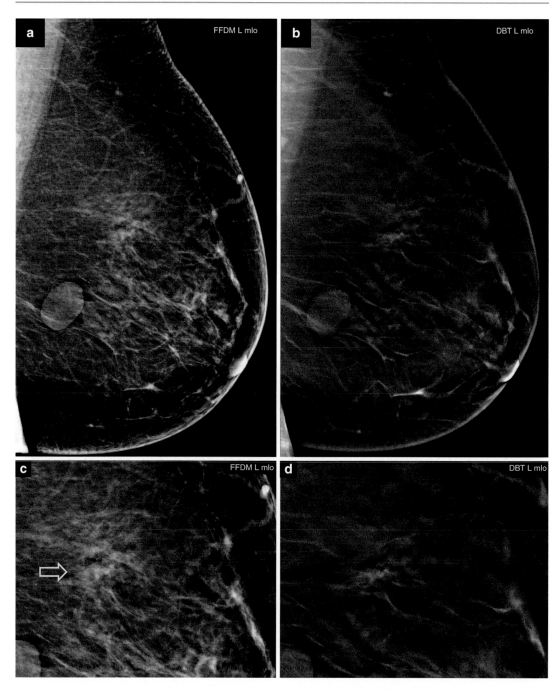

Fig. 4 (**a–d**) Screening mammography, left breast. (**a**) FFDM MLO shows a central, nonspecific asymmetric density. (**b**) DBT demonstrates a small spiculates mass. Zoomed images (**c** and **d**) clearly show a spiculated mass on DBT not seen on FFDM (arrow). Histology: Invasive lobular carcinoma, 8 mm

found that the screen reading time for DBT was about four times as long as for standard mammography (Houssami et al. 2019). Implementation of artificial intelligence (AI) in the future might not only improve diagnostic performance of screening programs but also shorten the DBT reading time (Conant et al. 2019a, b; Sechopoulos and Mann 2020).

Mammography Screening

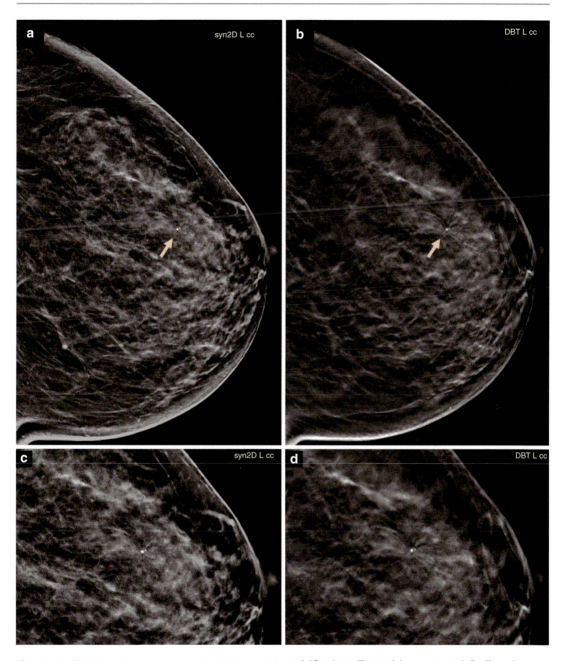

Fig. 5 (**a–d**) Screening mammography, 66-year-old woman. (**a**) Synthetic 2D shows only a benign small macrocalcification (arrow). (**b**) DBT clearly demonstrates spiculations (architectural distortion) around the small calcifications. Zoomed images (**c** and **d**): Even in retrospect a distortion is not visible on 2D. Histology revealed invasive lobular carcinoma, 6 mm

8.4 Other Imaging Modalities as Supplemental Screening

Several imaging modalities including molecular breast imaging, optical imaging, dedicated breast CT, contrast-enhanced mammography, and different hybrid and fusion techniques have the potential to improve cancer detection at early stage. Molecular breast imaging (MBI) is considered as one of the best supplemental imaging modalities to mammography in dense breasts if the radiotracer dosage can be reduced (Rhodes et al. 2015; Shermis et al. 2016). A nationwide Japanese study showed that combined FDG-PET scanning showed higher sensitivity and higher positive predictive values than mammography (Minamimoto et al. 2015). Fusion combining 3D automated breast ultrasound and breast tomosynthesis is of special interest (Schaefgen et al. 2018). However, these new advanced techniques and modalities are still under development and should be considered as work in progress.

9 Screening for Women at Higher Risk

Risk factors for breast cancer include genetic mutations of BRCA1 and BRCA2, family or personal history of breast cancer, young age at menarche, older age at menopause, no pregnancy or first pregnancy after age 30, dense breasts, oral contraceptives, hormone replacement therapy, previous radiation therapy, obesity, physical inactivity, increased consumption of alcohol, and high age (McPherson et al. 2000). Women at average risk for breast cancer (<15% lifetime risk) are in general invited to regular mammographic screening.

Breast density as an independent risk factor for breast cancer has been much discussed. The relative risk associated with dense breasts is about 3 for breasts that are 50–74% dense and about 4.5 for breasts that are 75% or more dense (Freer 2015). The increased breast cancer rates in women with dense breasts are attributable to increased relative risk as well as to the masking effect of dense tissue. Breast density remains an independent risk factor, although the relative risk of breast density is much smaller than that of other risk factors for breast cancer.

Supplemental screening in women with intermediate risk (15–20% lifetime risk) has been controversial, and this issue has been a "gray zone" regardless of breast density. Some countries have considered supplemental US or MRI screening to be appropriate, whereas other countries do not offer any adjunct screening for this group.

Women with high risk (lifetime risk >20%) for breast cancer are in general invited at an earlier age to annual, instead of biannual, screening. Due to higher risk and denser breast at younger age, these women (especially BRCA1 and BRCA2 mutation carriers) need to be offered supplemental screening, in general MRI. Some screening programs for high-risk women offer annual MRI, other programs include mammography plus MRI, and some programs include ultrasound between the annual MRI examinations. A large retrospective study of high-risk women undergoing both MRI and mammography (Sung et al. 2016) showed that invasive cancer is more likely to be detected with MRI, and most cancers detected with mammography were DCIS. There is for the time being no international consensus regarding guidelines for screening of high-risk women.

10 Adverse Effects of Mammography Screening

Adverse effects of mammographic screening include discomfort of the examination, radiation exposure, false-positive interpretations, false-negative results with interval cancers, and overdiagnosis with overtreatment.

10.1 Radiation Exposure

The radiation dose of mammographic examinations has decreased since the introduction of digital mammography (FFDM). Estimating the risk of radiation-induced cancer is a difficult topic, since this type of cancer is impossible to differentiate from spontaneously occurring malignancies. The potential harm of the small amount of radiation given in diagnostic imaging is based on the follow-up of individuals receiving much larger amount of radiation (nuclear bombs, radiation therapy), extrapolated to low doses by a no-threshold dose-response model. There is an ongoing discussion on whether the linear no-threshold can be applied to the low doses used in mammographic screening, and whether these doses have any potential at all to induce a cancer, especially in older women (Hendrick 2010). Based on the current knowledge, the risk of radiation-induced breast cancer due to mammographic screening of adult women is minimal (Kopans 2011; Hauge et al. 2014).

10.2 False Positives

A false-positive examination is when a woman is recalled from mammographic screening to further imaging and/or invasive diagnostic workup of a lesion that turns out to be benign. A review by L. E. Pace and N. L. Keating (2014) assessed the 10-year cumulative risk of at least one false-positive finding in 40- and 50-year-old women undergoing annual screening to around 61%, and that 7.0–9.8% of women had taken biopsy with benign result after 10 years of annual screening. In European population-based screening programs, with much lower recall rates than in the USA, the cumulative risk for a false-positive recall during a screening period of two decades has been estimated to be about 21%, and the cumulative risk of undergoing fine needle aspiration cytology and core needle biopsy with benign diagnosis is estimated to be 3.9% and 1.5%, respectively (Hofvind et al. 2004). The psychological effects associated with recalls and workup of a false-positive finding might be substantial for some women, but in general the recalls are associated with transiently increased anxiety, and after some weeks women are almost unanimously satisfied with their participation and would participate again (Schou Bredal et al. 2013). Most women prefer the inconvenience and anxiety associated with a higher recall rate if it results in the possibility of detecting breast cancer earlier (Ganott et al. 2006).

10.3 False Negatives and Interval Cancer

A false-negative examination is when a breast cancer is present but not diagnosed at screening interpretation. Retrospective review of previous screening examinations has shown that about 50% of interval cancers are visible on the previous mammograms, either representing "screening error" ("missed cancer") or the so-called minimal sign lesion (Van Dijck et al. 1993; Broeders et al. 2003). The reason for missing a cancer might be perception (detection) error or characterization (analysis) error. Explanation for overlooking a breast cancer at screening includes inexperienced reader, incomplete search of the images, heavy workload, distractions, or presence of very subtle small lesions. Very fine, small microcalcifications in women with dense breast parenchyma might represent a perception problem. Architectural distortion and non-spiculated, high-density masses on the mammograms prior to diagnosis are associated with potential benefit from an earlier diagnosis (Broeders et al. 2003). Subtle signs of such small cancers should therefore warrant extra attention at screening interpretation. We have to keep in mind the large variations in screening sensitivity and performance between countries (Tornberg et al. 2010).

Women between 40 and 50 years have a higher risk of developing rapid-growing cancer. The risk of interval cancer increases by time after the index screening examination, and about 70% of the interval cancers are diagnosed in the second year of the interval (Hofvind et al. 2006). In order to reduce the number of interval cancers, both the American Cancer Society and the American College of Radiology recommend annual screening for all women starting from 40 or 45 years. Shortening of the screening interval will reduce interval cancer, but will also increase the adverse effects of screening. The optimal length of screening intervals will depend on individual factors, but today most European population-based programs recommend biannual screening in order to achieve the best balance between cost and benefit. In the USA the interval is generally 1 year. The ongoing discussion on "personalized" screening will probably cause modifications of the intervals in Europe.

10.4 Overdiagnosis

Overdiagnosis (or overdetection) is usually defined as the diagnosis of a breast cancer as a result of screening that would neither have been diagnosed nor become symptomatic in a woman's lifetime in the absence of screening. The issue of overdiagnosis has been a topic of much interest and controversy. Overdiagnosis is an epidemiological concept, and it is not possible by histopathological examination to determine whether a screening-detected cancer has been overdiagnosed. Especially low-grade DCIS and small low-grade invasive cancers are considered to represent potential overdiagnosis in older women.

Implementation of advanced imaging techniques in breast cancer screening has the potential for overdiagnosis. The diagnosis of a breast cancer is brought forward in time by screening ("lead-time bias"). The time period during which a cancer is in the preclinical detectable phase and might be detected at screening ("sojourn time") varies considerably among malignant tumors. Detecting cancers earlier means that more cancers are diagnosed after implementation of a screening program. Mammography screening detects more slower growing cancers ("length-time bias") but may miss the faster growing tumors. Thus, mammography screening may detect slow-growing cancers that might never manifest clinically in a woman's lifetime, and overdiagnosis might be regarded as an extreme form of length-time bias.

The estimation of the amount of overdiagnosis is extremely difficult. Theoretically, at the end of a randomized screening trial, there should be a compensatory reduction of the incidence of cancer in the screened group, and comparison of the cumulative incidence in the screened and non-screened group should show a valid estimate of overdiagnosis ("cumulative incidence method").

There has, however, been a hot discussion whether to make adjustment and if then how to make adjustment for lead-time bias. Consequently, reports on overdiagnosis in mammography screening vary considerably among authors and methods applied, from less than 1% to more than 50% (Paci et al. 2004; Zahl et al. 2004; Duffy et al. 2005; Zackrisson et al. 2006; Olsen et al. 2006; Gøtzsche and Jørgensen 2013; Puliti et al. 2012). One study on overdiagnosis in relation to the benefit of screening concluded that 8.8 (Swedish cohort) and 5.7 (UK cohort) cases of breast cancer deaths were prevented per 1000 women participating in the screening program over a period of 20 years, indicating that between 2 and 2.5 lives are saved in the screening program for every overdiagnosed case (Duffy et al. 2010). An increasing percentage of overdiagnosis can be expected in the older population groups due to the shortened lifetime expectancy (Van Ravesteyn et al. 2015).

Overtreatment is occasionally confused with overdiagnosis. "There is no such thing as overdiagnosis: there is only correct, partially correct, or incorrect diagnosis. If abnormal findings are diagnosed correctly, there is only optimally managed, suboptimally managed, mismanaged, and possibly overtreated disease" (Gur and Sumkin 2013). And "Because the greatest harm of overdiagnosis is overtreatment, the key goal should not be less diagnosis but better treatment decision tools" (Morris et al. 2015).

11 The Future of Breast Cancer Screening

Breast cancer screening with mammography is the most validated and effective screening program worldwide, with a mortality reduction in the range of 15–45% (Smith 2003; Gabe et al. 2007; Olsen et al. 2005; Gotzsche and Nielsen 2011). Early detection of localized disease enables more gentle treatment and a better long-term prognosis. Nevertheless, for the time being there is a "never-ending debate" on the adverse effects of screening in which opponents of mammography screening are focusing more on adverse effects including overdiagnosis instead of the mortality benefit of screening.

Development of new advanced imaging technologies has shown that the quality of breast cancer screening programs may be improved. A main topic in the next years would probably be the challenge of moving from "one-size-fits-all" mammography to personalized screening based on individual risk factors including breast parenchyma density. Optimizing benefits-to-harms trade-offs will therefore be of much importance in the next years regardless of which imaging modality is applied.

An interesting theoretical question is how long we will still have imaging tests for breast cancer screening, and when imaging will be replaced by blood samples. Some years ago, a blood test based on gene expression profiling of peripheral blood cells for early detection of breast cancers showed an accuracy (measured by AUC, area under the ROC curve) which was comparable to mammography (Aaroe et al. 2010). A publication in Science on detection and localization of surgically resectable cancers with a multi-analyte blood test received much public attention (Cohen et al. 2018). Blood tests for breast cancer screening require not only a high sensitivity, but even more importantly a very high specificity. It will probably take several years for blood test (liquid biopsy) to replace imaging for breast cancer screening.

References

Aaroe J, Lindahl T, Dumeaux V, Saebo S, Tobin D, Hagen N, Skaane P, Lonneborg A, Sharma P, Borresen-Dale AL (2010) Gene expression profiling of peripheral blood cells for early detection of breast cancer. Breast Cancer Res 12:R7

Alonzo-Proulx O, Mawdsley GE, Patrie JT, Yaffe MJ, Harvey JA (2015) Reliability of automated breast density measurements. Radiology 275:366–376

Aujero MP, Gavenonis SC, Benjamin R, Zhang Z, Holt JS (2017) Clinical performance of synthesized two-dimensional mammography combined with tomosynthesis in a large screening population. Radiology 283:70–76

Azavedo E, Zackrisson S, Mejàre I, Heibert Arnlind M (2012) Is single reading with computer-aided detection (CAD) as good as double reading in mammog-

raphy screening? A systematic review. BMC Med Imaging 12:22

Bahl M, Gaffney S, McCarthy AM, Lowry KP, Dang PA, Lehman CD (2018) Breast cancer characteristics associated with 2D digital mammography versus digital breast tomosynthesis for screening-detected and interval cancers. Radiology 287:49–57

Baker LH (1982) Breast Cancer Detection Demonstration Project: five-year summary report. CA Cancer J Clin 32:194–225

Bakker MF, De Lange SV, Pijnappel RM, Mann RM, Peeters PHM, Monninkhof EM, Emaus MJ, Loo CE, Bisschops RHC, Lobbes MBI, De Jong MDF, Duvivier KM, Veltman J, Karssemeijer N, De Koning HJ, Van Diest PJ, Mali WPTM, Van Den Bosch MAAJ, Veldhuis WB, Van Gils CH (2019) Supplemental MRI screening for women with extremely dense breast tissue. N Engl J Med 381:2091–2102

Berg WA, Bandos AI, Mendelson EB, Lehrer D, Jong RA, Pisano ED (2016) Ultrasound as the primary screening test for breast cancer: analysis from ACRIN 6666. J Natl Cancer Inst 108:djv367

Bernardi D, Pellegrini M, Di Michele S (2012) Interobserver agreement in breast radiological density attribution according to BI-RADS quantitative classification. Radiol Med 117:519–528

Bernardi D, Macaskill P, Pellegrini M, Valentini M, Fantò C, Ostillio L, Tuttobene P, Luparia A, Houssami N (2016) Breast cancer screening with tomosynthesis (3D mammography) with acquired or synthetic 2D mammography compared with 2D mammography alone (STORM-2): a population-based prospective study. Lancet Oncol 17:1105–1113

Brem RF, Tabar L, Duffy SW, Inciardi MF, Guingrich JA, Hashimoto BE, Lander MR, Lapidus RL, Peterson MK, Rapelyea JA, Roux S, Schilling KJ, Shah BA, Torrente J, Wynn RT, Miller DP (2015) Assessing improvement in detection of breast cancer with three-dimensional automated breast US in women with dense breast tissue: the SomoInsight Study. Radiology 274:663–673

Broeders MJM, Onland-Moret NC, Rijken HJTM, Hendriks JHCL, Verbeek ALM, Holland R (2003) Use of previous screening mammograms to identify features indicating cases that would have a possible gain in prognosis following earlier detection. Eur J Cancer 39:1770–1775

Broeders M, Moss S, Nystrom L, Njor S, Jonsson H, Paap E, Massat N, Duffy S, Lynge E, Paci E (2012) The impact of mammographic screening on breast cancer mortality in Europe: a review of observational studies. J Med Screen 19(Suppl 1):14–25

Buchberger W, Geiger-Gritsch S, Knapp R, Gautsch K, Oberaigner W (2018) Combined screening with mammography and ultrasound in a population-based screening program. Eur J Radiol 101:24–29

Carney PA, Miglioretti DL, Yankaskas BC, Kerlikowske K, Rosenberg R, Rutter CM, Geller BM, Abraham LA, Taplin SH, Dignan M, Cutter G, Ballard-Barbash R (2003) Individual and combined effects of age, breast density, and hormone replacement therapy use on the accuracy of screening mammography. Ann Intern Med 138:168–175

Caumo F, Zorzi M, Brunelli S, Romanucci G, Rella R, Cugola L, Bricolo P, Fedato C, Montemezzi S, Houssami N (2018) Digital breast tomosynthesis with synthesized two-dimensional images versus full-field digital mammography: outcomes from the Verona screening program. Radiology 287:37–46

Ciatto S, Ambrogetti D, Risso G, Catarzi S, Morrone D, Mantellini P, Rosselli Del Turco M (2005a) The role of arbitration of discordant reports at double reading of screening mammograms. J Med Screen 12:125–127

Ciatto S, Houssami N, Apruzzese A (2005b) Categorizing breast mammographic density: intra- and interobserver reproducibility of BI-RADS density categories. Breast 14:269–275

Ciatto S, Houssami N, Bernardi D, Caumo F, Pellegrini M, Brunelli S, Tuttobene P, Bricolo P, Fanto C, Valentini M, Montemezzi S, Macaskill P (2013) Integration of 3D digital mammography with tomosynthesis for population breast-cancer screening (STORM): a prospective comparison study. Lancet Oncol 14:583–589

Cohen JD, Li L, Wang Y, Thoburn C, Afsari B, Danilova L, Douville C, Javed AA, Wong F, Mattox A, Hruban RH, Wolfgang CL, Goggins MG, Dal Molin M, Wang TL, Roden R, Klein AP, Ptak J, Dobbyn L, Schaefer J, Silliman N, Popoli M, Vogelstein JT, Browne JD, Schoen RE, Brand RE, Tie J, Gibbs P, Wong HL, Mansfield AS, Jen J, Hanash SM, Falconi M, Allen PJ, Zhou S, Bettegowda C, Diaz LA Jr, Tomasetti C, Kinzler KW, Vogelstein B, Lennon AM, Papadopoulos N (2018) Detection and localization of surgically resectable cancers with a multi-analyte blood test. Science 359:926–930

Collette HJ, Day NE, Rombach JJ, De Waard F (1984) Evaluation of screening for breast cancer in a non-randomised study (the DOM project) by means of a case-control study. Lancet 1:1224–1226

Comstock CE, Gatsonis C, Newstead GM, Snyder BS, Gareen IF, Bergin JT, Rahbar H, Sung JS, Jacobs C, Harvey JA, Nicholson MH, Ward RC, Holt J, Prather A, Miller KD, Schnall MD, Kuhl CK (2020) Comparison of abbreviated breast MRI vs. digital breast tomosynthesis for breast cancer detection among women with dense breasts undergoing screening. JAMA 323:746–756

Conant EF, Barlow WE, Herschorn SD, Weaver DL, Beaber EF, Tosteson ANA, Haas JS, Lowry KP, Stout NK, Trentham-Dietz A, Diflorio-Alexander RM, Li CI, Schnall MD, Onega T, Sprague BL (2019a) Association of digital breast tomosynthesis vs. digital mammography with cancer detection and recall rates by age and breast density. JAMA Oncol 5:635–642

Conant EF, Toledano AY, Periaswamy S, Fotin SV, Go J, Boatsman JE, Hoffmeister JW (2019b) Improving accuracy and efficiency with concurrent use of artificial intelligence for digital breast tomosynthesis. Radiol Artif Intell 1:e180096

De Waard F, Kirkpatrick A, Perry NM, Tornberg S, Tubiana M, De Wolf C (1994) Breast cancer screening in the framework of the Europe against Cancer programme. Eur J Cancer Prev 3(Suppl 1):3–5

del Moral Aldaz A, Aupee M, Batal-Steil S, Cecchini S, Chamberlain J, Ciatto S, Elizaga NA, Gairard B, Grazzini G, Guldenfels C et al (1994) Cancer screening in the European Union. Eur J Cancer 30a:860–872

Dinnes J, Moss S, Melia J, Blanks R, Song F, Kleijnen J (2001) Effectiveness and cost-effectiveness of double reading of mammograms in breast cancer screening: findings of a systematic review. Breast 10:455–463

Duffy SW, Agbaje O, Tabar L, Vitak B, Bjurstam N, Bjorneld L, Myles JP, Warwick J (2005) Overdiagnosis and overtreatment of breast cancer: estimates of overdiagnosis from two trials of mammographic screening for breast cancer. Breast Cancer Res 7:258–265

Duffy SW, Tabar L, Olsen AH, Vitak B, Allgood PC, Chen THH, Yen AMF, Smith RA (2010) Absolute numbers of lives saved and overdiagnosis in breast cancer screening, from a randomized trial and from the breast screening programme in England. J Med Screen 17:25–30

Duffy SW, Dibden A, Michalopoulos D, Offman J, Parmar D, Jenkins J, Collins B, Robson T, Scorfield S, Green K, Hall C, Liao XH, Ryan M, Johnson F, Stevens G, Kearins O, Sellars S, Patnick J (2016) Screen detection of ductal carcinoma in situ and subsequent incidence of invasive interval breast cancers: a retrospective population-based study. Lancet Oncol 17:109–114

Ekpo E, Ujong U, Mello-Thoms C, McEntee M (2016) Assessment of interradiologist agreement regarding mammographic breast density classification using the fifth edition of the BI-RADS Atlas. AJR Am J Roentgenol 206:1119–1123

Evans A, Clements K, Maxwell A, Bishop H, Hanby A, Lawrence G, Pinder SE (2010) Lesion size is a major determinant of the mammographic features of ductal carcinoma in situ: findings from the Sloane project. Clin Radiol 65:181–184

Ferlay J, Soerjomataram I, Dikshit R, Eser S, Mathers C, Rebelo M, Parkin DM, Forman D, Bray F (2015) Cancer incidence and mortality worldwide: sources, methods and major patterns in GLOBOCAN 2012. Int J Cancer 136:E359–E386

Fischer U, Korthauer A, Baum F, Luftner-Nagel S, Heyden D, Marten-Engelke K (2012) Short first-pass MRI of the breast. Acta Radiol 53:267–269

Freer PE (2015) Mammographic breast density: impact on breast cancer risk and implications for screening. Radiographics 35:302–315

Friedewald SM, Rafferty EA, Rose SL, Durand MA, Plecha DM, Greenberg JS, Hayes MK, Copit DS, Carlson KL, Cink TM, Barke LD, Greer LN, Miller DP, Conant EF (2014) Breast cancer screening using tomosynthesis in combination with digital mammography. JAMA 311:2499–2507

Gabe R, Tryggvadottir L, Sigfusson BF, Olafsdottir GH, Sigurdsson K, Duffy SW (2007) A case-control study to estimate the impact of the Icelandic population-based mammography screening program on breast cancer death. Acta Radiol 48:948–955

Ganott MA, Sumkin JH, King JL, Klym AH, Catullo VJ, Cohen CS, Gur D (2006) Screening mammography: do women prefer a higher recall rate given the possibility of earlier detection of cancer? Radiology 238:793–800

Garcia-Barquin P, Paramo M, Elizalde A, Pina L, Etxano J, Fernandez-Montero A, Caballeros M (2017) The effect of the amount of peritumoral adipose tissue in the detection of additional tumors with digital breast tomosynthesis and ultrasound. Acta Radiol 58:645–651

Geiger-Gritsch S, Daniaux M, Buchberger W, Knapp R, Oberaigner W (2018) Performance of 4 years of population-based mammography screening for breast cancer combined with ultrasound in Tyrol/Austria. Wien Klin Wochenschr 130:92–99

Gershon-Cohen J, Ingleby H (1958) Roentgen survey of asymptomatic breasts. Surgery 43:408–414

Gershon-Cohen J, Hermel MB, Berger SM (1961) Detection of breast cancer by periodic X-ray examinations. A five-year survey. JAMA 176:1114–1116

Giger ML, Inciardi MF, Edwards A, Papaioannou J, Drukker K, Jiang Y, Brem R, Brown JB (2016) Automated breast ultrasound in breast cancer screening of women with dense breasts: reader study of mammography-negative and mammography-positive cancers. AJR Am J Roentgenol 206:1341–1350

Gilbert FJ, Astley SM, Gillan MGC, Agbaje OF, Wallis MG, James J, Boggis CRM, Duffy SW (2008) Single reading with computer-aided detection for screening mammography. N Engl J Med 359:1675–1684

Giordano DL, Karsa LV, Tomatis M, Majek O, Wolf CD, Lancucki L, Hofvind S, Nystrom L, Segnan N, Ponti A (2012) Mammographic screening programmes in Europe: organization, coverage and participation. J Med Screen 19:72–82

Gold RH, Bassett LW, Widoff BE (1990) Highlights from the history of mammography. Radiographics 10:1111–1131

Gøtzsche PC, Jørgensen KJ (2013) Screening for breast cancer with mammography. Cochrane Database Syst Rev 2013(6):CD001877

Gotzsche PC, Nielsen M (2011) Screening for breast cancer with mammography. Cochrane Database Syst Rev (1):CD001877

Gur D, Sumkin JH (2013) Screening for early detection of breast cancer: overdiagnosis versus suboptimal patient management. Radiology 268:327–328

Hall FM (2008) The rise and impending decline of screening mammography. Radiology 247:597–601

Hauge IH, Pedersen K, Olerud HM, Hole EO, Hofvind S (2014) The risk of radiation-induced breast cancers due to biennial mammographic screening in women aged 50–69 years is minimal. Acta Radiol 55:1174–1179

Hendrick RE (2010) Radiation doses and cancer risks from breast imaging studies. Radiology 257:246–253

Hofvind S, Thoresen S, Tretli S (2004) The cumulative risk of a false-positive recall in the Norwegian Breast Cancer Screening Program. Cancer 101:1501–1507

Hofvind S, Bjurstam N, Sorum R, Bjorndal H, Thoresen S, Skaane P (2006) Number and characteristics of breast cancer cases diagnosed in four periods in the screening interval of a biennial population-based screening programme. J Med Screen 13:192–196

Hofvind S, Geller BM, Rosenberg RD, Skaane P (2009) Screening-detected breast cancers: discordant independent double reading in a population-based screening program. Radiology 253:652–660

Hofvind S, Ursin G, Tretli S, Sebuodegard S, Moller B (2013) Breast cancer mortality in participants of the Norwegian Breast Cancer Screening Program. Cancer 119:3106–3112

Hofvind S, Holen ÅS, Aase H, Houssami N, Sebuødegård S, Moger TA, Haldorsen IS, Akslen LA (2019) Two-view digital breast tomosynthesis versus digital mammography in a population-based breast cancer screening programme (To-Be): a randomised, controlled trial. Lancet Oncol 20:795–805

Houssami N, Lockie D, Clemson M, Pridmore V, Taylor D, Marr G, Evans J (2019) Pilot trial of digital breast tomosynthesis (3D mammography) for population-based screening in BreastScreen Victoria. Med J Aust 211:357–362

Irshad A, Leddy R, Ackerman S, Cluver A, Pavic D, Abid A, Lewis MC (2016) Effects of changes in BI-RADS density assessment guidelines (Fourth versus Fifth edition) on breast density assessment: intra- and inter-reader agreements and density distribution. Am J Roentgenol 207:1366–1371

Jemal A, Ward EM, Johnson CJ, Cronin KA, Ma J, Ryerson B, Mariotto A, Lake AJ, Wilson R, Sherman RL, Anderson RN, Henley SJ, Kohler BA, Penberthy L, Feuer EJ, Weir HK (2017) Annual report to the nation on the status of cancer, 1975–2014, featuring survival. J Natl Cancer Inst 109:djx030

Johnson K, Zackrisson S, Rosso A, Sartor H, Saal LH, Andersson I, Lång K (2019) Tumor characteristics and molecular subtypes in breast cancer screening with digital breast tomosynthesis: the Malmo breast tomosynthesis screening trial. Radiology 293:273–281

Kalra VB, Wu X, Haas BM, Forman HP, Philpotts LE (2016) Cost-effectiveness of tomosynthesis in annual screening mammography. Am J Roentgenol 207:1152–1155

Klompenhouwer EG, Weber RJ, Voogd AC, Den Heeten GJ, Strobbe LJ, Broeders MJ, Tjan-Heijnen VC, Duijm LE (2015) Arbitration of discrepant BI-RADS 0 recalls by a third reader at screening mammography lowers recall rate but not the cancer detection rate and sensitivity at blinded and non-blinded double reading. Breast 24:601–607

Kopans DB (2011) Just the facts: mammography saves lives with little if any radiation risk to the mature breast. Health Phys 101:578–582

Korhonen KE, Conat EF, Cohen EA, Synnestvedt M, McDonald ES, Weinstein SP (2019) Breast cancer conspicuity on simultaneously acquired digital mammographic images versus digital breast tomosynthesis images. Radiology 292:69–76

Kuhl CK, Schrading S, Bieling HB, Wardelmann E, Leutner CC, Koenig R, Kuhn W, Schild HH (2007) MRI for diagnosis of pure ductal carcinoma in situ: a prospective observational study. Lancet 370:485–492

Kuhl CK, Schrading S, Strobel K, Schild HH, Hilgers R-D, Bieling HB (2014) Abbreviated breast magnetic resonance imaging (MRI): first postcontrast subtracted images and maximum-intensity projection—a novel approach to breast cancer screening with MRI. J Clin Oncol 32:2304–2310

Kuhl CK, Strobel K, Bieling H, Leutner C, Schild HH, Schrading S (2017) Supplemental breast MR imaging screening of women with average risk of breast cancer. Radiology 283:361–370

Lang K, Andersson I, Rosso A, Tingberg A, Timberg P, Zackrisson S (2016) Performance of one-view breast tomosynthesis as a stand-alone breast cancer screening modality: results from the Malmo breast tomosynthesis screening trial, a population-based study. Eur Radiol 26:184–190

Lee W, Peters G (2013) Mammographic screening for breast cancer: a review. J Med Radiat Sci 60:35–39

Lee CI, Cevik M, Alagoz O, Sprague BL, Tosteson AN, Miglioretti DL, Kerlikowske K, Stout NK, Jarvik JG, Ramsey SD, Lehman CD (2015) Comparative effectiveness of combined digital mammography and tomosynthesis screening for women with dense breasts. Radiology 274:772–780

Lee EH, Kim KW, Kim YJ, Shin DR, Park YM, Lim HS, Park JS, Kim HW, Kim YM, Kim HJ, Jun JK (2016) Performance of screening mammography: a report of the alliance for breast cancer screening in Korea. Korean J Radiol 17:489–496

Lehman C, Holt S, Peacock S, White E, Urban N (2002) Use of the American College of Radiology BI-RADS guidelines by community radiologists: concordance of assessments and recommendations assigned to screening mammograms. AJR Am J Roentgenol 179:15–20

Lehman CD, Wellman RD, Buist DS, Kerlikowske K, Tosteson AN, Miglioretti DL (2015) Diagnostic accuracy of digital screening mammography with and without computer-aided detection. JAMA Intern Med 175:1828–1837

Lewin JM, Hendrick RE, D'Orsi CJ, Isaacs PK, Moss LJ, Karellas A, Sisney GA, Kuni CC, Cutter GR (2001) Comparison of full-field digital mammography with screen-film mammography for cancer detection: results of 4,945 paired examinations. Radiology 218:873–880

Lundgren B, Jakobsson S (1976) Single view mammography: a simple and efficient approach to breast cancer screening. Cancer 38:1124–1129

McDonald ES, McCarthy AM, Akhtar AL, Synnestvedt MB, Schnall M, Conant EF (2015) Baseline screening mammography: performance of full-field digital mammography versus digital breast tomosynthesis. AJR Am J Roentgenol 205:1143–1148

McDonald ES, Oustimov A, Weinstein SP, Synnestvedt MB, Schnall M, Conant EF (2016) Effectiveness of digital breast tomosynthesis compared with digital mammography. Outcomes analysis from 3 years of breast cancer screening. JAMA Oncol 2:737–743

McPherson K, Steel CM, Dixon JM (2000) Breast cancer—epidemiology, risk factors, and genetics. BMJ 321:624–628

Minamimoto R, Senda M, Jinnouchi S, Terauchi T, Yoshida T, Inoue T (2015) Detection of breast cancer in an FDG-PET cancer screening program: results of a nationwide Japanese survey. Clin Breast Cancer 15:e139–e146

Monticciolo DL, Newell MS, Hendrick RE, Helvie MA, Moy L, Monsees B, Kopans DB, Eby PR, Sickles EA (2017) Breast cancer screening for average-risk women: recommendations from the ACR Commission on Breast Imaging. J Am Coll Radiol 14:1137–1143

Morrell S, Taylor R, Roder D, Robson B, Gregory M, Craig K (2017) Mammography service screening and breast cancer mortality in New Zealand: a National Cohort Study 1999–2011. Br J Cancer 116:828–839

Morris E, Feig SA, Drexler M, Lehman C (2015) Implications of overdiagnosis: impact on screening mammography practices. Popul Health Manag 18(Suppl 1):S3–S11

Oberaigner W, Daniaux M, Geiger-Gritsch S, Knapp R, Siebert U, Buchberger W (2011) Introduction of organised mammography screening in Tyrol: results following first year of complete rollout. BMC Public Health 11:673

Olsen AH, Njor SH, Vejborg I, Schwartz W, Dalgaard P, Jensen MB, Tange UB, Blichert-Toft M, Rank F, Mouridsen H, Lynge E (2005) Breast cancer mortality in Copenhagen after introduction of mammography screening: cohort study. BMJ 330:220

Olsen AH, Agbaje OF, Myles JP, Lynge E, Duffy SW (2006) Overdiagnosis, sojourn time, and sensitivity in the Copenhagen mammography screening program. Breast J 12:338–342

Østerås BH, Martinsen ACT, Brandal SHB, Chaudhry KN, Eben E, Haakenaasen U, Falk RS, Skaane P (2016a) BI-RADS density classification from areometric and volumetric automatic breast density measurements. Acad Radiol 23:468–478

Østerås BH, Martinsen ACT, Brandal SHB, Chaudhry KN, Eben E, Haakenaasen U, Falk RS, Skaane P (2016b) Classification of fatty and dense breast parenchyma: comparison of automatic volumetric density measurement and radiologists' classification and their inter-observer variation. Acta Radiol 57:1178–1185

Østerås BH, Martinsen ACT, Gullien R, Skaane P (2019) Digital mammography versus breast tomosynthesis: impact of breast density on diagnostic performance in population-based screening. Radiology 293:60–68

Pace LE, Keating NL (2014) A systematic assessment of benefits and risks to guide breast cancer screening decisions. JAMA 311:1327–1335

Paci E, Warwick J, Falini P, Duffy SW (2004) Overdiagnosis in screening: is the increase in breast cancer incidence rates a cause for concern? J Med Screen 11:23–27

Palli D, Del Turco MR, Buiatti E, Carli S, Ciatto S, Toscani I., Maltoni G (1986) A case-control study of the efficacy of a non-randomized breast cancer screening program in Florence (Italy). Int J Cancer 38:501–504

Pattacini P, Nitrosi A, Rossi PG, Iotti V, Ginocchi V, Ravaioli S, Vacondio R, Braglia L, Cavuto S, Campari C (2018) Digital mammography versus digital mammography plus tomosynthesis for breast cancer screening: the Reggio Emilia tomosynthesis randomized trial. Radiology 288:375–385

Perry N, Broeders M, De Wolf C, Tornberg S, Holland R, Von Karsa L (2008) European guidelines for quality assurance in breast cancer screening and diagnosis. Fourth edition—summary document. Ann Oncol 19:614–622

Pisano ED, Gatsonis C, Hendrick E, Yaffe M, Baum JK, Acharyya S, Conant EF, Fajardo LL, Bassett L, D'Orsi C, Jong R, Rebner M (2005) Diagnostic performance of digital versus film mammography for breast-cancer screening. N Engl J Med 353:1773–1783

Posso MC, Puig T, Quintana MJ, Sola-Roca J, Bonfill X (2016) Double versus single reading of mammograms in a breast cancer screening programme: a cost-consequence analysis. Eur Radiol 26: 3262–3271

Puliti D, Duffy SW, Miccinesi G, De Koning H, Lynge E, Zappa M, Paci E (2012) Overdiagnosis in mammographic screening for breast cancer in Europe: a literature review. J Med Screen 19(Suppl 1):42–56

Rafferty EA, Durand MA, Conant EF, Copit DS, Friedewald SM, Plecha DM, Miller DP (2016) Breast cancer screening using tomosynthesis and digital mammography in dense and nondense breasts. JAMA 315:1784–1786

Redondo A, Comas M, Macia F (2012) Inter- and intraradiologist variability in the BI-RADS assessment and breast density categories for screening mammograms. Br J Radiol 85:1465–1470

Rhodes DJ, Hruska CB, Conners AL, Tortorelli CL, Maxwell RW, Jones KN, Toledano AY, O'Connor MK (2015) Molecular breast imaging at reduced radiation dose for supplemental screening in mammographically dense breasts. AJR Am J Roentgenol 204:241–251

Roberts MM, Alexander FE, Anderson TJ, Chetty U, Donnan PT, Forrest P, Hepburn W, Huggins A, Kirkpatrick AE, Lamb J et al (1990) Edinburgh trial of screening for breast cancer: mortality at seven years. Lancet 335:241–246

Sankatsing VD, Juraniec K, Grimm SE, Joore MA, Pijnappel RM, Dekoning HJ, Ravesteyn NT (2020) Cost-effectiveness of digital breast tomosynthesis in population-based breast cancer screening: a probabilistic sensitivity analysis. Radiology. https://doi.org/10.1148/radiol.2020192505

Schaefgen B, Heil J, Barr RG, Radicke M, Harcos A, Gomez C, Stieber A, Hennigs A, Von Au A, Spratte J, Rauch G, Rom J, Schutz F, Sohn C, Golatta M (2018) Initial results of the FUSION-X-US prototype combining 3D automated breast ultrasound and digital breast tomosynthesis. Eur Radiol 28:2499–2506

Schou Bredal I, Kåresen R, Skaane P, Engelstad KS, Ekeberg Ø (2013) Recall mammography and psychological distress. Eur J Cancer 49:805–811

Sechopoulos I, Mann RM (2020) Stand-alone artificial intelligence - the future of breast cancer screening? Breast 49:254–260

Shapiro S, Strax P, Venet L (1971) Periodic breast cancer screening in reducing mortality from breast cancer. JAMA 215:1777–1785

Shermis RB, Wilson KD, Doyle MT, Martin TS, Merryman D, Kudrolli H, Brenner RJ (2016) Supplemental breast cancer screening with molecular breast imaging for women with dense breast tissue. AJR Am J Roentgenol 207:450–457

Skaane P (2009) Studies comparing screen-film mammography and full-field digital mammography in breast cancer screening: updated review. Acta Radiol 50:3–14

Skaane P, Skjennald A (2004) Screen-film mammography versus full-field digital mammography with soft-copy reading: randomized trial in a population-based screening program—the Oslo II study. Radiology 232:197–204

Skaane P, Young K, Skjennald A (2003) Population-based mammography screening: comparison of screen-film and full-field digital mammography with soft-copy reading—Oslo I study. Radiology 229:877–884

Skaane P, Kshirsagar A, Stapleton S, Young K, Castellino RA (2007) Effect of computer-aided detection on independent double reading of paired screen-film and full-field digital screening mammograms. AJR Am J Roentgenol 188:377–384

Skaane P, Bandos AI, Gullien R, Eben EB, Ekseth U, Haakenaasen U, Izadi M, Jebsen IN, Jahr G, Krager M, Niklason LT, Hofvind S, Gur D (2013) Comparison of digital mammography alone and digital mammography plus tomosynthesis in a population-based screening program. Radiology 267:47–56

Skaane P, Bandos AI, Eben EB, Jebsen IN, Krager M, Haakenaasen U, Ekseth U, Izadi M, Hofvind S, Gullien R (2014) Two-view digital breast tomosynthesis screening with synthetically reconstructed projection images: comparison with digital breast tomosynthesis with full-field digital mammographic images. Radiology 271:655–663

Smith RA (2003) IARC handbooks of cancer prevention, Volume 7: Breast cancer screening. Breast Cancer Res 5:216–217

Sprague BL, Conant EF, Onega T, Garcia MP, Beaber EF, Herschorn SD, Lehman CD, Tosteson AN, Lacson R, Schnall MD, Kontos D, Haas JS, Weaver DL, Barlow WE (2016) Variation in mammographic breast density assessments among radiologists in clinical practice: a multicenter observational study. Ann Intern Med 165:457–464

Sung JS, Stamler S, Brooks J, Kaplan J, Huang T, Dershaw DD, Lee CH, Morris EA, Comstock CE

(2016) Breast cancers detected at screening MR imaging and mammography in patients at high risk: method of detection reflects tumor histopathologic results. Radiology 280:716–722

Tabar L, Tony Chen HH, Amy Yen MF, Tot T, Tung TH, Chen LS, Chiu YH, Duffy SW, Smith RA (2004) Mammographic tumor features can predict long-term outcomes reliably in women with 1–14-mm invasive breast carcinoma. Cancer 101:1745–1759

Tabár L, Tot T, Dean PB (2007) Breast cancer. Early detection with mammography. Casting type calcifications: sign of a subtype with deceptive features. Thieme, Stuttgart

Tabár L, Tot T, Dean PB (2008) Breast cancer-early detection with mammography. Crushed stone-like calcifications-the most frequent malignant type. Thieme, Stuttgart

Tagliafico AS, Calabrese M, Mariscotti G, Durando M, Tosto S, Monetti F, Airaldi S, Bignotti B, Nori J, Bagni A, Signori A, Sormani MP, Houssami N (2016) Adjunct screening with tomosynthesis or ultrasound in women with mammography-negative dense breasts: interim report of a prospective comparative trial. J Clin Oncol 34:1882–1888

Tornberg S, Kemetli L, Ascunce N, Hofvind S, Anttila A, Seradour B, Paci E, Guldenfels C, Azavedo E, Frigerio A, Rodrigues V, Ponti A (2010) A pooled analysis of interval cancer rates in six European countries. Eur J Cancer Prev 19:87–93

Van Dijck JA, Verbeek AL, Hendriks JH, Holland R (1993) The current detectability of breast cancer in a mammographic screening program. A review of the previous mammograms of interval and screen-detected cancers. Cancer 72:1933–1938

Van Ravesteyn NT, Stout NK, Schechter CB, Heijnsdijk EA, Alagoz O, Trentham-Dietz A, Mandelblatt JS, De Koning HJ (2015) Benefits and harms of mammogra-

phy screening after age 74 years: model estimates of overdiagnosis. J Natl Cancer Inst 107:djv103

Vedantham S, Karellas A, Vijayaraghavan GR, Kopans DB (2015) Digital breast tomosynthesis: state of the art. Radiology 277:663–684

Verbeek AL, Hendriks JH, Holland R, Mravunac M, Sturmans F, Day NE (1984) Reduction of breast cancer mortality through mass screening with modern mammography. First results of the Nijmegen project, 1975–1981. Lancet 1:1222–1224

Warner E, Heisey R, Carroll JC (2012) Applying the 2011 Canadian guidelines for breast cancer screening in practice. CMAJ 184:1803–1807

Winkler NS, Raza S, Mackesy M, Birdwell RL (2015) Breast density: clinical implications and assessment methods. Radiographics 35.316–324

Zackrisson S, Andersson I, Janzon L, Manjer J, Garne JP (2006) Rate of over-diagnosis of breast cancer 15 years after end of Malmo mammographic screening trial: follow-up study. BMJ 332:689–692

Zackrisson S, Lång K, Rosso A, Johnson K, Dustler M, Fornvik D, Fornvik H, Sartor H, Timberg P, Tingberg A, Anersson I (2018) One-view breast tomosynthesis versus two-view mammography in the Malmo breast tomosynthesis screening trial (MBTST): a prospective, population-based diagnostic accuracy study. Lancet Oncol 19:1493–1503

Zahl P-H, Strand BH, Mæhlen J (2004) Incidence of breast cancer in Norway and Sweden during introduction of nationwide screening: prospective cohort study. BMJ 328:921–924

Zuley ML, Guo B, Catullo VJ, Chough DM, Kelly AE, Lu AH, Rathfon GY, Lee Spangler M, Sumkin JH, Wallace LP, Bandos AI (2014) Comparison of two-dimensional synthesized mammograms versus original digital mammograms alone and in combination with tomosynthesis images. Radiology 271:664–671

Stereotactic Guided Breast Interventions

Daniela Bernardi and Vincenzo Sabatino

Contents

1	**Indications for Stereotactic Breast Biopsy**	70
2	**Stereotactic Biopsy Systems**	72
	2.1 Prone Biopsy Tables	72
	2.2 Add-On Biopsy Units	74
3	**Pre-biopsy Evaluations**	76
	3.1 Lesion Evaluation	76
	3.2 Needle Choice	76
	3.3 Patient Care	79
4	**Biopsy Technique**	80
	4.1 Patient Positioning	80
	4.2 Biopsy Preparations	80
	4.3 Lesion Targeting and Biopsy	80
	4.4 Technical Limitations and Potential Remedies	83
	4.5 Specimen Core Management	84
5	**Post-biopsy Measures**	85
	5.1 Clip Positioning	85
	5.2 Post-biopsy Mammography	85
	5.3 Patient Care and Follow-Up	86
	5.4 Pathological Result Management and Indications for Treatment	86
	5.5 Presurgical Localization	87
	5.6 Specimen Radiography	90
6	**Summary**	91
	References	91

D. Bernardi (✉)
Department of Biomedical Sciences,
Humanitas University, Via Rita Levi Montalcini,
Pieve Emanuele, Milan, Italy
e-mail: Daniela.Bernardi@hunimed.eu

V. Sabatino
A.P.S.S. Trento, Department of Radiology,
U.O. Senologia Clinica e Screening Mammografico,
Trento, Italia

Abstract

The use of screening mammography in asymptomatic women has increased the number of non-palpable suspicious breast abnormalities, which require histologic evaluation to define whether they are benign or malignant.

© Springer Nature Switzerland AG 2022
M. Fuchsjäger et al. (eds.), *Breast Imaging*, Medical Radiology Diagnostic Imaging,
https://doi.org/10.1007/978-3-030-94918-1_4

In the last decade, the introduction of digital breast tomosynthesis (DBT), a pseudo-three-dimensional mammographic application, has increased the diagnostic accuracy of digital mammography through the detection of abnormal findings that are seen only at DBT and which need to be assessed (Houssami et al., Breast 26:119–134, https://doi.org/10.1016/j.breast.2016.01.007, 2016).

Women with suspicious breast lesions identified on mammography or DBT are indicated for biopsy to obtain definitive tissue diagnosis. In these cases, needle biopsy should be the first option to avoid diagnostic surgical biopsies. A minimally invasive procedure offers better options compared to surgical biopsy: firstly, it reduces the physical and psychological stress of the patient, and secondly, it overcomes the problem of scarring after a surgical biopsy, which may impair future imaging (Yu et al., Breast Cancer Res Treat 120(2):469–479. https://doi.org/10.1007/s10549-010-0750-1, 2010). Consequently, open surgical biopsy is now obsolete for most indications.

Since it is well accepted, quick, readily accessible, and less costly, ultrasound-guided biopsy should be done for all lesions visible at ultrasound. Any lesions visualized at mammography (MX) or DBT but sonographically occult may instead undergo stereotactic biopsy, which should be guided by MX or DBT (Huang et al., Tech Vasc Interv Radiol 17(1):32–39. https://doi.org/10.1053/j.tvir.2013.12.006, 2014).

1 Indications for Stereotactic Breast Biopsy

Most of the abnormal mammographic findings, which undergo stereotactic biopsy, are calcifications and, less commonly, masses, asymmetries, and architectural distortions (Fig. 1). While there is no definitive consensus in the recent literature regarding detection and characterization of microcalcifications with DBT (Byun et al. 2017),

it has been shown that DBT improves the visualization of masses and architectural distortions not visible with other breast imaging modalities (e.g., mammography and/or ultrasound).

Breast abnormalities, detected on screening mammography or DBT, should be assessed prior to needle biopsy through clinical evaluation and additional mammographic or sonographic imaging to determine the degree of suspicion for malignancy. The assessment of the suspicious lesions detected only by DBT should include additional tomosynthesis views; in particular, tomosynthesis spot compressions can be helpful for radiologists in assigning the correct degree of suspicion for malignancy (Houssami et al. 2016) (Fig. 2).

The final assessment category depends on the different lexicons adopted by each individual center: the most widely used reporting system of mammographic examination is the Breast Imaging Reporting and Data System (BI-RADS) atlas of the American College of Radiology (ACR) (D'Orsi et al. 2013). According to the BI-RADS classification, lesions at mammography classified as category 4 (suspicious) or category 5 (highly suggestive of malignancy) require biopsy.

A second breast imaging classification is the one adopted in the UK by the Royal College of Radiologists Breast Group (RCRBG). In contrast to the American classification, the classification used in the UK indicates a need for biopsy not only for category 4 and 5 lesions but also for category 3 lesions (indeterminate/probably benign): this is because the standard UK RCRBG Score 3 has in terms of percentage a comparable cancer likelihood with BI-RADS 4a/b (Maxwell et al. 2009).

The Australian National Breast Cancer Centre (NBCC), in collaboration with the Royal Australian and New Zealand College of Radiologists, has developed a similar five-point system. This classification system also advocates needle biopsy for equivocal or probable benign (BI-RADS 3) findings to achieve a definitive diagnosis rather than recommending a short-term follow-up (The National Breast Cancer Centre (NBCC) 2007).

Stereotactic Guided Breast Interventions

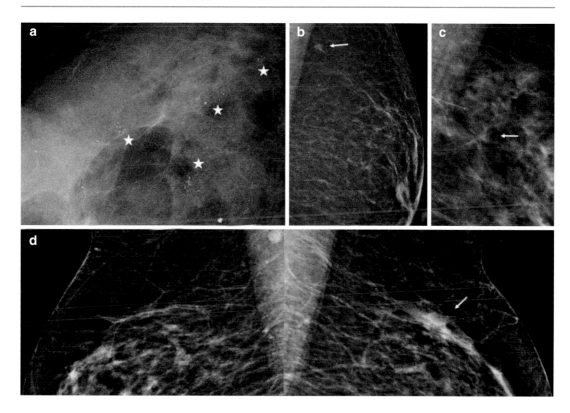

Fig. 1 Examples of breast abnormalities identified on standard mammography that should be referred for stereotactic guided biopsy. According to ACR BI-RADS® atlas: (**a**) grouped fine pleomorphic calcifications (stars) in extremely dense breast; (**b**) a small irregular mass with indistinct margins (arrow) completely surrounded by fatty tissue; (**c**) an architectural distortion manifested by thin radiating lines with primarily fatty tissue at the point of origin (arrow) located in the upper quadrants of a heterogeneously dense breast; (**d**) focal asymmetric dense tissue (arrow) in the upper quadrants of the left breast

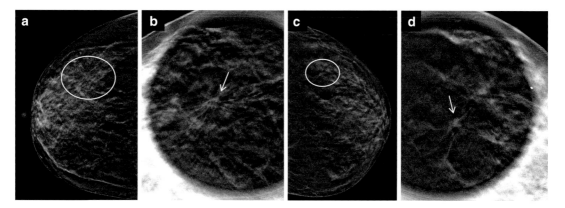

Fig. 2 (**a**) Example of mammographically occult architectural distortion with no definite mass, detectable by digital breast tomosynthesis. (**b**) The DBT spot compression view magnifies the central radiolucency at the point of origin with long and thin radiating spiculations (histology final exam: radial scar). (**c**) Example of a small spiculated mass identified by tomosynthesis. (**d**) The better tissue separation due to DBT spot compression results in a clear visualization of the lesion borders; their irregular appearance indicates sufficient suspicion of malignancy to justify a DBT-guided biopsy (histology final exam: IDC, low grade)

The effectiveness of the latter two classification systems demonstrated that also lesions classified as category 3 (probably benign) by the ACR BI-RADS classification might have indication for biopsy depending on the clinical suspicion, personal risk and patient or physician preference.

After the necessary evaluations, according to the judgment of the radiologist, mammographically identified lesions should undergo stereotactic biopsy; for lesions only or better visualized by DBT, tomosynthesis guidance is indicated.

2 Stereotactic Biopsy Systems

The first mammographically guided stereotactic biopsy was developed in Sweden in the late 1970s as a necessary alternative to follow-up or surgical biopsy. Fine needle aspiration cytology on non-palpable suspicious breast abnormalities was first performed using devices such as the one shown in Fig. 3. Using this equipment, Bolmgren et al. reported, for the first 21 cases with complete follow-up, strong diagnostic accuracy of the sampling procedures with a complete agreement between cytology and final histology (Bolmgren et al. 1977). The prone biopsy system in a short time became a reliable and safe method for tissue sampling, widely reducing indications for surgical excision and histological verification.

Over time upright devices added onto the mammography units have joined this biopsy guidance system; upright devices, which allow the execution of biopsies with patients standing or sitting, have been increasingly used after the introduction of digital imaging. Digital mammography has improved the accuracy and efficiency of the procedures, in both prone and upright positions, shortening—compared to screen-film mammography—the total time necessary for biopsy through the reduction of the interval between taking and viewing the check image pair during needle positioning. The acquisition of digital image pairs also allowed microcalcifications to be visualized and targeted more accurately by image post-processing facilities, including black-white inversion, contrast adjustment, and selective magnification. The advantage of shorter procedure times has been greater for upright stereotactic biopsies; however, the risk of having to stop the procedure for vasovagal reactions is higher in standing or sitting patients than in patients lying on a prone biopsy table.

After the introduction of DBT in breast imaging, new suspicious findings with no definitive mammographic or sonographic correlation have been identified; these suspicious lesions, represented in part by small cancers, and in part by benign lesions such as radial scars or stromal fibrosis (i.e., false-positive findings), needed to be biopsied to define their histology. To overcome this important limitation, dedicated guidance systems have been developed and installed as biopsy devices added onto DBT units. These devices can be used for both tomosynthesis-guided biopsies and "conventional" stereotactic biopsies; using in fact the DBT unit in stereotactic modality, the movement of the tomosynthesis arm is used to generate the pair of angulated stereotactic images.

For a significant period of time these add-on systems allowed biopsies with a DBT guide on patients sitting upright or recumbent, but not in prone position. Recently, a prone table with an integrated tomosynthesis detection system has been developed and is now in use.

2.1 Prone Biopsy Tables

The prone table system for interventions is a mammographic X-ray system especially designed for stereotactic localization of suspicious breast lesions.

During a prone stereotactic biopsy, the patient lies facedown (prone) on the table and the breast falls through a hole in the table. As shown in Fig. 4, using the prone table, several different approaches to biopsy are possible. The choice of the best biopsy approach depends partly on the skin-to-lesion distance and partly on other factors, such as the thickness of the breast. To guarantee accurate sampling of the lesions located inside the breast, there are two possible options for needle insertion: a vertical insertion (through the breast compression paddle, with the needle

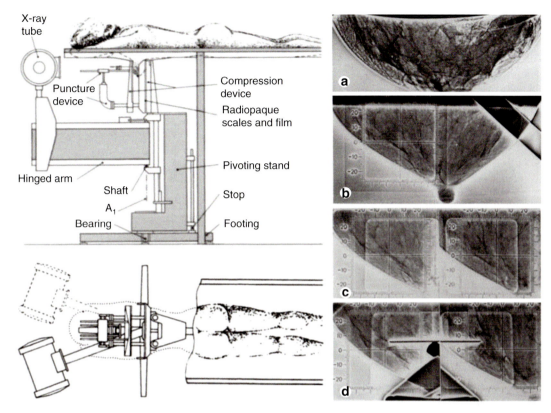

Fig. 3 The equipment used by Bolmgren and colleagues seen from above and from the side. In this prone-type table, the X-ray tube was angled to produce two views of the target lesion, typically at ±15° from the central axis. After the acquisition of a scout view (**a**), the position of the lesion in the breast was calculated from the movement relative to a fixed reference grid (**b**, **c**); the needle was placed within the lesion with direct confirmation of its position relative to the target abnormality on repeated pair of angulated X-ray views (**d**)

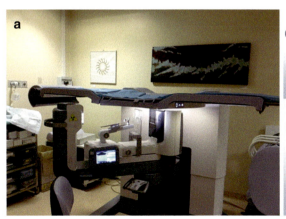

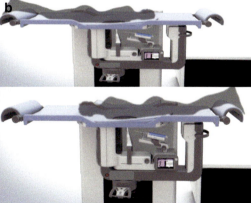

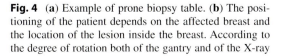

Fig. 4 (**a**) Example of prone biopsy table. (**b**) The positioning of the patient depends on the affected breast and the location of the lesion inside the breast. According to the degree of rotation both of the gantry and of the X-ray tube, various approaches are used for stereotactic or tomosynthesis-guided biopsies: cranial to caudal, medial to lateral, lateral to medial, or caudal to cranial

perpendicular to the mammography detector plate) and a lateral insertion (with the needle parallel to the compression paddle and mammography detector plate) (Fig. 5). As most of the prone units on the market only offer one option, biopsies are most commonly performed using the vertical approach. Doing DBT-guided biopsies, this approach will be burdened with wide artifacts in the tomo views acquired after needle insertion. For this reason the lateral approach is recommended for DBT-guided biopsies; if this is not possible after needle insertion, all additional views should be acquired by conventional mammography.

On average, a prone biopsy procedure takes about 20–45 min (Schrading et al. 2015; O'Flynn et al. 2010, Ohsumi et al. 2014), during which the woman should stay still and relaxed.

Compared to sitting, the prone position is usually better tolerated by the patient, who cannot see the biopsy needle, thus causing less anxiety (Tagliafico et al. 2015); in this position, there is less patient motion to interfere with accurate targeting. In addition, the radiologist and the technologist, working under the table, have more room to maneuver.

Although prone tables are effective, there are some limitations. One is the difficulty in lifting patients onto the table when they are unable to do so themselves. There are limitations in overweight patients, as prone tables have a patient weight limit between 136 and 158 kg; excess can lead to mechanical failure (Huang et al. 2014). Prone tables can only be used for biopsy, not for standard mammography; they require more space than standard mammography units, are more costly, and, sometimes, are underutilized due to low patient frequency.

2.2 Add-On Biopsy Units

Add-on biopsy devices are attached to the existing mammography or DBT units, converting them into a biopsy system (Fig. 6). During the procedure, the patient is generally sitting upright. However, using a "non-dedicated" bed or special reclining chair, the patient may lie in a lateral decubitus position: in this position, vasovagal reactions are greatly reduced compared to the sitting position (Sim and Kei 2008).

As with prone biopsies, several different approaches are also possible when using the add-on systems, including the use of the vertical—or lateral—needle insertion (Fig. 7).

It has been reported that stereotactic procedures using add-on systems take between 20 and 45 min (O'Flynn et al. 2010; Ohsumi et al. 2014); for biopsies performed using DBT guidance Schrading et al. reported reasonable reduction of the procedure time, on average 13 min per biopsy (Schrading et al. 2015).

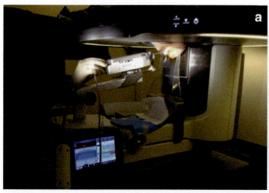
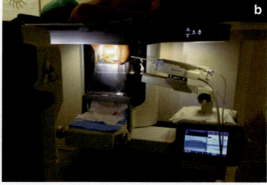

Fig. 5 (**a**) Vertical needle insertion using a prone-type device: the needle is inserted from above the breast compression paddle and perpendicular to the mammography detector plate. (**b**) Lateral needle insertion using a prone-type device: the needle is parallel both to the compression paddle and the mammography detector plate reducing any limitations due to breast size

Stereotactic Guided Breast Interventions

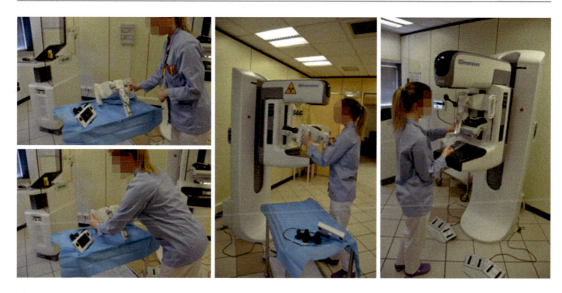

Fig. 6 An add-on biopsy device is installed onto a mammography unit, converting it to a biopsy system

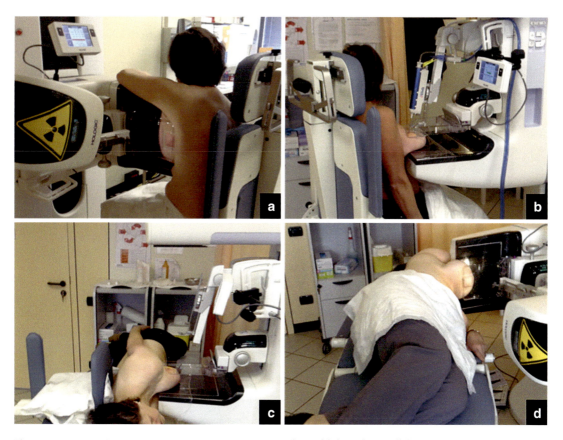

Fig. 7 Examples of biopsy approaches using an add-on system in combination with a reclining chair which allows the patient to stay in two different positions: sitting position, with lateral to medial (**a**) or cranial to caudal needle insertion (**b**); lying position and the needle inserted using a lateral to medial (**c**) or a caudal to cranial direction (**d**)

The upright biopsy technique is space-effective eliminating the need for a dedicated room or equipment for biopsy purposes only. Therefore, compared to prone systems, add-on biopsy units are also less costly, thereby equally accurate and safe for patients who usually tolerate it well. Still, the risk of vasovagal reactions, such as malaise, nausea, vomiting, and even fainting, may be increased when sampling is performed in the sitting position with the biopsy needle right in front of the patient's face. Concerning this risk, it is noteworthy that, while the first studies published on upright biopsies reported a high incidence of vasovagal reactions (with complication rates ranging between 20% and 37%) (Welle and Clark 1997; Welle et al. 2000), such reactions have been considerably reduced over time reaching the value of 7% published by Ohsumi et al. (2014). Furthermore, the experience of both the physician and the technologist involved in this kind of procedure plays a crucial role in minimizing the risk of suspending the procedure due to the effects of vasovagal reactions.

Another problem that may arise during upright procedures is patient motion, which can interfere with accurate targeting; using pillows to stabilize the patient can easily minimize this limitation.

3 Pre-biopsy Evaluations

Before proceeding with stereotactic guided biopsy, accurate evaluation has to be done. First the technical feasibility of the biopsy considering the lesion position has to be evaluated, and then according to the lesion pattern (e.g., microcalcifications rather than distortions or masses), the appropriate needle is selected. Finally, the best needle approach is determined.

3.1 Lesion Evaluation

The success of the biopsy procedure depends in part on lesion depth and location. Lesions located close to the chest wall cannot be biopsied using stereotactic guidance because they are difficult to access, both in prone and upright modes; these lesions should therefore be sent directly to surgery. Furthermore, lesions detected in very small breasts are also difficult to access; indeed, when the thickness of the compressed breast is less than 1 cm, both the vertical and the lateral insertion of the needle (see Sect. 3.1) is limited, and surgical biopsy should be performed. However, in case of very large breasts, considering target lesion position, needles of sufficient length are required.

In case of superficial calcifications, dermal calcifications have to be ruled in or out by placing a small metallic marker on the very skin site before starting the stereotactic localization.

3.2 Needle Choice

Fine needle aspiration cytology (FNAC), the original method of sampling, has been used for diagnosis since the 1950s. Then, since the early 1990s, due to the increasing number of women undergoing assessment for non-palpable lesions detected by mammographic screening, there has been a steady shift towards percutaneous biopsy techniques. FNAC was followed first by core needle biopsy (CNB), and then by vacuum-assisted biopsy (VAB). Both biopsy techniques have become widely practiced because of their proven high accuracy. The choice of the appropriate needle depends on several factors among which diagnostic accuracy is the most important.

3.2.1 Fine Needle Aspiration Cytology (FNAC)

Even though FNAC is the most basic and inexpensive form of sampling, this method is no longer recommended as routine technique for breast diagnosis because of certain important limitations.

The major limitation is in the sampling of cells and not of breast tissue. Consequently, FNAC is unable to diagnose some benign lesions and to distinguish definitive borderline breast lesions from malignant lesions. For example, pre-neoplastic lesions such as atypical ductal hyperplasia or in situ changes cannot be confidently diagnosed with FNAC, and the distinction between in situ and invasive malignancy is difficult if not impossible. Another limitation of the method is its highly variable range of sensitivity and diagnostic accuracy with a rate of inadequate samples between 8.5% and 46%. This is particularly noticeable in stereotactic guided samplings with a reported value at an unacceptable 39.9% (O'Flynn et al. 2010). For this reason, the potential diagnostic role of FNAC in the assessment of non-palpable breast abnormalities was markedly reduced.

3.2.2 Core Needle Biopsy (CNB)

Core needle biopsy, which is performed by using biopsy needle systems such as those shown in Fig. 8, has the advantages of higher sensitivity and specificity, higher negative and positive predictive values, and lower underestimation and re-biopsy rates compared to FNAC. However, false-negative results and/or underestimation of the presence of disease are reported; this occurs most commonly with lesions such as microcalcification or possible complex sclerosing lesions requiring stereotactic guidance (Wang et al. 2017).

The most common cause of false-negative results is inaccurate tissue sampling. This depends in part on repeated needle insertions and removals for obtaining breast specimens and is particularly important for stereotactic biopsy of lesions, such as microcalcifications rather than distortions, whose samples are frequently composed of blood because of the destruction of the breast architecture and focal hemorrhages.

A further limitation of stereotactic guided CNB samples is that, because of the smaller needle size (14 G), samples fail to provide a complete characterization of histological findings, thus frequently leading to an underestimation of disease. Reported underestimation rates for

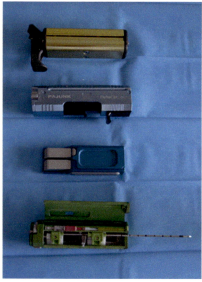
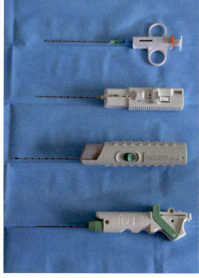

Fig. 8 Example of core biopsy needle systems available from many different vendors. On the left, four non-disposable models and on the right, four disposable models. For each of these models a variety of needle lengths and gauges are available. Most of these systems are automated biopsy systems and all of them work on the same basic two-phase firing mechanism: once fired, the core biopsy needle automatically advances through the breast parenchyma and the inner notched sheath advances forward. Almost immediately, a sharp outer cannula advances over the inner sheath, trapping a piece of tissue within the notch. The two systems on the top right are semiautomated cutting needles; using these kind of systems, the needle is manually inserted into the lesion; then the outer sheath is fired and a piece of tissue is trapped within the notch. Using core biopsy, the sampling needs repeated needle passes; for stereotactic or DBT-guided biopsies, using an introducer, radiologists can precisely obtain contiguous tissue specimens and reduce the procedure time

high-risk lesions range from 3.4% to 100%; in particular, atypical ductal hyperplasia (ADH) is frequently upgraded to ductal carcinoma in situ (DCIS) or invasive carcinoma in 56% of cases, after open surgery. Furthermore, when DCIS is diagnosed with core needle biopsy, the risk of upgrading to invasive cancer ranges between 16% and 55.5%. Underestimation by core needle biopsy has also been reported in radial scars, papillary lesions, lobular carcinoma in situ (LCIS), and phyllodes tumor (Sanderink and Mann 2017).

There has been much debate on the number of specimens necessary to achieve a reliable histological diagnosis, concluding that, for stereotactic CNB, diagnostic sensitivity is improved by increasing the number of cores to six or more (O'Flynn et al. 2010)

In daily practice usually 14 G needles are used. However, it has been shown that diagnostic accuracy improves significantly by increasing both needle size and number of specimens delivered to the pathologist.

3.2.3 Vacuum-Assisted Biopsy (VAB)

VAB was developed to overcome the limitations of CNB. In particular, VAB has proven to be advantageous compared to CNB as more tissue volume is obtained and therefore histological classification is more reliable (Preibsch et al. 2014). VAB has therefore replaced large core needle biopsy at several indications, becoming the method of choice to assess suspicious lesions without a relevant solid component (e.g., microcalcifications and distortions) using stereotactic guidance (Pfarl et al. 2002).

Currently several devices are available, each with their own minor technical differences. A double-lumen probe, powered by suction, and a rotating cutter characterize them all. Using the vacuum, multiple samples can be taken after a single insertion of the probe, as shown in greater detail in Fig. 9. At the end of the procedure, a metallic or gel-localizing clip can be placed through the VAB needle to mark the biopsy site. This is particularly useful for small lesions and microcalcification clusters that have been completely removed by percutaneous biopsy. If localization of the lesion is required for surgical excision, the marker can be visualized using ultrasound or mammography. In addition, the clip allows identification of the biopsy site on subsequent mammograms (O'Flynn et al. 2010).

Relative to core needle biopsy, VAB provides larger specimens, offers a higher sample retrieval rate, is less sensitive to targeting errors, and has lower re-biopsy and underestimation rates. In a systematic review, Yu et al. found that sensitivity of VAB ranged from 85% to 100%, and specificity from 96% to 100%. Underestimation rates, however, remain substantial with a pooled ADH and DCIS underestimation of 20.9% and 11.2%, respectively (Yu et al. 2010).

Because the purpose of VAB is to provide larger specimens than CNB, needles' diameters have increased over the years, and currently systems from 12 to 7 G are available. A comparison of 11 and 8 G needles at stereotactic core biopsy showed both better performance and increased accuracy for histologic diagnosis of 8 G versus 11 G needles (Venkataraman et al. 2012). Another advantage of increasing the needle caliber might be the shorter interventional time, as fewer specimens need to be obtained with larger needle sizes. From this perspective, the use of 7 G needles will most likely further decrease intervention time and achieve the same or an even higher diagnostic accuracy compared to smaller needle sizes (Preibsch et al. 2014).

Recently published national and international guidelines and results of consensus meetings provide different recommendations on the required number of tissue specimens, depending on the needle size and imaging method. Most of the recommendations, which refer to the 11 G needle, suggest taking 12 cores on a routine 360° rotation (Lomoschitz et al. 2004; Rageth et al. 2016).

During the procedure, any significant bleeding may be managed using vacuum to suck blood out of the biopsy cavity throughout the procedure, thereby reducing the chance of hematoma formation. As with other sampling methods, a learning curve is associated with performing VAB, and any operator needs to perform a certain number per year to maintain the competence.

Stereotactic Guided Breast Interventions

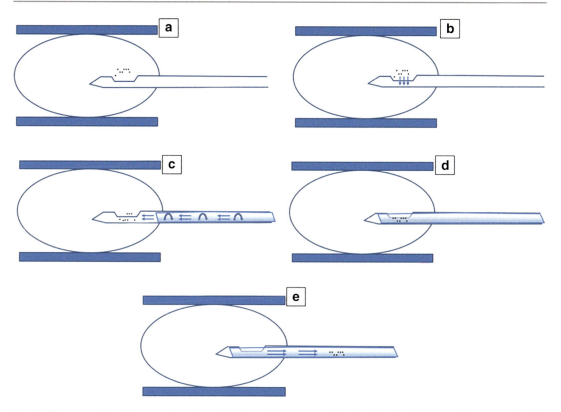

Fig. 9 Vacuum-assisted biopsy: after the positioning of the double-lumen needle-probe tissue at the target lesion site (**a**), tissue is sucked into the biopsy chamber (**b**) where it is separated from the surrounding breast tissue by an internal rotating trocar (**c, d**); the specimen is then transported to the site of collection without removing the needle from the biopsy site (**e**). By rotating the shaft of the needle, multiple samples can be taken after a single insertion of the probe

In practice, VAB, because of its safety, cost and efficacy, minimal complications, and high toleration from patients, is becoming even more widespread and represents, in most cases, a valuable alternative to open surgery.

3.3 Patient Care

A biopsy procedure can be emotionally distressing, not only because of the possibility of a subsequent cancer diagnosis, but also because the biopsy itself might potentially be painful; it is therefore highly recommended that the physician who performs the procedure has a preliminary meeting with the patient to provide all the necessary medical information. This should also include a description of the procedure and its associated risks (e.g., vasovagal reactions, bleeding, infection, adverse or allergic reaction to medications, latex, disinfectant solutions, and tape or adhesives). Patient-signed informed consent for breast interventional procedures is required.

Before the biopsy procedure, the physician should interview the patient about her medical history (especially bleeding disorders), allergy history (especially previous adverse reactions to local anesthetics, epinephrine, latex, disinfectant solutions, and tape or adhesives), and medication list (paying special attention to antiplatelet and anticoagulation medications because of the risk of bleeding). Biopsies can be performed on patients taking antiplatelet or anticoagulant medication with caution, and considering that the larger the needle and the higher the number of samples, the more the attention to be paid. Medicines such as aspirin, clopidogrel, and other antiplatelet agents (e.g., ticagrelor, prasugrel) should not be discontinued (also in case of VAB procedures) but patients should be informed of the increased risk of bleeding, bruising, and hematoma formation. Conversely, dual-antiplatelet therapy (such as aspirin plus clopidogrel, ticagrelor or prasugrel) needs to be discontinued 5 days before the procedure. For patients receiving anticoagulant agents, according to the national or local recommendations, the therapy may be discontinued some day before with different indications depending on the drug: anticoagulant agents like warfarin should be stopped 5 days before biopsy, while newer anticoagulant agents (such as rivaroxaban, dabigatran, apixaban, or edoxaban) may be discontinued 2 days before. Heparin bridge therapy should be planned, considering that also low-molecular-weight heparin should be discontinued 12 h before treatment. If in doubt, consultation with a hematologist and/or cardiologist (as appropriate) is recommended (Kulkarni and O'Connor 2015).

Because the patient is expected to remain immobile for at least 20–45 min with the breast compressed during biopsy, the physician should consider any physical limitations, such as limited range of motion of the neck or back which could compromise the patient's position. Taking into consideration these possible limitations as well as the patient's susceptibility to vasovagal reactions, the physician should choose the most appropriate approach to perform the biopsy (i.e., prone or, in case of an upright system, sitting versus decubitus position).

4   Biopsy Technique

4.1   Patient Positioning

Depending on whether the biopsy is carried out using a prone or an upright system, the patient rests in the prone position on the table or sits on the reclining chair, respectively. As previously reported, using an upright system, the woman can also lie in the lateral decubitus position, with the affected breast side up. For both systems, the cor-

rect target lesion approach mainly depends on the position of the lesion inside the breast. Because most of the biopsy systems currently on the market offer a large degree of access, up to 360° when the X-ray tube can rotate around itself, several different approaches are possible. The final choice should be made considering the shortest skin-to-lesion distance by ensuring that the needle does not go through the blood vessels.

4.2   Biopsy Preparations

After selection of the correct lesion approach, the breast is compressed between detector plate and compression paddle. The biopsy compression paddle has an open window allowing for access of the target lesion both during sampling and localization procedures.

The skin is then cleansed and disinfected with an aseptic solution and local anesthesia is given to obtain pain control during the procedure. Usually 5–10 mL of buffered 1% lidocaine is administered into the skin and subcutaneous tissue, with an additional 5 mL placed into deeper tissue when necessary. Because bupivacaine is longer acting, it can be used as an alternative to lidocaine especially when the latter does not work, but side effects, such as cardiotoxicity, should be considered. During stereotactic guided biopsy, adding epinephrine can be helpful to induce deeper breast parenchyma anesthesia although this is not recommended for the potential risks of skin necrosis (Fine and Bloom 2009).

4.3   Lesion Targeting and Biopsy

As already reported for a long time, targeting of mammographically suspicious lesions has only been possible using stereotactic guidance which allows its precise location to be determined in three dimensions. With the introduction of DBT, stereotactic guidance has been joined by a new localization technique, using a geometric principle very similar to the one applied to the stratigraphic technique. Today, both localization techniques provide correct lesion targeting, each with different indications depending on the type of lesion to be identified and biopsied.

4.3.1 Stereotactic Guided Biopsy

The image produced in any mammography projection, such as a craniocaudal (CC) or mediolateral oblique (MLO) view, is a two-dimensional representation of three-dimensional space. It follows that a suspicious lesion visible in one or both the mammograms has a location that can be described in terms of three specific coordinates: the x (which corresponds to the horizontal axis), the y (that matches the vertical axis), and the z (coinciding with the depth from the skin surface). Among these coordinates, the z is determined by the thickness of the breast under compression; to calculate it a pair of angled images ($15°$ from midline in both positive and negative directions) is acquired. After targeting the lesion on both the angled images, the computer determines its depth in the compressed breast, according to the principle of triangulation by calculating the apparent shift of the target lesion on the stereotactic images, compared with the target location on a reference view acquired at $0°$.

For this reason, during the stereotactic guided biopsy, after positioning the patient and breast, an initial scout image is obtained with the X-ray beam perpendicular to the compression plate ($0°$ angulation). In this scout image, which is used as a reference providing localization of the lesion in the x- and y-axes, the lesion should be located and positioned in the center of the biopsy window. Keeping the lesion in the center of the biopsy window, especially along its x coordinate (horizontal axis), is paramount to prevent it from moving out of the field of vision in subsequent angled images (Carr et al. 2001).

After checking that the lesion is properly localized in the biopsy paddle window, a pair of images with $30°$ of separation between projections is obtained through the controlled movement of the X-ray tube, as described above.

The pair of angled images is readily displayed on the console monitor; after identifying the target lesion on both views, it is marked on each of the images, thereby allowing the calculation of the coordinates. Once the computer coordinates have been determined the information is transferred from the computer to the stereotactic system, and the biopsy needle is moved into place.

When the biopsy needle is inserted into the calculated coordinates, another pair of stereotactic images is obtained to document the needle position. Retargeting and repositioning may be performed, if necessary. In this case, it is generally not necessary to create another skin incision. When the new target has been selected and transmitted to the equipment, the simple retraction of the needle until the tip is just beneath the skin is sufficient; the needle can then be moved to the newly targeted position. The repositioning may also be performed by adjusting the x-, y-, and z-axes of the needle position manually (Huang et al. 2014).

As shown in Fig. 10, using VAB needle devices, which represent the standard of care for stereotactic biopsy, a pair of stereotactic images is usually obtained to check the correct needle position just proximally to the target lesion. The needle is then manually inserted through the lesion rather than fired, so traversing it. Firing the needle through the lesion may be helpful for needle directional control in dense breast tissue: the amount of the needle advancement is chosen by the operator according to several factors: in primis the thickness of the compressed breast. A pair of angled views is then obtained to check the optimal final needle aperture position related to the target lesion. If accurate targeting is confirmed tissue sampling may be started, performing a turn of $360°$ around the needle axis in the lesion and taking at least 12 tissue sample cores. Sometimes, depending on the lesion size, selective samplings may be sufficient and performed mainly at the clock positions where the lesion is located, as identified on the postfire images.

At the end of the sampling biopsy, to check for adequate removal of the target lesion, post-biopsy angled images are obtained.

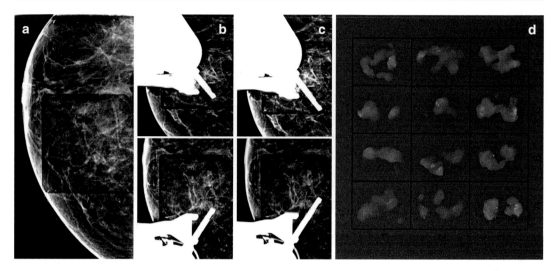

Fig. 10 Stereotactic guided vacuum-assisted biopsy: the position of the target lesion (in this case, grouped fine pleomorphic calcifications) within the biopsy window is checked by the acquisition of a digital scout mammogram (**a**). After inserting the biopsy needle, another pair of angulated views was obtained to document the needle position, respectively, in prefire (**b**) and postfire (**c**). The proper removal of adequate microcalcifications is documented by a radiography of the specimens (**d**)

When a second lesion needs to be biopsied, if it is included in the same biopsy window on both of the two angled views acquired for targeting the first lesion, the new mark can be directly placed on the second target lesion; otherwise, repositioning and new targeting will be required. After targeting, the new sampling can be started: the use of a new needle is mandatory to avoid the risk of tumor cell dissemination.

4.3.2 Digital Breast Tomosynthesis-Guided Biopsy

Using digital breast tomosynthesis (DBT) for guidance of non-palpable lesion biopsy, after the positioning of the patient and the breast compression, a DBT scout view is acquired. The reconstructed images are then displayed on the console monitor and the lesion location is determined by scrolling through the DBT thin sections. Indeed, depth information is provided without triangulation but only by placing a marker on the lesion in the appropriate DBT section. The selected section coincides with the depth (z-axis location) of the lesion inside the compressed breast. After targeting the lesion, the other coordinates (x and y) are easily determined and the information is sent to the biopsy unit.

The rest of the procedure is largely similar to the stereotactic one. As reported before (see Sect. 3.1), performing DBT-guided biopsy with a vertical approach, pre- and postfire control images should be obtained using standard mammography, acquiring a pair of angled stereotactic views for each step.

To check for the adequate removal of the target lesion at the end of sampling, unlike the two angled images necessary in the stereotactic mode, in DBT mode a single post-biopsy DBT image is acquired (Fig. 11).

Despite being introduced only recently, DBT-guided biopsy has shown to be a feasible and accurate method of obtaining a histologic sample of non-palpable breast abnormalities, offering several advantages compared to the stereotactic one.

The first obvious advantage is that lesions detectable by DBT only can be biopsied (Schrading et al. 2015; Freer et al. 2015). A second advantage is related to the possibility of localizing lesions without triangulation; this allows the one full detector size use for imaging, facilitating the identification of the target lesion and preventing the difficulties associated with the restricted imaging capabilities through the small biopsy window of conventional stereotactic

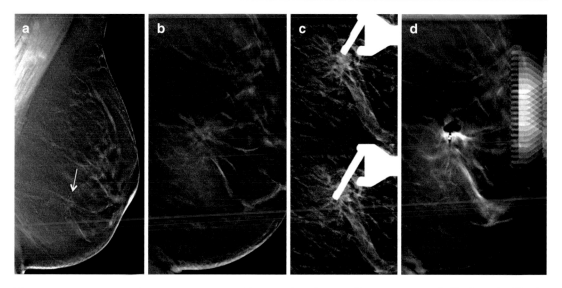

Fig. 11 Tomosynthesis-guided vacuum-assisted biopsy on a DBT-detected architectural distortion (arrow) (**a**): a DBT scout is firstly performed to reidentify the target lesion. The depth of the target lesions, which coincides with the z-axis, is determined by identifying the DBT section that yields the sharpest depiction of the target (**b**). After indicating the position of the target with a cursor, the other coordinates are automatically determined by the biopsy software system. A pair of pre- and postfire angulated views are then acquired to check the correct position of the needle (**c**). Finally a post-biopsy DBT image is acquired after releasing a marker clip to verify correct sampling (**d**)

systems. This is more significant for low-contrast lesions, such as noncalcified masses, architectural distortions, or asymmetric densities that can require multiple repositioning when working in stereotactic mode (Schrading et al. 2015).

Another benefit of using DBT as a guidance for biopsy comes with the inherent larger field of view: using both upright systems add-on to DBT devices and prone tables with tomosynthesis capability, the mammographic abnormality may be localized on a full-field detector (18 × 24 cm) versus the typical 5 × 5 cm biopsy window in the compression plate used for traditional biopsy systems. The larger field of view and the use of compression plates with larger biopsy window allow for sampling of more than one lesion without repositioning the patient even on lesions located at different depths, as long as they are placed inside the sampling window. As reported by Schrading et al., these technical advantages result in a significant reduction of time required for biopsy, both in terms of biopsy planning and total procedure execution, thereby improving patient care (Schrading et al. 2015).

4.4 Technical Limitations and Potential Remedies

Stereotactic biopsy, using both mammographic and DBT guidance, is limited when lesions are located deep inside and/or adjacent to the chest wall as well as for those lesions that are superficially located close to the skin.

For the lesions that are very deep and close to the chest wall, proper patient positioning is key to technical success. Using the prone biopsy table, to enable full access to these lesions, the patient's arm in addition to the targeted breast should be placed through the table aperture; this so-called arm-through-the-hole technique allows core biopsy or needle localization. Using this patient's position, it is also possible to biopsy lesions located in the axillary regions, which are usually difficult to reach (Soo et al. 1998).

To facilitate reaching these lesions using an upright biopsy system, a recumbent position of the patient (lying on one side) is mandatory; the detector should also be positioned at an oblique angle, to allow the compression paddle to be placed as close as possible up against the rib cage or sternum (O'Flynn et al. 2010).

For superficial lesions the greatest limitation is the difficulty in creating the vacuum in the probe, since the needle window comes out of the breast; as a result, the breast tissue cannot be sucked into and cut by the probe, which means the core sampling cannot be acquired. Moreover, during the sampling, the skin can be sucked and cut. To avoid these complications, the use of needles with a smaller biopsy aperture is recommended. Some probes are also complemented with plastic aperture sleeves that partially cover the probe aperture and prevent inadvertent skin sampling.

A last solution (but rarely adopted) may be the expansion of the subcutaneous tissue with an additional injection of local anesthetic or sterile saline to push the lesion deeper and away from the skin.

Another limitation of stereotactic biopsy is very small or thin breasts. However, several studies have reported that a biopsy might be successfully performed by adopting some precautions. Among these, in order to increase thickness, a first special maneuver is to position the breast so that more breast tissue gathers centrally and bulges through the biopsy rectangular aperture. If this is not sufficient, the use of the lateral approach (see Sect. 4.1), rather than the vertical one, is recommended; using this first approach, Myong et al. reported that biopsies were successful in breasts less than 3 cm thick, with a significant difference compared to the vertical approach, for which the mean breast thickness was 4 cm (Myong et al. 2013). Other studies have also reported that the lateral approach could be performed on thinner breasts of up to 1 cm of minimal breast thickness (Nakamura et al. 2010). In such cases, it may be necessary to increase the distance between the bottom of the breast and the mammography detector plate by placing a transparent spacer (usually made of plexiglass).

Despite the possible limitations using dedicated maneuvers and practical measures, most of the biopsies can be successfully performed, limiting surgery biopsy to only very few lesions.

4.5 Specimen Core Management

Specimen radiography should be performed to check for the presence of representative microcalcifications when biopsied lesions are purely microcalcifications rather than masses or distortions associated with calcifications. The samples are placed on a Petri dish or on a plexiglass plate and a magnification view is acquired using a mammography unit or other X-ray imaging systems, such as those specially designed for specimen imaging (see Fig. 10). The radiography of the specimens is done keeping the breast under the compression paddle, the needle inserted into the breast, and the biopsy system on standby, ready to perform additional samplings depending on the presence or absence of calcifications within the specimens.

The magnification view should be readily displayed on the console monitor, which must be of suitable quality. The time required for specimen radiographs should be as short as possible to ensure as much patient comfort as possible by limiting the time needed for the entire procedure.

To speed up biopsies, recently a new device, which allows for real-time imaging and instant verification of specimens, was introduced on the market: in contrast to the other biopsy devices, this one is equipped with an incorporated X-ray tube and a digital detector. During the sampling procedure, as every core is taken, it automatically travels through the biopsy needle and the plastic tube into a special cartridge. Once the sampling core arrives in the cartridge, it is X-rayed right away and the physician can quickly check the presence of microcalcifications, deciding whether to go further with the sampling or to stop.

The physician must ensure the presence of microcalcifications in at least three core specimens with, ideally, five calcifications per core, by performing a complete turn of the biopsy needle and obtaining at least 12 tissue samples. In case of small clusters of microcalcifications, it is recommended that the physician check a minimum 50% of the calcifications have been removed through a comparison between scout views, before and after the procedure (Wallis et al.

2007). Small lesions (e.g., less than 1 cm in size) may be completely removed (Bick et al. 2020).

A separation of calcified and noncalcified specimens, which may facilitate more focused interpretation from pathologists, is recommended: samples with calcifications and those without calcifications should be placed immediately into two separated formalin jars and sent to pathologists. Whenever possible, a radiological comment regarding the presence of representative microcalcification should be provided to the pathologist along with the specimen radiography image. In units using digital mammography, the pathologist must be able to view the core biopsy X-rays on a monitor of suitable quality.

For biopsy of noncalcified lesions, specimen radiographs are not required and samples, after being placed in a formalin fixative solution, may be sent directly to the laboratory.

5 Post-biopsy Measures

5.1 Clip Positioning

Once the specimen retrieval is completed, a localizing post-biopsy marker clip is placed at the biopsy site, which is then delivered into the biopsy cavity—depending on the biopsy system used—through the biopsy probe or the probe sheath. The first clips on the market, which were developed only for mammographic use, were all based on the basic design of a 2–3 mm metallic marker that was mainly either titanium or stainless steel. Over time, manufacturers have developed clip markers visible by ultrasound; these markers contain, in addition to the metallic radiopaque steel clip, an embedding material consisting of the collagen of bovine origin, polylactic acid, polyglycolic acid or starch pellets, and hydrogel. The embedding material offers some advantages: it fills the biopsy cavity, decreasing the risk of clip displacement and providing hemostatic effect through a direct pressure against the biopsy cavity walls. In addition, collagen activates the coagulation cascade and promotes platelet adhesion, aggregation, and activation, furthering hemostasis. One of the benefits in

using these kinds of markers is that, in the weeks following deployment, most embedding substances are easily identified by ultrasound allowing ultrasound-guided localization up to 6–8 weeks after the procedure (Thomassin-Naggara et al. 2012).

The marker clip positioning is helpful in various situations. For example, it facilitates accurate wire localization to guide excision in case of surgery. Moreover, when the mammographic monitoring of the biopsied area is sufficient, the clip placement facilitates future follow-up especially when most, if not all, of the target lesion has been removed by the biopsy procedure. It follows that the localization clip should be placed as close as possible to the biopsy site.

5.2 Post-biopsy Mammography

To ensure that the clip is correctly deployed, an image of the biopsied area is usually obtained when the breast is still under compression. This scout view will be acquired by standard mammography or DBT, depending on the guidance system used for biopsy. Then, because clip migration has been reported in up to 20% of cases (Chaveron et al. 2009; Yen et al. 2018), before preoperative wire localization, two-view mammography (including a craniocaudal and a mediolateral or lateromedial view) should be performed to assess its final position (Fig. 12). In case of DBT-guided biopsy, DBT post-procedure views are required.

It is recommended that these additional projections are not immediately acquired after the breast is released from the biopsy unit because repeated compressions and decompressions of the breast could contribute to clip migration. This kind of dislocation has been described by Thomassin-Naggara et al. as the "accordion effect" (Thomassin-Naggara et al. 2012), and it happens where structures that are not normally located adjacent to each other are brought closer in the compressed state. When the clip is deployed in this state, it may attach onto structures that are not at the biopsied site, and when the breast is released from compression, the clip will stay

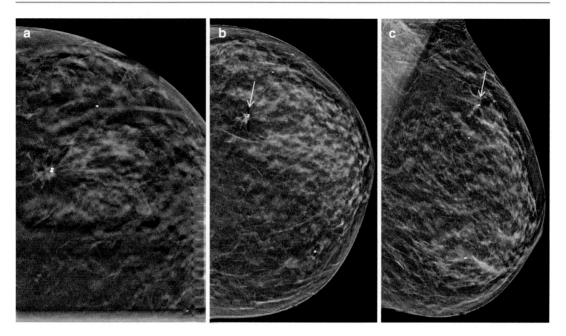

Fig. 12 (**a**) A DBT post-biopsy image acquired at the end of the sampling on an architectural distortion detected by tomosynthesis, and before releasing the breast compression. To check that the marker clip is still in the site of the biopsy (arrows), after decompression one craniocaudal (**b**) and one mediolateral (**c**) view is acquired

with the structure and be observed at a site distant from the biopsy cavity.

Other causes of clip displacement are migration within fatty tissue and/or post-procedure bleeding or hematoma formation.

Clip migration should be documented in the biopsy report.

5.3 Patient Care and Follow-Up

When the procedure is successfully completed and the needle is removed from the breast, manual compression of the biopsy site ensures adequate hemostasis. If persistent bleeding is noted immediately after the removal of the needle, it is helpful to keep the breast under the compression paddle, adding focal compression at the biopsy site. Continued bleeding after ten minutes of manual compression is considered prolonged bleeding and surgical evaluation can be helpful.

After hemostasis is achieved, the skin incision is closed, generally with thin adhesive strips; as the skin incision is a few millimeters, it is rarely necessary to close the skin with sutures. To ensure continued hemostasis a further compression may also be applied using an adhesive plaster. It is also helpful to place an ice pack at the biopsy site (O'Flynn et al. 2010).

As described above (see Sect. 5.2), to document the position of the clip marker, a few days after the sampling procedure, patients usually have a two-view mammography or tomosynthesis of the biopsied breast. For all patients, a clinical evaluation is also recommended to check possible complications such as hematomas or infections. There is little literature regarding infections following needle biopsy; the available data reported severe complications in less than 1% of all biopsies and need for antibiotic treatment in only 0.15% (Bruening et al. 2010).

5.4 Pathological Result Management and Indications for Treatment

The diagnostic accuracy of breast lesions depends on the correlation of clinical findings, imaging features, and pathology results.

While radiologists can discharge most patients with benign lesions, there are cases in which a re-evaluation is necessary to decide the next correct diagnostic and/or therapeutic proceedings.

When there is radiological-pathological discordance, a direct consultation with the pathologist is mandatory. For example, when the assessed lesions are microcalcifications and they are not described in the pathologist's report, the radiologist should request an additional evaluation of the tissue blocks (Huang et al. 2014); at the same time, a comparison between the mammograms of the samples and those carried out at the end of the biopsy should also be made to confirm the correct excision of microcalcifications during stereotactic or DBT-guided biopsy (O'Flynn et al. 2010). In case of lasting radiologic-pathologic discordance, re-biopsy or surgical excision is recommended, depending on the degree of the radiologist's suspicion.

A pathological diagnosis of lesions with uncertain malignant potential, such as the so-called B3 lesions including atypical ductal hyperplasia, flat epithelial atypia, classical lobular neoplasia, papillary lesions, benign phyllodes tumors, and radial scars, will require additional interventions. Because the evidence base for appropriate management of these B3 lesions is still limited and practice varies greatly from country to country, for these lesions a multidisciplinary team approach, including pathologists, radiologists, and surgeons, is required to form an individualized treatment plan (Huang et al. 2014; Rageth et al. 2016). A multidisciplinary approach to treatment is also mandatory for all the malignant lesions diagnosed by stereotactic or tomosynthesis-guided biopsies.

A final report, to share with the patient and the referring physician, should be issued describing radiologic-pathologic concordance or discordance, along with the final recommendation such as imaging follow-up and the need for a repeat biopsy rather than a surgical biopsy.

In case the patient does not have surgery, a mammography follow-up could be necessary. In the evaluation of the subsequent mammograms, it should be considered that scars may appear; scar formation has been reported with rates between 2% and 10%, depending on both the number of the excised cores and the needle used for biopsy (O'Flynn et al. 2010; Yazici et al. 2006; Zagouri et al. 2008).

5.5 Presurgical Localization

For patients with a biopsy-proven cancer and for those with a histologic diagnosis of high-risk lesion, surgical excision is indicated. A surgical biopsy is also required when the core needle biopsy fails to provide a definitive histological diagnosis (after potential re-biopsy) and in case of imaging pathological discordance. A last indication for surgery is the presence of non-palpable lesions considered suspicious and for which stereotactic and/or tomosynthesis-guided biopsy is technically not possible. In all these cases, presurgical localization is needed to enable intraoperative lesion localization and excision.

Among the different available methods, wire-guided localization (WGL) is considered the current gold standard. WGL consists of inserting—by stereotactic guidance—a hook wire into the lesion that needs surgery (Fig. 13). The targeting procedure is similar to the one used for stereotactic or DBT-guided biopsies. Using stereotactic guidance, the lesion depth is established through the acquisition of a scout view first and a pair of angled views later; however, when tomosynthesis is used, the acquisition of a DBT scout is enough to define the correct position of the lesion. Once this is satisfactory, the needle is inserted and, after a last radiological check to confirm that the needle tip is correctly located, the wire is advanced so that the hook anchors into the tissue. The needle is lastly withdrawn, leaving the wire in place. Finally a pair of orthogonal mammograms is performed to confirm that the wire tip is located ideally in or within 5 mm of the lesion. Although the wire-guided technique is a relatively simple and cost-effective, successful, and safe method for non-palpable breast lesion localization (Riedl et al. 2005), some disadvantages have been reported, such as wire rupture or migration, pneumothorax, or aesthetic complications (Kopans 1988). Furthermore, because the

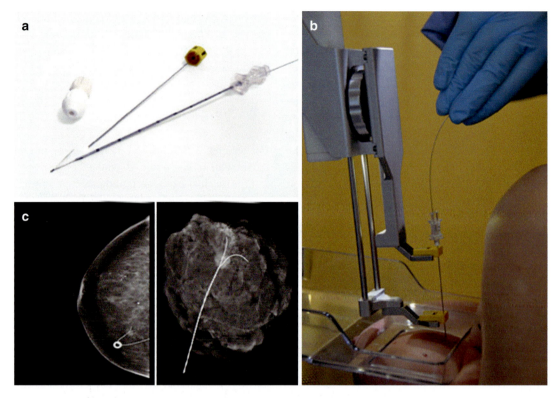

Fig. 13 Example of presurgical localization using a hook-wire (**a**). Using stereotactic or DBT guide, a wire is inserted into the breast, reaching the correct position of the non-palpable lesion; mammographic pictures are taken to check the needle position, adjusting it if required. Once the needle is in the correct position, a fine hook-wire is passed down the center of the needle and then the needle is removed, leaving the wire in place (**b**). A final mammogram is performed to show the surgeon where the tip of the wire lies in relation to the lesion that is to be removed; finally, a specimen radiography confirms the correct removal of the target lesion (**c**)

wire exits the patient's skin—to reduce the risk of hook-wire displacement—it is preferrable to perform the localization the same day of the scheduled surgery. This can create logistical challenges, limiting operating room efficiency.

Carbon-marking localization can be used as an alternative to the wire-guided technique in overcoming the abovementioned challenges. This localization method is based on the injection of sterile charcoal powder diluted with saline solution into the lesion that needs to be surgically removed. A charcoal trail is created from the lesion to the superficial layers of the breast, leaving a tattoo on the skin (Fig. 14). The subsequent surgical excision of the tumor is guided by the presence of the carbon suspension, which is removed with the lesion. Because of the stability of the charcoal powder, a delayed surgical intervention after the localization procedure is possible. A potential disadvantage of carbon marking is the possible obstruction of the needle tip during the injection due to precipitation of charcoal particles; moreover, in some cases, foreign-body giant-cell reactions mimicking malignancy have been reported after carbon marking (Ruiz-Delgado et al. 2008).

Both wire and carbon localization techniques are widely used as diagnostic and therapeutic tools, with their respective limitations as discussed above.

Other localization methods, developed over the years, have been able to overcome these limitations. Among them, radio-guided occult lesion localization (ROLL) described in 1999 by Luini et al. consists of a preoperative injection of particles of colloidal human serum albumin labeled

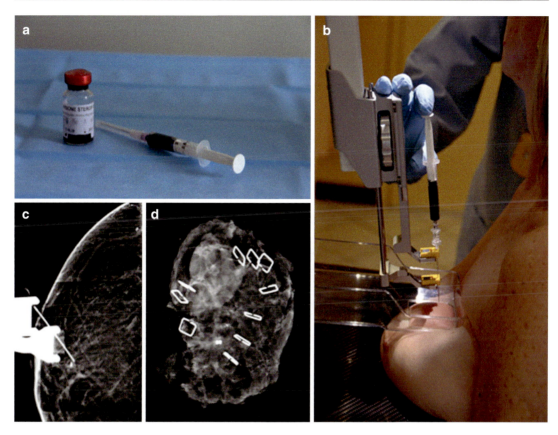

Fig. 14 (**a**) An aqueous suspension of carbon particles, (**b**) using a stereotactic or a DBT guide, is injected through a spinal needle (**c**). This trail gives precise guidance from the skin to the site of the lesion, facilitating the removal of a minimum volume of tissue (**d**). Dissection proceeds from the skin tattoo along the track towards the end of the charcoal trail; the latter represents the center of the lesion which is removed with adequate margins

with radioactive technetium (99mTc) into the tumor (Luini et al. 1999). The injection of isotope, such as that of charcoal, is done using the same modality described for wire localization. A scintigraphy scan of the breast is then obtained to check the correct inoculation of the tracer by comparison between its position and the localization of the lesion on mammograms. During the surgery, a gamma probe, directly used by the surgeon to verify the adequacy of excision, can detect the tumor. The ROLL technique, which requires careful communication and close collaboration among radiologists, nuclear medicine specialists, and surgeons, has proved to be highly effective in the preoperative and intraoperative localization of non-palpable breast lesions ensuring a reduction in the technical limitations of the two methods described before. The most significant potential complication of this procedure is the widespread dispersal of the isotope by accidental intraductal injection, which may cause a failure in identification of the lesion (Rampaul et al. 2003). Another concern with ROLL, which may limit its introduction, regards its cost: Medina-Franco et al. reported histological diagnosis at a total cost of $209 (USD) per procedure compared to $132 (USD) for wire-guided excision (Medina-Franco et al. 2007).

Other localization methods have been developed in the search for the most effective method in obtaining clear margins; to date, no single technique has proved to be better among the various ones described, because all of them have some advantages and disadvantages. In light of these results, each surgeon should adopt his/her most suitable localization or margin assessment technique, based on the team experience and on available skills and technologies.

5.6 Specimen Radiography

When non-palpable lesions are surgically removed, intraoperative specimen radiography is mandatory for the evaluation of the complete removal. According to the radiologist's indications, the surgeon should decide whether to complete the operation or extend the resection.

To ensure the correct evaluation of the specimen, the acquisition of two orthogonal radiograms is recommended. The greatest benefit provided by orthogonal specimen radiography, indeed, is in defining whether the lesion is located at the edge of the specimen or rather in the center with a respective safety margin; in such case, the surgery enlargement of the involved margin should be carried out. However, the diagnostic value of specimen radiography during breast-conservative surgery remains unclear. Multiple studies have evaluated the accuracy of specimen

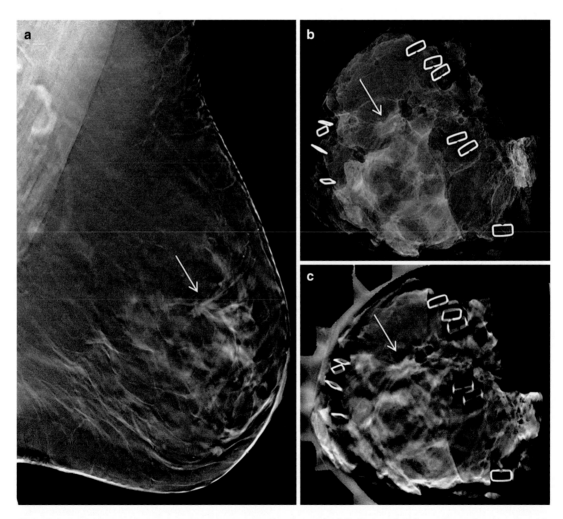

Fig. 15 (**a**) Mediolateral digital breast tomosynthesis demonstrating an architectural distortion (arrow) in the left upper quadrants (**a**). The distortion lesion is difficult to identify in the digital mammogram of the specimen (**b**). The DBT spot compression of the specimen shows clearly the excised lesion marked by a charcoal suspension (**c**). The surgeon has marked the specimen for orientation with one clip on the anterior surface of the specimen, two clips at the margin closest to the nipple, three clips at the superior margin, and four clips on the posterior margin

radiography in predicting margin involvement showing for conservative breast treatment (excluding surgical biopsies) sensitivity values variable between 27% and 76% (Rua et al. 2012; Versteegden et al. 2017). Such heterogeneity can be partly attributed to the different techniques adopted (such as digital vs. analogue imaging, and use of magnification) and partly to the type of intraoperative equipment employed. DBT is a promising modality in performing specimen analysis. As reported in recent publications, DBT significantly increases both the accuracy of specimen radiography, regarding identification of the closest margin, and the sensitivity, regarding margin status assessment compared to standard mammography (Urano et al. 2016; Amer et al. 2017). This results in a potential decrease in the number of second surgeries, especially in patients with invasive carcinomas.

It follows that specimen radiography by DBT, which is obviously recommended in the management of all the lesions detectable only by tomosynthesis (Fig.15), is also indicated for other lesions such as distortions, focal asymmetries, or small masses detectable by standard digital mammography. Urano et el. reported that DBT, reducing the influence of overlapping dense breast tissue, is superior to digital mammography in depicting and delineating entire lesions and their contours (Urano et al. 2016).

6   Summary

Stereotactic guided percutaneous needle biopsy represents a fundamental technique to characterize the nature of non-palpable suspicious mammographic abnormalities (i.e., calcifications, asymmetries, architectural distortion, and some masses). Over the years, this technique has constantly been improving: first new biopsy systems were introduced (passing from FNAC to CNB and finally to VAB), and then the stereotactic modality for biopsy guidance was joined by DBT. Stereotactic and DBT-guided percutaneous needle biopsy has replaced almost completely surgical biopsy and, to date, imaging plays a pivotal role not only in the early detec-

tion and diagnosis but also in the management of these non-palpable lesions. The choice of both the imaging modality for biopsy guidance (STX or DBT) and the sample system to use (CNB or VAB, limiting the use of FNAC to a few selected cases) depends on the equipment availability, expertise of the radiologist, lesion characteristics, and patient profile. Biopsies need to be carefully planned, thereby also considering potential side effects like bruising, bleeding, and mild pain. Serious side effects are very rare. After the biopsy, radiologic-pathologic correlation is crucial for an accurate and successful conclusion of the diagnostic procedure. In case of non-palpable lesions with indication to surgery for both diagnostic and therapeutic purposes, preoperative localization is recommended and available through ultrasound, mammography, or DBT.

References

Amer HA, Schmitzberger F, Ingold-Heppner B et al (2017) Digital breast tomosynthesis versus full field digital mammography-which modality provides more accurate prediction of margin status in specimen radiography? Eur J Radiol 93:258–264. https://doi.org/10.1016/j.ejrad.2017.05.041

Bick U, Trimboli RM, Athanasiou A, et al, for the European Society of Breast Imaging (EUSOBI), with language review by Europa Donna - The European Breast Cancer Coalition (2020) Image-guided breast biopsy and localisation: recommendations for information to women and referring physicians by the European Society of Breast Imaging. Insights Imaging 11:12. https://doi.org/10.1186/s13244-019-0803-x

Bolmgren J, Jacobson B, Nordenstrom B (1977) Stereotaxic instrument for needle biopsy of the mamma. AJR Am J Roentgenol 129(1):121–125

Bruening W, Fontanarosa J, Tipton K et al (2010) Systematic review: comparative effectiveness of core-needle and open surgical biopsy to diagnose breast lesions. Ann Intern Med 152:238–246. https://doi.org/10.1059/0003-4819-152-1-201001050-00190

Byun J, Lee JE, Cha ES et al (2017) Visualization of breast microcalcifications on digital breast tomosynthesis and 2-dimensional digital mammography using specimens. Breast Cancer (Auckl) 11:1178223417703388. https://doi.org/10.1177/1178223417703388. eCollection 2017

Carr JJ, Hemler PF, Halford PW et al (2001) Stereotactic localization of breast lesions: how it works and methods to improve accuracy. Radiographics 21(2):463–473

Chaveron C, Bachelle F, Fauquet I et al (2009) Clip migration after stereotactic macrobiopsy and presurgical localization: technical considerations and tricks. J Radiol 90(1 Pt 1):31–36

D'Orsi CJ, Sickles ES, Mendelson EB et al (2013) Mammography lexicon classification form. In: ACR BI-RADS® Atlas, Breast Imaging Reporting and Data System, 5th edn. Committee on BI-RADS® American College of Radiology, Reston, VA, pp 143–147

Fine RE, Bloom KJ (2009) Imaged-guided breast biopsy. In: Evans SRT (ed) Surgical pitfalls: prevention and management. Saunders Elsevier, Philadelphia, pp 433–442

Freer PE, Niell B, Rafferty EA (2015) Preoperative tomosynthesis-guided needle localization of mammographically and sonographically occult breast lesions. Radiology 275(2):377–383. https://doi.org/10.1148/radiol.14140515

Houssami N, Lång K, Bernardi D et al (2016) Digital breast tomosynthesis (3D-mammography) screening: a pictorial review of screen-detected cancers and false recalls attributed to tomosynthesis in prospective screening trials. Breast 26:119–134. https://doi.org/10.1016/j.breast.2016.01.007

Huang ML, Adrada BE, Candelaria R et al (2014) Stereotactic breast biopsy: pitfalls and pearls. Tech Vasc Interv Radiol 17(1):32–39. https://doi.org/10.1053/j.tvir.2013.12.006

Kopans DB (1988) Migration of breast biopsy localization wire. AJR Am J Roentgenol 151(3):614–615

Kulkarni T, O'Connor A (2015) Breast biopsy in patients on anti-coagulants: is new guidance needed? Breast Cancer Res 17(Suppl 1):P33. https://doi.org/10.1186/bcr3795

Lomoschitz FM, Helbich TH, Rudas M et al (2004) Stereotactic 11-gauge vacuum assisted breast biopsy: influence of number of specimens on diagnostic accuracy. Radiology 232(3):897–903. https://doi.org/10.1148/radiol.2323031224

Luini A, Zurrida S, Paganelli G et al (1999) Comparison of radioguided excision with wire localization of occult breast lesions. Br J Surg 86:522–525

Maxwell AJ, Ridley NT, Rubin G, et al Royal College of Radiologists Breast Group (2009) The Royal College of Radiologists Breast Group breast imaging classification. Clin Radiol 64(6):624–627. https://doi.org/10.1016/j.crad.2009.01.010

Medina-Franco H, Abarca-Pérez L, Ulloa-Gómez JL et al (2007) Radioguided localization of clinically occult breast lesions (ROLL): a pilot study. Breast J 13(4):401–405

Myong JH, Kang BJ, Yoon SK et al (2013) The clinical utility of a adding lateral approach to conventional vertical approach for prone stereotactic vacuum-assisted breast biopsy. Korean J Radiol 14(4):568–575

Nakamura Y, Urashima M, Matsuura A et al (2010) Stereotactic directional vacuum-assisted breast biopsy using lateral approach. Breast Cancer 17:286–289

O'Flynn EAM, Wilson ARM, Michell M (2010) Image-guided breast biopsy: state-of-the-art. Clin Radiol 65(4):259–270. https://doi.org/10.1016/j.crad.2010.01.008

Ohsumi S, Taira N, Takabatake D et al (2014) Breast biopsy for mammographically detected nonpalpable lesions using a vacuum-assisted biopsy device (Mammotome) and upright-type stereotactic mammography unit without a digital imaging system: experience of 500 biopsies. Breast Cancer 21(2):123–127. https://doi.org/10.1007/s12282-012-0360-3

Pfarl G, Helbich TH, Riedl CC et al (2002) Stereotactic needle breast biopsy: diagnostic reliability of various biopsy systems and needle sizes. Rofo 174(5):614–619

Preibsch H, Baur A, Wietek BM et al (2014) Vacuum-assisted breast biopsy with 7-gauge, 8-gauge, 9-gauge, 10-gauge, and 11-gauge needles: how many specimens are necessary? Acta Radiol 56(9):1078–1084. https://doi.org/10.1177/0284185114549224

Rageth CJ, O'Flynn EA, Comstock C et al (2016) First International Consensus Conference on lesions of uncertain malignant potential in the breast (B3 lesions). Breast Cancer Res Treat 59(2):203–213. https://doi.org/10.1007/s10549-016-3935-4

Rampaul RS, MacMillan RD, Evans AJ (2003) Intraductal injection of the breast: a potential pitfall radioisotope occult lesion localization. Br J Radiol 76(906):425–426

Riedl CC, Pfari G, Memarsadeghi M et al (2005) Lesion miss rates and false-negative rates for 1115 consecutive cases of stereotactically guided needle-localized open breast biopsy with long-term follow-up. Radiology 237(3):847–853. https://doi.org/10.1148/radiol.2373041391. Epub 2005 Oct 19

Rua C, Lebas P, Michenet P et al (2012) Evaluation of lumpectomy surgical specimen radiographs in subclinical, in situ and invasive breast cancer, and factors predicting positive margins. Diagn Interv Imaging 93(11):871–877. https://doi.org/10.1016/j.diii.2012.07.010

Ruiz-Delgado ML, Lòpez-Ruiz JA, Sàiz-Lòpez A (2008) Abnormal mammography and sonography associated with foreign-body giant-cell reaction after stereotactic vacuum-assisted breast biopsy with carbon marking. Acta Radiol 49(10):1112–1118

Sanderink WBG, Mann RM (2017) Advances in breast intervention: where are we now and where should we be? Clin Radiol. pii: S0009-9260(17)30513-5. https://doi.org/10.1016/j.crad.2017.10.018

Schrading S, Distelmaier M, Dirrichs T et al (2015) Digital breast tomosynthesis-guided vacuum-assisted breast biopsy: initial experiences and comparison with prone stereotactic vacuum-assisted biopsy.

Radiology 274(3):654–662. https://doi.org/10.1148/radiol.14141397

Sim LS, Kei PL (2008) Upright stereotactic vacuum-assisted needle biopsy of suspicious breast microcalcifications. J Med Imaging Radiat Oncol 52(4):358–364

Soo MS, Walsh R, Patton J (1998) Prone table stereotactic breast biopsy: facilitating biopsy of posterior lesions using the arm-through-the-hole technique. AJR Am J Roentgenol 171(3):615–617

Tagliafico A, Gristina L, Bignotti B et al (2015) Effects on short-term quality of life of vacuum-assisted breast biopsy: comparison between digital breast tomosynthesis and digital mammography. Br J Radiol 88(1056):20150593. https://doi.org/10.1259/bjr.20150593

The National Breast Cancer Centre (NBCC) (2007) Synoptic breast imaging report. https://canceraustralia.gov.au/publications-and-resources/cancer-australia-publications/synoptic-breast-imaging-report-update. Accessed 6 Apr 2018

Thomassin-Naggara I, Lalonde L, David J et al (2012) A plea for the biopsy marker: how, why and why not clipping after breast biopsy? Breast Cancer Res Treat 132(3):881–893. https://doi.org/10.1007/s10549-011-1847-x

Urano M, Shiraki N, Kawai T et al (2016) Digital mammography versus digital breast tomosynthesis for detection of breast cancer in the intraoperative specimen during breast-conserving surgery. Breast Cancer 23(5):706–711. https://doi.org/10.1007/s12282-015-0628-5

Venkataraman S, Dialani V, Gilmore HL et al (2012) Stereotactic core biopsy: comparison of 11 gauge with 8 gauge vacuum assisted breast biopsy. Eur J Radiol 81:2613–2619

Versteegden DPA, Keizer LGG, Schlooz MS et al (2017) Performance characteristics of specimen radiography for margin assessment for ductal carcinoma in situ: a systematic review. Breast Cancer Res Treat 166:669–679. https://doi.org/10.1007/s10549-017-4475-2

Wallis M, Tardivon A, Helbich T et al (2007) European Society of Breast Imaging, Guidelines from the European Society of Breast Imaging for diagnostic interventional breast procedures. Eur Radiol 17(2):581–588

Wang M, He X, Chang Y et al (2017) A sensitivity and specificity comparison of fine needle aspiration cytology and core needle biopsy in evaluation of suspicious breast lesions: a systematic review and meta-analysis. Breast 31:157–166. https://doi.org/10.1016/j.breast.2016.11.009

Welle GJ, Clark ML (1997) Adaptation of an add-on stereotaxic breast biopsy unit: use of a dedicated reclinable mammography chair. AJR Am J Roentgenol 169:1391–1393

Welle GJ, Clark M, Loos S et al (2000) Stereotactic breast biopsy: recumbent biopsy using add-on upright equipment. AJR Am J Roentgenol 175:59–63

Yazici B, Sever AR, Mills P et al (2006) Scar formation after stereotactic vacuum-assisted core biopsy of benign breast lesions. Clin Radiol 61:619–624

Yen P, Dumas S, Albert A et al (2018) Post-vacuum-assisted stereotactic core biopsy clip displacement: a comparison between commercially available clips and surgical clip. Can Assoc Radiol J 69(1):10–15. https://doi.org/10.1016/j.carj.2017.08.004

Yu YH, Liang C, Yuan XZ (2010) Diagnostic value of vacuum-assisted breast biopsy for breast carcinoma: a meta-analysis and systematic review. Breast Cancer Res Treat 120(2):469–479. https://doi.org/10.1007/s10549-010-0750-1

Zagouri F, Sergentanis TN, Kouloucheri D et al (2008) Vacuum-assisted breast biopsy: more cores, more scars? Clin Radiol 63:736–738

How to Use Breast Ultrasound

Boris Brkljačić, Gordana Ivanac,
Michael Fuchsjäger, and Gabriel Adelsmayr

Contents

1 Introduction 96

2 Equipment and Examination Technique 96

3 Sonographic Anatomy of the Normal Breast 98

4 Types of Breast Lesions and Their Sonographic Features as per the ACR BI-RADS Atlas 99
    4.1   BI-RADS Final Assessment Categories 102

5 Sonographic Features of Benign Breast Lesions 103

6 Sonographic Features of Breast Lesions 106

7 Sonographic Features of Malignant Breast Lesions 106

8 Further Ultrasound Applications: After Treatment, Screening, Intervention 108

9 Summary 110

References 110

B. Brkljačić (✉) · G. Ivanac
Department of Diagnostic and Interventional
Radiology, University Hospital "Dubrava",
Zagreb, Croatia

University of Zagreb School of Medicine,
Zagreb, Croatia
e-mail: boris@brkljacic.com; boris.brkljacic@mef.hr

M. Fuchsjäger · G. Adelsmayr
Division of General Radiology, Department of
Radiology, Medical University of Graz, Graz, Austria
e-mail: michael.fuchsjaeger@medunigraz.at

Abstract

Ultrasound technology has evolved remarkably over the last decades. High-resolution ultrasound enables the evaluation of breast lesions in great detail and provides excellent guidance modality for aspirations, biopsies, preoperative localization, and clip placements. A novel and promising field of use of breast ultrasound is minimally invasive therapeutic procedures (see Chapter "Minimal Invasive

© Springer Nature Switzerland AG 2022
M. Fuchsjäger et al. (eds.), *Breast Imaging*, Medical Radiology Diagnostic Imaging,
https://doi.org/10.1007/978-3-030-94918-1_5

Therapy"). Ultrasound is indicated as a primary imaging modality in young women; it is used as an adjunct to mammography to evaluate mammographically detected lesions, palpable abnormalities, and other breast symptoms, and after breast MRI as a targeted second-look examination. Furthermore, it is also used for the evaluation of the axilla. Grayscale or B-mode imaging is the most important ultrasound modality to evaluate breast lesions, but spatial compound imaging, harmonic imaging, color and power Doppler, 3D ultrasound, as well as sonoelastography and recently automated whole-breast ultrasound are routinely used. In this chapter, the technique of handheld ultrasound examinations of the breast and its normal sonographic morphology are dealt with; sonographic examples of the most common benign and malignant breast lesions are demonstrated.

1   Introduction

Current ultrasound (US) technology that uses high-frequency, high-resolution transducers enables visualization and highly accurate evaluation of the breast and breast lesions (Kremkau 2011; Stafford and Whitman 2011). Patients tolerate US examinations very well, and the technique is completely harmless for patients and staff, as there is no exposure to radiation. It is furthermore widely accessible and cheap and can be repeated whenever indicated (Brkljačić and Ivanac 2014). Due to all these advantages, the utilization of ultrasound has increased over the decades, and ultrasound is now an established modality for breast imaging. As a real-time, dynamic modality, ultrasound is very suitable for the guidance of fine needle aspirations, biopsies, and other interventional or minimally invasive procedures (Brkljačić and Ivanac 2014). Color Doppler is routinely used for the evaluation of lesion vascularization. There are many advanced techniques currently used, like 3D US, sonoelas-

Table 1 Indications for breast ultrasound

• Palpable lumps and other signs or symptoms
• Evaluations of suspicious lesion (at MX or MRI)
• Dense breast parenchyma (composition C or D)
• Screening of women at elevated risk for breast cancer
• Initial evaluation in young women or children
• Preoperative staging
• Axillary lymph nodes
• Occult primary cancer
• Targeted ultrasound after positive MRI examination
• Ultrasound guidance for interventions (FNA, biopsy, preoperative hook wire localization, minimally invasive therapy)

tography, and automated whole-breast ultrasound that will be dealt with in other chapters (Chapters "Breast Ultrasound: Advanced Techniques" and "Automated Breast Ultrasound"). In order to perform state-of-the-art breast ultrasound examinations, it is mandatory to select the proper equipment and transducer, to use the appropriate imaging technique, and to understand normal sonographic breast anatomy, as well as the sonographic features of benign and malignant breast lesions (Tables 1, 2, and 3).

2   Equipment and Examination Technique

It is reasonable and advisable to use the best scanners with the best transducers for breast ultrasound imaging. According to the American College of Radiology, the Royal College of Radiology, and the European Society of Breast Imaging, 10 MHz is the minimum frequency for a linear transducer used for breast imaging. High-frequency linear transducers today may well have a range up to 18 MHz. Resolution is better with higher frequencies, but consequently penetration of the sound beam decreases. The selection of optimal frequencies for specific parts of the breasts should be tailored individually, according to the position of the lesion and the breast size. Usual transducer apertures have a

Table 2 Ultrasound features for breast masses according to the "ACR BI-RADS atlas"

Shape	
	Round
	Oval
	Irregular
Margins	
	Circumscribed
	Non-circumscribed (indistinct, angular, microlobulated, spiculated)
Orientation	
	Parallel (wider than tall)
	Not parallel (taller than wide)
Echo pattern	
	Anechoic
	Hypoechoic
	Isoechoic
	Hyperechoic
	Heterogeneous
	Complex
Posterior features	
	None
	Enhancement
	Shadowing
	Combined
Associated features	
	Architectural distortion
	Skin changes
	Elasticity
	Duct changes
	Edema
	Vascularity

Table 3 Special cases according to the "ACR BI-RADS atlas" (= unique sonographic diagnosis or findings)

Simple cysts
Clustered microcysts
Masses in or on skin
Foreign bodies including implants
Intramammary and axillary lymph nodes
Vascular abnormalities (arteriovenous malformations/ pseudoaneurysms, Mondor's disease)
Postsurgical fluid collections
Fat necrosis

width of 4.5–6.5 cm, but wider transducers are also available on the market (Kremkau 2011).

Grayscale or brightness (B)-mode sonographic features are the basis for the interpretation of breast lesions, but current US systems routinely use compound and harmonic imaging, color and power Doppler, and strain or shear wave sonoelastography (Brkljačić and Ivanac 2014). Compound imaging is excellent for the evaluation of echotexture of breast lesions, since it uses multiple images obtained from different angles of insonation within the plane of imaging to create the final image. Harmonic imaging improves resolution further using harmonic frequencies to generate the image, while the original fundamental tissue echo frequencies are suppressed by phase inversion between two consecutive transmit pulses (Kremkau 2011; Stafford and Whitman 2011; Athanasiou et al. 2009). Vascularization of breast lesions can be evaluated by color and power Doppler using high Doppler frequencies (7 MHz or more) to visualize vessels within the lesions and to differentiate benign and malignant patterns; however, grayscale morphology is much more important than Doppler in the differentiation of benign and malignant breast lesions (Kremkau 2011; Stafford and Whitman 2011; Brkljačić and Ivanac 2014).

Ultrasound is considerably more operator dependent than other imaging methods, interobserver variability is high, and manual skills and experience are important factors in sonographic examination of the breast. Optimization of the examination technique is crucial, and all breast tissues have to be meticulously examined, in order to secure full detection. Examination should be performed both in the supine position of the patient and in the lateral oblique position, always with arms extended over the head. The latter position is optimal for the examination of outer breast quadrants, assuring that for the right breast the patient is placed to the left lateral oblique position (left flank), and for the examination of the left breast to the right lateral oblique position. In some cases, the examination may also be performed in sitting patient position. Extension of the arms over the head flattens breast tissue over the chest wall. Scanning can be performed using the radial technique, following radial and antiradial planes, centering the transducer at the nipple, and then stretching outwards, following breast lobes as per anatomy. Alternatively, scanning can be performed in parallel parasagittal planes, from top to the bottom, from lateral to medial and backwards (Kremkau 2011; Stafford and Whitman 2011; Brkljačić and Ivanac 2014; Athanasiou et al. 2009; Brkljačić et al. 2010). All detected lesions need to be visualized in at least two orthogonal planes. As per ACR guideline, even in the normal breast, it is recommended to document the axilla with at least one image.

One should take care to precisely focus the sound beam at the exact depth of the breast lesion, using electronic focusing. Tissue compression by the transducer should be uniform, to avoid scattering and absorption. Time-gain compensation is used to achieve homogeneous brightness and image intensity at different breast tissue depths. The gain settings are adjusted according to the echogenicity of the fatty tissue. Ultrasound is a real-time technique, and lesions can be dynamically examined regarding their mobility and delineation to neighboring tissues (Kremkau 2011; Stafford and Whitman 2011). The real-time nature of ultrasound is particularly important for performing ultrasound-guided fine needle aspirations and core or vacuum-assisted needle biopsies, because the needles' path through the parenchyma to the lesion can be constantly monitored and modified on the screen in real time, so that optimal positioning is achieved to obtain adequate specimens. The same applies for preoperative wire localization, clip placements, and minimally invasive procedures, like radiofrequency or cryoablations, that are performed under ultrasound guidance (Brkljačić et al. 2010).

3 Sonographic Anatomy of the Normal Breast

The adult female breast is composed of parenchyma, milk ducts, and fatty and connective tissue; the sonographic anatomy of the breast reflects its histologic composition. Detailed knowledge of normal sonographic anatomy is crucial to recognize pathologic changes. Breast cancers originate within the ductal epithelium (glandular tissue), including the accessory mammary tissue. Glandular tissue is predominant in the upper outer portion of the breast where approximately half of breast cancers originate; hence, this is the area that has to be examined meticulously by ultrasound. Glandular parenchyma is surrounded by fatty tissue and is supported by connective tissue or Cooper's ligaments inserting into the skin and prepectoral fascia, visualized by ultrasound. The breast consists of 15–20 lobes, arranged centripetally around the nipple. Ultrasound is the best imaging modality for depicting lobar breast anatomy and to evaluate cancer spread within the lobe. Individual lobes are organized around a lactiferous duct, and they converge into larger collecting ducts that open at the nipple. Lymph from the breast drains predominantly into the axillary lymph nodes, while lymph from the lower inner quadrants drains into internal mammary lymph nodes (Brkljačić and Ivanac 2014; Brkljačić et al. 2007).

When the breast is maturing, the echogenicity of the glandular tissue increases gradually. In the mature breast, glandular parenchyma is hyperechoic and bright, while the fatty tissue surrounding parenchyma and interspersed fat lobules appear hypoechoic and dark. Cooper's ligaments are visualized as fine linear hyperechoic bands that traverse the fat. They may produce shadowing due to the reflection of the sound beam, and careful compression and repositioning of the transducer are needed to eliminate these artifacts. The skin appears as thin, hyperechoic, bright, double-contour line, with thickness below 3 mm. Acoustic shadowing often impairs visualization of the retroareolar area because the retroareolar ducts reflect echoes away from the probe, since they run parallel to the beam direction (Brkljačić and Ivanac 2014; Hooley et al. 2013).

The higher the mammographic parenchyma density of the breast gets, the more important the role of ultrasound in the evaluation of the breast is. In mammographically very dense breasts, small lesions are hidden by the superposition of

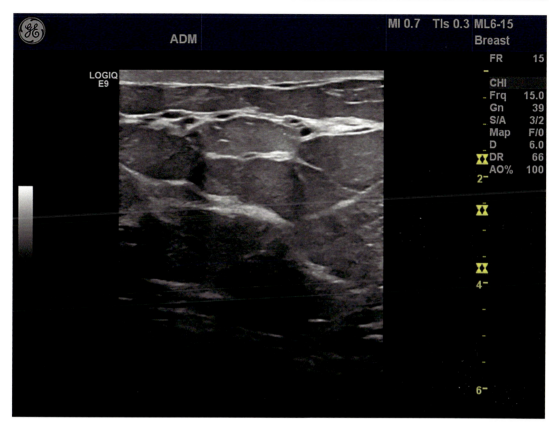

Fig. 1 Ultrasound image of the fatty breast, with dominantly hypoechoic fat lobules and Cooper's ligaments visible as hyperechoic linear bands that traverse the fat

the surrounding parenchyma. However, on ultrasound these lesions are often very clearly depicted because of the different acoustic impedance, and consequently different echogenicity between them and surrounding parenchyma (Crystal et al. 2003). With age, breast parenchyma undergoes involution and atrophy, and fatty tissue becomes predominate in the breast, which is hypoechoic, with only scarce echogenic patches of parenchymal tissue, while Cooper's ligaments remain hyperechoic. During pregnancy, echogenicity of the tissue decreases because of increased water content, hyperemia, fluid retention, and lobular hyperplasia. Hormone replacement therapy (HRT) causes proliferation of the breast parenchyma, and the breasts appear hyperechoic with increased volume of parenchyma (Hooley et al. 2013) (Figs. 1 and 2).

4 Types of Breast Lesions and Their Sonographic Features as per the ACR BI-RADS Atlas

Breast lesions may originate from the main lactiferous ducts (duct ectasia, main duct papilloma, intraductal carcinoma), small and terminal ducts (hyperplasia, peripheral duct papilloma, ductal carcinoma), lobules (cyst, fibroadenoma, adenosis, phyllodes tumor, lobular carcinoma), and stroma (sarcoma) or may have unclassified origin (radial scarring) (Tot et al. 2014). Ultrasound is used to evaluate palpable abnormalities and other breast symptoms, implants, changes detected by mammography or breast MRI, and axilla, as well as for supplemental screening, in addition to mammography. It is an excellent modality for the

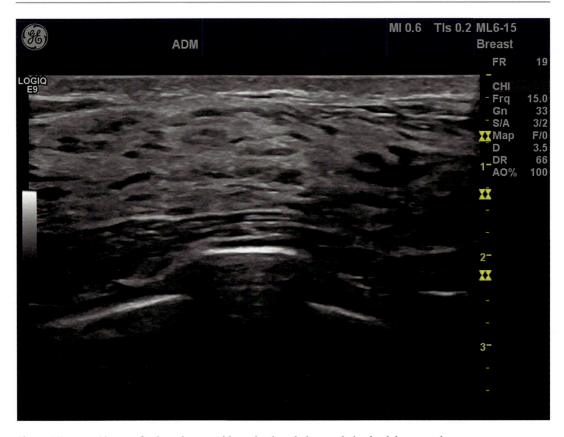

Fig. 2 Ultrasound image of a dense breast, with predominantly hyperechoic glandular parenchyma

guidance of fine needle aspirations, biopsies, and other interventional procedures (Brkljačić and Ivanac 2014; Berg et al. 2012a).

For ultrasound reporting, the most widely used terminology and classifications are those proposed by the American College of Radiology (ACR) Breast Imaging and Reporting Data System (BI-RADS) (Mendelson et al. 2013). Consistent terminology and assessment categorization ease the communication between experts from radiology and other medical senologic disciplines, dealing with breast diagnosis and treatment, and help to define the level of suspicion for malignancy. According to the fifth edition of the ACR BI-RADS Atlas, it is recommended to first define tissue composition, and then to describe abnormalities (masses, cysts, complex cystic and solid lesions, calcifications, associated features, and special cases). All these elements are a part of the structured report following a breast ultrasound examination.

Regarding tissue composition, the categorization is comparable to the variability seen on mammographic images. ACR BI-RADS differentiates homogeneous fatty background echotexture, homogeneous fibroglandular background echotexture, and heterogeneous focal or diffuse background echotexture.

A mass is a space-occupying three-dimensional lesion to be documented in two orthogonal planes. Shape, orientation, margins, echo pattern, and posterior acoustic features should be evaluated. The level of suspicion is to be based on the most worrisome feature. Regarding their shape, masses can be round, oval, or irregular. Oval and round lesions are usually benign and cancers usually irregular, but some cancers may be round and oval in shape, including very aggressive mucinous or triple-negative breast cancers (Mendelson et al. 2013). Orientation of the lesion (according to the axis of its longest diameter) in reference to the skin surface is unique for US examination. Parallel lesions ("wider than talle") are more likely benign, and vertical ("taller than wide") lesions are more likely to be malignant. Margins of a lesion can be circumscribed (well defined) or non-circumscribed. Non-circumscribed margins may be subdivided into indistinct, angular, microlobulated, or spiculated, and they raise the level of suspicion for malignancy.

Echo pattern is compared in reference to fatty and glandular tissue. Simple cysts are anechoic and therefore darker than fat. Hyperechoic lesions have the same or higher echogenicity as fibroglandular tissue and definitely a higher echogenicity than fat; hypoechoic lesions are less echogenic than fat; isoechoic lesions have the approximate echogenicity of the surrounding fat; and complex cystic and solid lesions contain an anechoic (cystic) and an echoic (solid) component. A mixture of echogenic patterns within a solid mass is called heterogeneous echo pattern. Distal acoustic phenomena should be observed: posterior shadowing, posterior enhancement, no changes in the posterior echogenicity, or combined patterns. Posterior enhancement suggests a benign lesion and it is rather typical for cystic lesions, but some carcinomas may also show enhancement. Posterior shadowing of different intensity suggests fibrosis, with or without an underlying malignancy. Areas of acoustic shadowing or enhancement not originating from focal lesions commonly appear in dense fibrous breasts; changing the transducer position shadowing originating from benign fibrous tissue or Cooper's ligaments may be eliminated (Mendelson et al. 2013).

Calcifications, including microcalcifications, can be seen with high-frequency transducers if carefully looked for, especially when specifically targeted, i.e., second-look ultrasound examinations, performed after mammography; the examiner exactly knows the location where to look for microcalcifications.

Calcifications larger than 0.5 mm usually present with dorsal acoustic shadowing. Microcalcifications are difficult to visualize on ultrasound and are too small to cause posterior shadowing. With high-frequency transducers however, they might be visible as echogenic foci, particularly when located in a mass. Microcalcification clusters present as multiple hyperechogenic foci within either masses or ducts. Calcifications should be classified as per location: in a mass, outside of a mass, or as intraductal. If the US correlate present is clearly a cluster, it can be subjected to US-guided biopsy (Fig. 3).

The fifth edition of the ACR BI-RADS further introduced associated features, like architectural distortion, duct changes, skin changes (thickening and retraction), edema, vascularity (absent, internal, rim vascularity), as well as elasticity assessment by sonoelastography (Berg et al. 2012b).

Special cases are those with a unique sonographic diagnosis or findings. These are simple cysts, clustered microcysts, complicated cysts, masses in or on the skin, foreign bodies including implants, intramammary and axillary lymph nodes, vascular abnormalities (arteriovenous malformations/pseudoaneurysms, Mondor's disease), postsurgical fluid collections, and fat necrosis (Mendelson et al. 2013).

Whenever possible, US should be correlated with mammographic and/or MRI findings and compared to previous examinations. Every report has to be ideally structured and should include the indication for the examination, patient history and clinical findings, technique of breast US examination performed, clear description of any important findings, composite reports (if more than one type of examination is performed concurrently), final assessment categories according to BI-RADS, and management recommendations. When correlating US with mammography and MRI, the examiner has to be aware that the patient's position affects the location of the lesion and it may differ considerably between ultrasound performed in supine or lateral oblique position and MRI performed in the prone position.

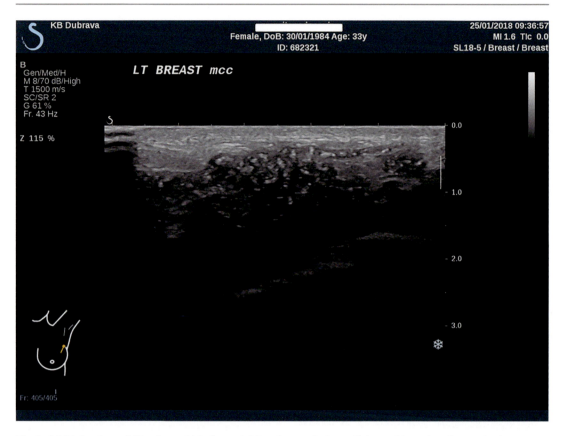

Fig. 3 Multiple microcalcifications within ducts visible as hyperechoic small dots, without dorsal acoustic phenomena. This 33-year-old woman had extensive DCIS, grade III

4.1 BI-RADS Final Assessment Categories

In Category 0 (incomplete assessment), additional imaging evaluation is needed; this should be reserved to the screening setting. Information should be provided on the exact additional imaging modality to be used, and it should be borne in mind that negative additional imaging should avoid biopsy.

Category 1 is for normal examinations, with no abnormalities.

Category 2 includes benign findings. Simple cysts are placed in this category, along with intramammary lymph nodes, breast implants, stable postsurgical fluid collections, and fibroadenomas, unchanged for at least 2 years.

Category 3 includes probably benign findings: a solid mass with circumscribed margins, oval shape, and parallel orientation, most likely to be a fibroadenoma, when described for the first time. The risk of malignancy is less than 2%, with furthermore isolated, nonpalpable complicated cysts. Clustered microcysts might also be placed in this category for short-interval (= 6-month) follow-up. If lesions are unchanged after 6 months, the next follow-up examination will be after another 6 months, and then after another 12 months. If lesions are stable over the course of 24 months, they are downgraded to BI-RADS Category 2. Elastographic features are also helpful, because cancers are usually stiff and benign lesions elastic (Berg et al. 2012b).

Category 4 is defined as suspicious lesions. The probability of cancer in this group is in a very wide range from 2% to 95%; therefore, a further subdivision into additional three groups (4A, 4B, and 4C) for risk stratification is possible. Those lesions require tissue sampling by needle biopsy providing histologic diagnosis.

Category 5 refers to lesions highly suggestive of malignancy, with a very high probability of 95% or higher.

Category 6 is reserved for lesions with biopsy proof of malignancy prior to definite (= surgical) therapy.

5 Sonographic Features of Benign Breast Lesions

More common benign breast lesions are cysts, fibroadenomas, duct ectasia, intraductal papillomas or papillomatosis, sclerosing adenosis, and epithelial hyperplasia involving lobules or larger ducts. Less common benign conditions are mastitis, lipomas, fat necrosis, foreign body granulomas, lactational mastitis, and sclerosing phlebitis (Mondor's disease) (Brkljačić and Ivanac 2014; Tot et al. 2014).

Cysts are very common and are found in approximately 50% of women in the age group between 30 and 40 years of age. Ultrasound can reliably depict microcysts measuring 1–2 mm in diameter, as well as simple or multiloculated macrocysts, not requiring further evaluation in this age group (Brkljačić et al. 2007; Hooley et al. 2013). Galactoceles are retention cysts filled with milk developing in pregnancy, while oil cysts, filled with necrotic material, may develop peripheral eggshell calcifications and are usually related to trauma or breast surgery. Simple cysts are easy to recognize sonographically, since they appear as round or oval, well-circumscribed anechoic lesions with clear visualization of their posterior wall, abrupt interface to the surrounding tissue, posterior acoustic enhancement, and lateral thin refraction shadows, without any internal color on sonoelastography. Complicated cysts may contain thin septa. Ultrasound-guided aspiration or tissue sampling may be needed to differentiate septa from solid intracystic vegetations (= complex cystic and solid lesions) suspicious for malignancy. Sonographic presentation of epithelial hyperplasia, focal fibrosis, adenosis, and pseudoangioma-

tous stromal hyperplasia is very diverse and inconsistent, with hypoechoic or irregular areas, solid and cystic lesions, and hyperechoic areas, and the diagnosis of these conditions is primarily through histopathology (Brkljačić and Ivanac 2014; Hooley et al. 2013; Berg et al. 2012b) (Figs. 4 and 5).

Radial scars are lesions that resemble invasive cancer on US and mammography because of their spiculated appearance. This is due to a focal tubular proliferation around a fibrous elastoid center; carcinomas can develop within a radial scar; therefore, it should be surgically excised (Adler 2000).

Focal fibrosis is a stromal proliferation occurring in younger women, which can potentially resemble malignancy if manifesting with hypoechoic focal lesions with acoustic shadowing (Brkljačić and Ivanac 2014; Brkljačić et al. 2007; Hooley et al. 2013).

Fibroadenomas are the most common benign breast tumors, typically occurring in young women with the highest incidence between 25 and 35 years; they are mixed fibroepithelial hyperplastic tumors of the lobular connective tissue (Brkljačić and Ivanac 2014; Hooley et al. 2013; Tot et al. 2014). Typical sonographic features of fibroadenomas are round or oval masses with circumscribed (= well-defined) margins, horizontal orientation, relatively homogeneous hypoechoic internal pattern, posterior enhancement, and soft appearance on sonoelastography (Brkljačić and Ivanac 2014; Hooley et al. 2013; Berg et al. 2012b). The incidence of fibroadenoma decreases after the age of 40 years. Fibroadenomas are usually solitary; however, multiple lesions are observed in 10% of patients. They typically measure 1–2 cm and rarely more than 4 cm in diameter. As stated above, the classical fibroadenoma appears as a mass lesion with benign features (horizontal orientation, oval shape, and circumscribed margins). If any of these features are not present, newly discovered solid lesions are to be placed into the BI-RADS 4 category and a biopsy is to be performed. In rare cases, grayscale features of some aggressive invasive

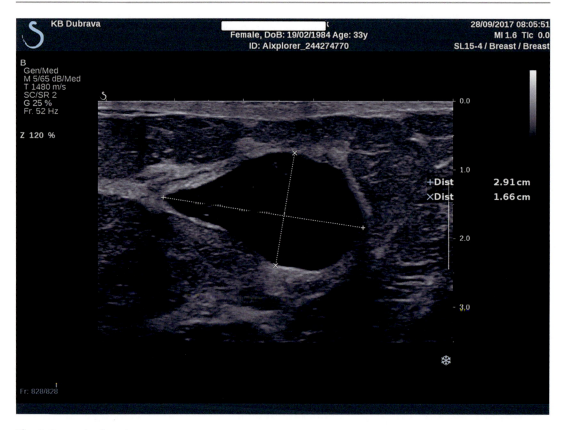

Fig. 4 Large simple cyst

breast cancers, like triple-negative invasive cancers, may resemble those of fibroadenomas, since they can present as a well-circumscribed, horizontally oriented lesions, but they typically are not as soft as fibroadenomas on sonoelastography (Yeo et al. 2018; Džoić et al. 2016) (Fig. 6).

Hamartomas are completely benign abnormal collections of tissues normally found in the breast (fat, parenchyma, and muscle), surrounded by a pseudocapsule, appearing on ultrasound as well-defined, horizontally oriented lesions with well-defined margins. The final diagnosis is established by core needle biopsy or excisional biopsy.

Papillomas are benign fibroepithelial tumors located within the milk ducts (Chapter "High-Risk Lesions of the Breast: Diagnosis and Management"). They are relatively rare and can present on sonography as intraductal, typically highly vascularized mass with or without ductal dilatation, or as intracystic mass and a predominantly solid pattern with the intraductal mass totally filling the duct. Reliable sonographic differentiation between benign papilloma and papillary carcinoma is not possible and yields further invasive diagnostic evaluation. Very frequently, papillomas become clinically apparent due to pathological nipple discharge.

Abscesses may be the consequence of inadequately treated acute mastitis. Ultrasound demonstrates skin thickening, changes in echogenicity of parenchyma and subcutaneous tissue, dilated ducts, as well as typical low-echogenicity lesions, irregularly circumscribed, with multiple internal echoes caused by pus, surrounded by a hyperechoic rim of edema. If the clinical presentation is not clear and any suspicious finding is present, tissue sampling is needed (Brkljačić and Ivanac 2014; Hooley et al. 2013).

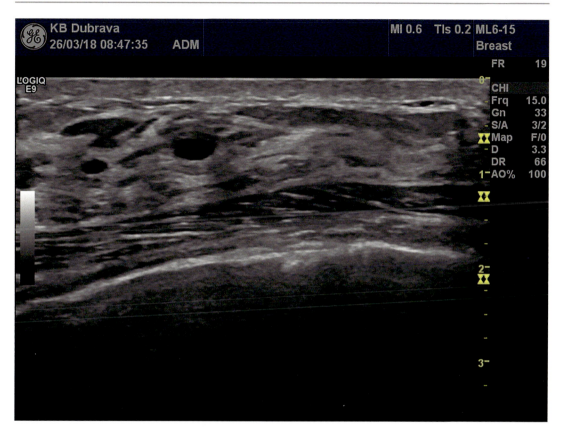

Fig. 5 Small cysts with typical sonographic features

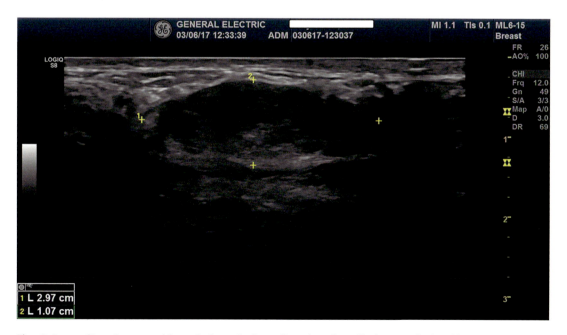

Fig. 6 Large fibroadenoma with oval shape horizontally oriented, well circumscribed, without distal acoustic phenomena

6 Sonographic Features of Breast Lesions

More than 25 years ago, Stavros in his landmark publication described grayscale sonographic features of malignant and benign breast lesions. Malignant features include vertical orientation (larger anteroposterior than laterolateral diameter), spiculation, distortion of breast tissue architecture, marked hypoechogenicity, angular margins, posterior acoustic shadowing, and microcalcifications, while benign features include gentle lobulations, ellipsoid shape, homogeneous echotexture, thin capsule, and horizontal orientation (larger laterolateral than anteroposterior diameter) (Stavros et al. 1995). Many carcinomas are stiff on sonoelastography examinations, while most benign lesions are soft (Brkljačić and Ivanac 2014).

7 Sonographic Features of Malignant Breast Lesions

The widespread use of mammographic screening has resulted in the considerable increase of diagnosed ductal carcinoma in situ (DCIS), on the basis of mammographically visible microcalcifications (Tot et al. 2014). Ultrasound and MRI are inferior to mammography in the detection of suspicious microcalcifications, but their role in the assessment of BI-RADS 4 and 5 mammographic microcalcifications should not be underestimated (Bennani-Baiti et al. 2017; Hrkać-Pustahija et al. 2018).

Carcinomas in situ are neoplasms that do not penetrate the ductal basement lamina; they carry an inherent risk for development of invasive cancer. Ductal carcinoma in situ (DCIS) develops from ductal epithelium of milk ducts and is often multifocal; several types of DCIS differ in the degree of differentiation and malignant potential. Comedo DCIS progresses into invasive carcinoma in approximately 50% of cases, while some higher differentiated types progress into invasive cancer less often (20–30%) (Tot et al. 2014). Sonographic features of DCIS include ductal abnormalities, predominantly ductal dilatation with intraductal content, usually with small echoic dots representing microcalcifications, architectural distortions, and less commonly hypoechoic irregular areas or masses. Sonographic features of DCIS most frequently are hypoechoic areas in the mammary gland according to a Japanese group (Watanabe et al. 2017), followed by solid masses and abnormalities of the ducts or mixed masses. Uncommon findings reported by the authors were distortions, clustered microcysts, and echogenic foci without a hypoechoic area. Calcifications in malignant breast tissue are more frequently visualized sonographically than benign calcifications. Moreover, in case of an invasive DCIS, ultrasound can be an adjunct method to detect associated masses and to assess axillary lymph nodes. The sonographic presentation of noncalcified DCIS is especially challenging, since its appearance is very heterogeneous, ranging from circumscribed round masses to clustered cysts (Wang et al. 2013). In our experience, in more than 70% of DCIS, hyperechoic foci can be found on ultrasound, either within a mass or within a duct, representing microcalcification clusters visible on mammography. If those changes are visible on ultrasound, an US-guided biopsy could be considered as an option (Brkljačić and Ivanac 2014; Hrkać-Pustahija et al. 2018; Uematsu 2012). Lobular cancer in situ (LCIS) is not recognizable on ultrasound; it arises in ductolobular units of the parenchyma. It has much lower malignant potential than DCIS and is considered as an epithelial atypia rather than a true carcinoma (Brkljačić and Ivanac 2014; Hooley et al. 2013) (Fig. 7).

Invasive breast cancers are classified into invasive ductal carcinoma (IDC), arising from ducts, with several subtypes, and invasive lobular carcinoma (ILC), arising from lobules. IDC is much more common than ILC and easier visualized with ultrasound (Brkljačić and Ivanac 2014; Tot et al. 2014). ILC accounts for roughly 10–15% of invasive breast cancers, often multicentric and bilateral, requiring preoperative MRI. Ultrasound can better evaluate multifocality, multicentricity, and intraductal spread than mammography, but is

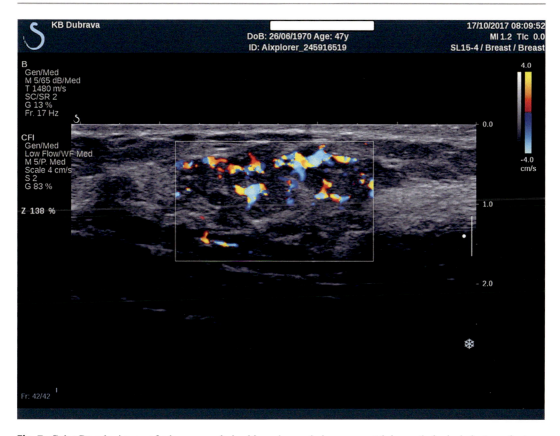

Fig. 7 Color Doppler image of a hypervascularized large hypoechoic area, containing pathological clusters of microcalcifications on mammography—core biopsy and final histopathologic diagnosis demonstrated pure DCIS

inferior to MRI (Brkljačić and Ivanac 2014; Hooley et al. 2013) (Fig. 8).

However, one needs to be very careful at differentiation between malignant and benign lesions, because the straightforward distinction on the basis of former Stavros categories is not completely accurate in every single case and there is a considerable overlap of sonographic features between benign and malignant (Stavros et al. 1995). Some very aggressive cancers, like triple-negative cancers, may demonstrate benign morphologic sonographic features (horizontal orientation and well-circumscribed, regular-shaped masses); correlation with mammography and MRI is needed, and image-guided biopsy is the best way to establish the accurate diagnosis (Džoić et al. 2016; Dogan and Turnbull 2012) (Fig. 9).

Some invasive cancers, invisible on mammography, may be visualized at ultrasound, especially in mammographically extremely dense breasts, and even small, nonpalpable carcinomas can be seen on ultrasound (Hooley et al. 2013; Crystal et al. 2003). Medullary and mucinous cancers often present as oval-shaped, well-circumscribed, hypoechoic masses that may look like complicated cysts with some internal echoes at ultrasound (Liu et al. 2011). Posterior acoustic shadowing is considered as an indicator for malignancy and is caused by extensive fibrotic reaction and fibrotic tissue absorbing the sound beam, although some carcinomas do not present posterior shadowing and may even have posterior enhancement, like some medullary and mucinous carcinomas (Liu et al. 2011).

Therefore, it should not be forgotten that breast US is primarily an adjunct modality and should, whenever possible, be evaluated together with mammography (and/or MRI) in combination with a clinical examination.

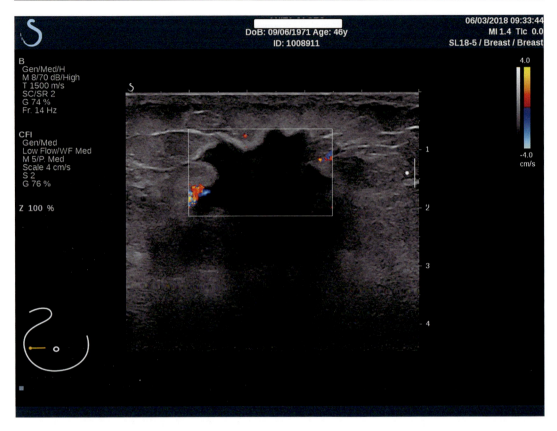

Fig. 8 Sonographic image of an irregular-shaped, ill-defined and spiculated, hypoechoic mass with dorsal shadowing—histopathologic diagnosis revealed invasive ductal cancer, cribriform type, luminal B

With the widespread use of breast MRI, targeted, second-look ultrasound for focused evaluation of lesions detected on contrast-enhanced MRI has become very important. Fifty-six percent of these lesions are visible on ultrasound and can be biopsied under ultrasound guidance. The larger the lesion on MRI, the higher the likelihood that it is visible on ultrasound (Brkljačić and Ivanac 2014; Candelaria and Fornage 2011).

8 Further Ultrasound Applications: After Treatment, Screening, Intervention

Postoperative scars after breast-conserving surgery as well as fat necrosis may resemble cancer, and appear irregular, hypoechoic, and spiculated, with varying degrees of dorsal acoustic shadowing. However, ultrasound is inferior to MRI in distinguishing postoperative scars from cancer (Chapter "Post-therapy Evaluation (Including Breast Implants)").

Postoperative seromas are fluid collections that may undergo secondary inflammation.

Aftereffects of radiation therapy include thickening of the skin, edema, and architectural distortions of breast parenchyma, which can be visualized by ultrasound. Ultrasound is also very helpful for the detection of implant pathology after oncoplastic surgery.

When biopsy is indicated, ultrasound is excellent as a guidance modality. Ultrasound can also be used to search for recurrence of cancer after surgery, including recurrence in the thoracic wall after mastectomy (Brkljačić and Ivanac 2014).

As already mentioned, mammography has considerable limitations in women with dense breasts. An additional 2.3–4.6 of mammographically

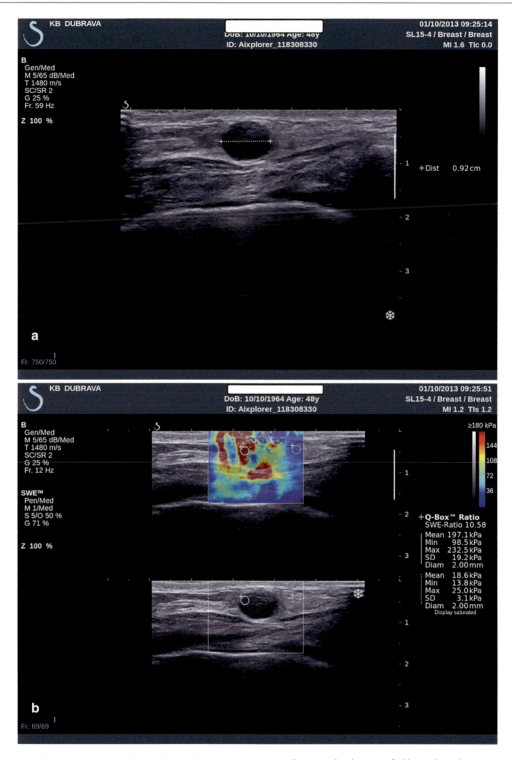

Fig. 9 (**a**) Grayscale image of a triple-negative invasive cancer with benign features—the lesion is oval shaped with well-defined margins, hypoechoic, horizontally oriented, and without dorsal shadowing. (**b**) Shear wave sonoelastography image of this patient demonstrates a stiff lesion. The histopathologic diagnosis was triple-negative invasive breast cancer

occult breast cancers per 1000 women can be diagnosed if ultrasound is added to mammography in women with dense breasts (Berg et al. 2012a). Some national mammographic screening programs in Europe, like in Austria or Croatia, recommend breast ultrasound to all women with ACR BI-RADS C and D density categories, and breast ultrasound examinations are mandatory and free of charge for these women, in the scope of the national health-care systems. Automated whole-breast ultrasound has been recently introduced as an alternative to handheld ultrasound for screening, but it will be covered in other chapters (Chapter "Automated Breast Ultrasound").

9 Summary

Ultrasound of the breast underwent rapid technical and application-related developments over the last years. Patients' toleration of examination, lack of radiation exposure, excellent spatial resolution, low costs, and consequently high availability render this method an ideal diagnostic option. Because of real-time imaging, interventional procedures like breast or axillary lymph node tissue sampling or minimally invasive breast therapies are routinely led by handheld ultrasound.

B(rightness) mode is the basis for breast evaluation, whereas color Doppler ultrasound and sonoelastography may add diagnostic value in selected cases. Automated three-dimensional breast ultrasound is a novel approach to make the examination less examiner dependent while depicting the whole breast.

The most widely used terminology and classifications in breast ultrasound are those proposed by the American College of Radiology (ACR) Breast Imaging Reporting And Data System (BI-RADS). Ultrasound has the potential to classify benign and malignant lesions and adds further value to mammography and MRI in evaluating the breast and axillary lymph nodes.

Limitations of standard handheld ultrasound in the detection and classification of breast lesions are especially its examiner dependence and the limited detectability of calcifications like in DCIS.

Nevertheless, breast ultrasound has over the years become one of the main pillars in diagnostic breast imaging and guidance for breast interventions alike, with promising applications for minimally invasive breast therapy. In the future, the extensive implementation of routine ultrasound in breast cancer screening may be considered in patients with dense breasts.

References

Adler DD (2000) Imaging evaluation of spiculated masses. In: Friedrich M, Sickles EA (eds) Radiological diagnosis of breast diseases. Springer, Berlin, pp 137–148

Athanasiou A, Tardivon A, Ollivier L, Thibault F, El Khoury C, Neuenschwander S (2009) How to optimize breast ultrasound. Eur J Radiol 69(1):6–13

Bennani Baiti B, Dietzel M, Baltzer PA (2017) MRI for the assessment of malignancy in BI-RADS 4 mammographic microcalcifications. PLoS One 12(11):e188679

Berg WA, Zhang Z, Lehrer D et al (2012a) Detection of breast cancer with addition of annual screening ultrasound or a single screening MRI to mammography in women with elevated breast cancer risk. JAMA 307(13):1394–1404

Berg WA, Cosgrove DO, Dore CJ et al (2012b) Shear-wave elastography improves the specificity of breast US: the BE1 multinational study of 939 masses. Radiology 262(2):435–449

Brkljačić B, Ivanac G (2014) Ultrasonography of the breast. Ultrasound Clin 9:391–427

Brkljačić B, Huzjan-Korunić R, Pavić L (2007) Ultrasound of the breast. In: Kurjak A, Chervenak F (eds) Donald school textbook of ultrasound in obstetrics and gynaecology. Jaypee Brothers Medical Publishers, New Delhi, pp 950–970

Brkljačić B, Čikara I, Ivanac G, Hrkać-Pustahija A, Žic R, Stanec Z (2010) Ultrasound-guided bipolar radiofrequency ablation of breast cancer in inoperable patients: a pilot study. Ultraschall Med 31:156–162

Candelaria R, Fornage BD (2011) Second-look US examination of MR-detected breast lesions. J Clin Ultrasound 39(3):115–121

Crystal P, Strano SD, Scharynski S, Koretz MJ (2003) Using sonography to screen women with mammographically dense breasts. AJR Am J Roentgenol 181(1):177–182

Dogan BE, Turnbull LW (2012) Imaging of triple-negative breast cancer. Ann Oncol 23:23–29

Džoić M, Ivanac G, Kelava T, Brkljačić B (2016) Elastographic features of triple negative breast cancers. Eur Radiol 26(4):1090–1097

Hooley RJ, Scoutt LM, Philpotts LE (2013) Breast ultrasonography: state of the art. Radiology 268(3): 642–659

Hrkać-Pustahija A, Ivanac G, Brkljačić B (2018) Ultrasound and magnetic resonance imaging in the evaluation of mammographic BI-RADS 4 and 5 microcalcifications. Diagn Interv Radiol 24(4): 187–194

Kremkau FW (2011) Sonography principles and instruments, 8th edn. Elsevier-Saunders, St Louis, MO

Liu H, Tan H, Cheng Y, Zhang X, Gu Y, Peng W (2011) Imaging findings in mucinous breast carcinoma and correlating factors. Eur J Radiol 80(3): 706–712

Mendelson EB, Bohm-Velez M, Berg WA et al (2013) ACR breast imaging reporting and data system. Ultrasound. American College of Radiology, Reston, VA, pp 1–145

Stafford RJ, Whitman GJ (2011) Ultrasound physics and technology in breast imaging. Ultrasound Clin 6(3):299–312

Stavros AT, Thickman D, Rapp CL, Dennis MA, Parker SH, Sisney GA (1995) Solid breast nodules: use of sonography to distinguish between benign and malignant lesions. Radiology 196(1):123–134

Tot T, Tabar L, Dean PB (2014) Practical breast pathology, 2nd edn. Thieme, New York, pp 50–66

Uematsu T (2012) Non-mass-like lesions on breast ultrasonography: a systematic review. Breast Cancer 19:295–301

Wang LC, Sullivan M, Du H, Feldman MI, Mendelson EB (2013) US appearance of ductal carcinoma in situ. Radiographics 33(1):213–228

Watanabe T, Yamaguchi T, Tsunoda H, Kaoku S, Tohno E, Yasuda H, Ban K, Hirokaga K, Tanaka K, Umemoto T et al (2017) Ultrasound image classification of ductal carcinoma in situ (DCIS) of the breast: analysis of 705 DCIS lesions. Ultrasound Med Biol 43(5):918–925

Yeo SH, Kim GR, Lee SH, Moon WK (2018) Comparison of ultrasound elastography and color doppler ultrasonography for distinguishing small triple-negative breast cancer from fibroadenoma. J Ultrasound Med 37(9):2135–2146

Breast Ultrasound: Advanced Techniques

Andy Evans

Contents

1   **Introduction** 113

2   **Elastography** 114
    2.1   Introduction 114
    2.2   Strain Elastography 114
    2.3   Shear Wave Elastography 114

3   **Ultrasound Assessment of Lesion Vascularity** 122
    3.1   Doppler 122
    3.2   Contrast-Enhanced Ultrasound 124
    3.3   Superb Microvascular Imaging 124

References 125

Abstract

Several additional techniques are now widely available when performing handheld breast US which may be helpful in routine clinical practice and others which show research potential. These include various forms of elastography including strain and shear wave techniques and Doppler assessment of vascularity with and without contrast. The most useful technique is shear wave elastography (SWE) which allows quantitative and repro-ducible analysis of tissue stiffness. Cancers tend to be stiff and benign lesions soft. SWE can be used successfully to differentiate benign from malignant lesions, monitor neo-adjuvant chemotherapy, and predict nodal metastasis and outcome. Superb vascular imaging is the most promising vascular modality and it may be useful in monitoring neoadjuvant chemotherapy and benign/malignant differentiation.

1   Introduction

A number of additional techniques are now widely available when performing handheld breast US which may be helpful in routine

---

A. Evans (✉)
University of Dundee, Dundee, Scotland, UK
e-mail: a.z.evans@dundee.ac.uk

© Springer Nature Switzerland AG 2022
M. Fuchsjäger et al. (eds.), *Breast Imaging*, Medical Radiology Diagnostic Imaging,
https://doi.org/10.1007/978-3-030-94918-1_6

2 Elastography

2.1 Introduction

Elastography is useful in the breast because most benign lesions are soft and most malignant lesions are stiff. The stiffness or softness of breast lesions is essentially due to the characteristics of the collagen these lesions contain or are surrounded by. Fibroadenomas have a large collagen content but the collagen is well ordered and has few cross-links making them soft at elastography. Malignant lesions, particularly invasive cancers, have cancer-associated fibroblasts (CAFs) both within and around the tumors. These CAFs produce abnormal collagen which is thicker, is disorganized in orientation, and has increased cross-links making the lesions and the surrounding stroma stiff (Shi et al. 2018). This stiff surrounding stroma is why clinical sizing of breast cancers is often overestimated. In a study where the size of the surrounding stiffness and the size of the grayscale abnormality were compared with the pathological size of the tumor, the grayscale size was often underestimated while the shear wave elastography (SWE) size was overestimated. The most accurate prediction was found when 50% of the SWE stiffness was added to the grayscale size (Mullen et al. 2014). This finding suggests that the area of stiffness surrounding the grayscale abnormality is a combination of tumor with stiff stroma immediately adjacent to the tumor and stiff stroma alone more peripherally. CAFs also secrete metalloproteinases which dissolve collagen as well as form collagen so this increased collagen turnover allows tumor invasion of stroma and creation of blood vessels, thus promoting tumor growth and metastasis.

2.2 Strain Elastography

Elastography is based on the fact that sound waves propagate through stiff tissue faster than soft tissue. Strain elastography (SE) is where the force is applied by the operator through the probe. SE has been available for many years. It is reliant on detecting the way the speckle within image moves, often with a tracking algorithm. This information is then used to form an image that is usually displayed in color.

There are three methods of interpreting SE: the elastographic-to-B-mode length ratio, a 5-point color scale, and the strain ratio (Barr et al. 2018). SE has been shown to aid benign/malignant differentiation of solid masses especially when used in conjunction with the Tsukuba criteria of stiffness within and around US visible lesions. This classification is based on the observations that malignant lesions are on average stiffer than benign lesions, that the stiffness of malignant lesions is most often seen at the edge of the cancer, and that this stiffness is also seen in the peritumoral stroma, making the elastographic lesion bigger than the grayscale abnormality. A lesion not stiffer than surrounding tissue is scored 1. Lesions with stiff areas are classified 2 or 3 while entirely stiff lesions are classified 4. A score of 5 indicates that the stiffness extends beyond the margins of the grayscale lesion. The drawbacks of strain elastography are poor reproducibility and lack of quantitative outputs.

2.3 Shear Wave Elastography

2.3.1 Technique

During shear wave elastography, the strain is produced by the ultrasound probe by means of an acoustic radiation force impulse (ARFI) which generates shear waves in the breast tissue and the speed of propagation of these waves is tracked by ultrafast ultrasound sequences. The speed of propagation is related to Young's modulus of elasticity. A similar technique called ARFI uses the amplitude of the displacement generated in the vicinity of the pushing beam rather than the generated shear waves.

During acquisition it is important that the probe is held still as the stiffness color map builds up in real time and that no pressure is applied as this will cause artifactual stiffness. Images should be obtained in orthogonal planes as many lesions display quite marked anisotropy. On average malignant lesions display greater anisotropy than benign lesions (Chen et al. 2018). There is no increased diagnostic information gained from using the ductal and anti-ductal planes compared to using any other orthogonal planes.

2.3.2 Number of Images

The use of four images rather than two has been shown to improve the reproducibility of SWE. The intra-class correlation coefficient for 4-image SWE taken by different operators is 0.85 which is nearly perfect (Evans et al. 2012). Similar agreement is found for quantitative data extracted from the same images by two people.

2.3.3 Region of Interest Size and Data Extraction

Once the color map image has been saved quantitative information can be obtained using a region of interest (ROI). This is normally 1 or 2 mm in diameter. This diameter gives optimal benign/malignant differentiation when using the parameters of maximum elasticity (Emax) and mean elasticity (Emean) (Moon et al. 2018).

The display also gives the standard deviation (SD) which is a measure of heterogeneity of the stiffness within the ROI. SD is a less useful parameter than Emean and Emax when using a small ROI (Fig. 1). However if a large ROI is used (>2 mm) then the performance of SD in benign/malignant differentiation improves to be similar to that of Emax and Emean. Acquiring of SWE images takes about 2 min and extraction of the quantitative data takes a similar time.

Currently quantitative data can only be extracted from the US machine. This means that quantitative information cannot be extracted once the images have fallen off the US machine. This limits the ease of performing multicenter studies and retrospective evaluation of SWE studies. However algorithms are being developed which will allow quantitative information to be extracted from images stored on PACS.

2.3.4 Qualitative Evaluation and Artifacts

Similarly to strain elastography, the pattern of stiffness can be useful in benign/malignant differentiation. The "ring sign" when a subtle halo of stiffness is seen around small, low-grade cancers is particularly useful as small low-grade cancers may not be stiff enough to reach the cut-off values used for Emax and Emean (Yoon et al. 2013) (Fig. 2). Stiffness which appears to arise from the skin or underlying pectoral muscle is often artifactual. Vertical bands of stiffness on the very edge of images are also often artifactual.

2.3.5 3D Shear Wave

3D SWE probes exist and this allows the volume of stiffness in and around a lesion to be measured. Extraction of the volumes requires freehand ROIs to be drawn on a number of slices taking about 4 min per lesion. 3D SWE has a similar diagnostic performance as 2D SWE in differentiating benign from malignant breast lesions (Lee et al. 2013) (Fig. 3). 3D SWE might be useful in assessing the response of cancers to neoadjuvant systemic therapy. However the use of 3D SWE in this context is hampered by the small probe footprint which often cannot capture the entire stiffness associated with the larger cancers which are often treated with neoadjuvant therapy.

The routine adoption of SWE into breast ultrasound examinations has been hampered by the small number of equipment manufacturers providing high-quality SWE technology. Those who did provide quality SWE images did not always have high-quality grayscale imaging as well. However in recent years these issues have been resolved.

2.3.6 Normal Breast Tissue

Normal breast tissue is soft on SWE with Emean values of around 10–30 kPa (Fig. 4). Surprisingly,

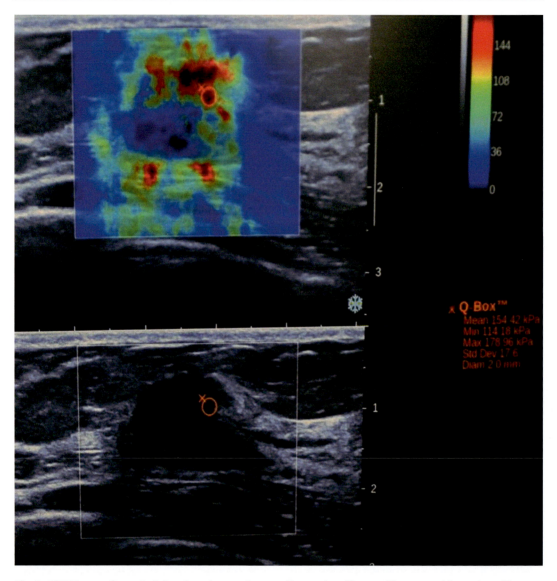

Fig. 1 SWE image of a grade 2 ductal carcinoma of no specific type in a 56-year-old woman with a region of interest. Readout on the right of the image shows the Emean, Emax, Emin, and SD readings

there are only minor differences in the stiffness of fatty breast tissue and dense breast issue. Dense breast tissue is however slightly stiffer than fatty tissue. This minor difference in stiffness is because dense breast tissue although having a high collagen content is made up of well-ordered, thin collagen fibers with low concentrations of cross-linking. Whether the stiffness of breast tissue carries any additional risk information beyond that found from mammographic density is unknown.

2.3.7 Benign Lesions at SWE

Most fibroadenomas are soft on SWE making SWE a useful technique in differentiating benign from malignant breast masses (Fig. 5). Larger fibroadenomas can be stiff, possibly due to pressure on the capsule from enlarging lesions (Elseedawy et al. 2016). Fibrocystic disease, hamartomas, and lipomas are usually soft. Fat necrosis, papillomas, and radial scars have variable stiffness while infection is usually very stiff. The "black hole" seen within cystic lesions can

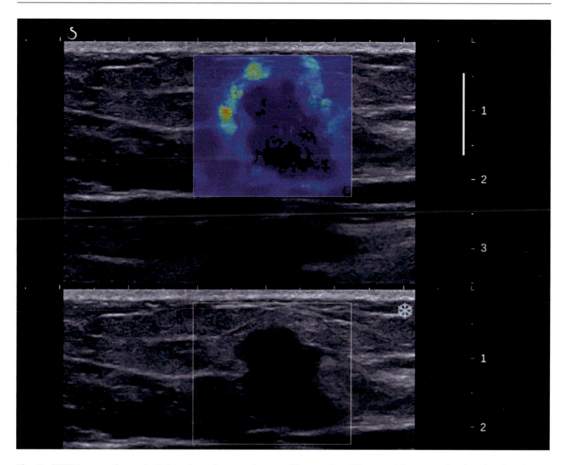

Fig. 2 SWE image of a grade 1 ductal carcinoma of no specific type in a 67-year-old woman showing the ring sign

be useful in differentiating cysts with echogenic contents from solid lesions.

2.3.8 Malignant Lesions at SWE

2.3.8.1 DCIS

About 50% of DCIS lesions are stiff and 50% are soft. DCIS is rarely very stiff and is much less stiff than invasive breast cancer. This is why SWE has been shown to be useful in predicting an invasive focus when an US-guided core biopsy has shown DCIS (Shin et al. 2019). SWE is very useful in identifying small invasive foci in large areas of DCIS. Encysted papillary cancers although classified as in situ disease are of similar stiffness to invasive cancers, suggesting that tumor stromal interactions in these tumors are akin to those seen with invasive cancer.

2.3.8.2 Invasive Cancer

Overall 95% of invasive cancers are stiffer than commonly used threshold values for SWE (Fig. 6). Around 98% of symptomatic invasive cancers are stiff compared to 75% of screen-detected cancers. This is why SWE is most useful in patients with symptoms compared to asymptomatic patients.

Stiffness at SWE has been shown to be associated with many pathological variables. The strongest association is with invasive size. Around a quarter of subcentimeter cancers are soft. Some have advocated using lower cutoff values for E_{mean} and E_{max} when assessing small lesions (Shang et al. 2019). High-grade cancers are stiffer than low-grade cancers even when correcting for size (Zhu et al. 2018a).

Ductal and lobular cancers have similar stiffness. This makes SWE particularly useful in detect-

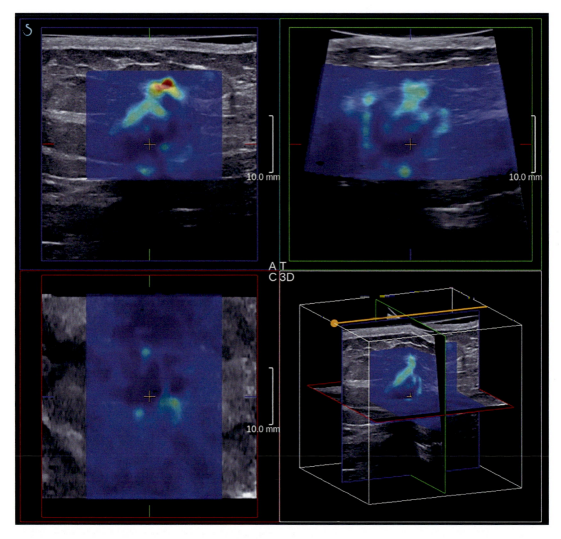

Fig. 3 3D SWE image of a grade 2 lobular cancer in a 76-year-old woman showing peripheral shell-shaped stiffness

ing lobular cancers as all other breast imaging modalities have poorer detection of lobular cancers compared to ductal cancers. It has been reported that SWE may have a role in sizing lobular cancers preoperatively. SWE has high sensitivity in the detection of lobular cancers in women with symptoms where negative US and mammographic findings are not uncommon (Sim et al. 2015).

Basal phenotype high-grade ductal cancers are particularly stiff. These are cancers which can be easily mistaken for fibroadenomas at gray-scale US examination as they often have well-defined margins and distal bright-up. This may be why US screening in BRCA 1 carriers has such poor sensitivity. Marked stiffness at SWE in these circumstances is often the finding leading to a correct diagnosis.

Many tubular cancers are soft which is why small screen-detected cancers are frequently soft (Evans et al. 2016). Many small low-grade cancers have a subtle halo of stiffness (the ring sign) which can alert suspicion even if the quantitative SWE parameters do not reach the threshold values to diagnose malignancy.

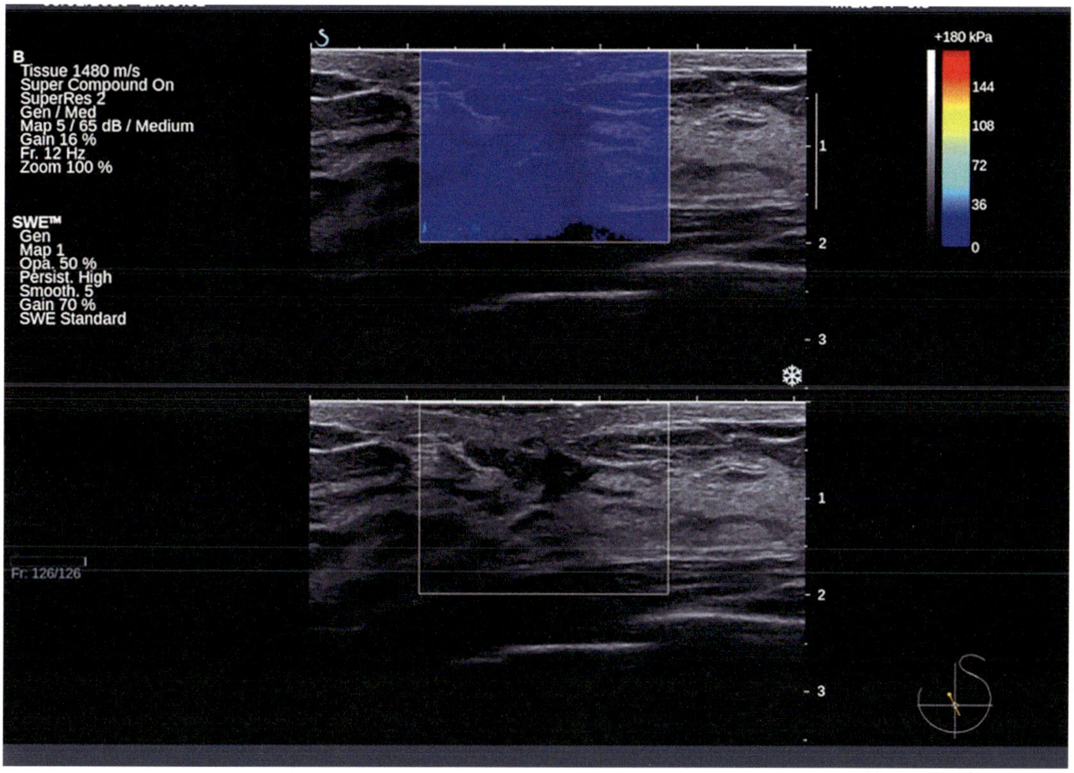

Fig. 4 SWE image of normal breast tissue in a 57-year-old woman. Note similar stiffness of fat and breast parenchyma

2.3.9 Benign Malignant Differentiation

The characteristic features on grayscale US of low-grade cancers and the stiffness of high-grade cancers on SWE mean that the two techniques are complementary in benign/malignant differentiation. The high-grade cancers missed by grayscale US are detected on SWE while the low-grade cancers missed on SWE are diagnosed on grayscale US.

In clinical practice SWE is most useful in upgrading BI-RADS 3 lesions to BI-RADS 4a and downgrading BI-RADS 4A lesions to BI-RADS3; this has been confirmed by a number of meta-analyses (Luo et al. 2018). If a lesion has BI-RADS3 grayscale appearances and is soft at SWE the malignancy rate is <1% and in a published series of over 700 symptomatic breast masses no cancers had benign grayscale and SWE features (Giannotti et al. 2016). Given these facts, short-term follow-up of BI-RADS 3 lesions which are also soft on SWE is not required and could bring about considerable saving of healthcare costs and be more convenient and reassuring for patients.

SWE has also been shown to be useful during second-look US after lesion detection on MRI, allowing a number of benign lesions to avoid biopsy (Au et al. 2019).

2.3.9.1 Nodal Metastasis and SWE

Nodal metastases from breast cancer are not much stiffer than normal nodal tissue probably due to the limited stromal reaction to tumor cells in lymph nodes. This makes SWE of axillary nodes in breast cancer patients less accurate than determining the nature of a primary breast lesion (Zhao et al. 2018).

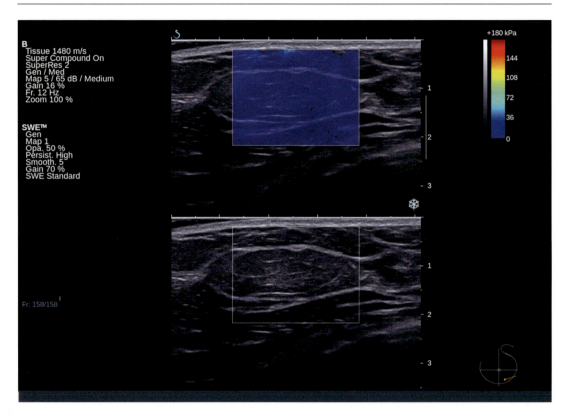

Fig. 5 Typical image of a fibroadenoma at SWE showing uniform soft appearance in a 26-year-old woman

The stiffness of the primary tumor on SWE is however a powerful predictor of nodal metastases even when corrected for tumor size, tumor grade, and vascular invasion status. The nodal metastasis rate in tumors which have a mean stiffness less than 50 kPa is only 5% while in tumors with a mean stiffness of over 200 kPa the nodal metastasis rate is around 40%. The reason why stiff tumors have a high rate of nodal metastasis is because the activated stroma seen in stiff tumors promotes neo-angiogenesis and stromal invasion which are required for nodal metastasis to occur (Evans et al. 2014). In the future stiffness of the primary tumor could be included in an algorithm to identify patients at very low risk of axillary metastasis who may be spared axillary surgery.

2.3.10 SWE Elastography in Women Receiving Neoadjuvant Chemotherapy (NACT)

A number of studies have shown that tumors which are stiff on SWE are more resistant to NACT than breast cancers which are soft. The association though definite is quite weak and patients should not be denied NACT because their cancer is stiff at SWE. The reason for this association is linked to the important part tumor stromal interactions have in defining the response of breast cancer to NACT. A number of studies have shown that stromal gene signatures are as important in predicting resistance to NACT as epithelial gene signatures. Given that stromal gene signatures influence collagen production, turnover, and structure, it is not surprising that stiffness at SWE has an association with response to NACT.

A number of studies have shown that changes in stiffness from baseline at interim and at the end of the treatment are helpful in predicting the response to NACT at the end of the treatment (Shin et al. 2019; Evans et al. 2018b) (Fig. 7). This is because tumor-free areas of fibrosis in women whose tumors have had a pathological complete response appear to be softer than

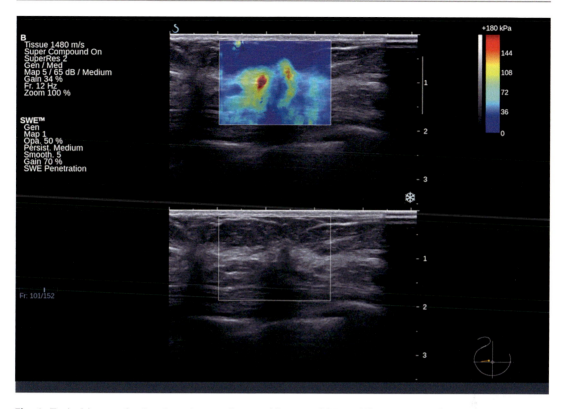

Fig. 6 Typical image of a ductal carcinoma of no specific type of SWE stiffness most marked at the tumor stromal border. The lesion was grade 3 and the patient was a 46-year-old woman

masses containing residual tumor. SWE is particularly helpful at interim scanning where it outperforms both grayscale US and standard MRI assessment in predicting final pathological response (Evans et al. 2018a). At the end of the treatment, MRI is the most useful in predicting response but a reduction in stiffness at SWE and US diameter combined is not statistically inferior to standard MRI assessment.

SWE also has the advantage over MRI in terms of cost, time, and convenience and availability.

2.3.11 SWE and Neoadjuvant Hormone Therapy

Little has been published on this topic but the author has found no relationship between the baseline stiffness of invasive breast cancer and its response to neoadjuvant hormone therapy. It is not clear whether SWE adds to the accuracy of response assessment by grayscale ultrasound.

2.3.12 SWE and the Prognosis of Breast Cancer

As has been previously mentioned increased stiffness of breast cancer is associated with many known poor prognostic factors such as large invasive size, nodal involvement, high histological grade, and lympho-vascular invasion. In addition stiffness at SWE is associated with resistance to chemotherapy.

Unlike these classical prognostic factors which are only fully available following resection of the cancer, stiffness at SWE is available preoperatively. It has recently been shown that stiffness at SWE is a strong prognostic factor and that it is independent of other preoperative prognostic indicators such as ultrasound size, core biopsy grade, preoperative nodal status, ER status, and presentation (screening or symptomatic) (Evans et al. 2018c) (Fig. 8). It is possible that stiffness at SWE could be part of a preoperative prognostic index which could be used when con-

2.3.13 Fibroepithelial Lesions

Whilst most fibroadenomas are soft, a proportion of particularly larger lesions are stiff. There is a gradual rise in average stiffness from fibroadenomas, through benign and indeterminate phyllodes tumors to malignant phyllodes tumors. Most breast sarcomas are very stiff.

2.3.14 Unusual Breast Malignancies

Metastases to the breast are less stiff than invasive breast cancers. Lymphoma and leukemia are also often soft or only slightly stiff. This is probably because these malignancies are associated with either no or minor stromal reactions.

3 Ultrasound Assessment of Lesion Vascularity

3.1 Doppler

Color and power Doppler are routinely used during breast US examinations. Their main use is to differentiate between a cyst with echogenic contents and a solid lesion which requires biopsy.

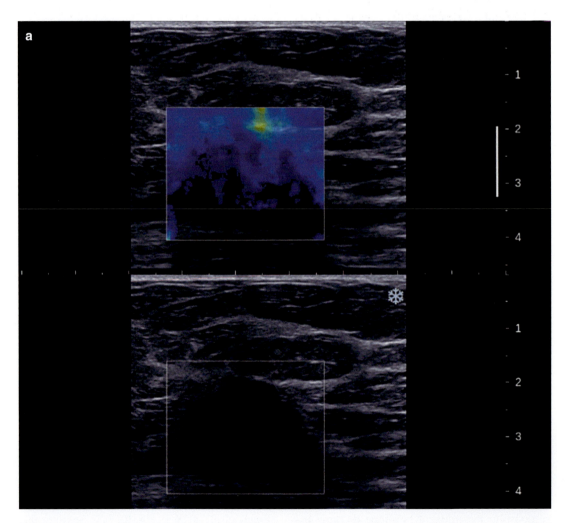

Fig. 7 (**a**) Pre-chemotherapy image of a grade 3 triple-negative carcinoma in a 53-year-old woman showing stiffness at SWE. (**b**) Interim SWE imaging after three cycles of chemotherapy showing a residual mass but no residual stiffness. At completion of chemotherapy the patient had a complete pathological response

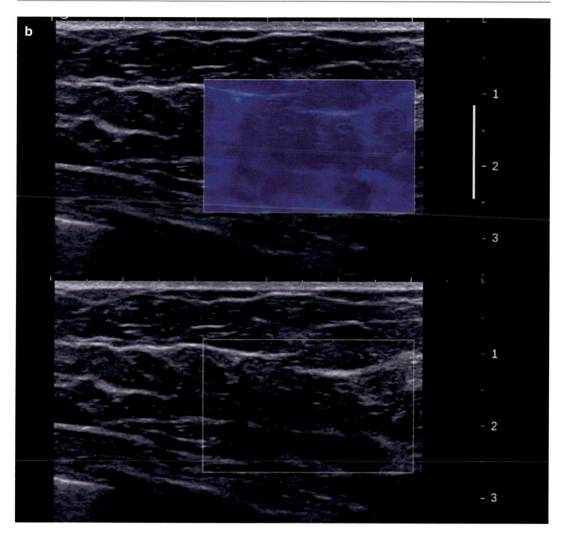

Fig. 7 (continued)

Other uses include differentiating a solid intracystic filling defect due to a cancer or papilloma from mass-like debris and identifying pus in women with breast infections prior to aspiration.

In the past, Doppler was used to aid benign/malignant differentiation of solid breast lesions as cancers have more central/penetrating vessels than fibroadenomas which often have vessels around the capsule of the lesion. A recent study showed that the sensitivity, specificity, PPV, and NPV of the presence of intratumoral penetrating vessels in predicting malignancy were 76.5%, 80.0%, 76.5%, and 80.0%, respectively (Ibrahim et al. 2016). Quantitative indices showing differences between malignant and benign lesions include peak blood flow velocity (Vmax), resistance index (RI), pulsatility index (PI), and blood flow classification (Song et al. 2020). Decreased RI and increased Vmax have been shown to be correlated with angiogenesis, proliferation, and tumor suppression in breast cancer (Niu et al. 2019).

A recent study showed that color Doppler had a sensitivity of 81.8% and specificity of 66.2% with AUC of 0.78. Color Doppler scoring detected malignant lesions with a diagnostic accuracy of 48.0% and did not improve on gray-scale assessment (Ranjkesh et al. 2020). The use

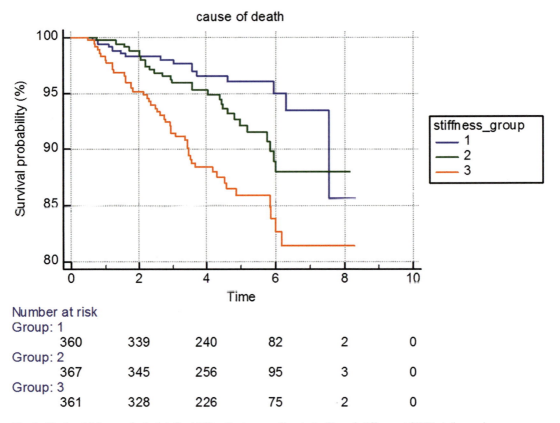

Fig. 8 Kaplan-Meier survival plots for 1100 patients according to tertiles of stiffness at SWE at diagnosis

of core biopsy and overlap of the Doppler features of benign and malignant breast lesions has meant a decline in the use of Doppler to aid benign/malignant differentiation.

3.2 Contrast-Enhanced Ultrasound

Contrast-enhanced ultrasound (CEUS) is a technique which uses a bolus intravenous injection of microbubble contrast agents to enhance vessel conspicuity of US examination. The use of contrast-specific examination modes and second-generation contrast agents has led to a resurgence of interest in CEUS and the breast. These low-solubility gases circulate in the blood with a more marked and longer signal enhancement, allowing more detailed evaluation. CEUS allows both quantitative and qualitative evaluation of lesion vascularity (Park and Seo 2018).

The use of CEUS has been shown to improve the diagnostic performance of breast ultrasound. Its use in detecting early response of breast cancer to neoadjuvant therapy looks encouraging (Jia et al. 2019).

3.3 Superb Microvascular Imaging

Superb microvascular imaging (SMI) is a new ultrasound technique which shows lesion vascularity with a similar clarity to that seen when using intravascular US contrast agents. SMI is a Doppler technique that adopts an advanced filter system to separate low-flow signals from artifacts. SMI provides two modes of vascular imaging: color and monochrome. It has been shown to improve benign/malignant differentiation of solid breast lesions and is complementary to the use of SWE (Zhu et al. 2018b).

Quantitative analysis of tumor vascularity recently became possible by calculating the vascular index. The vascular index is the ratio between the pixels for the Doppler signal and those for the entire lesion. Such quantification may be useful in determining the early response of cancer to neoadjuvant systemic therapy.

References

Au FW, Ghai S, Lu FI, Lu H (2019) Clinical value of shear wave elastography added to targeted ultrasound (second-look ultrasound) in the evaluation of breast lesions suspicious of malignancy detected on magnetic resonance imaging. J Ultrasound Med. https://doi.org/10.1002/jum.14936

Barr RG, De Silvestri A, Scotti V, Manzoni F, Rebuffi C, Capittini C, Tinelli C (2018) Diagnostic performance and accuracy of the 3 interpreting methods of breast strain elastography: a systematic review and meta-analysis. J Ultrasound Med. https://doi.org/10.1002/jum.14849

Chen YL, Gao Y, Chang C, Wang F, Zeng W, Chen JJ (2018) Ultrasound shear wave elastography of breast lesions: correlation of anisotropy with clinical and histopathological findings. Cancer Imaging 18(1):11

Elseedawy M, Whelehan P, Vinnicombe S, Thomson K, Evans A (2016) Factors influencing the stiffness of fibroadenomas at shear wave elastography. Clin Radiol 71(1):92–95

Evans A, Whelehan P, Thomson K, Brauer K, Jordan L, Purdie C, McLean D, Baker L, Vinnicombe S, Thompson A (2012) Differentiating benign from malignant solid breast masses: value of shear wave elastography according to lesion stiffness combined with gray scale ultrasound according to BI-RADS classification. Br J Cancer 107(2):224–229

Evans A, Rauchhaus P, Whelehan P, Thomson K, Purdie CA, Jordan LB, Michie CO, Thompson AM, Vinnicombe S (2014) Does shear wave ultrasound independently predict axillary lymph node metastasis in women with invasive breast cancer? Breast Cancer Res Treat 143(1):153–157

Evans A, Sim YT, Thomson K, Jordan L, Purdie C, Vinnicombe SJ (2016) Shear wave elastography of breast cancer: sensitivity according to histological type in a large cohort. Breast 26:115–118

Evans A, Whelehan P, Thompson A, Purdie C, Jordan L, Macaskill J, Henderson S, Vinnicombe S (2018a) Identification of pathological complete response after neoadjuvant chemotherapy for breast cancer: comparison of greyscale ultrasound, shear wave elastography, and MRI. Clin Radiol 73(10):910.e1–910.e6

Evans A, Whelehan P, Thompson AM, Purdie CA, Jordan LB, Macaskill EJ, Waugh S, Fuller-Pace F, Brauer K, Vinnicombe S (2018b) Prediction of pathological complete response to neoadjuvant chemotherapy for primary breast cancer comparing interim ultrasound, shear wave elastography and MRI. Ultraschall Med 39:422–431

Evans A, Sim Y, Pourreyron C, Thompson A, Jordan L, Fleming D, Purdie C, Macaskill J, Vinnicombe S, Pharoah P (2018c) Pre-operative stromal stiffness measured by shear wave elastography is independently associated with breast cancer-specific survival. Breast Cancer Res Treat 171(2):383–389

Giannotti E, Vinnicombe S, Thomson K, McLean D, Purdie C, Lee J, Evans A (2016) Shear wave elastography and grey scale assessment of palpable probably benign masses: is biopsy always required? Br J Radiol 89(1062):20150865

Ibrahim R, Rahmat K, Fadzli F et al (2016) Evaluation of solid breast lesions with power Doppler: value of penetrating vessels as a predictor of malignancy. Singapore Med J 57(11):634–640. https://doi.org/10.11622/smedj.2016001

Jia K, Li L, Wu XJ, Hao MJ, Xue HY (2019) Contrast-enhanced ultrasound for evaluating the pathologic response of breast cancer to neoadjuvant chemotherapy: a meta-analysis. Medicine 98(4):e14258. https://doi.org/10.1097/MD.0000000000014258

Lee SH, Chang JM, Kim WH, Bae MS, Cho N, Yi A, Koo HR, Kim SJ, Kim JY, Moon WK (2013) Differentiation of benign from malignant solid breast masses: comparison of two-dimensional and three-dimensional shear-wave elastography. Eur Radiol 23(4):1015–1026

Luo J, Cao Y, Nian W, Zeng X, Zhang H, Yue Y, Yu F (2018) Benefit of shear-wave elastography in the differential diagnosis of breast lesion: a diagnostic meta-analysis. Med Ultrason 1(1):43–49

Moon JH, Hwang JY, Park JS, Koh SH, Park SY (2018) Impact of region of interest (ROI) size on the diagnostic performance of shear wave elastography in differentiating solid breast lesions. Acta Radiol 59(6):657–663

Mullen R, Thompson JM, Moussa O, Vinnicombe S, Evans A (2014) Shear-wave elastography contributes to accurate tumour size estimation when assessing small breast cancers. Clin Radiol 69(12):1259–1263

Niu J, Ma J, Guan X, Zhao X, Li P, Zhang M (2019) Correlation between Doppler ultrasound blood flow parameters and angiogenesis and proliferation activity in breast cancer. Med Sci Monit 25:7035–7041. https://doi.org/10.12659/MSM.914395

Park AY, Seo BK (2018) Up-to-date Doppler techniques for breast tumor vascularity: superb microvascular imaging and contrast-enhanced ultrasound. Ultrasonography 37(2):98–106

Ranjkesh M, Hajibonabi F, Seifar F, Tarzamni MK, Moradi B, Khamnian Z (2020) Diagnostic value of elastography, strain ratio, and elasticity to B-mode ratio and color Doppler ultrasonography in breast lesions. Int J Gen Med 13:215–224. https://doi.org/10.2147/IJGM.S247980

Shang J, Ruan LT, Wang YY, Zhang XJ, Dang Y, Liu B, Wang WL, Song Y, Chang SJ (2019) Utilizing size-based thresholds of stiffness gradient to reclassify BI-RADS category 3-4b lesions increases diagnostic performance. Clin Radiol 74(4):306–313

Shi XQ, Li J, Qian L, Xue X, Li J, Wan W (2018) Correlation between elastic parameters and collagen fibre features in breast lesions. Clin Radiol 73(6):595.e1–595.e7

Shin YJ, Kim SM, Yun B, Jang M, Kim B, Lee SH (2019) Predictors of invasive breast cancer in patients with ductal carcinoma in situ in ultrasound-guided core needle biopsy. J Ultrasound Med 38(2):481–488

Sim YT, Vinnicombe S, Whelehan P, Thomson K, Evans A (2015) Value of shear-wave elastography in the diagnosis of symptomatic invasive lobular breast cancer. Clin Radiol 70:604–609

Song X, Liang B, Wang C, Shi S (2020) Clinical value of color Doppler ultrasound combined with serum CA153, CEA and TSGF detection in the diagnosis

of breast cancer. Exp Ther Med 20(2):1822–1828. https://doi.org/10.3892/etm.2020.8868

Yoon JH, Ko KH, Jung HK, Lee JT (2013) Qualitative pattern classification of shear wave elastography for breast masses: how it correlates to quantitative measurements. Eur J Radiol 82(12):2199–2204

Zhao Q, Sun JW, Zhou H, Du LY, Wang XL, Tao L, Jiang ZP, Zhou XL (2018) Pre-operative conventional ultrasound and sonoelastography evaluation for predicting axillary lymph node metastasis in patients with malignant breast lesions. Ultrasound Med Biol 44(12):2587–2595

Zhu YC, Zhang Y, Deng SH, Jiang Q, Wang DS (2018a) Correlation between histopathological grading and shear wave elastography in evaluating invasive carcinoma of no special type. Exp Ther Med 16(6):4700–4706

Zhu YC, Zhang Y, Deng SH, Jiang Q (2018b) Diagnostic performance of superb microvascular imaging (SMI) combined with shear-wave elastography in evaluating breast lesions. Med Sci Monit 24:5935–5942

Automated Breast Ultrasound

Ritse M. Mann

Contents

1   **Technique** 128

2   **Image Evaluation** 128
    2.1   Normal Findings and Artifacts 129
    2.2   Characteristics of Breast Lesions 131

3   **Potential in Screening** 132

4   **Potential in Staging and Therapy Monitoring** 134

5   **AI for ABUS** 136

6   **Future Perspectives** 138

References 138

Abstract

Automated breast ultrasound (ABUS) has primarily been developed as a screening tool for dense breasts. It makes use of a wide transducer and a standardized acquisition protocol in order to create reproducible evaluations of the breasts. This enables image acquisition by technicians and batch reading of screening examinations. The documented yield in a screening setting is between 2 and 7 per 1000 examinations. Unfortunately, using ABUS for screening will also yield substantial amounts of previously undetected benign lesions that are somewhat more difficult to classify than lesions observed on standard handheld ultrasound. It is therefore essential to use all available information to accurately classify a breast lesion in order to prevent too many false-positive examinations. ABUS can also be used to stage breast cancers, as it provides a very nice overview of the breast structure, commonly better showing the extent of a cancer than conventional ultrasound techniques. However, it should be noted that diffuse

R. M. Mann (✉)
Department of Medical Imaging, Radboud University
Medical Center, Nijmegen, The Netherlands

Department of Radiology, The Netherlands Cancer
Institute, Amsterdam, The Netherlands
e-mail: Ritse.Mann@radboudumc.nl

© Springer Nature Switzerland AG 2022
M. Fuchsjäger et al. (eds.), *Breast Imaging*, Medical Radiology Diagnostic Imaging,
https://doi.org/10.1007/978-3-030-94918-1_7

lesions and particularly extensive intraductal components are sometimes still hard to see on ABUS examinations. Finally, AI applications are under development to increase the ease of evaluation of ABUS studies. While they are currently not yet as good as human observers, they may already be used to increase the speed of evaluation without reducing the examination accuracy.

1 Technique

Automated breast ultrasound (ABUS) was developed as a method for systematic evaluation of the breast using ultrasound. It is a modification of handheld ultrasound that is primarily a targeted technique. Early implementations of this idea consist of a standard transducer in a bag of water that is moved over the breast by a mechanical arm. The first prototype systems were already developed by the late 1960s (Dempsey 2004).

Only recently ABUS systems have become commercially available. The major difference between the early systems and the currently available commercial systems is that the transducer has been adapted for the specific task of whole-breast evaluation (Shin et al. 2015).

To this end, the transducers have become much wider to cover a large section of the breast at once. In addition, one of the vendors has created a slightly convex transducer in order to better fit the breast shape. Most systems make use of a frame that is positioned on the breast with the woman in a supine or slightly rotated position in order to optimize the transducer-skin contact surface. The dedicated transducer is subsequently automatically moved within the frame. In order to ensure good skin contact a relatively fluid lotion (as opposed to the more sticky ultrasound gel) is used (van Zelst and Mann 2018).

To set the depth and focus of the ABUS machine the breast cup size is entered. The used high-frequency transducers (up to 14 MHz) provide decent image quality up to 6 cm in depth, which is sufficient for most breasts in this position.

Currently none of the ABUS techniques allows imaging of the whole breast in one sweep. Instead, several sweeps over the breast are required to image all tissue. Standard views include an anterior-posterior view, centered on the nipple; a lateral view, which includes the axillary tail; and a medial view (Fig. 1). It is advisable to include the nipple in all views as a point of reference, and also because the nipple-areolar complex may cause significant shadowing and consequently the breast area behind the nipple may be difficult to evaluate. In women with large or relatively firm breasts, the upper and lower central parts of the breast may not be entirely covered by the three views above, and consequently additional superior and/or inferior views may be obtained. Each obtained view consists of a volume of approximately 300–400 stacked transversal images of the breast, with a slice thickness of about 0.5 mm. Acquiring one view takes approximately 1 min. Hence a bilateral examination takes at least 6 min plus the time needed for positioning. However, the standardized protocols for the acquisition of bilateral ABUS allow image acquisition by nonradiologists after a short training course, which reduces interobserver variability and dependence of the technique on experience (Barr et al. 2017). It also enables current-prior comparison and allows for batch reading of screening examinations (Fig. 2). ABUS acquisition is in general well tolerated by women, and is regarded as being less uncomfortable than mammography by the majority of women (Smith et al. 2019), albeit particularly in very thin women the examination can still be painful.

2 Image Evaluation

To read ABUS images, the use of a dedicated workstation for image evaluation is strongly advised. This workstation should allow multiplanar reformatting of the volumetric views (van Zelst and Mann 2018). Especially the coronal plane has been shown very useful for image interpretation, speeding up the assessment and improving the differentiation between benign

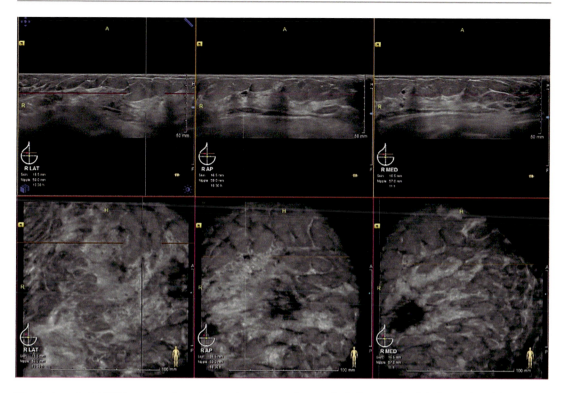

Fig. 1 A typical ABUS scan consists of three views per breast: a lateral, an anterior-posterior, and a medial view. Images are obtained axially and can be reconstructed in coronal and sagittal orientations. This image shows the three typical views of the right breast in axial (top) and coronal (bottom) orientation. There is a small cyst present visible in both the AP and medial views

and malignant lesions (Chae et al. 2015). The latter is mainly achieved by evaluating the relation of the lesion and the surrounding tissue; a desmoplastic reaction leading to spiculation, as commonly observed in malignant lesions, is relatively well depicted in this plane. Sagittal reconstructions are useful for the determination of tumor extent and the differentiation of real lesions and artifacts. After a short learning curve the reading time for a bilateral ABUS acquisition amounts to between 2 and 9 min per case (Chae et al. 2015; van Zelst et al. 2018; Skaane et al. 2015).

2.1 Normal Findings and Artifacts

ABUS enables an excellent overview of the breast composition and therefore allows determination of the amount of fibroglandular tissue within the breast in a similar fashion as breast MRI. While no formal categories for ABUS have been designated, these can be reported in analogy to the MRI lexicon (i.e., almost entirely fatty, scattered fibroglandular tissue, heterogeneous fibroglandular tissue, and extreme fibroglandular tissue) rather than using the terminology designed for handheld breast ultrasound that describes more a focal appearance of fibroglandular tissue in the evaluated portion of the breast (Moon et al. 2011a; Chen et al. 2016).

The composition of the breast also leads to some artifacts that are common in ABUS, and that one must learn to discern from true lesions. A common finding is strong shadowing behind the nipple-areolar complex. In handheld ultrasound angulating the transducer usually solves this. However, with ABUS that is obviously not possible. Consequently, assessment of this area in multiple views is mandatory to improve the sensitivity for lesions in this area (van Zelst and Mann 2018).

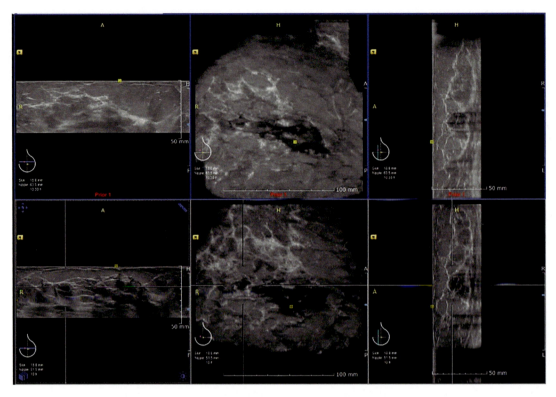

Fig. 2 When the same views are structurally obtained it is possible to compare ABUS scans to prior acquisitions easily. In this case the AP view of the left breast of the new ABUS acquisition is shown in the lower frames (axial, coronal, and sagittal from left to right), whereas the examination from 1 year ago is shown in the upper frames. The resemblance is remarkable

Likewise Cooper's ligaments may cause "wandering shadows" throughout the breast. These are caused by the tangential orientation of the ligaments to the transducer; shadows are strongest when the angle is approximately 45°. The shadows obviously follow the ligaments, and therefore "wander" through the breast, which can be used to differentiate them from true lesions. This phenomenon is also not common in handheld ultrasound, as the operator is usually capable of angulating the transducer in such a way that the ultrasound beam is perpendicular to the ligament.

Other typical artifacts of ABUS are caused by respiration, and may distort the dorsal coronal reconstructions, as the findings in these images may then in reality not be present at the same depth. This is best seen as a sort of sinusoidal wave pattern in the sagittal reconstructions. To avoid this type of artifact it is important to instruct women to breath shallowly during the acquisition, and avoid talking.

A particular problematic artifact that may sometimes be present is a skipped lesion (Fig. 3). This may occur when a relatively loose lesion in the breast is located relatively close to the skin. The motion of the transducer will push the lesion ahead of the transducer, since the surrounding tissue is easier to compress. At a certain point in time, the lesion cannot be pushed further and slips under the transducer to the other side. In the worst case, the lesion is subsequently not visualized at all, albeit this happens only rarely. Nonetheless one should be aware of the possibility and when a clearly palpable lesion is not seen repeat a handheld ultrasound examination of the palpable finding. In general the most common reason for non-detection of lesions is shadowing

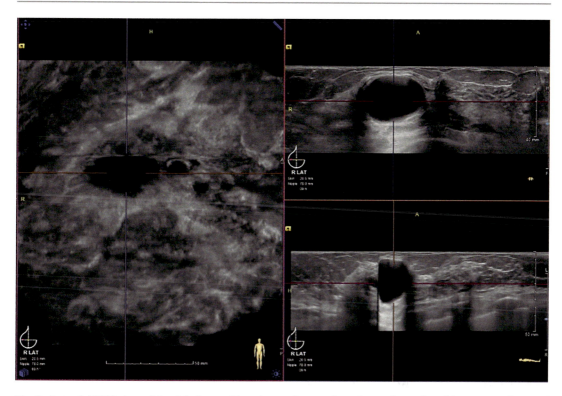

Fig. 3 Lateral ABUS view of the right breast. There is a large cyst present just subcutaneously. This has caused a "jump artifact." Due to the stiffness of the lesion, the transducer motion is temporarily blocked; subsequently, the transducer jumps forward, and hence a small part of the breast is not imaged. This effect is best seen in the sagittal view (lower right corner)

due to fibrotic tissue, or a very peripheral lesion location (van Zelst and Mann 2018; Grubstein et al. 2017).

2.2 Characteristics of Breast Lesions

Since ABUS is essentially just b-mode ultrasound, lesions can be evaluated in a similar manner as when using conventional breast ultrasound (Figs. 4, 5, and 6). Lesions are evaluated by their shape, margin, internal echo pattern, orientation, presence of an echogenic halo, and effect on the surrounding tissue (Choi et al. 2018; Vourtsis and Kachulis 2018).

In ABUS, large numbers of small, oval, circumscribed horizontally oriented lesions with a relatively uniform hypoechoic internal ultrasound pattern are present. These lesions correspond to small cysts that appear not entirely black due to the simple fact that the imaging settings are not optimized for their specific evaluation. Hence, they may be either present in a tangential orientation or imaged just out of focus. Albeit it is impossible to recall all these tiny cysts, some small, but highly aggressive, cancers may have a similar appearance, and may therefore potentially be overlooked. Close evaluation of morphological features (e.g., shape and orientation) may facilitate accurate lesion classification (van Zelst et al. 2017a).

The coronal plane also provides handholds for improving the accuracy of lesion classification. In this plane the effect of a lesion on the surrounding tissue is well appreciated. Malignant lesions are in general attached to the surrounding tissue and consequently a spiculation and retraction pattern are typically observed around malignant lesions, whereas this is not present around

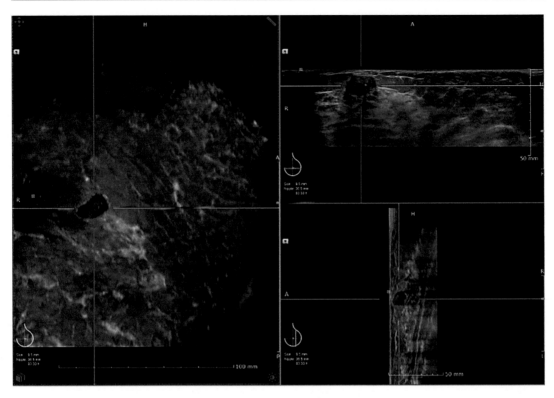

Fig. 4 Lateral view of the left breast of a 53-year-old woman. There is an oval, sharp, homogeneous mass present within the crosshair. This is a typical (biopsy-proven) fibroadenoma. Note the resemblance with the typical appearance of fibroadenomas on handheld ultrasound

benign lesions (Van Zelst et al. 2015; Zheng et al. 2015) (Fig. 6).

It should be noted that such a retraction pattern is most visible in relatively indolent tumors; that is, it is strongest in luminal A cancers, and least strong in triple-negative cancers, leading to a lower sensitivity for more aggressive cancers than that for more indolent cancers, as is also commonly reported for other anatomy-based imaging techniques (in particular mammography) (Zheng et al. 2017; van Zelst et al. 2017b). Larger cysts, which present as well-circumscribed oval black lesions and fibroadenomas (oval hypoechoic well-circumscribed masses), usually show no retraction at all. Obviously, a very strong retraction pattern is observed around scars (Fig. 7). However, in general there should be no central mass in pure scars, and it should be possible to follow the lesion to the skin (usually very well visible in the most anterior coronal slice).

The accuracy of lesion classification using ABUS has been reported to be similar to that of handheld ultrasound (Barr et al. 2017; Choi et al. 2018; Golatta et al. 2013), albeit in some studies the classification properties of ABUS seem even better than those of handheld ultrasound, likely due to the visualization of architectural distortion in the coronal plane (Vourtsis and Kachulis 2018; Zhang et al. 2018).

3 Potential in Screening

ABUS is primarily designed as a supplemental screening tool for women in whom mammographic screening is insufficient. In particular women with a relatively large amount of fibroglandular tissue, i.e., dense breasts (mostly younger women), are at risk of having breast cancer that is not recognized during mammographic

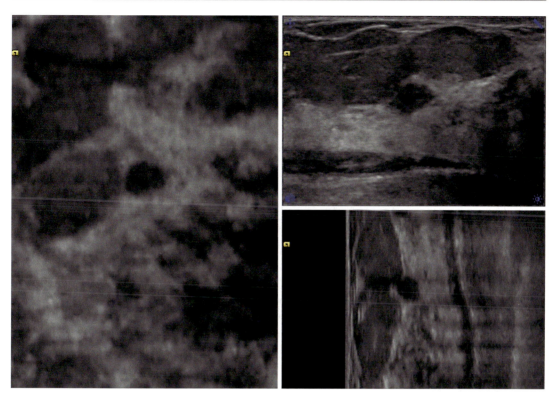

Fig. 5 Thirty-seven-year-old woman presenting with a palpable lump in the right breast. This is a zoomed-in AP view of the symptomatic area showing a small oval mass with slightly angulated margins and no posterior acoustic features. Note that in the coronal view there is no effect of the lesion on the surrounding breast parenchyma. This turned out to be a small fibroadenoma on biopsy

screening (Wanders et al. 2017a; Weigel et al. 2017). Large compact patches of fibroglandular breast tissue may mask underlying breast cancers on a two-dimensional mammogram (Wanders et al. 2017b). The sensitivity of population-based mammographic screening in women with extremely dense breasts is reported to be as low as 61% with an interval cancer rate of 4.4% compared to 85.7% and 0.7%, respectively, for women with fatty breasts in the population of women at average risk for the development of breast cancer (Wanders et al. 2017b).

There is mounting evidence that supplemental breast US detects two to five mammography occult early-stage breast cancers per 1000 screens in asymptomatic women with dense breasts at various risk levels in a wide range of ages (Berg et al. 2008; Ohuchi et al. 2016; Buchberger et al. 2018; Kolb et al. 2002). In addition, early reports indicate that detecting mammographically occult cancers with breast US reduces the number of interval cancers in subsequent screening rounds in women with dense breasts (Ohuchi et al. 2016; Corsetti et al. 2011). Similar to handheld breast US, supplemental ABUS screening has also been shown to detect mammographically occult early-stage breast cancers (2–7 per 1000 screening rounds) (Vourtsis and Kachulis 2018; Wilczek et al. 2016; Brem et al. 2015; Choi et al. 2014; Giuliano and Giuliano 2013) (Fig. 8). The large advantage of ABUS over handheld ultrasound in this setting is that the examinations can be obtained by a radiographer and read-in batches, improving the efficiency of ultrasound screening, as initial studies reported approximately 31-min evaluation time for bilateral handheld ultrasound in screening (Berg et al. 2008). The systematic evaluation of the breast also allows much easier comparison of

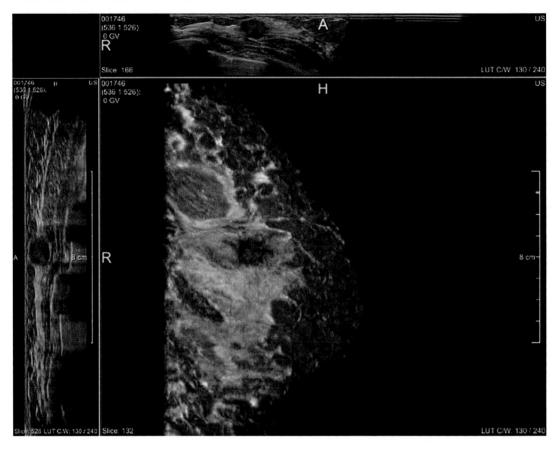

Fig. 6 Lateral view of the right breast of a 62-year-old woman with heterogeneously dense breasts. She presented with a palpable mass. There is an oval mass with irregular margin visualized at the location of the abnormality. Note the spiculation within the surrounding tissue, which is most evident at the coronal view. This turned out to be a 2 cm Her2+ invasive ductal carcinoma

obtained acquisitions to prior images, although the actual value of this in clinical practice has not yet been shown. It has been reported that supplemental ABUS reduces the frequency of advanced cancers, when compared to mammography screening alone (31% vs. 40% reduction as compared to no screening, respectively) (Grady et al. 2017). The downside of supplemental screening with either handheld US or ABUS is that it also leads to an increase in recalls for benign abnormalities (Vourtsis and Kachulis 2018; Wilczek et al. 2016; Brem et al. 2015; Choi et al. 2014; Giuliano and Giuliano 2013). In this respect it should be noted that supplemental ultrasound screening, either by hand or with ABUS, appears to have very limited value in women screened with MRI, as it mainly leads to an increase in false-positive recalls (Mann et al. 2019).

4 Potential in Staging and Therapy Monitoring

The helicopter view of the breast that is provided by ABUS also enables capturing large cross sections of cancer in one plane, which can be used for the estimation of disease extent. In initial pilot studies the performance of ABUS for size and volumetric assessment is as good as that of breast MRI (Clauser et al. 2014; Lagendijk et al. 2018), although a larger and more recent study showed that ABUS improved upon handheld ultrasound

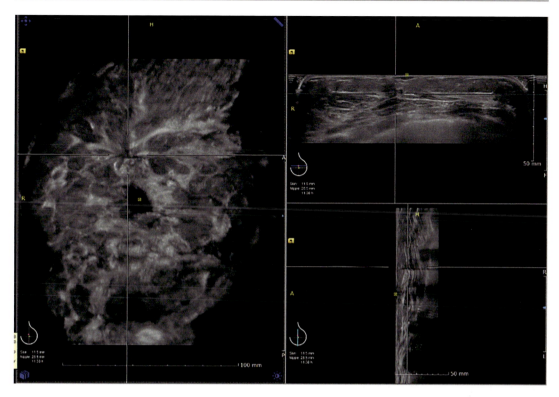

Fig. 7 AP view of the left breast in three directions. This 46-year-old woman had a history of prior breast surgery for a T1c invasive ductal carcinoma 3 years earlier. There is a clear scar present, which is most evident in the coronal reconstruction as it gives particularly in this direction a large architectural distortion. Note that there is no central mass, as such a retraction phenomenon is also commonly seen in lower grade malignant lesions

(ICC 0.85 vs. 0.75), but was still worse than breast MRI (ICC 0.93) (Girometti et al. 2018a). ABUS may miss additional tumor foci and extensive intraductal components, as these are less evident in ultrasound acquisitions, even when combined with digital breast tomosynthesis (Girometti et al. 2018b). However, in one study it was stated that ABUS is significantly better for the evaluation of the extent of pure ductal carcinoma in situ lesions than handheld ultrasound (Huang et al. 2016). In addition, there are certain advantages in ABUS for cancer staging as the acquisition position resembles the positioning of the patient at surgery, and therefore the findings are easier to transfer to the surgical plan than findings from breast MRI.

The overview of the breast also enables the use of ABUS for therapy monitoring and response prediction in women with breast cancer treated with some form of primary systemic therapy. Available studies are currently very small, but it was reported that mid-treatment response evaluations can quite accurately predict eventual pathological complete response, with best results using the product of perpendicular diameters in the axial or coronal plane. A reduction of 50% or more has a sensitivity of 85% predicting pCR (Wang et al. 2016). The correlation of ABUS and MRI measurements in this setting was shown to be good (van Egdom et al. 2018), whereas patients seemed to prefer ABUS over MRI for follow-up. However, contradictory results were reported in other recent studies in which MRI still outperformed ABUS, as well as digital breast tomosynthesis and mammography (Park et al. 2018; D'Angelo et al. 2019). Overall, it seems of paramount importance that more data becomes available. At this point in time it seems however safe to presume that ABUS is a viable alternative to MRI when there are clear contraindications for the latter.

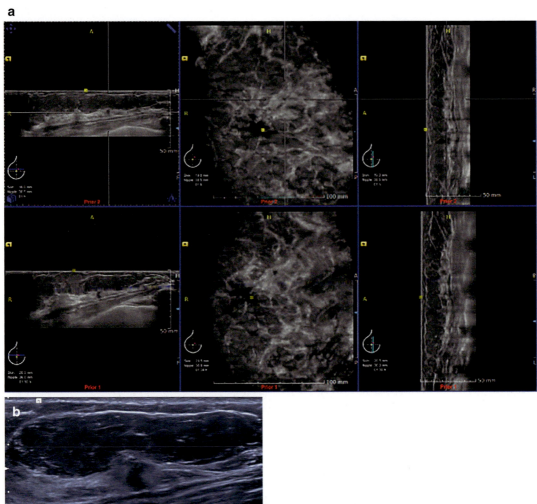

Fig. 8 Forty-three-year-old woman with very dense breasts screened because of familial risk with mammography and supplemental ABUS. (**a**) The AP view of the left breast is shown. The top row shows the exam from 1 year ago, and the lower row shows the current examination (labeled prior 1, because there is also an additional handheld examination in the system). In the upper outer quadrant of the left breast there is a small irregular mass, taller than wide, that seems to distort the surrounding tissue. The lesion has clearly grown since the last examination (in which it was not recalled). This turned out to be a 12 mm invasive ductal carcinoma. In (**b**) the corresponding handheld ultrasound image is shown, which strongly resembles its ABUS appearance

5   AI for ABUS

The reading of ABUS can be done behind a computer station and in recent studies takes no more than approximately 2–3 min per case (van Zelst et al. 2018; Huppe et al. 2018); still for breast screening this is substantial as the time needed to read one screening mammogram is below 1 min. This is due to the fact that there are still a lot of images that need to be read. Moreover, the presence of artifacts and the detection of many benign abnormalities such as small cysts make the reading of ABUS error prone. Unsurprisingly, many studies therefore have focused on the development of automated lesion detection and classification techniques for ABUS. Initial studies were mainly aimed at the classification of lesions detected by radiologists (i.e., CADx), and showed that shape and spiculation features can be used for accurate automated discrimination between benign and malignant lesions (Moon et al. 2011b, 2012; Tan et al. 2012). Other studies aimed at automatically segmenting the chest wall from ABUS images (Tan et al. 2013; Huisman and Karssemeijer 2007). This has the advantage that from the remaining volume a minimum-intensity projection can be made, in which cancers, that are in general hypoechoic in ultrasound images, stand out as dark spots (Fig. 9). Several other more recent studies focused on the automated detection and segmentation of lesions in ABUS volumes, showing high sensitivities at acceptable false-positive rates (Golatta et al. 2016; Sreekumari et al. 2016; Kozegar et al. 2018; Liu et al. 2018). In one study automated analysis of breast density obtained from ABUS images was compared to acquisitions from breast MRI, showing a strong correlation between these two methods, thus confirming that whole-breast density can be inferred from these kind of images (Chen et al. 2016). Furthermore a classification system for the automated detection of ABUS acquisitions of inferior quality was presented (Schwaab et al. 2016). Most computer-aided detection and diagnosis systems are based upon handcrafted features, as the small datasets available have prevented extensive use of the currently much more successful deep learning techniques. An initial study using deep learning

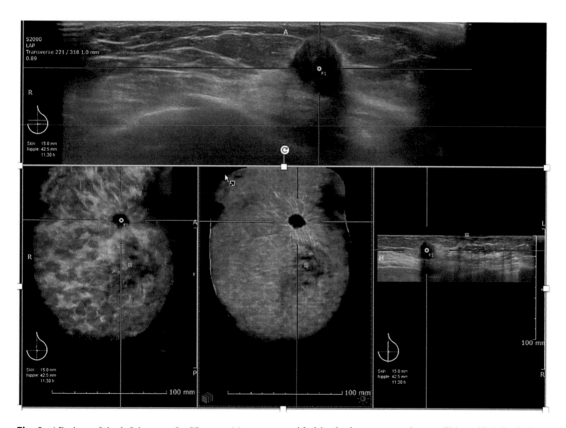

Fig. 9 AP view of the left breast of a 57-year-old woman with a large triple-negative breast cancer. The lesion is clearly recognizable in all views. However, to facilitate reading an AI-based minimum-intensity projection is provided in the lower center image. This artificially darkens relevant findings and shows all relevant findings of the entire image stack in one image, thus allowing faster evaluation

was recently published showing improvement in lesion detection over more conventional approaches and also released the images for further use by the community in order to enable further development of such deep learning-based systems (Yap et al. 2018, 2019). Another deep learning system was developed to prioritize findings in ABUS in order to allow radiologists to read the most suspicious findings first (Chiang et al. 2019). So far, however, most artificial intelligence approaches for ABUS have not yet left the research field. Still, some studies using a commercially available system that creates intelligent minimum-intensity projections using several of the abovementioned (feature based) techniques have been published. These studies unequivocally show that using such a CAD system currently already allows for a reduction of the reading time while preserving accuracy (van Zelst et al. 2018; Jiang et al. 2018; Xu et al. 2018).

6 Future Perspectives

Since ABUS is a relatively new modality, despite its long history, there is still a lot of ongoing development in this field. For example, recently a prone device was evaluated in which a mounted ultrasound probe scans the compressed breast in a clockwise fashion. Albeit the sensitivity was excellent the false-positive rate appears relatively high compared to handheld ultrasound (Farrokh et al. 2018). It also appears possible to use plane waves instead of line-by-line acquisition to dramatically speed up the image acquisition process, allowing for a single view to be obtained in seconds rather than the current acquisition time of about a minute (Hollander et al. 2016).

To enhance specificity several improvements are proposed. Already in 2008 the acquisition of 3D power Doppler volumes was proposed (Hsiao et al. 2008, 2009). Modern approaches combining this with ultrasensitive Doppler may allow for the creation of tumor vascular maps (Rocher et al. 2018). Likewise, integrating elastography, either by adjusting the compression force or by using shear waves, may improve the specificity of ABUS and reduce the recall rate for benign

findings (Sigrist et al. 2017). Several prototypes have been presented to enable this using automated breast ultrasound machines (Hendriks et al. 2016; Wang et al. 2017), albeit currently these studies are still phantom based.

A novel technique that has already been tested in patients is fusion of digital breast tomosynthesis and ABUS (Schaefgen et al. 2018; Larson et al. 2018). For this, dedicated compression paddles consisting of an US transparent membrane have been designed, which allow movement of the transducer over the compressed breast. The hybrid technique has the advantage that spatial co-registration of DBT and ABUS findings is ensured, and allows for example immediate dismissal of cysts detected on DBT that otherwise might have led to recall. Likewise mammographic patches of dense breast tissue may be scrutinized in detail for breast cancers that might otherwise be masked. Current issues, however, are that the compressed breast may be somewhat thicker than in a supine patient and ultrasound penetration might therefore be somewhat limited. Moreover compression is prolonged due to the slow motion of the US transducer. In addition, due to the curvature of the breast, some areas are not entirely covered by the US probe. Consequently, further developments are required before this technique can become clinically feasible.

References

Barr RG, DeVita R, Destounis S, Manzoni F, De Silvestri A, Tinelli C (2017) Agreement between an automated volume breast scanner and handheld ultrasound for diagnostic breast examinations. J Ultrasound Med 36(10):2087–2092

Berg WA, Blume JD, Cormack JB et al (2008) Combined screening with ultrasound and mammography vs mammography alone in women at elevated risk of breast cancer. JAMA 299(18):2151–2163

Brem RF, Tabar L, Duffy SW et al (2015) Assessing improvement in detection of breast cancer with three-dimensional automated breast US in women with dense breast tissue: the SomoInsight Study. Radiology 274(3):663–673

Buchberger W, Geiger-Gritsch S, Knapp R, Gautsch K, Oberaigner W (2018) Combined screening with mammography and ultrasound in a population-based screening program. Eur J Radiol 101:24–29

Chae EY, Cha JH, Kim HH, Shin HJ (2015) Comparison of lesion detection in the transverse and coronal views on automated breast sonography. J Ultrasound Med 34(1):125–135

Chen JH, Lee YW, Chan SW, Yeh DC, Chang RF (2016) Breast density analysis with automated whole-breast ultrasound: comparison with 3-D magnetic resonance imaging. Ultrasound Med Biol 42(5):1211–1220

Chiang TC, Huang YS, Chen RT, Huang CS, Chang RF (2019) Tumor detection in automated breast ultrasound using 3-D CNN and prioritized candidate aggregation. IEEE Trans Med Imaging 38(1):240–249

Choi WJ, Cha JH, Kim HH et al (2014) Comparison of automated breast volume scanning and hand-held ultrasound in the detection of breast cancer: an analysis of 5,566 patient evaluations. Asian Pac J Cancer Prev 15(21):9101–9105

Choi EJ, Choi H, Park EH, Song JS, Youk JH (2018) Evaluation of an automated breast volume scanner according to the fifth edition of BI-RADS for breast ultrasound compared with hand-held ultrasound. Eur J Radiol 99:138–145

Clauser P, Londero V, Como G, Girometti R, Bazzocchi M, Zuiani C (2014) Comparison between different imaging techniques in the evaluation of malignant breast lesions: can 3D ultrasound be useful? Radiol Med 119(4):240–248

Corsetti V, Houssami N, Ghirardi M et al (2011) Evidence of the effect of adjunct ultrasound screening in women with mammography-negative dense breasts: interval breast cancers at 1 year follow-up. Eur J Cancer 47(7):1021–1026

D'Angelo A, Rinaldi P, Belli P et al (2019) Usefulness of automated breast volume scanner (ABVS) for monitoring tumor response to neoadjuvant treatment in breast cancer patients: preliminary results. Eur Rev Med Pharmacol Sci 23(1):225–231

Dempsey PJ (2004) The history of breast ultrasound. J Ultrasound Med 23(7):887–894

Farrokh A, Erdonmez H, Schafer F, Maass N (2018) SOFIA: a novel automated breast ultrasound system used on patients in the prone position: a pilot study on lesion detection in comparison to handheld grayscale ultrasound. Geburtshilfe Frauenheilkd 78(5):499–505

Girometti R, Zanotel M, Londero V, Linda A, Lorenzon M, Zuiani C (2018a) Automated breast volume scanner (ABVS) in assessing breast cancer size: a comparison with conventional ultrasound and magnetic resonance imaging. Eur Radiol 28(3):1000–1008

Girometti R, Tomkova L, Cereser L, Zuiani C (2018b) Breast cancer staging: combined digital breast tomosynthesis and automated breast ultrasound versus magnetic resonance imaging. Eur J Radiol 107:188–195

Giuliano V, Giuliano C (2013) Improved breast cancer detection in asymptomatic women using 3D-automated breast ultrasound in mammographically dense breasts. Clin Imaging 37(3):480–486

Golatta M, Franz D, Harcos A et al (2013) Interobserver reliability of automated breast volume scanner (ABVS) interpretation and agreement of ABVS findings with hand held breast ultrasound (HHUS), mammography and pathology results. Eur J Radiol 82(8):e332–e336

Golatta M, Zeegers D, Filippatos K et al (2016) LECANDUS study (LEsion CANdidate Detection in UltraSound Data): evaluation of image analysis algorithms for breast lesion detection in volume ultrasound data. Arch Gynecol Obstet 294(2):423–428

Grady I, Chanisheva N, Vasquez T (2017) The addition of automated breast ultrasound to mammography in breast cancer screening decreases stage at diagnosis. Acad Radiol 24(12):1570–1574

Grubstein A, Rapson Y, Gadiel I, Cohen M (2017) Analysis of false-negative readings of automated breast ultrasound studies. J Clin Ultrasound 45(5):245–251

Hendriks GA, Hollander B, Menssen J, Milkowski A, Hansen HH, de Korte CL (2016) Automated 3D ultrasound elastography of the breast: a phantom validation study. Phys Med Biol 61(7):2665–2679

Hollander B, Hendriks GA, Mann RM, Hansen HH, de Korte CL (2016) Plane-wave compounding in automated breast volume scanning: a phantom-based study. Ultrasound Med Biol 42(10):2493–2503

Hsiao YH, Kuo SJ, Liang WM, Huang YL, Chen DR (2008) Intra-tumor flow index can predict the malignant potential of breast tumor: dependent on age and volume. Ultrasound Med Biol 34(1):88–95

Hsiao YH, Huang YL, Kuo SJ, Liang WM, Chen ST, Chen DR (2009) Characterization of benign and malignant solid breast masses in harmonic 3D power Doppler imaging. Eur J Radiol 71(1):89–95

Huang A, Zhu L, Tan Y et al (2016) Evaluation of automated breast volume scanner for breast conservation surgery in ductal carcinoma in situ. Oncol Lett 12(4):2481–2484

Huisman H, Karssemeijer N (2007) Chest wall segmentation in 3D breast ultrasound using a deformable volume model. Inf Process Med Imaging 20:245–256

Huppe AI, Inciardi MF, Redick M et al (2018) Automated breast ultrasound interpretation times: a reader performance study. Acad Radiol 25(12):1577–1581

Jiang Y, Inciardi MF, Edwards AV, Papaioannou J (2018) Interpretation time using a concurrent-read computer-aided detection system for automated breast ultrasound in breast cancer screening of women with dense breast tissue. AJR Am J Roentgenol 211(2): 452–461

Kolb TM, Lichy J, Newhouse JH (2002) Comparison of the performance of screening mammography, physical examination, and breast US and evaluation of factors that influence them: an analysis of 27,825 patient evaluations. Radiology 225(1):165–175

Kozegar E, Soryani M, Behnam H, Salamati M, Tan T (2018) Mass segmentation in automated 3-D breast ultrasound using adaptive region growing and supervised edge-based deformable model. IEEE Trans Med Imaging 37(4):918–928

Lagendijk M, Vos EL, Ramlakhan KP et al (2018) Breast and tumour volume measurements in breast cancer patients using 3-D automated breast volume scanner images. World J Surg 42(7):2087–2093

Larson ED, Lee WM, Roubidoux MA et al (2018) Preliminary clinical experience with a combined automated breast ultrasound and digital breast tomosynthesis system. Ultrasound Med Biol 44(3):734–742

Liu L, Li K, Qin W et al (2018) Automated breast tumor detection and segmentation with a novel computational framework of whole ultrasound images. Med Biol Eng Comput 56(2):183–199

Mann RM, Kuhl CK, Moy L (2019) Contrast-enhanced MRI for breast cancer screening. J Magn Reson Imaging 50(2):377–390

Moon WK, Shen YW, Huang CS et al (2011a) Comparative study of density analysis using automated whole breast ultrasound and MRI. Med Phys 38(1):382–389

Moon WK, Shen YW, Huang CS, Chiang LR, Chang RF (2011b) Computer-aided diagnosis for the classification of breast masses in automated whole breast ultrasound images. Ultrasound Med Biol 37(4):539–548

Moon WK, Lo CM, Chang JM, Huang CS, Chen JH, Chang RF (2012) Computer-aided classification of breast masses using speckle features of automated breast ultrasound images. Med Phys 39(10):6465–6473

Ohuchi N, Suzuki A, Sobue T et al (2016) Sensitivity and specificity of mammography and adjunctive ultrasonography to screen for breast cancer in the Japan Strategic Anti-cancer Randomized Trial (J-START): a randomised controlled trial. Lancet 387(10016):341–348

Park J, Chae EY, Cha JH et al (2018) Comparison of mammography, digital breast tomosynthesis, automated breast ultrasound, magnetic resonance imaging in evaluation of residual tumor after neoadjuvant chemotherapy. Eur J Radiol 108:261–268

Rocher L, Gennisson JL, Ferlicot S et al (2018) Testicular ultrasensitive Doppler preliminary experience: a feasibility study. Acta Radiol 59(3):346–354

Schaefgen B, Heil J, Barr RG et al (2018) Initial results of the FUSION-X-US prototype combining 3D automated breast ultrasound and digital breast tomosynthesis. Eur Radiol 28(6):2499–2506

Schwaab J, Diez Y, Oliver A et al (2016) Automated quality assessment in three-dimensional breast ultrasound images. J Med Imaging (Bellingham) 3(2):027002

Shin HJ, Kim HH, Cha JH (2015) Current status of automated breast ultrasonography. Ultrasonography 34(3):165–172

Sigrist RMS, Liau J, Kaffas AE, Chammas MC, Willmann JK (2017) Ultrasound elastography: review of techniques and clinical applications. Theranostics 7(5):1303–1329

Skaane P, Gullien R, Eben EB, Sandhaug M, Schulz-Wendtland R, Stoeblen F (2015) Interpretation of automated breast ultrasound (ABUS) with and without knowledge of mammography: a reader performance study. Acta Radiol 56(4):404–412

Smith B, Woodard S, Chetlen AL (2019) Patient perception of automated whole-breast ultrasound. Breast J 25(1):180–182

Sreekumari A, Shriram KS, Vaidya V (2016) Breast lesion detection and characterization with 3D features. Conf Proc IEEE Eng Med Biol Soc 2016:4101–4104

Tan T, Platel B, Huisman H, Sanchez CI, Mus R, Karssemeijer N (2012) Computer-aided lesion diagnosis in automated 3-D breast ultrasound using coronal spiculation. IEEE Trans Med Imaging 31(5):1034–1042

Tan T, Platel B, Mann RM, Huisman H, Karssemeijer N (2013) Chest wall segmentation in automated 3D breast ultrasound scans. Med Image Anal 17(8):1273–1281

van Egdom LSE, Lagendijk M, Heijkoop EHM et al (2018) Three-dimensional ultrasonography of the breast; an adequate replacement for MRI in neoadjuvant chemotherapy tumour response evaluation? - RESPONDER trial. Eur J Radiol 104:94–100

van Zelst JCM, Mann RM (2018) Automated three-dimensional breast US for screening: technique, artifacts, and lesion characterization. Radiographics 38(3):663–683

Van Zelst JCM, Platel B, Karssemeijer N, Mann RM (2015) Multiplanar reconstructions of 3D automated breast ultrasound improve lesion differentiation by radiologists. Acad Radiol 22(12):1489–1496

van Zelst JCM, Mus RDM, Woldringh G et al (2017a) Surveillance of women with the BRCA1 or BRCA2 mutation by using biannual automated breast US, MR imaging, and mammography. Radiology 285(2):376–388

van Zelst JCM, Balkenhol M, Tan T et al (2017b) Sonographic phenotypes of molecular subtypes of invasive ductal cancer in automated 3-d breast ultrasound. Ultrasound Med Biol 43(9):1820–1828

van Zelst JCM, Tan T, Clauser P et al (2018) Dedicated computer-aided detection software for automated 3D breast ultrasound; an efficient tool for the radiologist in supplemental screening of women with dense breasts. Eur Radiol 28(7):2996–3006

Vourtis A, Kachulis A (2018) The performance of 3D ABUS versus HHUS in the visualisation and BI-RADS characterisation of breast lesions in a large cohort of 1,886 women. Eur Radiol 28(2):592–601

Wanders JOP, Holland K, Karssemeijer N et al (2017a) The effect of volumetric breast density on the risk of screen-detected and interval breast cancers: a cohort study. Breast Cancer Res 19:67

Wanders JO, Holland K, Veldhuis WB et al (2017b) Volumetric breast density affects performance of digital screening mammography. Breast Cancer Res Treat 162(1):95–103

Wang X, Huo L, He Y et al (2016) Early prediction of pathological outcomes to neoadjuvant chemotherapy in breast cancer patients using automated breast ultrasound. Chin J Cancer Res 28(5):478–485

Wang Y, Nasief HG, Kohn S et al (2017) Three-dimensional ultrasound elasticity imaging on an automated breast volume scanning system. Ultrason Imaging 39(6):369–392

Weigel S, Heindel W, Heidrich J, Hense HW, Heidinger O (2017) Digital mammography screening: sensitivity of the programme dependent on breast density. Eur Radiol 27(7):2744–2751

Wilczek B, Wilczek HE, Rasouliyan L, Leifland K (2016) Adding 3D automated breast ultrasound to mammography screening in women with heterogeneously and extremely dense breasts: report from a hospital-based, high-volume, single-center breast cancer screening program. Eur J Radiol 85(9):1554–1563

Xu X, Bao L, Tan Y, Zhu L, Kong F, Wang W (2018) 1000-Case reader study of radiologists' performance in interpretation of automated breast volume scanner images with a computer-aided detection system. Ultrasound Med Biol 44(8):1694–1702

Yap MH, Pons G, Marti J et al (2018) Automated breast ultrasound lesions detection using convolutional neural networks. IEEE J Biomed Health Inform 22(4):1218–1226

Yap MH, Goyal M, Osman FM et al (2019) Breast ultrasound lesions recognition: end-to-end deep learning approaches. J Med Imaging (Bellingham) 6(1):011007

Zhang X, Lin X, Tan Y et al (2018) A multicenter hospital-based diagnosis study of automated breast ultrasound system in detecting breast cancer among Chinese women. Chin J Cancer Res 30(2):231–239

Zheng FY, Yan LX, Huang BJ et al (2015) Comparison of retraction phenomenon and BI-RADS-US descriptors in differentiating benign and malignant breast masses using an automated breast volume scanner. Eur J Radiol 84(11):2123–2129

Zheng FY, Lu Q, Huang BJ et al (2017) Imaging features of automated breast volume scanner: correlation with molecular subtypes of breast cancer. Eur J Radiol 86:267–275

Ultrasound-Guided Interventions

Eva Maria Fallenberg

Contents

1　**Indications** 144

2　**Biopsy Guidance Method** 145
  2.1　Role of a Second-Look Ultrasound 145

3　**Types of Biopsy Procedures** 146
  3.1　Cytological Sampling 146
  3.2　Histological Sampling 147

4　**Considerations Regarding Lesion Type** 148
  4.1　Cystic Lesions 148
  4.2　Solid Lesions 149
  4.3　Calcifications 149

5　**Patient Information** 151
  5.1　Patient History 152
  5.2　Allergy 152
  5.3　Anticoagulation Medication and Handling ... 152
  5.4　Endocarditis Prophylaxis 152

6　**Preparation of the System and Material** 153

7　**Patient Preparation** 153
  7.1　Local Anesthesia 153

8　**Biopsy Technique** 156
  8.1　Indications for Clip Marking 158
  8.2　Preoperative Wire Localization 158

9　**Reporting and Probe Handling and Pathology Information** 159

10　**Radiological-Histopathological Correlation** ... 160

11　**Summary** 161

References 162

E. M. Fallenberg (✉)
Klinikum Rechts der Isar of the Technical University,
Munich, Germany
e-mail: eva.fallenberg@tum.de

© Springer Nature Switzerland AG 2022
M. Fuchsjäger et al. (eds.), *Breast Imaging*, Medical Radiology Diagnostic Imaging,
https://doi.org/10.1007/978-3-030-94918-1_8

Abstract

With increased numbers of screening examinations and awareness of women regarding suspicious clinical findings, the number of lesions requiring further assessment increases. In addition, the average size of a detected lesion decreases, and reliable imaging modalities for guiding further procedures are required.

After the successful detection of a lesion of concern in various modalities for breast imaging like US, MRI, mammography, tomosynthesis, or contrast-enhanced mammography, a histological proof of the nature of this lesion is necessary.

As open surgical biopsy has been the method of choice in former days, minimally invasive procedures have come into focus and are recommended now for providing histological proof and information for operative or neoadjuvant therapy planning (Wallis et al., Eur Radiol 17(2):581–588, 2007; Perry et al., European guidelines for quality assurance in breast cancer screening and diagnosis, 2006; Helbich et al., Eur Radiol 14(3):383–393, 2004; Bick et al., Insights Imaging 11(1):12, 2020).

Due to different approaches in the treatment of breast cancer, surgery is no longer always the first line of treatment. Preoperative minimally invasive assessment of a carcinoma is requested to get further information about the molecular subtype of a lesion in order to tailor treatment and avoid unnecessary damage and scarring, or further anxiety due to additional general anesthesia (Wallis et al., Eur Radiol 17(2):581–588, 2007; Perry et al., European guidelines for quality assurance in breast cancer screening and diagnosis, 2006).

Additionally, minimally invasive approaches are less expensive and are performed in an outpatient setting (Gruber et al., Eur J Radiol 74(3):519–524, 2010; Abbate et al. Breast 18(2):73–77, 2009).

Ultrasound is a cheap and widely available technique, in addition it is quite comfortable for women and therefore the working horse in the field of breast biopsies. Furthermore, it plays a major role in preoperative localization of non-palpable lesions and is used more and more often to guide vacuum-assisted removal of benign lesions and other tumor ablation techniques.

In this chapter, we explain how to manage ultrasound-guided interventions and provide tips and tricks to successfully plan and perform ultrasound-guided procedures.

1 Indications

Before starting any interventional breast procedure, the complete imaging workup including clinical examination and reviewing all available images (e.g., mammography, additional views, MRI) has to be finalized.

If an imaging finding results in a BI-RADS 4 or 5 assessment category, the probability of malignancy is above 2% and a histological diagnosis is recommended.

Following the EUREF guidelines, a minimally invasive biopsy should be performed in a minimum of 70% of the cases, and open biopsies should be avoided. Also, the number of unnecessary surgical procedures should be limited (the benign/malignant ratio should be less than 1; possibly less than 0.5) (Wallis et al. 2007; Perry et al. 2006). Obtaining the diagnosis of malignancy before surgery has several advantages:

- The confirmation of the diagnosis makes it easier for the patient to accept therapeutic proposals.
- Initial surgical or medical treatment can be decided upon.
- Neoadjuvant chemotherapy or hormone therapy can be initiated.
- Surgery can be optimized regarding initial volume of resection and number of reoperations.
- The management of sentinel lymph nodes can be planned.

In case of a BI-RADS category 3, usually, according to guidelines, a 6-month follow-up is recommended.

A biopsy of a BI-RADS 3 lesion is recommended if new in a breast cancer staging examination, in high-risk patients, discordant images, early pregnancy, or monitoring difficulties.

Also, if the patient is very anxious about having breast cancer, a biopsy can be considered, but the deviation from the usual protocol as the last resort has to be documented.

Furthermore, the lesion has to be clearly identifiable with the imaging method used for guiding the intervention.

2 Biopsy Guidance Method

Even if initially detected by screening mammography or MRI, 50%+ lesions are detectable by ultrasound, in a second-look examination, and therefore suitable for ultrasound-guided interventions/biopsies (Meissnitzer et al. 2009; Spick and Baltzer 2014; Park et al. 2013).

2.1 Role of a Second-Look Ultrasound

Ultrasound is not necessarily the first imaging modality used to detect suspicious lesions. Especially in asymptomatic women above the age of 50, lesions are usually detected at mammography screening. Younger women will usually get an ultrasound first, especially if they have suspicious clinical findings. In the high-risk population, lesions are mostly detected by MRI (Peter et al. 2016; Altobelli and Lattanzi 2014; Murphy et al. 2008; Perry et al. 2008; Wockel et al. 2018).

Therefore, before deciding whether ultrasound-guided intervention is appropriate, a careful re-examination of the patient is performed correlating initial imaging findings with ultrasound. In up to 60% of cases, it will be able to correlate lesions primarily detected by MRI for example, if you know where to look, even if the initial US exam was negative (Park et al. 2013; Shin et al. 2007).

2.1.1 Visible at Ultrasound

Findings clearly visible at ultrasound should only be biopsied under ultrasound guidance.

2.1.2 Visible at Ultrasound and Mammography

Lesions visible at mammography and ultrasound can be biopsied with either guidance technique. The decision depends on the exact localization, lesion features, breast shape, availability of consumables (needles, etc.), costs involved, and experience of the examiner. As ultrasound is radiation free, it should be preferred over mammography guidance due to the ALARA principle avoiding any unnecessary radiation (European Society of Radiology 2011).

2.1.3 Visible at MRI

Lesions detected by MRI should always undergo second-look ultrasound examination and additional mammography workup first. If there is a clear correlation with the MRI finding, the biopsy procedure can be switched. This is quite often the case in mass lesions detected by MRI. If the target lesion at MRI is non-mass enhancement, correlation with ultrasound can be difficult. Additional mammography can be helpful to find microcalcifications indicating DCIS without corresponding US findings. Using more advanced US techniques like Doppler and elastography (Chapter "Breast Ultrasound: Advanced Techniques") can be of benefit as well (Plecha et al. 2014). In general, very small masses, non-mass enhancement, invasive lobular cancers (ILC), and DCIS are less likely to have an US correlate. If the lesion cannot be identified by ultrasound, biopsy has to be performed under MRI guidance (Park et al. 2013; Peter et al. 2016).

2.1.4 Very Small or Subtle Correlating Findings at Ultrasound

If there is a subtle US correlation for an MRI-detected lesion, or a huge area of microcalcifications at mammography and calcifications, dilated ducts, or architectural distortions visible at ultrasound in the corresponding breast area, ultrasound-guided biopsy can be considered in certain circumstances (e.g., no access to the appropriate biopsy method to avoid delay in diagnosis). Such an approach should only be followed by highly experienced multimodality breast radiologists.

In all cases with diffusely distributed findings, vacuum-assisted biopsies (VAB) with large core needles can be advantageous due to a lower underestimation rate compared to regular core needle biopsies (Suh et al. 2012; Bae et al. 2015).

To be able to prove that the correct lesion was biopsied, clip marking of the biopsied lesion is mandatory. This will help at follow-up examinations and serve as the localizer in case of an unclear pathological-clinical correlation. A specimen X-ray can help to identify microcalcifications, if this was the target.

In addition, very small lesions (5 mm and smaller) are likely to be removed at least partially during biopsy, or masked by bleeding thereafter, so that the area is difficult to reidentify in the follow-up.

In all of these cases, clip marking is necessary to verify that the correct target lesion was biopsied, in, e.g., a follow-up MRI exam, or to enable preoperative localization. As most lesions, except non-mass enhancement, quite often have a corresponding finding on non-enhanced images, non-enhanced follow-up MRI verifying the clip position can be considered (Lee et al. 2018).

It is mandatory to clearly inform the patient about an increased risk of missing the target lesion and potential subsequent repeat biopsies, if the target lesion is only subtly visible at US. Guidelines and approaches may vary from country to country; therefore, the patient has to be informed and it should be documented.

3 Types of Biopsy Procedures

There is a great variety of different biopsy devices and procedures available to biopsy lesions and assess samples. Depending on the examiner's experience and the expertise of the involved pathologist, recommended techniques may vary.

3.1 Cytological Sampling

3.1.1 Fine Needle Aspiration (FNA): Cytological Sampling

Fine needle aspiration is a very quick and cheap procedure, but it requires a highly experienced team of radiologists and pathologists working side by side in the same room, to keep the number of insufficient samples low. FNA results in a cytological diagnosis. Hence, due to disintegration of cells, differentiation between invasive and in situ cancer is not possible. FNA is not at all suitable for assessing microcalcifications.

With a needle of a diameter of less than 1 mm (18–27 G) a collection of single cells is sampled from a suspicious mass. This can be done either by the so-called capillary technique or the aspiration technique. With the "capillary technique," a needle is put into the lesion, then moved back and forth, and rotated around its own axis. In the "aspiration technique," a needle is connected to a syringe and is put into the lesion, and active aspiration is performed. With these procedures, cells are detached from the surrounding tissue, harvested, and then directly spread onto a glass slide. The cells are immediately assessed by the cytopathologist. Within minutes, information about the dignity of the lesion is obtained. Further assessment and information about immune-histochemical features of the samples are not possible.

Fine needle aspiration is mainly used for cysts or cyst-like lesions. Nevertheless, some important points have to be kept in mind, to be described later. Aspiration of symptomatic cysts can offer the patient quick pressure and pain relief.

If liquid is obtained, the aspirate should at all times be sent for analysis to exclude malignancy or infection. If there was a suspicion of a breast implant-associated anaplastic large-cell lymphoma (BIA-ALCL), due to a newly developed severe seroma more than 1 year after operation, all of the fluid, not only parts of it, should be sent in to give the cytopathologist the opportunity to collect cell blocks for proper diagnosis (Kricheldorff et al. 2018).

3.2 Histological Sampling

Histological sampling enables taking tissue cylinders with various calibers and lengths depending on the equipment used. Especially for microcalcifications, the diagnostic accuracy improves with increasing tissue volume taken. Opposite to fine needle aspiration, core needle biopsy requires local anesthesia, the histological workup needs more time, and diagnosis is not immediate. Even if the procedure is more invasive, it is generally well or very well tolerated.

Tissue samples should be handled very carefully and manipulated as little as possible. Ideally, tissue samples can be placed into pathology cassettes immediately and fixed in formalin. The pathological workup includes embedding the specimen into paraffin, then slicing, and applying different staining for diagnosis of type of tumor, differentiation, grading, receptor status, and immunological or genetic markers. This comprehensive pathological information enables the best treatment choice for each individual patient; this is the biggest advantage compared to FNA. False positives happen very rarely.

3.2.1 Core Needle Biopsy: Histological Sampling

Core needle biopsy is the standard and most frequent percutaneous biopsy method, first reported in the late 1970s and increasingly used since the first study of Parker et al. in 1993 (Roberts et al. 1975; Parker et al. 1993). Different needle systems usually with diameters between 14 and 12 G are used.

These special needle systems consist of an internal component which has a notch to collect the tissue and a sharp outer hollow part cutting the tissue into the needle (see Fig. 1).

Sensitivity increases proportionally with core needle size. Also, the length of the specimen correlates with the sensitivity increase (Lai et al. 2013). The general recommendation is to use a minimum of 14 G needles and length of core of 20 mm.

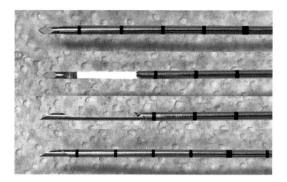

Fig. 1 Typical core biopsy needle with open and closed notch

Recommendations for the number of samples vary and depend on the authors. Some consider two specimens to be sufficient, while others recommend at least five. On average, 3–6 samples are optimal depending on the quality of the samples; an intact specimen of at least 1 cm is considered adequate (Evans et al. 2018). Diffusely growing lesions need more samples than compact growing ones. The most important thing is that the samples are representative (Perry et al. 2008; Liberman 2000).

The cutting is done automatically or semiautomatically.

The semiautomatic approach can be advantageous if you want to have perfect control of your needle tip. Especially if the lesion is located very close to the chest wall or in the axilla, the biopsy needle can be prepared to be put half-tensioned and half-open directly into the lesion to get the sample without shooting the needle uncontrolled. In addition, it is possible to optimize the notch position after firing only the inner part of the needle first, before cutting the tissue (see Fig. 2).

The equipment is relatively cheap and the examination quick; in experienced hands, it lasts for approximately 15 min.

Even if this method is causing more tissue damage than fine needle aspiration, it is the current standard of care because it allows for nearly the whole pathological workup, including immunhistochemistry (e.g., receptor status), thus optimizing therapy planning.

The bleeding risk is judged as low (Patel et al. 2012).

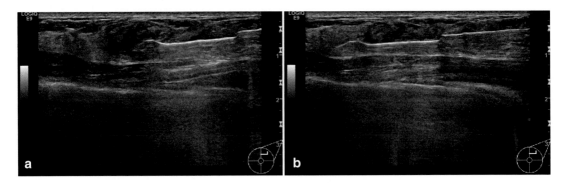

Fig. 2 Notch repositioning: Needle tip just at the border of the lesion in **a**; after pushing forward under image control, correct notch position with centered suspicious lesion (**b**). Especially in very hard lesions, it can happen that they are pushed away and the biopsy is not sufficient as a result

3.2.2 Vacuum-Assisted Biopsy: Histological Sampling

In the last decade, the role of vacuum-assisted biopsy (VAB) has become more and more important (Hahn et al. 2012; Parker and Klaus 1997).

Needles used for vacuum-assisted biopsies show larger dimensions—usually in the 7–13 G range—even larger than the ones used for core needle biopsy. Using vacuum needles, the tissue is sucked into a cavity and then cut by a rotating hollow external needle part. Through the internal needle part, the specimen is taken out and collected without removing the needle. By rotating the needle 360°, a much bigger area of tissue can be sampled. The total amount of tissue collected depends on the size and type of the lesion, if it is very stiff or soft and flexible.

With this procedure, it is possible to completely remove small lesions and also biopsy lesions that are growing in a discontinuous pattern. The trauma and bleeding caused by this type of procedure are bigger than those with simple core needles as described before. Therefore, a compression bandage is recommended after the procedure.

Regarding the consensus guidelines for peri-procedural management of coagulation status and hemostasis, the risk in percutaneous image-guided extra-abdominal and extrathoracic interventions is low. The bleeding risk of VAB is not clearly described in most of the guidelines, but most likely it is still a procedure with a low bleeding risk (perhaps due to the large needle size and greater volume, it comes closer to medium bleeding risk). Therefore, risk management of low and medium bleeding risks should be considered depending on the clinical situation (see Tables 1 and 2). The bleeding risk of axillary lymph node biopsy is judged medium to high by the British society of breast imaging due to the proximity of axillary vessels and difficulties of compression after the procedure and therefore using no more than 14G needle is recommended.

4 Considerations Regarding Lesion Type

4.1 Cystic Lesions

Simple cysts are without any risk of cancer and therefore usually not a target for any intervention, but some large tender cysts can be very painful. In this circumstance, a FNA is possible and offers immediate pain release.

Complicated cystic lesions and clustered microcysts exhibit a very low risk of malignancy, and usually a follow-up (BI-RADS 3) is recommended (Greenwood et al. 2017).

Table 1 Minimally invasive breast biopsy: Management of patients receiving anticoagulation medication (adapted from Patel et al. 2012; Jaffe et al. 2015; Patel et al. 2013)

Procedures with low risk of bleeding, easily detected and controllable	Procedures with moderate risk of bleeding
Preprocedural laboratory testing	
INR: routinely recommended for patients receiving warfarin anticoagulation or known or suspected liver disease	INR: recommended
aPTT: routinely recommended for patients receiving intravenous unfractionated heparin	
Platelet count: not routinely recommended	
Hematocrit: not routinely recommended	
Management	
INR: correct to <2.0	INR: correct to <1.5
aPTT: no consensus	aPTT: no consensus (trend towards correcting for values >1.5 × control)
Hematocrit: no recommended threshold for transfusion	
Platelets: transfusion recommended for counts <50,000/µL	
Clopidogrel: withhold for 5 days before procedure	
Aspirin: do not withhold	
LMWH (therapeutic dose): withhold one dose or 12 h before procedure	

Management recommendations assume that there is no combination of different coagulation defects or anticoagulation drugs
Abbreviations: *aPTT* activated partial thromboplastin time, *FFP* fresh frozen plasma, *INR* international normalized ratio, *IVC* inferior vena cava, *LMWH* low-molecular-weight heparin, *PICC* peripherally inserted central catheter

In the case of so-called complex cystic and solid lesions, containing liquid and solid parts, the biopsy device has to be chosen wisely. If the solid part of the lesion differs significantly from the surrounding tissue and would still be visible, after the liquid part is gone, a simple CNB can be considered. Nevertheless, as intracystic lesions are quite often papillomatous lesions, the pathologist could have difficulties in judging the real architecture of the lesion just getting small parts after CNB. Therefore, solely open biopsy for

these lesions was recommended up until recently. VAB is increasingly taking over though, as it allows for sampling nearly the whole lesion with bigger samples. If a minimally invasive procedure is done, keep in mind to put a clip marker to enable locating the area again in the case of a malignant or premalignant histopathology result (Rogers 2005).

4.2 Solid Lesions

The most frequent and cost-effective way of using ultrasound-guided biopsy is the further assessment of unclear imaging findings preventing surgery in case of benign histopathology. This mainly refers to solid BI-RADS category 4 lesions with a 2% to <95% percentage of malignancy. On average, the amount of malignancies in these groups varies between 15% and 25% depending on the examiner, and therefore open surgical biopsies under general anesthesia can be prevented in approximately 80% of patients.

The biopsy of such a lesion should be done using core needles to maintain the integrity of the peritumoral environment and still enable a good size estimation of the lesion at final pathology (Rogers 2005; Charles et al. 2003).

Findings of the BI-RADS category 3 usually undergo short-term follow-up after 6 months. By definition, the malignancy rate is below 2%.

4.3 Calcifications

Fine pleomorphic or linear calcifications usually do not have any ultrasound correlate and should be biopsied under mammographic guidance. If they are slightly larger, or associated with small masses or dilated ducts, they can be found at ultrasound as well and therefore US-guided biopsy is possible. Due to the discontinuous growth of these lesions, VAB is recommended to reduce underestimation rate (Suh et al. 2012;

Table 2 Recommendations for withdrawal time and reinsertion of anticoagulants and antiplatelet medications (adapted from Jaffe et al. 2015)

Medication	Interval between last dose and procedure		Resumption after procedure		Comments
	Low bleeding risk	Medium bleeding risk	Low bleeding risk	Medium bleeding risk	
Anticoagulants					
Warfarin	5 days	5 days	12 h	12 h	
UFH (IV)	1 h	4 h	1 h	1 h	
UFH (SQ)	4 h	4 h	Immediate	Immediate	
LMWH (SQ)	12 h	12 h	6 h	6 h	
Dabigatran	24 h	48 h	24 h	48 h	
Rivaroxaban	24 h	48 h	24 h	48 h	
Apixaban	24 h	48 h	24 h	48 h	
Fondaparinux	24 h	36 h	6 h	6 h	
Acova	None	4 h	1 h	1 h	
Desirudin	None	4 h	1 h	1 h	
Bivalirudin	None	4 h	1 h	1 h	
Antithrombotic					
ASA, low dose	None	None	Immediate	Immediate	
ASA, high dose	None	5 days	Immediate	Immediate	
ASA and dipyridamole	2 days	5 days	Immediate	Immediate	
NSAIDs	None	None	Immediate	Immediate	Interval before procedure
Cilostazol	None	None	Immediate	Immediate	
Clopidogrel	5 days	5 days	Immediate	Immediate	
Prasugrel	5 days	5 days	24 h	24 h	
Ticagrelor	5 days	5 days	24 h	24 h	
Tirofiban	No consensus	No consensus	No consensus	No consensus	Recent surgery is a contraindication (within 4 weeks)
Eptifibatide	No consensus	No consensus	No consensus	No consensus	Recent surgery is a contraindication (within 6 weeks)
Abciximab	NR	NR	No consensus	No consensus	Recent surgery is a contraindication (within 6 weeks)

Abbreviations: *UFH* unfractionated heparin, *SQ* subcutaneous, *LMWH* low-molecular-weight heparin, *ASA* acetylsalicylic acid (aspirin), *NSAIDs* nonsteroidal anti-inflammatory drugs, *NR* not recommended

Bae et al. 2015; Cho et al. 2009; Soo et al. 2003; Kim et al. 2008). In general, the likelihood of malignancy is higher in microcalcifications with an US finding. This has to be kept in mind for imaging-pathology correlation (Bae et al. 2015; Soo et al. 2003). If findings are subtle, a marker has to be placed to be able to relocate the area, especially if the lesion could have been removed completely with the procedure. Specimen radiography has to be performed to demonstrate adequate sampling results with representative microcalcifications within the specimens (see Fig. 3) (Liberman et al. 1994). A careful dose reduction of the orthogonal two-view control mammography, that does not completely blur calcifications, can be possible due to the high contrast of the clips (Riedl et al. 2005). Looking for calcifications at pathology only is not enough, as it could contain calcifications not even visible in imaging (<100 μm) and therefore it could be a false-negative biopsy even if containing calcifications (Rosen et al. 2002).

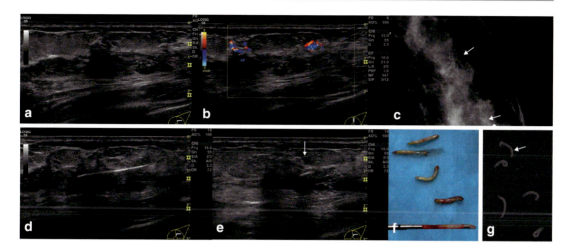

Fig. 3 Correlation of calcification-containing lesions. Hypoechoic area with slight distortion and bright speckles (**a**) with hyperperfusion (**b**) as US correlate for an area of mammographic suspicious fine linear segmental calcifications (**c**). US-guided biopsy with needle documentation in two orthogonal views (**d**, **e**). Corresponding heterogeneous specimens with dense (white) and fatty tissue (**f**). Calcifications in specimen radiography (**g**)

5 Patient Information

Depending on national/local legal requirements, usually the most common side effects and possible problems and complications that can occur during a biopsy have to be discussed with the patient, documented in written form, and signed prior to the procedure. In general, complications in minimally invasive biopsies are rare, occurring in about 1:1000 procedures (Evans et al. 2018). Usually, the information about the procedure can be processed on the same day (Vosshenrich et al. 2013).

The patient has to be informed about the advantages and disadvantage of the chosen approach as well as about possible alternatives, especially if using a method that is not part of the clinical routine. Some exceptions that can be justified by the experience of the examiner and the circumstances, like doing an ultrasound-guided biopsy of calcification due to lack of examination time on stereotactic devices and to avoid delay of treatment. In this case, the patient has to be informed that it is not the usual procedure and that there is a possibility of a repeat biopsy due to undersampling or missing the target lesion at all (Suh et al. 2012; Lai et al. 2013; Yu et al. 2015).

The patient has to be informed that after local anesthesia, there will not be anymore pain, but that there may still be some sensation. Also, inform patients that the biopsy procedures come with a special noise when harvesting the samples.

Depending on your local/national regulations, the most common complications you have to disclose are:

- Bleeding
- Bruises
- Pain, esp. if you biopsy close to the nipple
- Infection
- Allergic reaction on any material (disinfection, local anesthetics, latex)
- Fainting
- Possibility of damage to the chest wall (pneumothorax), heart, or axillary nerve and vessel structure
- Clip placement and chance of migration (if necessary)
- Possibility of complete removal of a very small lesion by core
- Tumor seeding (but no evidence of clinical significance) (Liebens et al. 2009; Santiago et al. 2017)

In general, careful information of the patient about the upcoming procedure and management as well as time interval until the final results will greatly reduce and improve the patient's cooperation (Humphrey et al. 2014).

5.1 Patient History

Before performing any biopsy, careful patient history has to be taken, to prevent any side effects or abnormal bleeding that could compromise further assessment of lesion size or additional lesions and to facilitate imaging-pathological correlation and judgment.

5.2 Allergy

It is of special importance getting information on potential prior allergic reactions or medications of the patient that could influence the outcome of our procedure. Allergies to latex or iodine or local anesthetics result in a change of material used in your daily routine like different gloves and covers for the ultrasound probe and iodine-free disinfection liquid. In addition, some allergies against metals or proteins have to be cleared if you plan to place a clip.

If there is any prior reaction or allergy to aminoglycosides, xylocaine can be replaced by articaine.

Be prepared prior to starting.

5.3 Anticoagulation Medication and Handling

Before starting a biopsy, some contraindications have to be kept in mind. These belong mainly to blood coagulation.

Elderly people frequently take aspirin or other blood-thinning medications due to cardiac problems or other comorbidities, which have to be evaluated before biopsy. Some of these medications do not compromise blood clotting suffi-

ciently that they should be paused prior to an intervention, but others do.

Patients with an increased risk of thromboembolism like arterial fibrillation are usually treated with warfarin or new-generation anticoagulation medication. Patients with arterial venous disease are treated with ASS or clopidogrel, and sometimes also with heparin. Patients with a disease desiring anticoagulation therapy are usually aware of the increased bleeding risk due to their medication. Patients taking aspirin for headaches are usually not aware of this risk. Therefore, a dedicated questioning for anticoagulation therapy, or medication that could result in thinning of the blood, is mandatory.

The aim of taking this respective history is to prevent any danger to the patient due to bleeding complications. Likewise, the time to intervention should not be prolonged unnecessarily. Moreover, the damage to a patient from thrombotic or embolic complications due to an unnecessary pausing of anticoagulation therapy should be avoided.

The most common anticoagulating medications and the recommendations of the peri-interventional management including blood tests and respective pausing intervals prior to biopsy are listed in Tables 1 and 2.

In rare cases, blood tests and special medication preventing bleeding become necessary.

If there are no diseases and no medication requiring anticoagulation, usually a laboratory test of the coagulation status can be avoided.

For patients with decreased renal function (GFR <50 mL/min) and patients over the age of 75, 12-h longer time intervals for suspension of factor Xa or direct thrombin inhibitor should be considered.

5.4 Endocarditis Prophylaxis

If you have patients suffering from defective or replaced heart valves, antibiotic prophylaxis is necessary. This is usually documented in the device pass and known by the patient.

6 Preparation of the System and Material

Not only the patient but also the ultrasound probe has to be prepared before biopsy for two reasons: first to prevent infections and second to prevent the probe from being damaged by the disinfection liquid. Therefore, the probe has to be covered by a plastic or latex cover that is sterile or can be disinfected (Nyhsen et al. 2017).

All the materials used during the procedure should be prepared in advance and arranged (in a consistent manner on a table), to allow for a quick and smooth procedure. If, during the procedure, the technologist has to fetch missing items, unnecessary patient anxiety can be the result; this, of course, should be avoided.

7 Patient Preparation

After obtaining proper patient history and providing information, and before starting any patient preparation regarding the biopsy, make sure that the suspicious lesion can be adequately localized. Sometimes, findings are subtle on ultrasound as mentioned above. If so, it has to be made clear to the patient that there is a chance of missing the lesion. In addition, it is necessary to do a marker localization to be sure that samples have been taken from the suspicious region and to be able to correlate the biopsied area with the prior imaging.

Patient positioning is as in a diagnostic ultrasound examination. Usually, the patient lies in supine position with the arms comfortably elevated above the head. Make sure that the patient is able to keep this position for about 20 min.

Depending on the localization of the lesion, it can be helpful to lift one or the other side of the torso to get better lesion access. Support with a towel or special wedge-shaped positioning devices can make it easier for the patient to keep position.

Prior to disinfection, make sure that the suspicious lesion can be adequately localized and find a position where you can hold the probe immobile without "losing" the lesion. In addition, think about the biopsy direction and make sure that the lesion can be reached with the needle without being compromised by any obstacle like the belly or the examination bed. It is also important that the examiner is positioned comfortably using an adjustable chair being able to control the biopsy device as well as the ultrasound screen and the patient without turning back and forth.

Sometimes, excess fat or the patient's ribs can obstruct the intended path to the lesion and increase the risk of complications, like a puncture of the chest wall. The access path has to be clearly defined prior to the application of local anesthesia, since repetitive application may cause unnecessary pain and skin damage to the patient.

After lesion access is established, it can be helpful to place a small skin mark before disinfection, to better retrieve the exact localization for the local anesthesia application. I recommend to do this marking with a plastic needle cap as this does not disappear after disinfectant washing.

In general, always make sure that needle and puncture area of the skin remain sterile. Due to the circumstances using contact liquid and need of a bigger uncovered area of the skin to securely display the lesion, sterile covers with only a small hole are usually not adequate. To cover the rest of the abdomen, simple sterile towels are the best choice.

7.1 Local Anesthesia

There is a variety of local anesthetics that can be used for biopsies; xylocaine is the most common. The combination with adrenaline can be helpful in large-core biopsy to minimize bleeding risk. If anesthetic medication is combined with adrenaline, be aware of direct injection into any vessel!

Careful preparation of the needle and syringe is necessary. Air in the syringe or needle will be injected into the breast and can severely compromise US image quality or even completely obscure the lesion (see Fig. 4). Staff has to be properly trained in syringe preparation.

At core needle biopsy, anesthesia of the skin "entrance" and the actual biopsy area are most important; the needle track to the lesion only needs a small amount of local anesthetics. Usually, a maximum of 10 mL is sufficient. Carefully control the needle when injecting local anesthesia to avoid punctur of a feeding vessel resulting in bleeding and lesion masking. During this procedure, you can also get an idea of the tissue composition of your target by indirect palpation (very hard, very soft) providing extra information that can be useful in later correlation with histopathology results.

If the lesion is located centrally or directly behind the nipple, extra care has to be taken in this sensitive area to avoid pain when applying local anesthesia.

In VAB, a greater area around the lesion should be anesthetized with up to 15–20 mL to avoid any pain (Park et al. 2011).

If the lesion is very close to the chest wall, biopsy can be a little bit more difficult. By injecting some of the local anesthetics directly behind the far side of the lesion, preferably into the pectoral muscle, you can create a little more distance between chest wall and lesion making biopsy easier. This additional injection into the breast tissue, either between skin and lesion or between lesion and chest wall, can create extra space and security, esp. if VAB is performed (see Figs. 5, 6, 7).

For an easy insertion of the biopsy needle, a 2–3 mm skin incision is made with a scalpel blade cutting the superficial fascia. In general, always define your access point optimized for cosmesis and accurate targeting before doing a damage to the patient's skin.

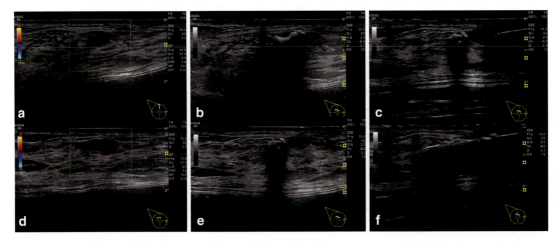

Fig. 4 Air masking the lesion. Air bubbles after injection of not carefully evacuated anesthetic syringe result in nearly complete masking of the lesion (only due to proper fixation of the probe during the procedure and orientation according to other anatomic landmarks, the biopsy was still possible). Clearly visible lobulated mass (**a**, **d**), air bubbles masking the lesion (**b**, **e**), needle before and after firing, lesion still not visible (**c**, **f**)

Ultrasound-Guided Interventions 155

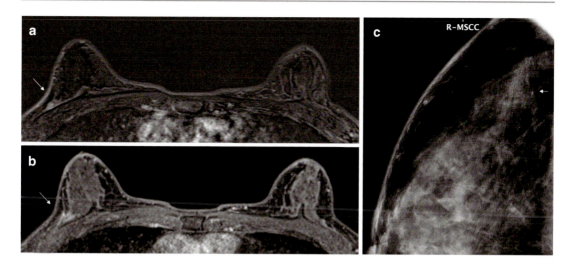

Fig. 5 Enlarged space: Suspicious mass close to the chest wall (**a**) with adjacent non-mass enhancement (**b**) at MRI. Corresponding segmental amorphous microcalcification in magnification mammography (**c**)

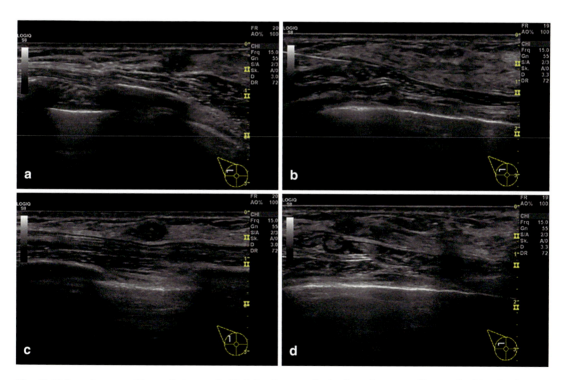

Fig. 6 Enlarged space: Hypoechoic, oval, ill-defined mass lesion close to the pectoralis muscle, with 1 cm distance from skin to chest wall (**a, c**). Injection of local anesthetics into the pectoralis muscle (**b**) enlarging the space to 1.5 cm (**d**)

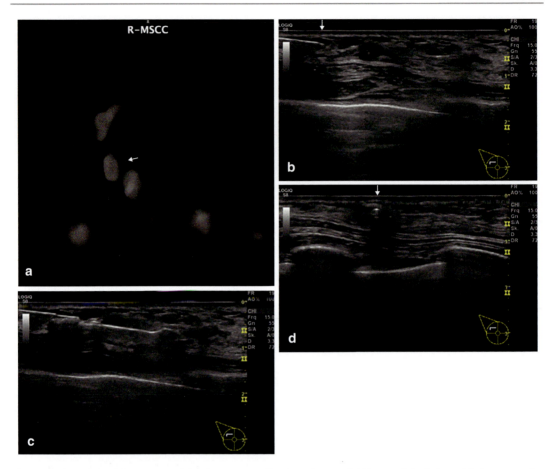

Fig. 7 (**a**) Specimen radiography positive for microcalcifications. Successful biopsy of the lesion with documentation of the needle positioning prefire (**b**) and in two orthogonal views postfire (**c, d**)

8 Biopsy Technique

Independently of performing fine needle aspiration, core needle biopsy, or vacuum-assisted biopsy, safe placement of the needle is necessary to avoid any complications.

A minimum number of 25 intervention procedures under supervision with histological verification should be performed before operating independently. Also, a minimum number of 25 interventions per year are judged to be necessary to maintain competence (Wallis et al. 2007; Liberman et al. 2001; Schulz et al. 2003).

To ensure that the needle is fully visible, some typical reflection and breaking features of ultrasound have to be kept in mind. The needle is best visible, if it is oriented parallel to the probe. If it is imaged at an angle, visibility of the needle and esp. the needle tip gets poor. This is independent from needle type and thickness (Figs. 8 and 9).

The tissue layer between ultrasound probe and chest wall is usually only 2–4 cm thick. Consequently, a steep angle approach increases the risk of complications, such as chest wall penetration. Furthermore, correct needle positioning is barely possible.

It is preferable to place the probe in a way that the target lesion is 1–2 cm beside the image edge. Due to the convex nature of the breast and the possibility of deformation, nearly horizontal biopsy, parallel to the ultrasound probe and chest wall, is possible. Inserting the needle in a flat angle gives you optimal control during the whole biopsy procedure (see Fig. 10a). Furthermore, even if you lose sight of your needle or of the lesion in the image, there is no risk of damaging the thorax wall or the intrathoracic structures.

It is important that the needle is exactly positioned below the middle and in-line with the long axis of the ultrasound probe covering the whole length of the needle (see Figs. 8 and 9). If the nee-

Ultrasound-Guided Interventions

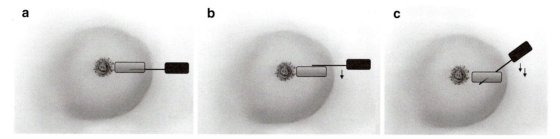

Fig. 8 The probe should be fixed in the position, where the lesion is displayed best. After that, ideally only the needle should be adapted. The needle should be in-line with the probe visible over the full length of the needle track (**a**), giving the examiner full control of the needle during the firing procedure. If this is not the case, needle orientation must be adapted with parallel movement (**b**) or correction of the angle between probe and needle (**c**). (Illustration courtesy of Sophie von Stockhausen)

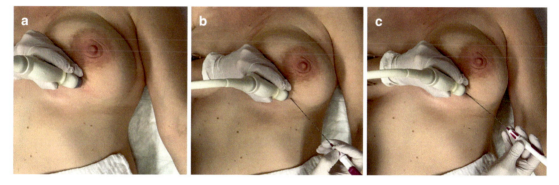

Fig. 9 Needle orientation. Intracutaneous wheal of anesthetics close to the probe in optimal fixed position for imaging the lesion (**a**). Inserting the biopsy or clip containing needle (**b**) adjusting the needle orientation parallel to the direction of the probe (**c**)

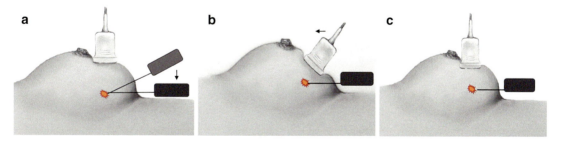

Fig. 10 Needle and probe angulation. The needle should be parallel to the probe and chest wall to be best visualized and to avoid any damage to intrathoracic structures. Therefore, the needle should be flattened after short-distance insertion (**a**). If the needle cannot be flattened anymore due to the belly or chest wall (**b**), the probe can be adapted as well with different angulation due to the softness of the breast tissue (**c**). (Illustration courtesy of Sophie von Stockhausen)

dle is inserted eccentrically or strides across the imaging plane transversally, it will not be imaged in total, especially with regard to the needle tip. Therefore, the chance of missing the lesion is high.

Even if properly positioned, the needle may still sometimes be difficult to be seen. Most of the time, the angle relation between the needle and the probe has become too steep and therefore the needle does not create sufficient reflection. To overcome such issues, lower the external parts of the needle/biopsy device to try to orientate probe and needle more parallelly. If there is no more space left to lower the needle, adjusting the probe accordingly can be the solution (see Fig. 10b, c).

After identifying the lesion and displaying it at US, the ultrasound probe should be fixed in this position. Try not to move it during insertion of the needle; then you should be able to follow the needle to the lesion. If you cannot visualize the needle, do not move the ultrasound probe, but move the needle parallel up and down to the probe until you see it again (Fig. 8b).

If you are able to visualize the needle tip along the whole track, you should position the needle just in front of the lesion you aim to biopsy. Fire the needle from this position. It is recommended to use a semiautomatic approach, fire first the inner part of the needle, and then control the positioning of the notch; if this is correctly placed with the lesion centered, then fire. All this should be done under imaging control. Also, check the needle localization by an orthogonal view, to confirm that the needle is correctly positioned in both planes (see Fig. 7b–d). Especially with advanced US techniques like compound imaging, it can happen especially in small lesions, where the needle appears to be centrally located in the lesion but in fact it is behind or in front of the lesion!

After fully firing the device, the needle is withdrawn, and the specimen is collected and fixated. If you use the shortest lesion access, a coaxial guidance needle system is not necessary.

After finishing the core needle biopsy, the whole area including the needle track should be compressed for a minimum of 5 min. After vacuum-assisted biopsy, compression should last for 15 min and an additional pressure dressing should be applied for 3–6 h.

The patient should get a written information about behavioral precautions after biopsy.

8.1 Indications for Clip Marking

There are two main indications for lesion clip marking after biopsy. First, if lesions are very small, they could be masked by bleeding or just disappear due to the loss of the main tissue portion during biopsy (Evans et al. 2018). Secondly, make sure that you can find the lesion or the area again after neoadjuvant chemotherapy with partial or complete tumor response (Association of Breast Surgery at Baso 2009).

There are different opinions regarding clip marking. Some authors recommend putting a clip in all biopsied lesions, while others only at some of them. Clip marking mainly depends on lesion size, with the resulting possibility that the lesion is masked due to bleeding and might not be detectable although needed for planned treatment (e.g., surgery).

8.2 Preoperative Wire Localization

After successful minimally invasive diagnosis of malignancy, depending on tumor type, surgery will follow directly or after neoadjuvant chemotherapy.

In case of a non-palpable lesion, either the lesion itself or the clip after chemotherapy is marked to guide the surgeon during the operation. The classical method is a wire localization. A flexible wire with hook(s) is placed either into the breast lesion or closest to the clip. The placement should be adapted to the planned surgical approach. Ideally, the wire is directly placed in the lesion with the branches just outside. If a direct placement is not possible, the distance to the lesion should not exceed 1 cm. Localization of the incision and planned amount of tissue removal should be kept in mind as well. Therefore, a close collaboration with the surgeon is necessary.

Recently developed markers, like radioactive or magnetic seeds, can also be used to guide the surgeon, who uses a detector probe, like during the sentinel node procedure. The magnetic procedure is quite simple, but keep in mind, that the magnetic particle can severely compromise follow up MR-imaging. The seeds can be placed during biopsy or before neoadjuvant chemotherapy. The radioactive seeds should be placed shortly before the operation. Some additional requirements for radiation protection and colleting of the seeds have to be fulfilled rendering the workflow more complex. Such procedures are not necessary for magnetic seeds.

After all marking procedures, mammography in two orthogonal planes is recommended for

Ultrasound-Guided Interventions

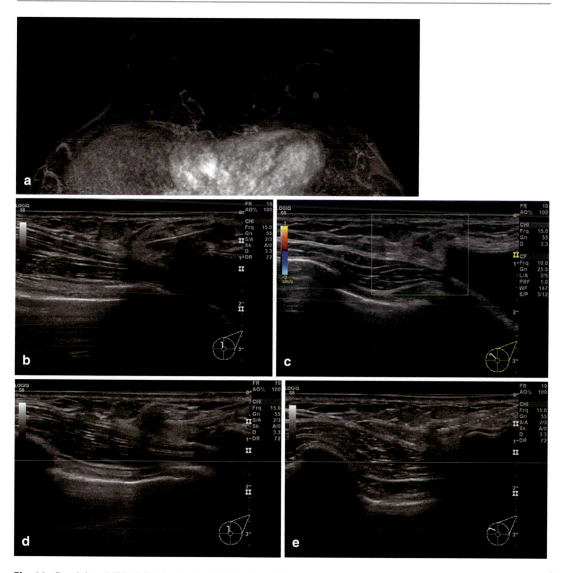

Fig. 11 Suspicious MRI-visible lesions in a BRCA1-positive patient after augmentation of the left breast due to micromastia (**a**) with corresponding US lesions at 12 o'clock (**b, d**) and 10 o'clock (**c, e**)

correlation of lesion and clip. If the lesion was only detectable at US and MRI, a control MRI examination after applying a MRI-compatible wire may be helpful (see Figs. 11 and 12).

9 Reporting and Probe Handling and Pathology Information

To provide proper interpretation of core biopsy results, details of patient history as well as clinical and radiological findings should be provided to the pathologist, ideally on a standardized request form.

This should contain clinical information, a detailed description of the radiology findings (e.g., mass, architectural distortion, microcalcifications and respective classification), level of suspicion (e.g., BI-RADS final assessment score), laterality, and exact lesion location within the breast.

The specimen X-ray should be available for the pathologist. Information on representative sampling, number of cores, and separation of cores containing microcalcifications should be provided. Ideally, probes with and without calcifications should be sent in using different containers.

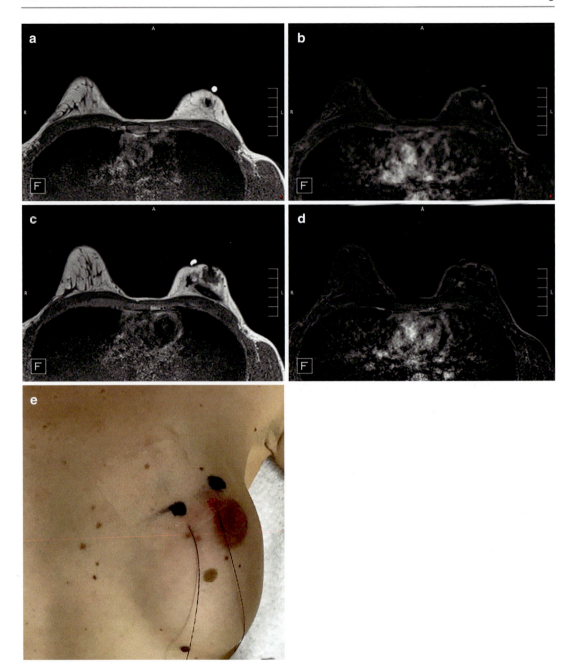

Fig. 12 MRI control images of correct wire positioning in T1 unenhanced (**a**, **c**) and post-contrast subtracted images (**b**, **d**). (**e**) Wire localization in patient with additional marking of the lesion location on the skin

For specimens with biopsies from multiple sites, separate containers and separate reports should be used for each lesion.

Furthermore, the type of sampling (CNB versus VAB) and the type of biopsy guidance (US, stereotaxis, MRI) should be recorded.

10 Radiological-Histopathological Correlation

Even if the false-negative rate of core needle and vacuum-assisted biopsy is very low, they are not zero and most of the times the reason for the false negatives is discordance between imaging findings and histopathology results. The false-negative rate ranges from 0.1% to 2.5% in core needle biopsy using a 14 G needle and 0.1% to 1% in vacuum-assisted biopsy using a needle with a diameter of 11 or 8 G (Huang et al. 2017; Schueller et al. 2008; Youk et al. 2008, 2010; Zhang et al. 2012; Jung et al. 2014, 2018).

In addition, there is an underestimation rate of high-risk lesion by ultrasound-guided core needle biopsy within a range from 24.5% to 65%, mainly attributed to atypical ductal hyperplasia lesions (Kim et al. 2008; Huang et al. 2017; Schueller et al. 2008; Youk et al. 2008; Jang et al. 2008; Ahn et al. 2016; Atkins et al. 2013; Rageth et al. 2016, 2019). Every radiologist performing image-guided breast biopsy should therefore not only know exactly how to technically perform the biopsy procedure, but also be aware of the possibility of a false-negative diagnosis or underestimation of lesions. He/she should therefore know how to ensure a correct radio-pathological correlation and appropriate strategies to manage the patient, if there are any respective uncertainties (e.g., lesions with unclear potential of malignancy).

For every biopsy performed, make sure that you have targeted the correct lesion. In addition to image control of the needle position, also check the composition of the specimen you sampled and look out if there are different tissues combined in the samples. Also, the consistence of a specimen, being rather stiff (tumor tissue) or soft (fatty tissue), when putting into formalin can give you a hint, if you hit the right target. At last, check if the specimen is floating on the formalin surface or if it sinks. If it sinks, it is highly likely that you sampled the right lesion.

Secondly, you have to do a proper correlation with the pathologist whether the findings of the microscopes fit with the findings in imaging. This is especially important if you have a malignant-looking lesion in the imaging and benign finding in pathology.

In his/her report, the pathologist will assign a certain B category according to the histopathology result of the lesion specimens. The B categories are as follows (Perry et al. 2006):

- B1 (Normal)
- B2 (Benign)
- B3 (Uncertain malignant potential with epithelial atypia)
- B3 (Uncertain malignant potential without epithelial atypia)
- B4 (Suspicious)
- B5a (Malignant in situ)
- B5b (Malignant invasive)
- B5c (Malignant not assessable)

If the lesion was associated with microcalcifications, it should be checked that the pathologist saw calcifications of the same size as at initial imaging and specimen X-rays.

For obvious imaging finding like a hypoechoic mass or clearly dilated ducts and calcifications, the histopathology B1 category is not adequate and represents a noncorrelation of radiology and histopathology; in these cases, biopsy is to be repeated.

Further management of B3 lesions depends on its exact histopathology. Some of these have to be further assessed by open or vacuum-assisted excision to be able to safely exclude malignancy before final therapeutic surgery, and others can be handled with 6-month follow-up.

B4 lesions have to be cleared by getting more tissue before the definite therapeutic surgery. B5 lesions usually result in a therapy recommendation such as surgery or neoadjuvant chemotherapy (Ellis et al. 2004; Lee et al. 2016).

11 Summary

Ultrasound-guided minimally invasive procedures are cheap, reliable, and safe for the assessment of suspicious lesions in any diagnostic setting. FNA provides immediate diagnosis, whereas CNB offers far more detailed pathological information about tumor type, grading, or receptor status allowing for a personalized therapy plan for each patient. In addition, preoperative localization of non-palpable lesions is quickly performed by ultrasound-guided wire localization, preventing multiple reoperations due to unclear lesion location or extent.

References

Abbate F et al (2009) Ultrasound-guided vacuum assisted breast biopsy in the assessment of C3 breast lesions by ultrasound-guided fine needle aspiration cytology: results and costs in comparison with surgery. Breast 18(2):73–77

Ahn HS et al (2016) Diagnosis of columnar cell lesions and atypical ductal hyperplasia by ultrasound-guided core biopsy: findings associated with underestimation of breast carcinoma. Ultrasound Med Biol 42(7):1457–1463

Altobelli E, Lattanzi A (2014) Breast cancer in European Union: an update of screening programmes as of March 2014 (review). Int J Oncol 45(5):1785–1792

Association of Breast Surgery at Baso (2009) Surgical guidelines for the management of breast cancer. Eur J Surg Oncol 35(Suppl 1):1–22

Atkins KA et al (2013) Atypical lobular hyperplasia and lobular carcinoma in situ at core breast biopsy: use of careful radiologic-pathologic correlation to recommend excision or observation. Radiology 269(2):340–347

Bae S et al (2015) Breast microcalcifications: diagnostic outcomes according to image-guided biopsy method. Korean J Radiol 16(5):996–1005

Bick U et al (2020) Image-guided breast biopsy and localisation: recommendations for information to women and referring physicians by the European Society of Breast Imaging. Insights Imaging 11(1):12

Charles M et al (2003) Effect of stereotactic core needle biopsy on pathologic measurement of tumor size of T1 invasive breast carcinomas presenting as mammographic masses. Cancer 97(9):2137–2141

Cho N et al (2009) Ultrasound-guided vacuum-assisted biopsy of microcalcifications detected at screening mammography. Acta Radiol 50(6):602–609

Ellis IO et al (2004) Best Practice No 179. Guidelines for breast needle core biopsy handling and reporting in breast screening assessment. J Clin Pathol 57:897–902

European Society of Radiology (2011) White paper on radiation protection by the European Society of Radiology. Insights Imaging 2(4):357–362

Evans A et al (2018) Breast ultrasound: recommendations for information to women and referring physicians by the European Society of Breast Imaging. Insights Imaging 9(4):449–461

Greenwood HI et al (2017) Clustered microcysts on breast ultrasound: what is an appropriate management recommendation? AJR Am J Roentgenol 209(6):W395–W399

Gruber R, Walter E, Helbich TH (2010) Cost comparison between ultrasound-guided 14-g large core breast biopsy and open surgical biopsy: an analysis for Austria. Eur J Radiol 74(3):519–524

Hahn M et al (2012) Interdisciplinary consensus recommendations for the use of vacuum-assisted breast biopsy under sonographic guidance: first update 2012. Ultraschall Med 33(4):366–371

Helbich TH, Matzek W, Fuchsjager MH (2004) Stereotactic and ultrasound-guided breast biopsy. Eur Radiol 14(3):383–393

Huang ML et al (2017) Comparison of the accuracy of US-guided biopsy of breast masses performed with 14-gauge, 16-gauge and 18-gauge automated cutting needle biopsy devices, and review of the literature. Eur Radiol 27:2928–2933

Humphrey KL et al (2014) Percutaneous breast biopsy: effect on short-term quality of life. Radiology 270(2):362–368

Jaffe TA et al (2015) Management of anticoagulant and antiplatelet medications in adults undergoing percutaneous interventions. AJR Am J Roentgenol 205(2):421–428

Jang M et al (2008) Underestimation of atypical ductal hyperplasia at sonographically guided core biopsy of the breast. AJR Am J Roentgenol 191:1347–1351

Jung HK et al (2014) Benign core biopsy of probably benign breast lesions 2 cm or larger: correlation with excisional biopsy and long-term follow-up. Ultrasonography 33:200–205

Jung I et al (2018) Ultrasonography-guided 14-gauge core biopsy of the breast: results of 7 years of experience. Ultrasonography 37:55–62

Kim HS et al (2008) US-guided vacuum-assisted biopsy of microcalcifications in breast lesions and long-term follow-up results. Korean J Radiol 9(6):503–509

Kricheldorff J et al (2018) Breast implant-associated lymphoma. Dtsch Arztebl Int 115(38):628–635

Lai HW et al (2013) Differences in accuracy and underestimation rates for 14- versus 16-gauge core needle biopsies in ultrasound-detectable breast lesions. Asian J Surg 36(2):83–88

Lee AHS, Anderson N et al (2016) Guidelines for non-operative diagnostic procedures and reporting in breast cancer screening. Royal College of Pathologists, London

Lee AY et al (2018) Sonographic-MRI correlation after percutaneous sampling of targeted breast ultrasound lesions: initial experiences with limited-sequence unenhanced MRI for postprocedural clip localization. AJR Am J Roentgenol 210(4):927–934

Liberman L (2000) Clinical management issues in percutaneous core breast biopsy. Radiol Clin North Am 38(4):791–807

Liberman L et al (1994) Radiography of microcalcifications in stereotaxic mammary core biopsy specimens. Radiology 190(1):223–225

Liberman L et al (2001) Learning curve for stereotactic breast biopsy: how many cases are enough? AJR Am J Roentgenol 176(3):721–727

Liebens F et al (2009) Breast cancer seeding associated with core needle biopsies: a systematic review. Maturitas 62(2):113–123

Meissnitzer et al (2009) Targeted ultrasound of the breast in women with abnormal MRI findings for whom biopsy has been recommended. AJR Am J Roentgenol 193(4):1025–1029. https://doi.org/10.2214/AJR.09.2480

Murphy CD et al (2008) The American Cancer Society guidelines for breast screening with magnetic resonance imaging: an argument for genetic testing. Cancer 113(11):3116–3120

Nyhsen CM et al (2017) Infection prevention and control in ultrasound - best practice recommendations from the European Society of Radiology Ultrasound Working Group. Insights Imaging 8:523–535

Park JM et al (2011) Core biopsy of the breast lesions: review of technical problems and solutions: a pictorial review. Can Assoc Radiol J 62(1):73–82

Park VY et al (2013) Second-look US: how to find breast lesions with a suspicious MR imaging appearance. Radiographics 33(5):1361–1375

Parker SH, Klaus AJ (1997) Performing a breast biopsy with a directional, vacuum-assisted biopsy instrument. Radiographics 17(5):1233–1252

Parker SH et al (1993) US-guided automated large-core breast biopsy. Radiology 187(2):507–511

Patel IJ et al (2012) Consensus guidelines for periprocedural management of coagulation status and hemostasis risk in percutaneous image-guided interventions. J Vasc Interv Radiol 23(6):727–736

Patel IJ et al (2013) Addendum of newer anticoagulants to the SIR consensus guideline. J Vasc Interv Radiol 24(5):641–645

Perry N, Broeders M, de Wolf C, Törnberg S, Holland R, von Karsa L (2006) European guidelines for quality assurance in breast cancer screening and diagnosis, 4th edn. Office for Official Publications of the European Communities, Luxembourg

Perry N et al (2008) European guidelines for quality assurance in breast cancer screening and diagnosis. Fourth edition—summary document. Ann Oncol 19(4):614–622

Peter P et al (2016) MRI screening-detected breast lesions in high-risk young women: the value of targeted second-look ultrasound and imaging-guided biopsy. Clin Radiol 71(10):1037–1043

Plecha DM et al (2014) Addition of shear-wave elastography during second-look MR imaging-directed breast US: effect on lesion detection and biopsy targeting. Radiology 272(3):657–664

Rageth CJ et al (2016) First International Consensus Conference on lesions of uncertain malignant potential in the breast (B3 lesions). Breast Cancer Res Treat 159:203–213

Rageth CJ et al (2019) Second International Consensus Conference on lesions of uncertain malignant potential in the breast (B3 lesions). Breast Cancer Res Treat 174(2):279–296

Riedl CC et al (2005) Potential of dose reduction after marker placement with full-field digital mammography. Invest Radiol 40:343–348

Roberts JG et al (1975) The 'tru-cut' biopsy in breast cancer. Clin Oncol 1(4):297–303

Rogers LW (2005) Breast biopsy: a pathologist's perspective on biopsy acquisition techniques and devices with mammographic–pathologic correlation. Semin Breast Dis 8(3):127–137

Rosen EL et al (2002) Imaging-guided core needle biopsy of papillary lesions of the breast. AJR Am J Roentgenol 179(5):1185–1192

Santiago L et al (2017) Breast cancer neoplastic seeding in the setting of image-guided needle biopsies of the breast. Breast Cancer Res Treat 166(1):29–39

Schueller G et al (2008) US-guided 14-gauge core-needle breast biopsy: results of a validation study in 1352 cases. Radiology 248(2):406–413

Schulz K-D, Kreienberg R, Fischer R, Albert U-S (2003) Stufe-3-Leitlinie Brustkrebs-Früherkennung in Deutschland. Onkologe 9:394–403

Shin JH et al (2007) Targeted ultrasound for MR-detected lesions in breast cancer patients. Korean J Radiol 8(6):475–483

Soo MS, Baker JA, Rosen EL (2003) Sonographic detection and sonographically guided biopsy of breast microcalcifications. AJR Am J Roentgenol 180(4):941–948

Spick C, Baltzer PAT (2014) Diagnostic utility of second-look US for breast lesions identified at MR imaging: systematic review and meta-analysis. Radiology. https://doi.org/10.1148/radiol.14140474

Suh YJ et al (2012) Comparison of the underestimation rate in cases with ductal carcinoma in situ at ultrasound-guided core biopsy: 14-gauge automated core-needle biopsy vs 8- or 11-gauge vacuum-assisted biopsy. Br J Radiol 85(1016):e349–e356

Vosshenrich R, Kühn S, Reimer P (2013) Aufklärung in der Radiologie. Radiologie up2date 13(02):145–155

Wallis M et al (2007) Guidelines from the European Society of Breast Imaging for diagnostic interventional breast procedures. Eur Radiol 17(2):581–588

Wockel A et al (2018) Interdisciplinary screening, diagnosis, therapy and follow-up of breast cancer. Guideline of the DGGG and the DKG (S3-Level, AWMF Registry Number 032/045OL, December 2017) - Part 1 with Recommendations for the screening, diagnosis and therapy of breast cancer. Geburtshilfe Frauenheilkd 78:927–948

Youk JH et al (2008) Sonographically guided 14-gauge core needle biopsy of breast masses: a review of 2,420 cases with long-term follow-up. AJR Am J Roentgenol 190:202–207

Youk JH et al (2010) Analysis of false-negative results after US-guided 14-gauge core needle breast biopsy. Eur Radiol 20(4):782–789

Yu CC et al (2015) Predictors of underestimation of malignancy after image-guided core needle biopsy diagnosis of flat epithelial atypia or atypical ductal hyperplasia. Breast J 21(3):224–232

Zhang C et al (2012) The negative predictive value of ultrasound-guided 14-gauge core needle biopsy of breast masses: a validation study of 339 cases. Cancer Imaging 12:488–496

Breast MRI: Techniques and Indications

Francesco Sardanelli, Luca A. Carbonaro, Simone Schiaffino, and Rubina M. Trimboli

Contents

1 Introduction 166

2 The Standard Acquisition Protocol 168

3 Post-processing: Image Subtraction and MIP Reconstructions 171

4 Post-processing: Dynamic Analysis 173

5 Diffusion-Weighted Imaging 174

6 Abbreviated CE Protocols 176

7 High-Risk Screening 177
    7.1 Assessing the Response to Neoadjuvant Therapy (NAT) 181
    7.2 Preoperative 187
    7.3 Occult Primary Breast Cancer 195

8 Equivocal/Inconclusive Findings at Conventional Imaging Including
   Suspicion of Breast Cancer Recurrence 196

9 Evaluation of Breast Implant Integrity 199

10 Pathologic Nipple Discharge 201

11 Borderline (B3) Lesions at Mammography/US-Guided Needle Biopsy 202

12 Conclusions 203

References 205

F. Sardanelli (✉)
Department of Biomedical Sciences for Health,
Università degli Studi di Milano, Milan, Italy

Unit of Radiology, IRCCS Policlinico San Donato,
Milan, Italy
e-mail: francesco.sardanelli@unimi.it

L. A. Carbonaro · S. Schiaffino
Unit of Radiology, IRCCS Policlinico San Donato,
Milan, Italy

R. M. Trimboli
Department of Biomedical Sciences for Health,
Università degli Studi di Milano, Milan, Italy

Abstract

This chapter summarizes technical protocols and clinical indications for magnetic resonance imaging (MRI) of the breast. The established protocol used in the last two decades worldwide, essentially composed of an unenhanced T2-weighted sequence and a contrast-enhanced T1-weighted dynamic study, is firstly described. Thereafter, the new

© Springer Nature Switzerland AG 2022
M. Fuchsjäger et al. (eds.), *Breast Imaging*, Medical Radiology Diagnostic Imaging,
https://doi.org/10.1007/978-3-030-94918-1_9

approaches allowed by diffusion-weighted imaging, currently integrated into routine clinical protocols, with a brief mention also of abbreviated contrast-enhanced protocols, are discussed. The following well-recognized indications for breast MRI are considered: screening of women at high risk for breast cancer; assessment of response to neoadjuvant therapy; search for occult primary breast cancer; and evaluation of implant integrity (with dedicated unenhanced sequences). Preoperative breast MRI is discussed describing the limitations of past studies and the new evidences regarding the cooperation between radiologists and surgeons to avoid unnecessary mastectomies and to tailor a conserving personalized treatment. The limited role of MRI in characterizing equivocal findings identified on mammography and/or ultrasound is also illustrated. In addition, the increasing role of MRI in the setting of nipple discharge and its potential for decision-making when lesions with uncertain malignant potential (B3) are found at mammography- or ultrasound-guided biopsy are outlined.

Abbreviations

2D	Two-dimensional
3D	Three-dimensional
ACR	American College of Radiology
ADC	Apparent diffusion coefficient
AUC	Area under the curve
BC	Breast cancer
BI-RADS	Breast Imaging Reporting and Data System
CE	Contrast-enhanced
CI	Confidence interval
DBT	Digital breast tomosynthesis
DCIS	Ductal carcinoma in situ
DWI	Diffusion-weighted imaging
EBM	Evidence-based medicine
EUSOBI	European Society of Breast Imaging
EUSOMA	European Society of Breast Cancer Specialists
Fat-sat	Fat saturation
GBCA	Gadolinium-based contrast agent
Gd	Gadolinium
HER2	Human epidermal growth factor receptor 2
MIP	Maximum-intensity projection
MRI	Magnetic resonance imaging
NAT	Neoadjuvant therapy
NPV	Negative predictive value
pCR	Pathological complete response
PET	Positron-emission tomography
PPV	Positive predictive value
RCT	Randomized controlled trial
RECIST	Response evaluation criteria in solid tumors
ROI	Region of interest
SPAIR	Spectral attenuated inversion recovery
SPIR	Spectral inversion recovery
STIR	Short tau inversion recovery
US	Ultrasound

1 Introduction

Over the last three decades, magnetic resonance imaging (MRI) has entered the clinical field of detection and management of breast cancer (BC). This was due to the introduction of contrast-enhanced (CE) sequences, firstly reported in 1986 by S. Heywang and coworkers (1986).

The availability of specialized multichannel radiofrequency coils and of powerful gradient systems allowed getting both good image quality and sufficient temporal resolution, playing in favor of an increasing use of breast MRI. The technique was early recognized as a top-level sensitivity tool thanks to the new CE approach, based on lesion vascularization (Kaiser 1989). While initially regarded as a third option after mammography and ultrasound (US), breast MRI has progressively gained an independent position in specific settings such as high-risk screening and neoadjuvant therapy (NAT) assessment thanks to its very high sensitivity and intrinsic multiparametric nature.

As for many innovations in medicine, a generalized application of a new technique mainly depends on the standardization of technical protocols and clinical interpretation. This also happened for breast MRI.

On the technical side, although some variations were applied by different groups, reproducibility across centers was mainly reached by adopting a protocol essentially composed of an unenhanced T2-weighed sequence and of T1-weighted sequences acquired before and after the intravenous administration of gadolinium-based contrast agent (GBCA), with repetitions of the post-contrast sequence to get information about the dynamics of contrast uptake (Sardanelli et al. 2010). In the last decade, diffusion-weighted imaging (DWI) has been added to the standard protocol in many centers with the aim of a better lesion characterization (Sardanelli et al. 2016a) while abbreviated protocols, originally composed by only one pre- and one post-contrast T1-weighted sequence (Kuhl et al. 2014), were proposed with the aim of reducing acquisition and reading time in the screening setting.

On the side of clinical interpretation, in 2003, the inclusion of MRI in the Breast Imaging Reporting and Data System (BI-RADS) by the American College of Radiology (ACR) (American College of Radiology 2003), updated in 2013 (D'Orsi et al. 2013), established common descriptors and diagnostic categories all over the world. This was a great achievement in terms of good clinical practice and clarity of reporting, also allowing comparisons among studies and building of secondary evidence by meta-analyses.

The discussion about indications for breast MRI started very soon, taking into account its very high sensitivity but also the possibility of false positives, opening the discussion on the so-called *low specificity of breast MRI*. Although the specificity of MRI compared favorably with that of mammography or US, this myth delayed the clinical adoption of the technique. Indeed, during the first 15 years of clinical use of CE breast MRI, the reported specificity was highly variable, depending on clinical settings and methods of interpretation. For example, in 1993 it was reported to be as low as 37% (with 94% sensitivity) in a small study on 30 breasts with 47 malignant and 27 benign lesions (Harms et al. 1993),

while in 1994 it was reported to be as high as 97% (with 98% sensitivity) in a large study on 2053 examinations (Kaiser 1994). But those studies that reported a low specificity had a much greater impact than those that reported an intermediate to high specificity.

However, we should admit that in those years, false positives on MRI implied a special weakness: the lack of systems allowing MRI guidance for biopsy and pre-surgical localization. Breast radiologists were able to enroll breast US as a second (targeted) look for assessing and performing biopsy of suspicious MRI-detected lesions (Linda et al. 2008a; Spick and Baltzer 2014), only leaving the task of characterizing not otherwise visible suspicious findings, a minority of cases also in the high-risk screening setting, to MRI-guided procedures (Peter et al. 2016). Devices for MRI-guided interventions started to become clinically available during the 1990s (Fischer et al. 1994). Thereafter, MRI-compatible vacuum-assisted systems were introduced in clinical practice (Heywang-Köbrunner et al. 1999) and its use was established as a standard of care (Heywang-Köbrunner et al. 2009). This was the sign of maturity of the technique: what was visible on MRI could be pathologically characterized and, if necessary, localized for surgical removal. Thus, was this a way open for a generalized use of breast MRI? Which was the context?

When evaluating the introduction of breast MRI in clinical practice we should take into account a complex social and medical context given by the presence of organized and spontaneous screening mammography programs (Lauby-Secretan et al. 2015); the established preference of conserving surgery plus radiation therapy instead of mastectomy (Veronesi et al. 2002; Fisher et al. 2002); the discovery of *BRCA1* and *BRCA2* genes determining hereditary predisposition to BC (Miki et al. 1994; Wooster et al. 1995); the evolution of medical treatments from only chemotherapy to more complex and effective approaches including biologically targeted drugs (Saadatmand et al. 2015a); the general acceptance of methods of evidence-based medicine (EBM) for evaluating the effectiveness of any medical option (Sackett et al. 1996); and the decrease of health-care spending (Budhdeo et al. 2015). Successes and difficulties of breast MRI can be understood only considering this historical background. Of course, all this was not only a matter of science.

The aim of this chapter is to provide a general knowledge about technical requirements, scheduling, protocols, and post-processing for breast MRI (Table 1) as well as to give an overview of its clinical indications (Table 2). Special techniques such as T1-weighted CE ultrafast sequences, T2* weighted perfusion, or intravoxel incoherent motion DWI as well as magnetic resonance spectroscopy will not be considered, being currently outside of routine clinical protocols.

Table 1 Breast MRI: technical requirements, scheduling, standard protocol, and postprocessing

Technical requirements	
Intensity of magnetic field	≥1.5T
Gradient power	≥20 mT/m
Channels of dedicated coil	≥4
Scheduling in premenopausal women	
Days of the menstrual cycle	7–14
Standard protocol	
One of the three T2-weighted sequences (axial or sagittal):	
• Fast/turbo spin-echo ± fat-sat or	
• Short tau inversion recovery (STIR) or	
• Spectral presaturation with inversion recovery (SPIR)	
Contrast dose	0.1 mmol/kg (equal to 0.2 mL/kg for 0.5 M concentration)
Dynamic study (2D or 3D T1-weighted gradient-echo sequence ± fat-sat, axial or sagittal)	
• Slice thickness	≤3 mm
• Spatial in-plane resolution	≤1.5 mm² (preferably ≤1 mm²)
• Temporal resolution	≤120 s
• Duration	6 min
Postprocessing	
Non-fat-sat dynamic studies	
• Image subtraction (enhanced minus unenhanced) of the first or second frame	
• Maximum-intensity projections (MIPs)	
Dynamic analysis	
• ROI based or	
• Color code mapping (dedicated software)	

2D two-dimensional, 3D three-dimensional, ROI region of interest

Table 2 Breast MRI: clinical indications

Established indications
High-risk screening
Assessment of response to neoadjuvant therapy
Search for primary breast cancer occult to mammography and US
Characterization of equivocal findings at mammography and/or US
Evaluation of breast implant integrity (unenhanced study)
Debated indication
Preoperative assessment
Emergent indications
Nipple discharge
Borderline (B3) lesions at mammography/US-guided needle biopsy

US ultrasound

2 The Standard Acquisition Protocol

As explained in Sect. 1, a standard protocol for breast MRI was practically established during the 1990s, when sufficiently advanced MRI systems were available. Technical recommendations were issued by different bodies such as the European Society of Breast Cancer Specialists (EUSOMA) (Sardanelli et al. 2010), the European Society of Breast Imaging (EUSOBI) (Mann et al. 2008, 2015), and the ACR (American College of Radiology 2018). We summarize here the most important issues to be considered.

Breast MRI must be performed using magnets with ≥1.5T intensity field and ≥20 mT/m power gradients, equipped with bilateral dedicated multichannel coils, with a minimum of four channels.

In premenopausal women, even if taking oral contraceptives, it is important to schedule the examination between days 7 and 14 of the menstrual cycle to avoid superimposition of moderate or marked background parenchymal enhancement, possibly determining false-positive and false-negative results (Baltzer et al. 2011) (Fig. 1). In the preoperative staging, exceptions to this rule can be necessary to avoid delay in treatment (Sardanelli et al. 2010). A specific scheduling is not required for postmenopausal women even if taking hormone

Breast MRI: Techniques and Indications

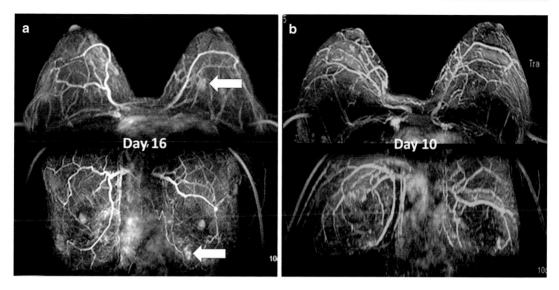

Fig. 1 Effect of scheduling breast MRI in relation to the menstrual cycle. A 36-year-old women with negative family history, pregnancy, and breast-feeding for 8 months at age 23, breast implants at age 30 presented with a palpable lump in the right breast, negative at mammography and US. Breast MRI was firstly performed on day 16 of the menstrual cycle. (**a**): Axial (above) and coronal (below) MIP reconstructions of the first dynamic phase showed a suspicious enhancement in the left internal lower quadrant; no suspicious findings in the right breast at analysis of the whole MRI examination. MRI was repeated on day 10 of the menstrual cycle. (**b**): The finding in the left breast completely disappeared. Both examinations were performed at 1.5T with the same equipment, with 0.1 mmol/kg of gadobenate dimeglumine and the same 3D spoiled gradient-echo sequence (time resolution 120 s). Note that on day 10, more vessels are visible with less pronounced enhancement, in the absence of the suspicious finding

replacement therapy, recently reported to not consistently affect the background parenchymal enhancement (Hegenscheid et al. 2012). In the case of irregular menses, premenopausal hysterectomy, or any difficulty in establishing a correct timing for the MRI examination, a blood sampling for serum progesterone (Ellis 2009) may be helpful to identify the optimal phase.

After gaining a venous access, usually through a medial cubital vein, the patient is placed in the prone position with the arms along the body and the breast pending in the coil. Due to the higher incidence of movement artifacts on the side of the injection, contrast injection should be performed, whenever possible, on the opposite side to that of the breast potentially harboring the most relevant finding(s) (Schiaffino et al. 2018).

After scout-view sequences, the standard breast MRI protocol usually includes the following (Sardanelli et al. 2010):

1. A bilateral (with the exception of prior mastectomy) morphological study using at least one unenhanced T2-weighted fast/turbo spin-echo with or without fat saturation (fat-sat), short tau inversion recovery (STIR), or spectral presaturation with inversion recovery (SPIR) sequences (Fig. 2a).
2. A bilateral (with the exception of prior mastectomy) two-dimensional (2D) or three-dimensional (3D) gradient-echo T1-weighted dynamic sequence, with or without fat-sat (slice thickness ≤3 mm, spatial in-plane resolution ≤1.5 mm^2 (preferably ≤1 mm^2), temporal resolution ≤120 s) (Fig. 2b–d).

For both sequences, the scan plane is chosen by the radiologist according to personal preference, local habit, or individual clinical needs. Currently, axial and sagittal planes are mostly used. For the sake of brevity, we do not enter here into further technical details of these standard sequences (such as advantages and disadvantages

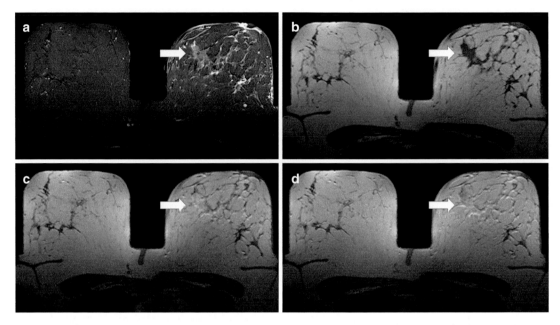

Fig. 2 The breast MRI standard protocol. 1.5T preoperative MRI in a 44-year-old woman with a newly diagnosed invasive ductal cancer at upper inner quadrant of the left breast. The same slice best demonstrating the index lesion is shown for four axial sequences: STIR (**a**); 3D spoiled gradient-echo T1-weighted sequence, unenhanced (**b**), 2 min (**c**) and 8 min (**d**) after injection of 0.1 mmol/kg of gadobenate dimeglumine. The spiculated lesion (arrow on each panel) appears to be slightly hyperintense in **a**, hypointense in **b**, and clearly enhancing in **c** (but reaching a signal intensity only close to that of the surrounding fat), with its anterior part showing a washout in the late phase (**d**)

of the fat-sat approaches) that the reader can find in book chapters (Kaiser 1993; Heywang-Köbrunner and Beck 1996; Hylton 2005; Hendrick 2010) and articles (Kuhl 2007; Melsaether and Gudi 2014). As a general note, when a compromise has to be fixed between spatial and temporal resolution for the dynamic study, the former has to be preferred (Gutierrez et al. 2012).

For the dynamic study, 6 min is sufficient for evaluating the contrast uptake (i.e., the wash-in and washout kinetics). In fact, when the dynamic acquisition is prolonged over 6 min, misleading late washout can be appreciated in benign lesions (Tannaphai et al. 2012). A final acquisition with a spatial resolution higher than that of the dynamic study can be useful in the case of suboptimal spatial resolution in the standard study, in particular when a ductal carcinoma in situ (DCIS) is suspected, either pure or associated to an invasive cancer.

The use of two-compartment (vascular/interstitial) GBCAs is recommended at the standard dose of 0.1 mmol/kg, with an injection rate of 2–3 mL/s, followed by saline flushing (20–30 mL at 2–3 mL/s), using an automatic injector. Given the recent evidence of Gd accumulation/retention in the brain after multiple administration of GBCA and the debate on the distinction between linear and macrocyclic agents (Kanal 2017), the standard dose (0.1 mmol/kg) has to be considered as the maximal dose for all GBCAs, independently of their chemical structure and of the magnetic field intensity. Due to regulations issued by the European Medicines Agency in 2017 (European Medicines Agency 2017), in the European Union the use of linear GBCAs—gadobenate dimeglumine (Gd-BOPTA, MultiHance), gadodiamide (Gd-DTPA-BMA, Omniscan), gadopentetate dimeglumine (Gd-DTPA, Magnevist), and gadoversetamide (Gd-DTPA-BMEA, OptiMARK)—has been suspended, so that only the macrocyclic GBCAs—gadobutrol (Gd-BT-DO3A, Gadovist or Gadavist), gadoterate (Gd-DOTA, Dotarem), or gadoteridol (Gd-HP-DO3A, ProHance)—can be used.

For GBCAs with the standard concentration (0.5 M), the dose to be administered is obtained by doubling the kg of body weight divided by 10 (e.g., 14 mL for a woman with 70 kg of body weight). This works for all GBCAs with the only exception of the gadobutrol that has a 1 M concentration. In that case, the final doubling has to be skipped (e.g., 7 mL for a woman with 70 kg of body weight). Attention must be paid in reporting the contrast dose, carefully distinguishing between mmol and mL (for the standard 0.5 M concentration, 0.1 mmol/kg is equivalent to 0.2 mL/kg of body weight). Confusion on this aspect is sometimes encountered also in published articles.

When MRI is requested for the evaluation of breast implant integrity, a dedicated protocol composed of multiplanar unenhanced special sequences must be performed (see below).

3 Post-processing: Image Subtraction and MIP Reconstructions

If non-fat-sat dynamic sequences are used, *temporal subtraction* is mandatorily performed on a pixel-by-pixel basis (post-contrast images minus pre-contrast images, all of them being the *primary images*) for each of the dynamic phases. Image subtraction works here as a way for suppressing the high-fat signal and also the signal from all the other tissues that do not enhance. This implies the advantage of isolating the enhancing structures (mainly vessels and enhancing lesions) on a black background (Fig. 3a, b). We could name these subtracted images as *secondary images*, produced by the software for all dynamic phases, a post-processing that doubles the number of the enhanced images, contributing to a total number of images for an individual breast MRI examination up to 1200 (Fausto et al. 2007) and more, depending

on the breast size and the adopted through-plane image resolution, i.e., the slice thickness. When using fat-sat dynamic sequences, temporal subtraction is not mandatory but could be useful for getting a higher conspicuity of enhancing lesions.

The subtracted dataset obtained for one of the dynamic phases is used for generating *tertiary images* by means of maximum-intensity projection (MIP) 3D reconstructions, obtained for the total volume or only for part of them (partial MIP). MIPs are usually presented as bilateral axial, bilateral coronal, and unilateral sagittal views, so summarizing the examination in few images comparable to mammograms (Fig. 3c–f). These images are easy to be understood also by members of the multidisciplinary team who are not radiologists, especially surgeons with whom the surgical planning has to be defined. For this aim, we should remember that in breast MRI the patient is studied in the prone position with the arms along the body while she will be operated in the supine position, with the arm abducted. Notably, the change from prone to supine position implies a lesion displacement along the three spatial dimensions from 3 to 6 cm (Fig. 4) with lesion-to-skin and lesion-to nipple displacements smaller than 1 cm, even though the nipple displacements are similar or larger than those of lesions (the lesion-to-nipple distance remains the most reliable measure to be used for targeted US after MRI) (Carbonaro et al. 2012).

The choice of the dynamic phase to be used for generating MIPs depends on temporal resolution, contrast injection rate, and saline flushing as well as on physiological parameters such as blood pressure and heart rate. Usually, using a temporal resolution from 90 to 120 s, the first phase is the best one, avoiding high superimposition of background parenchymal enhancement; in the case of 60 s or less, the first or the second phase may be the best one. Anyway, a visual check has to be made.

In the case of patient movements, in particular between pre- and post-contrast sequences, subtracted images can be heavily burdened by mis-

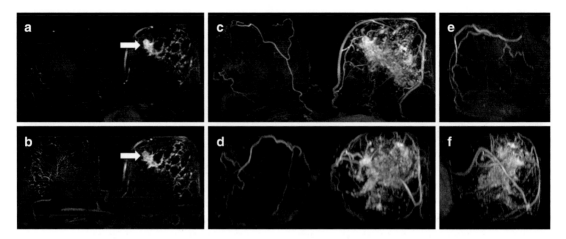

Fig. 3 Breast MRI postprocessing: image subtraction and MIP reconstructions. Same patient and examination shown in Fig. 2. Subtraction of the unenhanced from the CE 2-min image (**a**) and from the CE 8-min image (**b**). Both subtracted images show with high conspicuity a 24 mm mass enhancement (arrow) at the upper inner quadrant of the left breast (with enhancement lower in **b** than in **a**, showing a washout) but also non-mass enhancement extended in the outer part of the breast. MIP reconstructions of the 2-min subtracted images from the entire 3D dataset: bilateral axial (**c**), bilateral coronal (**d**), and unilateral sagittal right (**e**) and left (**f**). These 3D reconstructions show the whole extent of an invasive ductal carcinoma with an associated extensive DCIS component, confirmed on pathological examination of mastectomy specimen

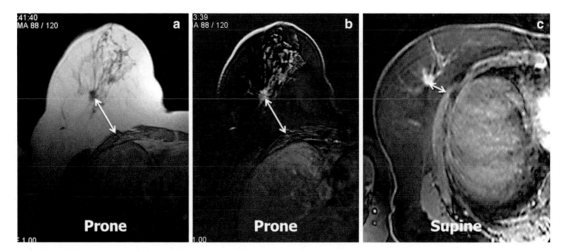

Fig. 4 Prone versus supine breast MRI. Spatial displacement of a 14-mm invasive ductal cancer in the central region of the right breast (1.5T magnet, 0.1 mmol/kg of gadobenate dimeglumine). Axial spoiled 3D gradient-echo T1-weighted unenhanced sequence (**a**) and CE-subtracted sequence (**b**), obtained with the patient in standard prone position; axial T1-weighted fat-sat volumetric interpolated breath-hold sequence (VIBE) obtained with the patient in supine position as a final phase of the examination (**c**). The large spatial displacement of the spiculated tumor can be appreciated evaluating the distance between the lesion and the pectoral muscle (double-ended arrow in **a**, **b**, and **c**): in **c** the lesion is much closer to the thoracic wall and in a more lateral position than in **a** and **b**. (From Carbonaro et al. (2012), with permission from the publisher)

registration artifacts leading to both false-negative and false-positive results as well as to misleading results of the dynamic analysis. The presence of artifacts, also including inhomogeneous fat-sat or ghost artifacts on the phase axis, obliges to a careful visual evaluation of native (i.e., unsubtracted) images, comparing pre- and post-contrast phases, slice by slice (Fig. 5).

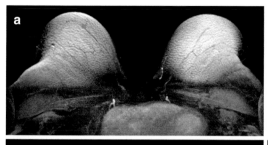
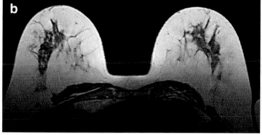
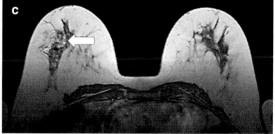

Fig. 5 Misregistration artifacts. Preoperative breast MRI in a 57-year-old woman (1.5T magnet, 0.08 mmol/kg of gadobutrol). The MIP 3D reconstruction of the first post-contrast dataset (**a**) was nondiagnostic due to strong misregistration artifacts caused by patient's movement in between unenhanced and enhanced sequences, implying that subtracted images were unreliable. Only by visual comparing, slice-by-slice, unenhanced images (**b**) with the corresponding CE images (**c**) a non-mass enhancement (arrow in **c**) corresponding to a high-grade DCIS can be identified

4 Post-processing: Dynamic Analysis

Clinical interpretation should be based on the integration of morphology (including signal analysis on unenhanced T1- and T2-weighted images) and kinetic analysis of the dynamic study, for a total of 147 signs, as described by Werner A. Kaiser in his historical book (Kaiser 2008).

Dynamic analysis can be performed visually or using dedicated software. The second option is performed by positioning regions of interest (ROIs) inside the lesion under consideration using post-processing tools available on every MRI workstation or by color-coded mapping provided by dedicated software (Dorrius et al. 2011). In the former case, attention should be paid to include only those parts of the lesion which show high signal on the first (or second, see above) dynamic phase, avoiding the inclusion of internal necrosis or fibrosis as well as of tissues outside the lesion (Sardanelli et al. 2004a). For the sake of robustness, we advise to obtain a graph including at least a "control" curve, for example on the pectoral muscle (Fig. 6), the aorta, or the left ventricle.

The shape of the signal-to-time curve includes (1) the initial signal increase from the pre-contrast measurement to the maximum value within the first 3 min after injection; (2) the post-initial behavior from the maximum peak within the first 3 min to the sixth minute. The initial increase (wash-in) can be low, intermediate, or high, historically defined (Heywang-Köbrunner and Beck 1996) as up to 50%, 50–100%, and >100% for ROI-based measurements, respectively. Three types of post-initial curves are basically identifiable (Heywang-Köbrunner and Beck 1996; Kuhl et al. 1999; Baum et al. 2002):

1. *Continuous increase* (type 1 curve), with a signal increase >10% in comparison to the peak reached within the first 3 min (Fig. 6a, b)
2. *Plateau* (type 2 curve), with maximum deviation between +10% and −10% in comparison to the peak reached within the first 3 min (Fig. 6c, d)

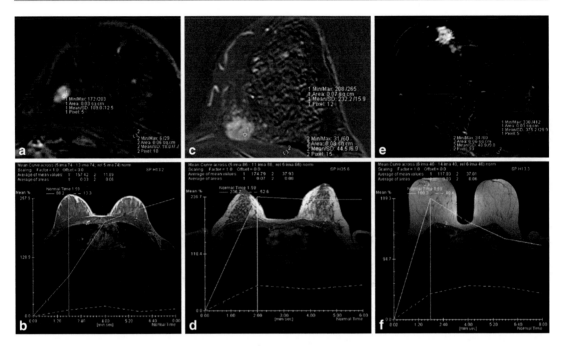

Fig. 6 Dynamic analysis (1.5T magnet, 0.1 mmol/kg of gadobenate dimeglumine). Fibroadenoma (**a**) with moderate initial enhancement and post-initial continuous increase: type 1 curve (**b**). Invasive lobular carcinoma (**c**) with high initial enhancement and post-initial plateau: type 2 curve (**d**). Invasive ductal carcinoma (**e**) with high initial enhancement and post-initial washout: type 3 curve (**f**). Same protocol of Fig. 3; images **a**, **c**, and **e** are magnified subtracted images of the first dynamic phase, images under the curves in **b**, **d**, and **f** are the unsubtracted CE whole images of the first dynamic phase. Note on the bottom of the graphs the "control" curves (dotted lines) obtained with ROIs positioned on the pectoral muscles

3. *Washout* (type 3 curve), with a decrease >10% in comparison to the peak reached within the first 3 min (Fig. 6e, f)

The three curves are associated with different probabilities of malignancy, depending—as is for any positive predictive value (PPV)—on disease (cancer) prevalence (Sardanelli and Di Leo 2009a). C.K. Kuhl and coworkers (1999) reported the following distributions of curve types: for BCs, 9% (type 1), 34% (type 2), and 57% (type 3); for benign lesions 83%, 12%, and 6%, respectively. Anyway, kinetics *per se* does not make the diagnosis. For differential diagnosis, morphology and kinetics have to be combined: a benign lesion such as an intramammary lymph node can exhibit a type 3 curve while a DCIS can exhibit a type 1 curve. On the other hand, when a morphologically benign lesion is seen, a type 1 curve makes the exclusion of malignancy more confident.

5 Diffusion-Weighted Imaging

Among the unenhanced sequences, DWI is the most promising approach for routine clinical use.

The basic principle underlying DWI is totally different from that of standard unenhanced morphological sequences or of CE studies. The signal intensity is here mainly correlated with the freedom of movement of water molecules in the tissue and partly with the perfusion effects. Pulsed gradients are switched on and off during the acquisition of an echo-planar sequence, with a b factor (depending on the strength, duration, and spacing of pulsed gradients), expressed as s/mm^2, driving the weight of diffusion dependence of the signal intensity: the higher the b-value, the higher the dependence on diffusivity. A larger b-value is obtained by increasing the gradient amplitude and duration and by widening the interval between gradient pulses. The reader can

Breast MRI: Techniques and Indications

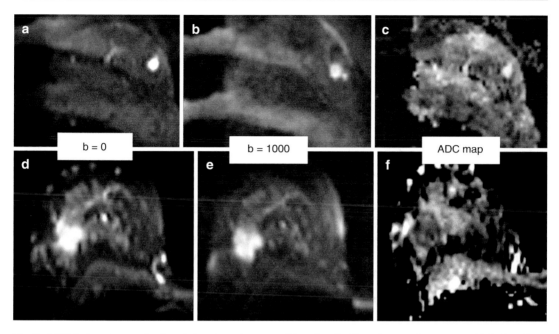

Fig. 7 DWI lesion characterization. Echo planar images obtained at 1.5T with $b = 0$ s/mm^2 and with $b = 1000$ s/mm^2, and ADC map for a 17-mm fibroadenoma in a 46-year-old woman (**a**, **b**, and **c**) and for an invasive ductal cancer (pT2, G3, ER/PgR positive, HER2 negative, Ki-67 >15%) in a 45-year-old woman (**d**, **e**, and **f**, respectively). Note that the fibroadenoma shows a very high signal in **a**, a reduction in signal intensity in **b**, and a still relatively high signal in **c** while the ductal cancer has high signal in **d** and **e** but low signal in **f** (reduced diffusivity): the ROI-based mean ADC was 1.83 and 1.12 × 10^{-3} mm^2/s, respectively

find details on specialized book chapters and articles (Hendrick 2010; Melsaether and Gudi 2014) or on websites (Elster 2018).

The relation between high tumor cellularity and low water diffusivity is the rationale for interpreting the main products of a DWI acquisition (Fig. 7):

1. An image obtained with $b = 0$, which is substantially a T2-weighted image
2. A high b-value image, usually obtained with $b = 700$–1000 s/mm^2
3. A map of the apparent diffusion coefficient (ADC), obtained by combining data from images 1 and 2 and expressed as mm^2/s

Since a restriction in diffusivity determines a high signal on DWI with high b-value while the ADC map represents a high tissue diffusivity with a high signal and a low tissue diffusivity with low signal, a cancer mostly appears hyperintense on high-b-value images and hypointense on the ADC map. Conversely, a benign lesion (which typically has tissue diffusivity lower than that of the normal gland but higher than that of an invasive cancer) appears as relatively hyperintense on high-b-value images as well as on the ADC map (see Fig. 7).

An evaluation of the secondary evidence, i.e., of systematic review and meta-analyses, showed a substantial robustness of the technique: the pooled sensitivities ranged from 84% to 91%, and the pooled specificities from 75% to 84% (Sardanelli et al. 2016a). These levels of performance favorably compare with those of screening mammography. Initial experiences showing a potential for DWI in cancer detection were published (Kazama et al. 2012; Trimboli et al. 2014; Belli et al. 2016; McDonald et al. 2016).

However, the main challenge to DWI is standardization, with the aim of a higher reproducibility of results, in particular for a quantitative biomarker as ADC (Spick et al. 2016a). Methods for gradient nonlinearity corrections were proposed in the framework of the ACR Imaging Network 6698 (Newitt et al. 2015).

The EUSOBI DWI Club tried to set technical guidelines and to contribute for making DWI included in the BI-RADS atlas. During the EUSOBI Annual Scientific Meeting held in Berlin in September 2017, representatives of 25 centers in 15 countries agreed on the following first general recommendations (Baltzer et al. 2020): axial scan plan; in-plane resolution of 2×2 mm^2 or better; slice thickness ≤ 4 mm; field of view to cover both breasts; and mandatory fat suppression, with spectral attenuated inversion recovery (SPAIR) as the recommended technique. The echo-planar imaging sequence should include a minimum of two b-values: the one as close as possible to 0 s/mm^2, not higher than 50 s/mm^2, and the other one equal to 800 s/mm^2. Additional suggested b-values are 200 s/mm^2, to handle intravoxel incoherent motion effects, and above 1200 s/mm^2, to handle non-Gaussian diffusion effects. Two or more excitations are suggested at the lowest b-value, three or more excitations at $b = 800$ s/mm^2 (and optional $b = 200$ s/mm^2), and five or more for $b \geq 1200$ s/mm^2. Whenever possible, those numbers of excitations should be adjusted to warrant a minimum level for signal-to-noise ratio at the highest b-value. The minimum value of echo time allowed by the MRI system for the highest b-value is recommended, as well as the minimum value of the repetition time to allow multislice coverage of both breasts.

The ADC, estimated by ROI or at voxel-by-voxel level, is calculated as

$$\ln\left(S_{\text{low}} / S_{\text{high}} \right) / \left(b_{\text{high}} - b_{\text{low}} \right)$$

where S_{low} and S_{high} are the image signal values obtained with the low and the high b-values, respectively.

The issue of defining cutoffs for ADC values to characterize breast lesions will be illustrated in Sect. 8. Notably, GBCA injected before performing DWI does not negatively impact the diagnostic performance (Dorrius et al. 2014), allowing DWI to be performed after the dynamic study during its post-processing.

6 Abbreviated CE Protocols

Abbreviated protocols for CE breast MRI were recently proposed, the original one by C.K. Kuhl and coworkers (2014), composed by only one T1-weighted gradient-echo sequence before GBCA injection, repeated after injection, for a total acquisition time of only 3 min. When reading sessions using only MIPs are used, the reading time is reduced to 3 s for a dichotomous outcome (positive versus negative, i.e., recall versus non-recall), typical of a screening setting. In this study, the intraindividual comparison with the full protocol (implying 17 min of acquisition time and 28 s of reading time) showed no change in sensitivity (100% for both, based on 11 cancers) and specificity (94% for both).

Thereafter, many studies (for example, Mango et al. 2015; Grimm et al. 2015; Harvey et al. 2016; Machida et al. 2017; Oldrini et al. 2018) confirmed the diagnostic performance of abbreviated protocols without statistically significant difference compared to a standard full protocol, however, with reading time always drastically reduced. The usefulness of this approach has also been shown for screening women with a personal BC history (Choi et al. 2018).

Abbreviated protocols can be an interesting way for reducing MRI costs for acquisition and reading time in the screening setting. The advantages can be well appreciated in the case of breast MRI sessions dedicated to screening only. Otherwise, the reduction in the acquisition time would not impact so much the MRI room time that includes positioning, venous access connection, scout-view images, patient's get off the magnet, etc. Similarly, the reduction of the reading time has to be considered in comparison with time required for information systems to upload any MRI study. A substantial advantage is foreseeable in the case of reading sessions composed of only breast MRI screening examinations.

Future prospective large studies will clarify the scenarios for the usage of abbreviated CE MRI protocols in the screening setting, also in comparison/combination with DWI as a non-contrast option (Yamada et al. 2018). An issue deserving accurate evaluation is the diagnostic performance of abbreviated protocols for the evaluation of known BCs not only for the detection/characterization of already known cancer lesions (Heacock et al. 2016), but also for the detection of additional ipsilateral or contralateral invasive cancers, DCIS associated to invasive cancers, and ipsilateral or contralateral pure DCIS lesions.

The readers will find an extensive review on abbreviated protocols for breast MRI in the Chapter "Abbreviated Breast MRI: Short and Sweet?".

7 High-Risk Screening

A high risk of BC pertains to women:

1. Being carriers of deleterious *BRCA1* or *BRCA2* mutations, or their untested first-degree relatives who have a 50% probability to be a carrier (Saslow et al. 2007)
2. Being affected with Li-Fraumeni (*TP53*), Cowden (*PTEN*), or Bannayan–Riley–Ruvalcaba syndromes, or their untested first-degree relatives (Saslow et al. 2007)
3. Having a lifetime risk of 20–25% or greater (Saslow et al. 2007) as defined by risk assessment tools such as those incorporating familial and personal risk factors (Tyrer et al. 2004; IBIS Breast Cancer Risk Evaluation Tool 2018)
4. Previously treated with chest radiation therapy before 30 years of age (Saslow et al. 2007; Henderson et al. 2010; Mariscotti et al. 2016)

Of note, while the first, the second, and also the fourth categories are associated with a very-high-risk profile (over 40–50% of lifetime risk), the third category includes women with substantially lower risk, even though at least about double if compared to that of the general population. A practical approach is to consider genetically untested women with a strong family history of BC as being at high risk when three or more events occurred in first- or second-degree rela-

tives in either the maternal or the paternal line, including female BC under 60 years of age, ovarian cancer, or male BC at any age (Sardanelli et al. 2007, 2010, 2011). Radiologists should evaluate personal and family history of women they encounter in screening or diagnostic practice in order to use risk modeling software and, importantly, to refer to genetic counselling those women potentially being at high risk.

However, thresholds of lifetime risk for defining a high-risk profile vary across countries. For instance, while the American Cancer Society (Saslow et al. 2007) and the ACR (American College of Radiology 2012), both from the USA, agree upon a $\geq$20% lifetime risk, the National Institute for Clinical Excellence, from the UK, proposes a $\geq$30% lifetime risk (National Institute for Clinical Excellence 2013).

Breast MRI has been largely demonstrated to outperform conventional imaging (i.e., mammography and/or US) for screening high-risk women (Fig. 8). Evidence from three individual patient data meta-analyses suggests that:

1. Screening *BRCA* mutation carriers with mammography and MRI improves sensitivity, relative to mammography alone, not only in women aged <50 years but also $\geq$50 years, thus indicating that there are no reasons to stop MRI screening over 50 (Phi et al. 2015).
2. In *BRCA1* and *BRCA2* mutation carriers, the relative contribution of mammography compared to MRI is not significant even though, especially in *BRCA2* mutation carriers $\leq$40 years, mammography can detect some DCIS with microcalcifications occult to MRI (Phi et al. 2016).
3. When considering only women with a strong family history of BC, without a known gene mutation (i.e., excluding from analysis all mutation carriers), the incremental diagnostic power of MRI remains impressive, with sensitivity going from 55% (mammography alone) to 89% (MRI alone) to 98% (MRI plus mammography), even though with an (acceptable) trade-off in terms of specificity (94%, 83%, 79%, respectively) (Phi et al. 2017).

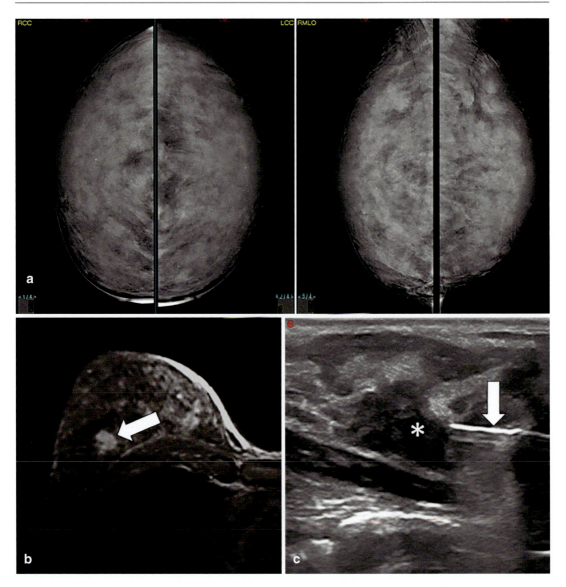

Fig. 8 High-risk screening. Forty-one-year-old woman with *BRCA1* mutation. Negative bilateral mammography, with extremely dense pattern (ACR class, *d*) (**a**). First-look bilateral US (not shown) was negative. 1.5T MRI (0.08 mmol/kg of gadobutrol) showed a 10-mm suspicious enhancing lesion in the right breast in typical prepectoral location (arrow in **b**), corresponding, at second-look targeted US, to a hypoechoic suspicious lesion (asterisk in **c**, where the needle for the core biopsy sampling is also visible, arrow). Pathology revealed a triple-negative grade 2 invasive ductal carcinoma

To note, the high statistical power of individual patient data meta-analysis methodology allowed by data sharing among the authors of original studies who accepted to contribute (Sardanelli et al. 2018a) permitted to clarify these important aspects of the application of breast MRI to the screening of high-risk women. Of course, this cannot overcome limitations of the original studies incorporated in the meta-analyses, such as the relatively low MRI sensitivities obtained by the first studies. The MRISC study from the Netherlands (Kriege et al. 2004) reported an MRI sensitivity of 71% overall and only 17% for DCIS, the Canadian study (Warner et al. 2004) 77% and 67%, and the MARIBS study from the UK (Leach et al. 2005) 77% and 50%, respectively.

Interestingly, looking at the data of multiple studies, the 2007 paradigm of the American Cancer Society (*MRI as an adjunct to mammography*) for screening high-risk women (Saslow et al. 2007) has been reverted, investigating on *mammography as an adjunct to MRI* to verify the possibility to avoid screening mammography in this particular population. This possibility was already evident from the EVA (Kuhl et al. 2010) and the HIBCRIT (Sardanelli et al. 2007, 2011) studies that showed a very low (and not significant) additional value of mammography and/or US when MRI is performed. Importantly, the EVA trial (Kuhl et al. 2010) showed this also when US is performed every 6 months. More recent studies confirmed that in the high-risk screening setting, when MRI is performed, the additional diagnostic contribution of mammography is negligible or strongly limited to low-grade DCIS (Chiarelli et al. 2014; Obdeijn et al. 2014; Riedl et al. 2015; Lo et al. 2017).

Notably, this *residual role, if any, of mammography* in the high-risk screening has to be discussed also for radioprotection concerns, especially important for *BRCA* mutation carriers. An increasing evidence for a word of caution is available (Colin et al. 2017). Mammography should not be performed in high-risk women below 35 years as there is no evidence that benefits outweigh risks and, in particular, it should be avoided in *TP53* mutation carriers at any age. If the additional value, even if low, of mammography has to be added, e.g., in *BRCA2* mutation carriers (Phi et al. 2016), one solution can be to perform only one (mediolateral oblique) view (Colin and Foray 2012). When a salpingo-oophorectomy is opted, MRI surveillance should not be discontinued as the BC risk decreases but still remains to be high (Fakkert et al. 2012). In the presence of prophylactic or therapeutic mastectomy, annual clinical breast examination and US are suggested.

However, even though no doubts exist on the diagnostic performance of MRI for screening women with hereditary BC predisposition, asso-ciated with either identified deleterious mutations or only strong family history, the demonstration of an impact of MRI on patient outcome is more difficult to achieve due to the combined effect of early diagnosis and modern therapies. In fact, in all studies where a non-randomized controlled design is adopted, advanced treatments act as a confounding factor for assessing the effect of the early diagnosis (Sardanelli and Di Leo 2009b). From this viewpoint, the comparison of historical cohorts (i.e., of groups of women who had not only different screening but also different treatments) (Evans et al. 2014) is interesting but not conclusive. The better outcome (i.e., survival) of high-risk women who had MRI screening compared to those who had mammography, and of the latter compared to those who were not screened at all, showed a positive historical trend (Evans et al. 2014): both imaging techniques and therapies improved during the years but the relative contribution of each of the two factors is not discernible (Santoro et al. 2014).

Interestingly, S. Saadatmand and coworkers (2015b) reported on survival benefit from the Dutch MRI Screening (MRISC) study for a median follow-up of 9 years (range 0–14). They matched (1:1 ratio) 93 patients (with 97 BCs) who received MRI <2 years before breast cancer diagnosis during the study with controls, unscreened if <50 years, and screened with biennial mammography if ≥50 years, taking into account risk category (*BRCA1/2* mutation carriers, familial risk), year, and age of diagnosis. MRISC patients showed the following significant results when compared to controls: smaller BCs (<T2 stage, 87% versus 52%); more often node-negative nodal status (69% versus 44%); less chemotherapy (39% versus 77%) and hormonal therapy (14% versus 47%); lower frequency of diagnosis of metastases (9% versus 23%); and longer metastasis-free survival (hazard ratio 0.36), even after lead time correction (hazard ratio 0.40). The overall survival was nonsignificantly higher in MRISC patients (hazard ratio 0.51). The authors concluded that the addition of annual MRI to screening mammography improves metastasis-free survival in these patients.

Another viewpoint has been offered by F. Podo and coworkers (2016) who analyzed survival data of triple-negative BCs and non-triple-negative BCs from the HIBCRIT-1 study. They showed that annual screening including MRI is associated with a 5-year overall survival not significantly different between non-triple-negative BCs (86% ± 9%) and triple-negative BCs (93% ± 5%). A similar trend was found for the 5-year disease-free survival (77% ± 12% versus 76% ± 8%, respectively). This data show that in high-risk women, by combining an MRI-including annual screening with adequate treatment, the gap in outcome between triple-negative and non-triple negative BCs, reported to be very high in the average-risk population (Dent et al. 2007) (hazard ratio 2.6 for distant recurrence and 3.2 for death), can be reduced. However, the outcome results of the HIBCRIT study have to be tempered with the evidence for a better response to neoadjuvant therapy (NAT) in *BRCA* mutation carriers than in noncarriers, with an odds ratio of 2.5 for pathologic complete response (pCR) (Wunderle et al. 2018).

Considering the ethical impossibility to propose any randomized controlled trial (RCT) for comparing patient outcome in high-risk women receiving or not receiving MRI screening, the relative contribution of the MRI-determined earlier diagnosis to the good outcome for these women remains an issue deserving further investigation.

The fourth category of high-risk women we are considering here is composed of patients who have been treated with chest radiation therapy, typically lymphoma survivors. The cumulative BC incidence in women who underwent chest radiation therapy is not substantially different from that of *BRCA* mutation carriers (Henderson et al. 2010; Mariscotti et al. 2016). Importantly, BCs in these women show different phenotypes from those we observe in women with hereditary BC predisposition. Indeed, MRI sensitivity is lower (63–80%) and that of mammography higher (67–70%) than that observed in women with hereditary predisposition, due to a higher incidence of DCIS with microcalcifications and low neo-angiogen-

esis, with the latter probably related to the previous radiation therapy. A sensitivity close to 95% can be obtained only using *mammography as an adjunct to MRI*.

Considering the available evidence, women who underwent chest radiation therapy before 30 receiving a cumulative dose ≥10 Gy should be invited after 25 (or, at least, 8 years after chest radiation therapy) to have annual MRI using the same protocol recommended for women with hereditary predisposition and annual bilateral two-view full-field digital mammography or tomosynthesis with synthetic 2D reconstructions (Mariscotti et al. 2016).

While breast MRI is a well-accepted screening tool for high-risk women, the indication for women at intermediate risk is a matter for discussion. This condition, the intermediate risk, needs to be defined accurately due to the wrong perception that is in the middle between the high risk and the average risk. This is not true. Many high-risk women enrolled in many studies are *BRCA* mutation carriers or belong to families with a strong history of breast/ovarian cancer, implying a lifetime risk equal to 40–50% or greater. Thus, BC incidence in intermediate-risk women should be substantially lower than that in women at high risk. The distinction between *women at high risk* and *women at elevated ("higher-than-average") risk* should be kept clear, with the latter being a much larger category including the former one.

For example, women with heterogeneously or extremely dense breasts at mammography, with previous diagnosis of BC or personal history of some types of B3 lesions (such as atypical ductal hyperplasia, atypical lobular hyperplasia, and lobular carcinoma in situ), should be considered at intermediate risk. Recently, the ACR (Monticciolo et al. 2018) recommended annual MRI screening for women with a personal BC history and dense tissue or diagnosed by age 50. The authors also advice to consider screening MRI for women with personal BC history not included in the previous category and for women who were diagnosed with atypical ductal hyperplasia or lobular neoplasia.

In our opinion, also considering the issue of GBCA brain accumulation/retention, RCTs comparing mammography and US versus MRI (alone or as supplemental tool) in intermediate-risk women is the best way to get a high level of evidence. Women with a personal history of BC could be offered with dedicated sessions including annual mammography or digital breast tomosynthesis (DBT), starting from the year after treatment and lasting up to 74 years of age, under the organization of population-based screening programs (Bucchi et al. 2016). Regarding women with extremely dense breasts (class *d*), the results of the DENSE trial (Bakker et al. 2019) changed the scenario. The authors showed that screening women with density *d* with contrastenhanced breast MRI results into an additional breast cancer detection of 16.5‰ and a 50% reduction of the interval cancer rate, from 5.0‰ with mammography only to 2.5‰ when MRI is added. Cost-efficacy analysis resulted favorable to MRI screening of women with d breast density (Geuzinge et al. 2021). This perspective has been embraced by recent EUSOBI recommendations (Mann et al. 2022).

7.1 Assessing the Response to Neoadjuvant Therapy (NAT)

In the last years, clinical indications to NAT for BC have dramatically expanded including not only locally advanced breast cancers less than 5 cm in diameter with regional, skin, or chest wall involvement, but also tumors larger than 2.5 cm in diameter and triple-negative or human epidermal growth factor receptor 2 (HER2)-positive and node-negative tumors where the excision might be suboptimal or not feasible (Slanetz et al. 2017).

The primary aim of NAT pertains to reducing tumor burden allowing for conserving surgery; secondary aims are treating (occult) metastatic disease present in nearly 70% of women with locally advanced disease (Cox et al. 2013) and optimizing therapeutic protocols by getting early information on the responder versus nonresponder condition. Importantly, patients who

achieve a pCR to NAT have an improved disease-free survival (Dialani et al. 2015).

Indeed, the role of imaging is crucial before, during, and after NAT. Digital mammography and DBT, most often in conjunction with US, represent the usually performed modalities (Slanetz et al. 2017; Dialani et al. 2015). Their limitations can occur in early prediction of response and in assessing residual tumor after NAT. Relying mainly on morphologic characteristics, these methods may be unable to reflect changes in tumor metabolism and vascularization, which can be the only appreciable early signs of NAT effect, thus being not predictive for pathologic response.

MRI, as per its highly resolved tomographic and multiparametric approach including functional assessment, overcomes this hurdle and ranks as the modality of choice in monitoring NAT. V. Dialani and coworkers (2015) reported a 90% accuracy for MRI in assessing residual tumor size compared to 32% for mammography and 60% for US. Importantly, MRI has been shown to be more accurate than mammography also when residual microcalcifications are visible on the post-NAT mammograms (Kim et al. 2016; Um et al. 2018).

The aims of imaging, especially of MRI as the best option, in the NAT setting can be summarized as follows:

1. *Pretreatment prediction of response to NAT*
2. *Early prediction of response during NAT*, after only 1–2 therapy cycles (Fig. 9), potentially inducing changes of NAT regimens
3. *Assessment of residual tumor, if any, after NAT*, i.e., pre-surgical prediction of response—of note, a special case of preoperative breast MRI (Fig. 10), guiding surgical decision-making (mastectomy versus conserving surgery)
4. *Prognostic prediction* as a contribute to clinical decision-making during the follow-up

Up to now, these aims were partially exploited in clinical practice. High-quality research is still needed, in particular for aims 2 and 3, where only coordinated multidisciplinary efforts can

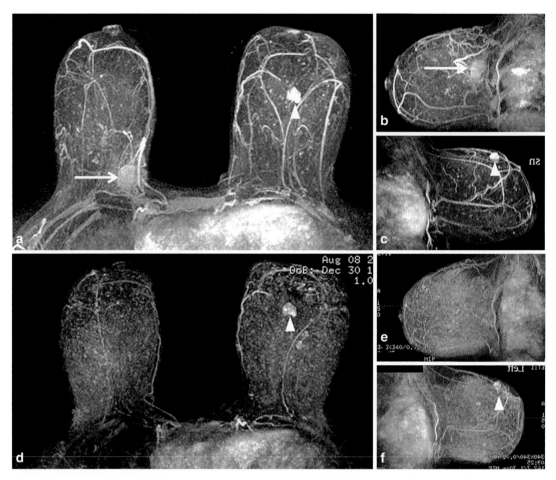

Fig. 9 Early response to neoadjuvant therapy (NAT). A 37-year-old woman with right breast invasive ductal carcinoma and left breast known fibroadenoma. Breast MRI MIP reconstructions of the first CE sequence before and during NAT (3T magnet, 0.1 mmol/kg of gadobenate dimeglumine): axial (**a**, **d**), right sagittal (**b**, **e**), and left sagittal (**c**, **f**). Before NAT, at the right inner quadrants (arrow in **a** and **b**), a 20 mm mass enhancement corresponding to the invasive ductal carcinoma, at the left upper quadrants, a 13 mm mass enhancement corresponding to the known fibroadenoma (arrowhead in **a** and **c**). After two cycles of NAT, MIP reconstructions (same technique as before NAT) showed no residual contrast enhancement in the right breast (**d**, **e**), and at the left upper quadrants, the known fibroadenoma (**d** and **f**, arrowhead). Note that NAT also strongly reduced the visibility of both breasts and the enhancement of the fibroadenoma. The patient underwent conservative surgery and the pathology of the specimen did not find any residual invasive or in situ cancer. (Courtesy of Dr. Massimo Calabrese, Breast Radiology, Ospedale Policlinico San Martino, Genoa, Italy)

conduct observational and, at the best, RCTs to clarify the role of imaging for tailoring treatment in the NAT setting. Of note, at all four steps, quantitative MRI-derived parameters such as volumetric measurements, kinetic analysis, and ADC measurement of the tumor as well as of the ipsilateral and contralateral apparently healthy gland can give in vivo diagnostic and prognostic information. Aim 4 is currently only a perspective and has been rarely explored (Heldahl et al. 2010), going also beyond the specific topic of NAT.

With regard to aim 1 (pretreatment prediction of response to NAT), only few studies are available. For CE-MRI, tumor washout was shown to be a predictor of pCR (Dongfeng

Breast MRI: Techniques and Indications

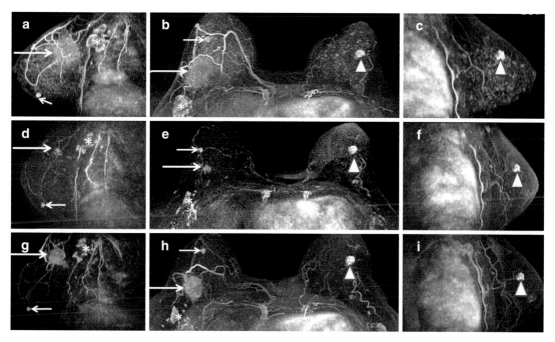

Fig. 10 Early partial response and finally nonresponse to NAT. A 47-year-old woman with an invasive ductal carcinoma in the right upper outer quadrant and two small fibroadenomas, one at the right lower outer quadrant and one at the left upper quadrant. MIP reconstructions of the first contrast-enhanced sequence (3T magnet, 0.1 mmol/kg of gadobenate dimeglumine) before (**a**, **b**, and **c**), during (**d**, **e**, and **f**), and after (**g**, **h**, and **i**) NAT: right sagittal (**a**, **d**, **g**), axial (**b**, **e**, **h**), and left sagittal (**c**, **f**, **i**). Before NAT, at the right inner quadrants, a 48-mm mass enhancement corresponding to the invasive ductal carcinoma (long arrow in **a** and **b**), with metastatic axillary involvement (asterisk in **a** and **b**), at the lower outer quadrant, an 8 mm enhancing mass corresponding to a fibroadenoma (short arrow in **a** and **b**). At the left upper quadrants, a 13 mm mass enhancement corresponding to a fibroadenoma (arrowhead in **a** and **c**). Note also the marked asymmetry of the whole-breast vascularization, increased on the tumor side. After two cycles of NAT, on the right side a strong reduction of the enhancing tumor, from 48 to 13 mm in diameter (partial response, long arrow in **d** and **e**), can be observed; the metastatic axillary involvement (asterisk in **d** and **e**) is also reduced; the whole-breast vascularization is markedly reduced. The fibroadenoma on the right breast is reduced in conspicuity, probably as an effect of the reduced whole-breast vascularization (short arrow in **d** and **e**), while the fibroadenoma on the left side is unchanged (arrowhead in **e** and **f**). However, after the end of NAT, on the right side the tumor mass has increased again, up to 27 mm (long arrow in **g** and **h**) in association with a re-increased axillary nodal involvement (asterisk in **g** and **h**) and ipsilateral vascularization, while the two fibroadenomas remained unchanged (short arrow and arrowhead in **g**, **h**, and **i**) in comparison to the examination after 2 NAT cycles. Pathology of right mastectomy confirmed a residual 36 mm invasive ductal carcinoma. (Courtesy of Dr. Massimo Calabrese, Breast Radiology, Ospedale Policlinico San Martino, Genoa, Italy)

et al. 2012); radiomics such as intratumoral/peritumoral parameters (Braman et al. 2017), texture analysis (Giannini et al. 2017; Fan et al. 2017), or tumor perfusion and background parenchyma enhancement of contralateral breast (Lee et al. 2018) were investigated with interesting results. For DWI, studies on pretreatment ADC as a predictor of response gave conflicting results (Park et al. 2010; Richard et al. 2013; Bufi et al. 2015) while interesting results were obtained using texture analysis (Teruel et al. 2014).

Considering aims 2 (early prediction of response during NAT) and 3 (assessment of residual tumor size after NAT), many studies were published but the evaluation of the evidence is a complex matter for several reasons. First, several studies did not report any details of MRI and postprocessing technique adopted, thus heavily limiting the reproducibility of results; second, there is a lack of consistency in the pathological reference standard, mainly related to the inclusion or noninclusion of residual DCIS in the context of the pCR, making the comparison of results difficult (Marinovich et al. 2012, 2013a).

We summarize here the results available in the literature from systematic review published on this topic.

The secondary evidence on MRI for early prediction of response to NAT was firstly presented by M.L. Marinovich and coworkers (2012). They included 13 studies totaling 605 subjects. The technique considered was the dynamic CE-MRI, typically performed after 1–2 cycles of anthracycline-based or anthracycline/taxane-based NAT, compared to a pre-NAT baseline scan. Although heterogeneity in MRI methods and reference standard precluded statistical meta-analysis, descriptive data showed that sensitivity/specificity pairs for early prediction of pathologic response were highest in studies measuring reductions in K_{trans}, early contrast uptake, and tumor volume, at high thresholds (typically >50% of reduction), while lower sensitivity/specificity pairs were evident in studies measuring reductions in unidimensional or 2D tumor size.

The same group evaluated the role of CE-MRI in detecting residual tumor after NAT (Marinovich et al. 2013a). They included 44 studies totaling 2050 patients. The overall area under the curve (AUC) at receiver operator characteristic analysis for MRI was 0.88 (0.83 for standard definitions of pCR, 0.90 for "less clearly described" pCR, and 0.91 for "near pCR"). Specificity was significantly higher when negative MRI was defined as contrast enhancement less than or equal to normal tissue versus no enhancement (AUC 0.83 and 0.54, respectively), without significantly different sensitivity (AUC 0.83 and 0.87, respectively). When direct comparisons were obtained, MRI was significantly more accurate than mammography (AUC 0.95 versus 0.89). Weak evidence was found ($p = 0.10$) for MRI (AUC 0.89) to be more accurate than clinical examination, while the difference between MRI (AUC 0.93) and US (AUC 0.90) was not significant.

Focusing on the agreement between MRI after NAT and pathologic tumor size, again the same group (Marinovich et al. 2013b) extracted data from 19 studies for 980 patients. The percentage agreement between MRI and pathology was greater than that of comparator tests, but measurement errors may be large enough to be clinically significant. A deeper insight was obtained using the method of individual patient data meta-analysis (Marinovich et al. 2015). Data from 300 patients shared by the authors of 8 studies allowed to estimate the mean difference between MRI and pathology to be 0.0 mm (with limits of agreement of ±3.8 cm); US underestimated the pathologic size by -0.3 cm; mammography had similar mean difference from pathology as MRI but with wider limits of agreement; and clinical examination underestimated tumor size (-0.8 cm), with also wider limits of agreement. The authors concluded that MRI performance was generally superior to that of mammography, US, and clinical examination and that *MRI may be considered the most appropriate test in this setting*. However, MRI under- and overestimation of tumor size has to be always considered as a possibility in a non-negligible fraction of patients.

In the same years (2012), L.M. Wu and coworkers (2012) meta-analyzed 34 studies totaling 1932 patients to investigate the role of DWI and CE-MRI in predicting the pathological response after NAT. For DWI, sensitivity was 0.93, specificity 0.82, positive likelihood ratio 5.09, and negative likelihood ratio 0.09; for CE-MRI, the same data were 0.68, 0.91, 7.48, and 0.36. Although the authors considered their results to be only "tentative," data showed the potential of DWI in the NAT setting and that of a combined use of both techniques.

Thereafter, other two meta-analyses confirmed the ability of DWI in predicting pCR after NAC. W. Chu and coworkers (2017) included 15 studies totaling 1181 patients and obtained pooled sensitivity of 0.88, specificity 0.79, positive likelihood ratio 4.1, negative likelihood ratio 0.16, and AUC 0.91. W. Gao and coworkers (2018) included 20 studies totaling 1490 patients and obtained pooled sensitivity of 0.89, specificity 0.72, and AUC 0.91. The similarity of the results of these two recent meta-analyses plays in favor of the high diagnostic performance of DWI in the preoperative NAT setting.

However, in the NAT setting, also positron-emission tomography (PET) (using the standard ^{18}F-FDG tracer) has been evaluated and compared to MRI. Y.L. Gu and coworkers (2017) concluded that after NAT, CE-MRI has high specificity and DWI high sensitivity, CE-MRI is more accurate than US or mammography, and PET/CT is valuable in this setting, so that CE-MRI, combined with PET/CT or DWI, might allow for a precise assessment of pCR. Two meta-analyses specifically aiming at comparing PET/CT and MRI in this setting gave specular results. Q. Liu and coworkers (2016) included 6 studies totaling 382 patients. Pooled sensitivity, specificity, and AUC were 0.65, 0.88, and 0.84 for MRI, and 0.86, 0.72, and 0.88 for PET/CT. More recently, another meta-analysis (Li et al. 2018) evaluated 13 studies totaling 575 patients who had MRI and 618 who had PET/CT: sensitivity, specificity, and AUC were 0.88, 0.69, and 0.88 for MRI, and 0.77, 0.78, and 0.84 for PET/CT. The more innovative approach, the hybrid PET/MRI examination, was used in a single-center study on 26 patients (Cho et al. 2018): the combination of total lesion glycolysis at PET/CT and signal enhancement ratio at dynamic CE-MRI allowed to reach 100% sensitivity but only 71% specificity in predicting pCR.

At present, considering the advantages of MRI in comparison to PET (lower cost, no radiation exposure) and the double technical possibility offered by MRI (CE dynamic study and DWI), two questions are open. First, could DWI be performed as a stand-alone technique in the NAT setting, offering a very fast MRI approach to be repeated before, during (also more than one time), and after NAT, avoiding multiple GBCA injections? Second, which is the best approach for the combined interpretation of CE-MRI and DWI to maximize the diagnostic performance in predicting pCR? These questions deserve further research, for example evaluating the combined use of CE-MRI and DWI before and after NAT and of DWI alone during the treatment.

Trying to summarize the available evidence, we can say that *MRI is the best we can propose to patients undergoing NAT for BC*, combining a CE study with DWI.

Some practical recommendations should be considered:

1. MRI should always be performed using *a fixed repeatable sequence protocol possibly on the same magnet*, before, during, and after NAT in order to allow comparisons between examinations (unless in the case of research investigating the role of DWI alone during the NAT).
2. After NAT, MRI should be preferably performed 2 weeks after the end of the treatment and within 2 weeks before surgery.
3. The same criteria of interpretation should be systematically adopted when evaluating the response, for the CE study, with reference to the response evaluation criteria in solid tumors (RECIST 1.1) (Eisenhauer et al. 2009; Semiglazov 2015) or more advanced approaches taking into consideration K_{trans}, early contrast uptake, and tumor volume (Marinovich et al. 2012), possibly measured with software reducing the subjectivity of the human operator (Sardanelli et al. 2012).
4. To avoid false-negative results, i.e., the false diagnosis of pCR when invasive cancer is still present, even low enhancement areas located at the primary tumor site should be considered a sign for residual disease; in a recent study (Santamaría et al. 2017), the absence of late contrast enhancement allowed to predict pCR after NAT with an AUC of 0.85, in correlation with an increase in ADC.
5. An important distinction should be made between concentric shrinkage and tumor fragmentation, both during and after NAT, with important implications for early prediction of response (more frequent with the presence of concentric pattern (Ballesio et al. 2017)) and for guiding the choice between conserving surgery and mastectomy (contraindicated by the fragmented pattern).
6. Consider the differences in imaging performance according to BC molecular subtypes. Triple-negative and HER2-positive BCs are more assessable with MRI than luminal tumors (McGuire et al. 2011; Moon et al. 2013; Koolen et al. 2013; Park et al. 2016;

Fatayer et al. 2016; Schaefgen et al. 2016; De Los Santos et al. 2013); this also holds for PET/CT (Koolen et al. 2013; Schmitz et al. 2017). In the case of monitoring response during NAT, MRI was found to be more accurate than PET/CT for HER2-positive tumors and equivalent to PET/CT in triple-negative tumors while for estrogen receptor-positive tumors MRI combined with PET/CT was better than MRI alone, although not significantly (Schmitz et al. 2017). A study (Fukuda et al. 2016) found that MRI closely predicts pCR in triple-negative subtype, not true in luminal subtypes (where the absence of enhancement cannot be considered a predictor if pCR and visible residual lesions are reliable markers of non-pCR). Another recent study (Kim et al. 2018) showed that CE-MRI (delayed phase) underestimates the size of lobular cancers in comparison with ductal cancers and that of HER2-negative cancers in comparison with HER2-positive cancers and triple-negative cancers.

7. Thresholds for reading MRI after NAT could be more effective if adjusted for pathological subtypes (Lo et al. 2016), a task that every center should be performed for the MRI unit, the sequence protocol, the GBCA type, and the postprocessing software used.

8. Be cautious in MRI interpretation when patients are treated with taxane-containing (Charehbili et al. 2014) or bevacizumab-containing (Etxano et al. 2015) regimens (in this setting, the lack of CE is a less sure marker for pCR).

9. A standardized definition of pCR should be always adopted, including the possibility of the presence of DCIS (Ogston et al. 2003), as a necessary homogeneous ground of truth for comparison of clinical and research results.

Finally, the use of MRI in the NAT setting should be still considered an evolving matter for several reasons:

1. Indications to NAT are expanding also in not locally advanced BCs (Slanetz et al. 2017).

2. Further optimization of MRI techniques can be reached, especially combining CE-MRI and DWI with interpretation thresholds taking into account BC molecular subtypes.

3. Prospective, possibly randomized controlled, studies are needed to show how MRI can:
   (a) Guide a change from first-line NAT to a second-line NAT on the basis of MRI after 1 or 2 NAT cycles, as already shown in a retrospective study (Fatayer et al. 2016)
   (b) Guide the choice between mastectomy and breast-conserving surgery after NAT
   (c) Exploit the negative predictive value (NPV) of MRI, also in combination with directed core biopsy, with the golden aim to avoid surgery in the cases of negative CE-MRI, DWI, and core biopsy, referring the patient directly to radiation therapy

At any rate, for both clinical routine and research MRI examinations in the NAT setting, only a great cooperation of the multidisciplinary BC team can exploit the potential for a better patient outcome, especially reducing overtreatment. For this strategic aim, oncologists and surgeons will have to increase their confidence in MRI, depending on the ability of radiologists to show how to make the best use of it. For instance, when considering surgical treatment, the team will have to overcome the old propensity of surgeons to opt for mastectomy also in case of excellent response to NAT (Chen et al. 2009).

This propensity has been confirmed by a recent study (McGuire et al. 2015) reporting on surgical patterns in patients receiving NAT and MRI in eight centers in the USA. Of 759 patients, 45% received conserving surgery and 55% mastectomy. Mastectomy was significantly more frequent in the case of incomplete MRI response *versus* complete (58% versus 43%). At multivariate analysis, positive estrogen receptor status, incomplete MRI response, higher baseline T, younger age, and institution were independent mastectomy predictors. In patients with incomplete response at MRI only, a highly significant trend for mastectomy with increasing baseline T was observed. Importantly, among women with complete response on MRI, 43% underwent mastectomy. The authors rightly concluded that *receptor status, T stage at diagnosis, young age, and treating institution are more significant determinants of surgical treatment choice than MRI response data.*

Finally, we should not forget that while MRI has been clearly demonstrated to outperform mammography in the NAT setting, its superiority to US resulted to be less pronounced also in meta-analyses. A study (Vriens et al. 2016) showed US to be equivalent to MRI in assessing the residual tumor size after NAT in 123 patients.

7.2 Preoperative

The preoperative setting is the most debated breast MRI indication.

To understand the complexity of the discussion, we have to firstly place the topic within the historical context of BC therapy evolution. Since many years, breast-conserving treatment composed of limited surgery (lumpectomy/quadrantectomy) and whole-breast irradiation has been accepted as the preferred option for operable BCs, being comparable to mastectomy in terms of overall survival as shown by long-term studies (Veronesi et al. 2002; Fisher et al. 2002). Nevertheless, it is associated with a non-negligible incidence of locoregional recurrences and new primary ipsilateral or contralateral BCs, from 1.0% to 1.5% per year during 15–20 years (Bucchi et al. 2016). In addition, a meta-analysis of 21 studies totaling 14,571 patients (Houssami et al. 2010) reported a 26% pooled rate of positive or close margins at pathology examination of surgical specimens, associated with an odds ratio for local recurrence of 2.42 compared to patients with negative margins. A study on surgical outcome of 1648 women having conserving surgery for screen-detected BCs (Kurniawan et al. 2008) reported a rate of close (≤1 mm) margins of 16% and of positive margins of 14%, which prompted re-excision in 17% of the women, of whom 33% had residual disease.

The second point is the unparalleled sensitivity of CE-MRI for BC lesions, in particular in the case of multifocal and multicentric disease. When MRI was compared to double-reading mammography using 5-mm slicing mastectomy specimens as a reference standard in 99 breasts of 90 women in a multicenter study, its sensitivity for 188 malignant lesions was significantly higher (81%) than that of mammography (66%), with a PPV not significantly different (69% versus 79%, respectively) (Sardanelli et al. 2004b). Thus, the performance of preoperative MRI is out of discussion, as also recently shown by the report regarding two international multicenter studies for a total of 903 patients (Sardanelli et al. 2016b), where local investigators obtained up to 96% sensitivity and 97% specificity.

On this basis, MRI has been advocated as a method for tailoring, i.e., personalizing, the surgical treatment, anticipating the diagnosis of contralateral cancers, improving the surgical outcome, and reducing the rate of re-excision for positive margins, with a potential for improving disease-free survival. However, it is not easy to verify these expectations in the context of the usual approach to BC treatment, mostly including mastectomy (per guidelines still indicated for any case of multifocal or multicentric cancer) or conserving surgery and whole-breast radiation therapy. The discussion is far from being concluded, with arguments in favor (Sardanelli 2010a, b; Mann and Boetes 2010; Sardanelli and Trimboli 2012) and against (Morrow and Harris 2009; Solin 2010; Houssami and Solin 2010; Jatoi and Benson 2013) preoperative breast MRI.

The third point deals with methodological problems in the application of EBM (Oxford Centre for Evidence-based Medicine 2009) to preoperative breast MRI. In fact, with this examination we explore three clinical issues at once (Fig. 11):

1. The size of the known index lesion (the T parameter)
2. The possible presence of additional cancers in the ipsilateral breast

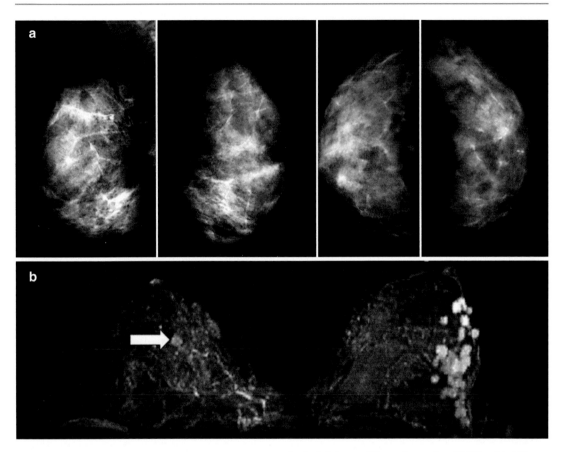

Fig. 11 Preoperative MRI: tailored treatment or overtreatment? A 36-year-old woman with palpable nodules at the left lower outer quadrant had inconclusive mammography with an extremely dense pattern (**a**). US (not shown) detected three hypoechoic nodules suspected for malignancy. MRI (1.5T magnet, 0.1 mmol/kg of gadobenate dimeglumine) detected 22 suspicious lesions (**b**, axial MIP reconstruction), all of them in the left external lower quadrant and a suspicious lesion (arrow) in the right breast, not visible at second-look US. US-guided biopsy confirmed multifocal disease (invasive ductal carcinomas) in the left breast. The patient refused MRI-guided biopsy of lesion at the right breast. Left mastectomy was performed and more than 20 malignant lesions at the lower outer quadrant were confirmed as invasive ductal cancers at pathology. Systemic therapy was administered. Up to 2 years after the end of treatment, no enhancing suspect lesion was visible in the right breast. This case shows the contemporary high performance of MRI for local ipsilateral staging but also the potential for overdiagnosis and overtreatment in the preoperative setting in the same patient

3. The possible presence of additional cancers in the contralateral breast

According to EBM rules (Oxford Centre for Evidence-based Medicine 2009), the definition of T (issue 1) is a *diagnostic task* for which tests can be validated by cohort studies with reference standards independent of the test and applied blindly or objectively to all patients. In other words, non-randomized prospective (intraindividual) studies enable us to choose the test with the best sensitivity/specificity, without needing RCTs. No doubt that a state-of-the-art breast MRI is the best option for this diagnostic task. On the other hand, searching for cancers in the contralateral breast (issue 3) is a screening in a high-risk breast. However, any screening before being implemented in clinical practice should be demonstrated to be effective in terms of patient outcome by RCTs (Oxford Centre for Evidence-based Medicine 2009; The Council of the European Union 2003). Searching for additional cancers in the ipsilateral breast (issue 2) can be considered in the middle, allowing for a comprehensive evaluation of the T parameter, beyond the size, especially when they are nearby the known index lesion, thus being associated to the issue 1 (disease "extent" beyond the pure size), not needing RCTs before implementation. But they could also be thought to be the results of screening a high-risk tissue (the apparently healthy ipsilateral breast), thus being associated to the issue 3, needing RCTs before implementation. Breast MRI gives information on all the three issues at the same time, while one would like to evaluate separately each of them in terms of outcome—a "mission impossible."

The fourth point is given by the difficulties in transferring the knowledge on disease extent obtained by preoperative MRI from the radiologist to the surgeon considering that breast MRI is performed in prone position while the patient will be operated in supine position, as explained above in this chapter (Carbonaro et al. 2012). Pre-surgical localization by US or MRI guidance should be performed in all complex situations such as the need of additional excision in the context of a conserving surgery. A learning curve by the surgeons is obvious and experience in cooperation by the team is necessary for getting optimal results.

If we take these four preliminary points into account, we can understand the debate on preoperative breast MRI.

The frequency of additional cancers detected by preoperative breast MRI has been shown to be 16% in a meta-analysis published in 2008 (Houssami et al. 2008) and 20% in a meta-analysis published in 2012 (Plana et al. 2012). MRI has also been shown to detect additional BCs in the contralateral breast, in 3.1% in a large prospective study (Lehman et al. 2007), and in 4.1% (Brennan et al. 2009) and 5.5% (Plana et al. 2012) of patients in meta-analyses. These results were somehow expected in consideration of the relatively high frequency of multifocal and multicentric nature of BCs, as already shown by old pathological studies on mastectomy specimens (Holland et al. 1985). The clinical relevance of additional cancers detected at breast MRI has been investigated (Iacconi et al. 2016), showing, among patients with MRI-detected additional

malignant lesions, lesions larger than the index cancer in 23% and more biologically relevant in 5% of the cases. However, we should consider that many of the studies published (and meta-analyzed) suffer from a selection bias because those patients who are referred for preoperative breast MRI have a higher probability of additional disease than those who are not. This is a bias that frequently limits the external validity of those studies that consider *a consecutive series of patients who had a disease AND a diagnostic test* (Houssami and Ciatto 2010).

Only few RCTs on preoperative breast MRI were performed, using the reduction of re-intervention rate as a proxy of clinical effectiveness. They gave conflicting results (two studies in favor of breast MRI (Sakakibara et al. 2008; Gonzalez et al. 2014), two studies against (Turnbull et al. 2010; Peters et al. 2011)), not allowing for drawing reliable conclusions (Sardanelli and Trimboli 2012).

We should note that the first study (Sakakibara et al. 2008) was only a small single-center study showing the advantage of supine MRI guidance for tailoring the conserving surgical treatment of relatively localized DCIS versus mammography guidance on a total of 52 patients: the average volume of pathologic specimens in the supine MRI group was significantly smaller than that in the conventional group (27.5 cm^3 versus 57.6 cm^3), and the positive margin rate significantly lower (12.5% versus 39.3%). So, it was a special study, anyway showing an interesting way to be run.

The second study in favor of MRI (Gonzalez et al. 2014) was a multicenter trial including 440 breast cancer patients under 56 years of age. Patients randomized to MRI group had an observed higher percentage of planned breast-conserving surgery compared with the control group, with a change from suggested breast conservation to mastectomy in 23 of 153 (15%) patients. The breast reoperation rate was significantly lower in the MRI group: 11 of 220 (5%) versus 33 of 220 (15%) in the control group. The rate of mastectomies and axillary reoperations did not differ significantly between the groups.

We need here to comment the two large studies that gave results against MRI, taking into account that they strongly contributed to the following meta-analyses. In the COMICE trial (Turnbull et al. 2010), over 1800 women with a newly diagnosed BC were randomized to MRI or no MRI. The reoperation rate resulted to be 19% in both groups, and total mastectomy rate 13% and 9%, respectively. The additional MRI cost was not significant. We should note at least that (1) many centers had low or very low experience with preoperative breast MRI; (2) imaging-guided (including MR-guided) needle biopsy was not systematically performed; and (3) concern on randomization can be raised by the difference in terms of local recurrence rate 3 years after randomization between the MRI group (6.1%) and the non-MRI group (4.5%).

In the MONET trial (Peters et al. 2011), the effect of preoperative 3T MRI for non-palpable lesions was evaluated. From 626 eligible patients (including also those with benign lesions), the randomized comparison for cancer staging was done only between 74 patients (MRI arm) and 75 patients (non-MRI arm), about half of each arm being affected with DCIS detected as microcalcifications at mammography. No significant difference was found for the rate of mastectomy, but the reoperation rate after conserving surgery resulted significantly higher in the MRI arm (34%) than in the non-MRI arm (12%), an unexpected result explained arguing that "patients with DCIS which could not be reproduced on MRI were treated with smaller lumpectomy specimens during the initial BCS [breast conserving surgery] procedure." Sensitivity of 3T MRI *for index lesions* was suboptimal (lower than 85%), raising reasonable doubts on the reliability of the study results.

Of note, these studies (and other old studies, especially when reporting unnecessary mastectomies for false-positive MRI findings) were criticized for the lack of specific experience, in particular regarding targeted US and MRI guidance for biopsy/localization. Both procedures are now considered a *must* for a good clinical practice in breast MRI, in particular in the preoperative setting where suspicious additional finding

should be handled firstly with targeted US (Spick and Baltzer 2014) or with digital breast tomosynthesis (Clauser et al. 2015), leaving to MRI-guided procedures (Peter et al. 2016; Spick et al. 2016b), with the cases not solved otherwise, as already mentioned in Sect. 1.

In this context, we can appreciate the results of meta-analyses on surgical outcomes of preoperative breast MRI. These studies tried to overcome the intrinsic limitations of previous meta-analyses that had considered observational studies not having a control group (Houssami et al. 2008; Brennan et al. 2009) which implied an overestimation of the surgical impact of MRI, as admitted by the same authors' group (Houssami et al. 2013).

Thus, a first new meta-analysis including studies with control group (Houssami et al. 2013) reported data for 3112 patients from 9 studies (2 RCTs and 7 comparative cohorts). Pooled comparisons between the MRI group and the no-MRI group were presented using odds ratio, not adjusted and adjusted for study-level median age and, where appropriate, for temporal effect. The initial mastectomy rate was significantly higher for the MRI group (16%) than for the no-MRI group (8%), even when adjusted for confounding factors; the re-excision after initial breast conservation was not significantly different (12% versus 11%, respectively); the overall mastectomy rate was significantly higher for the MRI group (26% versus 18%, respectively), even when adjusted for confounding factors. In 766 patients with invasive lobular histology, the initial mastectomy rate was 31% versus 25% (significantly different after adjustment); re-excision after initial breast conservation 11% versus 18% (not significantly different after adjustment, but with a $p = 0.09$); and overall mastectomy rate 43% versus 40% (significantly different after adjustment). The authors concluded for a significant increase of mastectomy rate associated with MRI and for unfavorable harm-benefit ratio for routine use of preoperative MRI. The evidence for the reduction of re-excision rate of lobular BCs was considered only weak and associated with a trade-off of increased mastectomies.

An individual patient data meta-analysis published in 2014 (Houssami et al. 2014) (3180 affected breasts in 3169 patients from 4 studies) showed that the 8-year local and distant recurrence-free survival did not significantly differ between patients locally staged with and without MRI. A more recent meta-analysis (Houssami et al. 2017) (19 studies, 85,975 patients) did not find any evidence for preoperative MRI to improve surgical outcomes such as re-excision or positive margins. A significant odd for ipsilateral mastectomy (odds ratio 1.39) and contralateral prophylactic mastectomy (odds ratio 1.91) was reported. In the subgroup with invasive lobular histology, preoperative MRI was not associated with an increase in mastectomy rate (odds ratio 1.0) while the odd for re-excision was reduced (odds ratio 0.65), even though not significantly.

The crucial point for interpreting the results of these researches is that, also when using the strongest approach, i.e., the *individual patient data* approach, meta-analyses cannot overcome the above-described general background and the limitations of the original studies included, both the problems of the two RCTs which obtained results against MRI and the limitations of the observational cohort studies in particular the selection bias, as we will explain below. As anyone can understand, the debate is far from being closed.

In fact, the current scenario is characterized by two opposite tendencies. On the one side, the American Society of Breast Surgeons, in the context of a *Choosing Wisely* campaign (American Society of Breast Surgeons 2018), suggests: "Don't routinely order breast MRI in new breast cancer patients." This statement was based on the "lack of evidence that routine use of MRI lessens cancer recurrence, death from cancer, or the need for reoperation after lumpectomy surgery" while it is "associated with an increased need for subsequent breast biopsy procedures, delays in time to treatment, and higher cost of care." They also added that "increased mastectomy rates can occur if the MRI finds additional cancers or indeterminate findings cause patient anxiety, leading to patient requests for mastec-

tomy" (American Society of Breast Surgeons 2018).

On the other side, preoperative breast MRI is increasingly applied. Its use is highly variable worldwide depending on local policies and surgeons' confidence, primarily. Interestingly, a survey of the same American Society of Breast Surgeons (Parker et al. 2013) showed that of 1012 surgeons who responded (45.5% of a total of 2274), 41% declared a routine breast MRI use for newly diagnosed patients with higher rates among surgeons from high-volume practice, high specialization, and private practice and in the case of high mammographic density, strong family history of breast cancer, and invasive lobular carcinoma. Another survey among surgeons in the USA (Lee et al. 2017a) reporting data from 289 surgeons (154 breast surgeons and 135 general surgeons) showed a propensity for requesting preoperative breast MRI in the case of (decreasing order) *BRCA* mutations; familial or personal breast cancer history; extremely dense breasts; age below 40; axillary nodal involvement; mammographically occult tumor; multifocal or multicentric disease at conventional imaging; invasive lobular pathology; triple-negative BC; T2 or T3 stage; patient candidate to mastectomy requesting conserving surgery; and radiologist's recommendation. In addition, breast surgeons referred to MRI more than general surgeons for BRCA mutation carriers and tumors smaller than 1 cm, less than general surgeons for multifocal/multicentric disease. The authors rightly concluded that *selection bias could affect analyses of observational studies regarding preoperative breast MRI* (Lee et al. 2017a).

In this complex context, the definition of indications for preoperative breast MRI is not an easy task. The authors of this chapter are personally in favor of offering breast MRI to all women newly diagnosed with a BC, *if a well-established relation does exist between the radiologist and the surgeon*, possibly in a structured breast unit where the surgical planning is a result of the multidisciplinary panel discussion. If selective criteria have to be adopted for any reason, useful suggestions still come from the multidisciplinary

EUSOMA recommendations (Sardanelli et al. 2010) in favor of MRI in the following four cases:

1. Patients newly diagnosed with an invasive lobular cancer
2. Patients at high BC risk newly diagnosed with a BC with mammography/US
3. Patients under 60 years of age with discrepancy in size >1 cm between mammography and US with expected impact on treatment decision
4. Patients eligible for partial breast irradiation on the basis of clinical breast examination and mammography/US

As a matter of fact, if we consider carefully the discussion of the meta-analysis on surgical outcomes from preoperative MRI by N. Houssami and coworkers (2013), all the first three EUSOMA indications are at least partially confirmed by those authors. The fourth (eligibility for partial breast irradiation) can be considered a special case, due to the not generalized use of this reduced radiation therapy approach.

The first indication (invasive lobular histology), even if only a *weak* evidence was found at meta-analyses, has been confirmed by a retrospective study (Mann et al. 2010) at two tertiary centers in the Netherlands on a consecutive series of 257 patients with invasive lobular cancer, showing a significant reduction in reoperation rate in the MRI group (9%) versus the non-MRI group (27%) and a decrease in mastectomy rate (48% versus 59%, respectively). A second retrospective study at two district general hospitals in the UK (Derias et al. 2016) was performed on 126 patients with invasive lobular histology, and 46 patients had MRI. MRI showed multicentric unilateral disease occult on US/mammogram in 17 patients who underwent mastectomy, with confirmed multifocal disease in 16 of them. MRI showed a contralateral lesion in 9 patients, 4 of which were malignant and had bilateral surgery. MRI also downgraded 3 patients to unifocal disease with reported multifocal appearances on mammography/US, and these patients underwent conserving surgery. More recently, another retrospective study from the Netherlands (Lobbes et al. 2017) reported on 36,050 patients, 10,740 of them with MRI (30%). Patients with invasive ductal cancer with MRI were significantly more likely to undergo primary mastectomy than those without MRI (OR 1.30). Patients with invasive lobular cancer with MRI were significantly less likely to undergo primary mastectomy than those without MRI (OR 0.86). A significantly lower risk of positive surgical margins after conserving surgery was only seen in patients with lobular cancer with MRI as compared to those without MRI (OR 0.59) and, consequently, a lower risk of secondary mastectomy (OR 0.61). Patients with MRI were almost four times more likely to be diagnosed with contralateral cancer (OR 3.55). A third retrospective study (Ha et al. 2018) reported on 603 patients with invasive lobular cancer, 369 of them (61%) with MRI. At propensity score-matched analysis, MRI was associated with significantly lower odds of repeat surgery (OR 0.14) and similar likelihood of initial mastectomy (OR 0.87) and final mastectomy (OR 0.74).

The second indication (high-risk patient) is overcome by the general acceptance of MRI as a screening tool for high-risk women (see above). The third indication has been confirmed by a retrospective study, showing a higher probability of additional cancers with mammography/US size discrepancy >1 cm, without age limitations (Bernardi et al. 2012; Sardanelli 2013). The fourth indication has been confirmed by a meta-analysis (Di Leo et al. 2015) showing, on the basis of 3136 patients from 6 studies, that MRI prompted ineligibility for PBI in 6–25% of patients who were initially deemed eligible or in 2–20% if calculated on the overall number of patients initially screened. The pooled percentage of patients eligible at mammography/US but ineligible after MR imaging was 11%, suggesting that MRI should be used to select patients for partial breast irradiation.

An indirect support to this indication comes from a very recent study (Wang et al. 2018), based on the Surveillance, Epidemiology and End Results-Medicare dataset of women aged 67–94 diagnosed during 2004–2010 with stage I/II BC who received conserving surgery (24,379 patients, 19% of them receiving preoperative

MRI). While adjusted rates of subsequent mastectomy and BC mortality were not significantly different in the MRI group versus the no-MRI group overall, for those patients who received conserving surgery alone (i.e., without radiation therapy), in the MRI group the risks of subsequent mastectomy and BC mortality were significantly lower (adjusted hazard ratio 0.60 and 0.57, respectively). This means that, if radiation therapy is not given, MRI strongly improves the patient outcome. The logic consequence of these results is that we are not able to see an effect of MRI on patient outcome if we continue to give whole-breast radiation therapy to all women treated with conserving surgery, which implies overtreatment in part of them. One first exit way from this situation is to use MRI in all new BC cases for selecting those patients who can undergo partial breast irradiation and, potentially, those patients who could avoid radiation therapy at all. Studies are needed for exploring this perspective.

Other potential indications may be nonfatty breasts, i.e., ACR density categories *b*, *c*, and *d* (Seely et al. 2016), especially if multifocal/multicentric/bilateral disease is suspected at clinical examination and/or conventional imaging, Paget's disease (Morrogh et al. 2008), skin- or nipple-sparing mastectomy (Bahl et al. 2016; Chan et al. 2017; Malya et al. 2018; Mariscotti et al. 2018), and positive margins after breast-conserving surgery (Krammer et al. 2017). The list of all these indications is reported in Table 3.

In this scenario, one interesting way for deeper insights is the comparison between concurrent cohorts of women newly diagnosed with BC who have or do not have preoperative MRI.

This approach has been proposed retrospectively by J.S. Sung and coworkers (2014). They compared the cases of 174 women with stage 0, I, or II BC who underwent preoperative MRI between 2000 and 2004 with a control group of 174 patients who did not undergo preoperative MRI before breast-conserving therapy, matched by age, histopathologic finding, stage, and surgeon. Patients with MRI were significantly more likely to have extremely dense breasts (28% versus 6%) and mammographically occult cancers

Table 3 Indications to preoperative breast MRI when it is not offered to all patients with newly diagnosed breast cancer

EUSOMA indications[a]
1. Patients newly diagnosed with an invasive lobular cancer
2. Patients at high BC risk newly diagnosed with a BC with mammography/US
3. Patients under 60 with discrepancy in size >1 cm between mammography and US
4. Patients eligible for partial breast irradiation on the basis of clinical examination and mammography/US
Additional indications[b]
5. Nonfatty breasts
6. Paget's disease
7. Skin- or nipple-sparing mastectomy
8. Positive margins after conserving surgery

[a]Sardanelli et al. (2010)
[b]Sakakibara et al. (2008), Gonzalez et al. (2014), Turnbull et al. (2010), Peters et al. (2011), Clauser et al. (2015)

(24% versus 9%). The two groups had identical rates of final negative margins, lymph node involvement, lympho-vascular invasion, extensive intraductal component status, positive hormone receptor results, and systemic adjuvant therapy. While the re-intervention rate for positive margins was significantly lower in the MRI group (29% versus 45%), no significant difference in locoregional recurrences or disease-free survival was observed after a median follow-up of 8 years. This means that MRI may be able to reduce the re-intervention rate but would not impact long-term patient outcome.

An international group of radiologists developed the idea of a large prospective observational multicenter study to be performed at highly qualified high-volume institutions aimed at verifying the impact of preoperative breast MRI: *Preoperative Breast MRI in Clinical Practice: Multicenter International Prospective Analysis (MIPA) of Individual Woman Data* (Sardanelli et al. 2020). The MIPA study results (Sardanelli et al. 2022) were recently reported. Of 5896 analyzed patients, 2763 (46.9%) had conventional imaging only (noMRI group), and 3133 (53.1%) underwent MRI that was performed for diagnosis, screening, or unknown purposes in 692/3133 women (22.1%), with preoperative intent in

2441/3133 women (77.9%, MRI group). Patients in the MRI group were significantly younger, had denser breasts, more cancers ≥ 20 mm, and a higher rate of invasive lobular histology than patients of the noMRI group. Mastectomy based on conventional imaging was planned significantly more frequently in the MRI group (22.4%) than in the noMRI group (14.4%). The additional planned mastectomy rate in the MRI group was 11.3%. The overall performed first- plus second-line mastectomy rate was significantly higher for the MRI group (36.3%) than for the noMRI group (8.0%). In women receiving conserving surgery, MRI group had a significantly lower reoperation rate (8.5% versus 11.7%). The authors concluded that preoperative breast MRI was requested for women with a higher a priori probability of receiving mastectomy and that MRI was associated with 11.3% additional mastectomies, partially counteracted by 3.2% fewer reoperations in the breast conservation subgroup.

Importantly, we highlight here that something is changing in the consideration of the type of studies needed for building the evidence for the best choices in clinical practice. Since the late 1940s, RCTs have become the standard in clinical research on drugs and therapies. In the last years, experts and regulatory bodies have acknowledged important limitations of RCTs, including high costs, extensive resource requirements, long timelines, and lack of generalizability of the results obtained in the trial population to larger populations faced in clinical practice. As recently pointed out in the JAMA by J. Corrigan-Curay and coworkers from the Drug Evaluation and Research, Food and Drug Administration (Corrigan-Curay et al. 2018), the real-world data from observational studies and the real-world evidence coming from them are currently re-evaluated. They state: *The increasing accessibility of digital health data, spurred in large part by the transition to electronic health records, together with rising costs and recognized limitations of traditional trials, has renewed interest in the use of real-world data to enhance the efficiency of research and bridge the evidentiary gap between clinical research and practice.* The MIPA study

is an attempt to explore this way for preoperative MRI.

Notwithstanding the abovementioned intrinsic limitations for studies (RCTs or observational cohort studies) aimed at assessing the potential of preoperative breast MRI for a reduction of the recurrence rate after conserving surgery, some researchers had interesting results on long-term follow-up after conserving surgery and radiation therapy. M.K. Gervais and coworkers (2017) reported on a cohort of 470 women treated from 1999 and 2005. Of them, 27% underwent MRI and 73% did not. After a median follow-up of 97 months, 10-year in-breast recurrence rate was 3.6% overall, lower but not significantly for the MRI group (1.6%) than for the no-MRI group (4.2%). However, patients with triple-negative and HER2-positive cancers had a significantly higher in-breast recurrence rate (9.8%) than all others (1.7%) and in the no-MRI group in-breast recurrence rate reached 11.8%, significantly higher than in the remainder (1.8%). The authors concluded that the triple-negative/HER2-positive population showed an increased in-breast recurrence rate, more marked in the no-MRI group, and acknowledged that the small population size could have prevented from reaching the statistical significance for the association between performing preoperative MRI and reducing the in-breast recurrence rate in the triple-negative/HER2-positive subgroup, even when the difference was high: only 3.3% in the MRI group and 11.8% in the no-MRI group (Gervais et al. 2017). The ongoing Alliance A011104/ACRIN 6694 study (NCT01805076) will provide data on the role of preoperative MRI in recurrence outcomes in triple-negative and HER2-positive patients.

On the other hand, Tracy Onega and coworkers (2018) followed a cohort of 4454 women with nonmetastatic stage I–III BC diagnosed from February 2005 through June 2010 in five registries of the United States Breast Cancer Surveillance Consortium. Of these women, 917 (21%) had preoperative MRI. The authors did not find significant difference in the cumulative probability of specific mortality. The hazard ratio of all-cause mortality during the follow-up after adjusting for sociodemographic and clinical factors for the MRI group was not significantly different from that of the no-MRI group (hazard ratio 0.90). However, these authors did not perform a subgroup analysis taking into consideration estrogen/progesterone receptor and HER2 status of the tumors.

Anyway, we are convinced that preoperative breast MRI will remain a conundrum for many years. In this context, practical recommendations for preoperative MRI should include:

1. Clear patient information, possibly using a dedicated informed consent form
2. High-quality MRI examination technique
3. Mandatory verification of MRI additional findings with potential impact on surgical treatment using second-look (targeted) US, second-look mammography/digital breast tomosynthesis, or MRI guidance
4. Biopsy/localization of suspicious findings with impact on surgical treatment under US, mammography/digital breast tomosynthesis, or MRI guidance
5. Treatment delay due to MRI no longer than 1 month
6. Decision on changes of treatment planning by a multidisciplinary team
7. Attention paid to methods for transferring MRI 3D information on disease extent from radiology to the operating theatre

High-quality research is still warranted and specific multidisciplinary guidelines for treating breast cancer when preoperative MRI is performed are welcome.

7.3 Occult Primary Breast Cancer

Occult primary breast cancer presents as a metastatic disease consistent with breast cancer in the absence of any clinical and primary breast tumor identifiable with mammography and US. This rare condition mainly refers to axillary adenopathy (pT0N+) and occurs in less than 1% of breast cancer cases (Macedo et al. 2016; McCartan et al. 2017; Fayanju et al. 2013). Breast MRI has become the standard of care for this condition, reporting suspicious findings in 43–86% of cases and a cancer yield higher than 70% (Macedo et al. 2016; He et al. 2012) (Fig. 12). Depending on the whole-body staging of the disease, the identification of the primary tumor can be crucial, allowing for breast preservation.

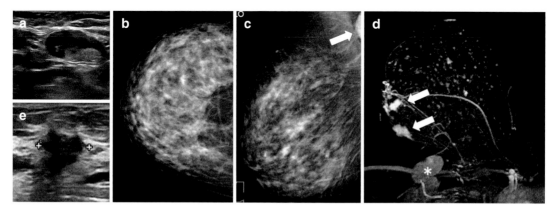

Fig. 12 Search for primary BC occult at conventional imaging. Forty-nine-year-old woman with palpable lymphadenopathy in the right axilla, confirmed at US (**a**). Right mammography (**b**, **c**) shows an enlarged dense axillary lymph node (arrow in the mediolateral oblique view, **c**). Both mammography and first-look US did not find the primary lesion. Breast MRI (1.5T magnet, 0.1 mmol/kg of gadobenate dimeglumine): the axial MIP of the right breast (**d**) shows two mass-enhancing lesions at upper outer quadrant of the right breast (arrows in **d**), associated with non-mass enhancement as well as the axillary lymphadenopathy (asterisk in **d**). Second-look targeted US (**e**) detected only one of the two mass lesions allowing for US-guided percutaneous biopsy. Mastectomy proved multifocal invasive ductal carcinoma, associated with DCIS

The widespread adoption of breast MRI for the management of occult primary breast cancers suggested limiting this definition to those cases presenting with nodal or distant metastases without clinical, mammographic, US, and MRI evidence of breast disease, accounting for less than 0.3% of cases (McCartan et al. 2017; Fayanju et al. 2013). When also MRI does not detect the cancer, a therapeutic dilemma exists between the historically applied modified radical mastectomy and the recent less invasive approaches including axillary lymph node dissection with or without whole-breast radiation therapy. In fact, in patients with a negative clinical and comprehensive radiographic workup, ipsilateral mastectomy specimens are positive for cancer in only 20–33% of cases (Barton et al. 2011). A meta-analysis (Macedo et al. 2016) showed no difference in survival outcomes between mastectomy with axillary lymph node dissection versus combined axillary lymph node dissection and whole-breast radiation therapy in patients with occult primary carcinoma. Moreover, radiotherapy turned out to improve locoregional recurrence and possibly mortality rates in patients undergoing axillary lymph node dissection. Authors concluded that combined nodal dissection and adjuvant radiation therapy should be considered as the primary modality of treatment in this relatively rare condition.

8 Equivocal/Inconclusive Findings at Conventional Imaging Including Suspicion of Breast Cancer Recurrence

The well-cut established definition for equivocal/inconclusive finding is not available. In clinical practice it refers to the inability to reach a conclusive diagnosis when conventional imaging and breast examination findings, alone or in combination, are not suggestive to define the presence or absence of breast cancer. However, this can imply a wide spectrum of BI-RADS assessment categories (D'Orsi et al. 2013), including BI-RADS 0, 3, and 4. What we will describe in the following

paragraphs also applies to suspicion of cancer recurrence.

A meta-analysis concluded for an excellent diagnostic performance of MRI in the case of noncalcified equivocal breast findings detected with conventional imaging (Bennani-Baiti et al. 2016). Based on 14 studies totaling 2316 lesions, pooled sensitivity was 99% (95% CI, 93–100%), NPV 100% (95% CI, 99–100%), specificity 89% (95% CI, 85–92%), and PPV 56% (95% CI, 42–70%).[1] Authors asserted breast MRI to be able to rule out malignancy in most cases but admitted that "considering the substantial heterogeneity with regard to prevalence of malignancy, problem-solving criteria need to be better defined." In our opinion, this means that the generalizability of this performance is limited.

The same group of authors also recently evaluated the role of MRI for characterizing calcified findings. They firstly assessed mammographic calcifications categorized as BI-RADS 3, 4, or 5 (Bennani-Baiti and Baltzer 2017) and then focused on BI-RADS 4 microcalcifications (Bennani-Baiti et al. 2017). The first paper (Bennani-Baiti and Baltzer 2017) was a meta-analysis including 20 studies totaling 1843 findings. For all lesions, pooled sensitivity was 87% and specificity 81%; for invasive lesions, 95% and 61%; for BI-RADS 3 lesions, 57% and 32%; for BI-RADS 4 lesions 92% and 82%; and for BI-RADS 5 lesions, 95% and 66%, respectively. They concluded that MRI is not recommended for BI-RADS 3 and 5 microcalcifications, but can be considered for BI-RADS 4 microcalcifications. Importantly, they suggest the use of dichotomous criterion (i.e., presence or absence of enhancement) as the diagnostic criterion to rule out malignancy on MRI in this setting. The second paper (Bennani-Baiti et al. 2017) reported on a single-center retrospective study that used the abovementioned dichotomous diagnostic criterion, i.e., the author rightly lowered maximally the sensitivity of the CE technique, not using standard morphologic and dynamic BI-RADS criteria. The cases were 107 malignant

---

[1] We reported here the 95% confidence intervals due to their relevance for this topic.

and 141 benign microcalcifications, with malignancy rates of 18.3% for BI-RADS 4a, 42% for BI-RADS 4b, and 95% for BI-RADS 4c findings. Sensitivity was 96% (95% CI, 91–99%), specificity 82% (95% CI, 75–88%), PPV 81% (95% CI, 73–87%), and NPV 97% (95% CI, 92–99%).[2] The 4 false negatives were 1 invasive cancer and 3 DCIS (2 BI-RADS 4c, 1 BI-RADS 4b on mammography). The authors concluded that MRI may be helpful to avoid unnecessary biopsies in BI-RADS 4a and 4b lesions. BI-RADS 4c microcalcifications should be biopsied irrespective of MRI findings.

Here the crucial question is: Is there any real advantage in performing a MRI study for an equivocal finding at mammography and/or US, when a needle biopsy can solve the problem with minimally invasive procedure (and also relatively cheap, if performed under US guidance)? To do this, we should reach at least an NPV over 98% (i.e., to stay under the 2% of probability of malignancy, thus being enabled to reclassify a lesion as a BI-RADS 3 finding). Considering that predictive values strongly depend on malignancy prevalence (Sardanelli and Di Leo 2009a), which is highly variable (see above the heterogeneity reported in the meta-analysis on MRI for noncalcified equivocal findings (Bennani-Baiti et al. 2017)), only a sure sensitivity of 100% (impossible, due to the biological variability of BCs, especially of DCIS) could guarantee this result. There is still a non-negligible probability to miss a cancer using MRI when the pretest probability is high as it is for suspicious/equivocal findings at conventional imaging. In fact, to make a simple numerical example, hypothesize to have an MRI sensitivity of 98% (using the dichotomous diagnostic criterion, etc.) and a malignancy prevalence of 70%, then your NPV will be "only" 97%. After a negative MRI (no enhancement), you should perform biopsy (Fig. 13).

A special comment has to be deserved to the use of DWI for the characterization of breast findings.

Several meta-analyses were published on this topic. We consider here two of them. R.Y. Shi and coworkers (2018) reported on 4778 patients and 5205 breast lesions from 61 studies: pooled sensitivity of DWI was 90%, specificity 86%, and AUC 0.94. Interestingly, for the 44 1.5T studies, sensitivity was 91% and specificity 86%, and for the 17 3.0T studies, 88% and 84%, respectively, without significant difference, confirming that state-of-the-art breast MRI can be performed on standard 1.5T magnets. L. Zhang and coworkers (2016) reported on 1140 patients with 1276 lesions from 14 studies: sensitivity and specificity were 93% and 71% for CE-MRI, 86% and 76% for DWI, and 92% and 86% for DCE-MRI combined with DWI.

An interesting report (Ding et al. 2016) on 1097 cases (928 invasive ductal 169 DCIS) from nine studies showed that ADC value in IDC is significantly lower than DCIS; however, stratifying by ethnicity, this difference was confirmed in Asian population, not in Caucasians. These results indirectly show an intrinsic difficulty for differentiating DCIS from benign lesions. In addition, ethnicity as a hidden and forgotten variable for quantitative MRI comes to the stage making the entire picture more complex and deserving further research.

One important point is what cutoff should be adopted for differentiating malignant from benign lesion based on ADC values and the role of b-value in determining the diagnostic performance. One relevant contribution on this topic has been given by M.D. Dorrius et al. (Dorrius et al. 2014) who proposed a meta-analysis including 26 studies for a total of 2111 patients and 2151 lesions (60% of them malignant and 40% benign). In the group of b-values ≤ 600 s/mm^2, the mean ADC threshold was 1.50×10^{-3} mm^2/s (range 1.29–1.81) with 91% sensitivity, 75% specificity, and 0.92 AUC. In the group of b-values >600 s/mm^2, the mean cutoff was 1.23×10^{-3} mm^2/s (range 0.90–1.60) with 89% sensitivity, 84% specificity, and 0.93 AUC. Of note, the median ADC was significantly higher than for the latter group for both benign (+13%) and malignant (+35%) lesions. The highest differentiation of benign versus malignant lesions was obtained with a combination of b-value = 0 and 1000 s/mm^2. However, overall nonsignificant differences in sensitivity and specificity were observed between the two groups.

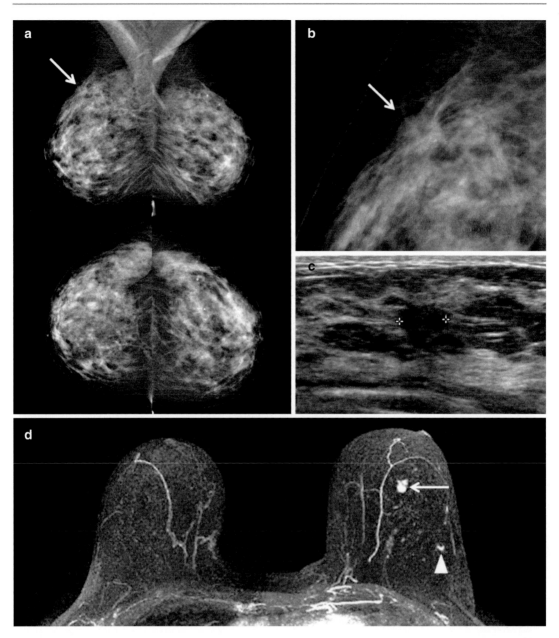

Fig. 13 Breast MRI, false negative. Fifty-year-old asymptomatic woman with extremely dense breast. Bilateral mammography (**a**) showed a small nodular mass associated with distortion in the right upper quadrants, only in the mediolateral oblique view (arrow in **a** and in the electronic magnification, **b**). Handheld US did not find any correlate of the mammographic finding in the right breast but identified a 7 mm inhomogeneous solid nodule in the central region of left breast (calipers in **c**), which was biopsied under US guidance and turned out to be an invasive ductal carcinoma. Contrast-enhanced MRI was performed (3T magnet, 0.1 mmol/kg of gadobenate dimeglumine). Axial MIP reconstruction of the first post-contrast sequence (**d**) showed no findings in the right breast, identified an enhancing lesion with one spiculation in the left breast, corresponding to the US finding (arrow in **d**), and revealed a second enhancing lesion (**c**, arrowhead in **d**), which was diagnosed as invasive ductal carcinoma by MRI-guided vacuum-assisted biopsy. Skin-sparing bilateral mastectomy was performed, and histopathology revealed a multicentric invasive ductal carcinoma in the left breast and an 8-mm invasive ductal carcinoma in the right breast, false negative at MRI. (Courtesy of Dr. Massimo Calabrese, Breast Radiology, Ospedale Policlinico San Martino, Genoa, Italy)

At any rate, the sensitivity of DWI can be considered to be at the best around 90%, insufficient for the goal of avoiding biopsy. We note here that sensitivity is the most relevant metrics to be taken into consideration when the disease prevalence is high, as is in any case of suspicious lesion already identified on mammography/US or CE-MRI (Sardanelli and Di Leo 2009a). Of note, also the so-called *relative ADC* (calculated as a ratio of the lesion ADC to the ADC of the surrounding healthy gland parenchyma), supposed to be unaffected by the menstrual cycle, failed to be shown to have any superior performance than the standard ADC. E. Yılmaz and coworkers (2018) studied 81 patients with 88 lesions (37% malignant, 63% benign). Using standard ADC (cutoff 1.04×10^{-3} mm²/s), sensitivity was 88% and specificity 87%, and using relative ADC (cutoff 0.639×10^{-3} mm²/s), 82% and 83%, respectively.

Overall, considering CE-MRI, DWI, or also their combination, *MRI should not be used to characterize suspicious/equivocal findings found at conventional imaging*. Only large specifically designed studies, prospectively applying predefined diagnostic criteria, will be able to define a clinical role of MRI for this setting as a real alternative to biopsy. This concept has also been reinforced by the introduction of tomosynthesis-guided biopsy which has been shown to reduce radiation exposure as well as duration and complexity of the procedure (Schrading et al. 2015).

Therefore, we confirm the recommendation from the EUSOMA working group (Sardanelli et al. 2010) that in the case of equivocal findings at conventional imaging, including the suspicion of recurrence, MRI can be considered only when needle biopsy cannot be performed. Also the 2013 edition of the ACR BI-RADS atlas (D'Orsi et al. 2013) states that breast MRI is not an appropriate follow-up measure for minimal or equivocal findings.

Practically, we suggest that CE-MRI (integrating DWI in the protocol) can be performed only in special cases such as the following: (1) patient refusal of needle biopsy; (2) impossibility to perform needle biopsy in particular locations (e.g., mammography-only findings very close to the chest wall); (3) difficulty to define the site for needle biopsy (e.g., numerous suspicious findings); and (4) suspicious findings at clinical examination (typically palpable lumps), with negative mammography and US. A further indication for MRI, however, not supported by evidence in the literature, may be the case of radio-pathologic discordance, which is typically a negative pathological report for a highly suspicious mammography/US finding. In that situation, after a pathologic review and second opinion, MRI could be considered as an alternative to repeat biopsy.

9 Evaluation of Breast Implant Integrity

Breast implant augmentation represents the most common cosmetic surgical procedure performed in developed countries. The American Society of Plastic Surgeons (2018) reported 300,378 breast augmentation procedures for the year 2017, with an increase of 3% to 2016 and of 41% to 2000. Moreover, advancements in surgical conserving techniques prompted a widespread use of implants for oncoplastic reconstruction.

Breast US is the first-line method for evaluating implant integrity (Evans et al. 2018): if an implant rupture is suspected at US, the probability of a true rupture is high. But it is not so sensitive: it cannot reliably exclude the presence of a rupture.

Breast MRI is the most accurate method for evaluating implant integrity. The implant evaluation requires dedicated protocols: axial silicone-selective sequences (with fat and water suppression, where silicone alone appears bright) are usually combined with axial and coronal fast spin-echo T2-weighted and/or axial STIR sequences with water saturation and silicone suppression; sagittal sequences can also be added (Fig. 14). For further details on the MRI technical protocols, see dedicated articles (Seiler et al. 2017; Green et al. 2018).

A meta-analysis published in 2011 (Song et al. 2011) reported for MRI 87% sensitivity and 89% specificity for implant rupture, the same data being 61% and 76% for US. Significant heterogeneity

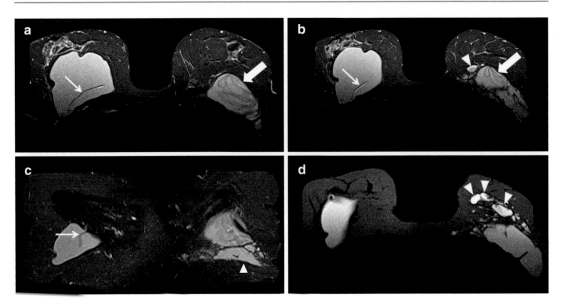

Fig. 14 Implant rupture. A 66-year-old woman, who had breast augmentation at 51, presented with symptoms of implant failure on the left side. Unenhanced MRI was performed at 1.5T. The linguine sign in the left implant (large arrows in axial STIR images, **a** and **b**) and multiple siliconomas external to the implant (the largest of them being indicated by arrowheads in **b**, **c**, and **d**), hyperintense in both STIR (**b**) and water-suppressed STIR (**d**), suggested the diagnosis of intra- and extracapsular rupture of the left implant. Only radial folds were visible as hyper/hypointense lines in the right implant on two planes (axial STIR, **a** and **b**; coronal STIR, **c**)

was found across studies and the accuracy of MRI was much higher in symptomatic than in asymptomatic/screening setting. A study (Maijers et al. 2014) including 107 women with Poly Implant Prothèse implants who underwent explantation reported for MRI 93% sensitivity, 93% specificity, 77% PPV, and 98% NPV, along with an excellent interobserver agreement (κ 0.92).

In 2006, at the time of the reintroduction of silicone breast implants into the US market, the Food and Drug Administration of the USA recommended MRI screening 3 years after implantation and every 2 years thereafter (U.S. Food and Drug Administration 2017). Nevertheless, this recommendation is not widely accepted.

Special attention should be paid to the possibility of a newly described clinicopathologic entity, the implant-associated anaplastic large-cell lymphoma, whose only sign can be a peri-implant effusion for which MRI has been shown to have an 82% sensitivity, but where PET/CT can be more sensitive for mass detection (64% versus 50% of MRI) (Adrada et al. 2014).

Indications for breast MRI in this setting are the following (Sardanelli et al. 2010):

1. Patients with symptoms suggestive for implant rupture (pain, asymmetry, change in shape, etc.) and inconclusive conventional imaging (unenhanced MRI with dedicated protocol)
2. Augmented patients with symptoms of parenchymal disease (e.g., breast lump) and inconclusive conventional imaging (unenhanced MRI with dedicated protocol and contrast-enhanced MRI)

For the first indication, the only purpose is implant integrity assessment; for the second one, the aims are implant integrity assessment and search for parenchymal lesions, both in case of cosmetic implants and oncologic reconstruction. In the case of implant rupture confirmed or newly diagnosed with MRI for which surgical removal is indicated, CE sequences should be performed to exclude malignant lesions that could be surgically removed during the same intervention.

10 Pathologic Nipple Discharge

Nipple discharge is one of the most common breast symptoms, experienced by at least 80% of women during their life. *Lactational* (milk secretion), *physiologic* (white, green, or yellow), and medication-related discharges usually derive bilaterally from multiple ducts and do not require breast imaging. The same applies for cases depending on non-breast pathologies such as a pituitary prolactinoma. Conversely, pathologic nipple discharge presents spontaneously from a single duct, commonly unilateral, clear, serous, or bloody. Intraductal papilloma and ductal ectasia are the most common causes but in 4–29% of patients pathological discharge is caused by a malignancy (Panzironi et al. 2018). After physical examination and nipple discharge cytology (strongly limited by a false-negative rate of over 50%), mammography is performed from 40 years of age, but its sensitivity has been reported to range only from 7% to 26%, while the sensitivity of US, preferred as first-line examination under 40, is highly variable (63–100%) (Panzironi et al. 2018; Lee et al. 2017b). Mammography/digital breast tomosynthesis can be performed in men regardless of age, given the high incidence of breast cancer with pathologic nipple discharge (Panzironi et al. 2018; Lee et al. 2017b). Of note, in case of negative clinical examination and conventional imaging, the probability of malignancy is reported to be higher than 2% (Sardanelli et al. 2010; Bahl et al. 2017), thus needing further workup.

Unless surgery is preferred as direct therapeutic option, after negative mammography and US, in the presence of pathological nipple discharge, MRI should be considered as a good alternative to both galactography and ductoscopy. A standard CE protocol should be adopted and partial MIP reconstructions of T2-weighted fat-suppressed images can be useful to obtain images similar to galactography (Fig. 15).

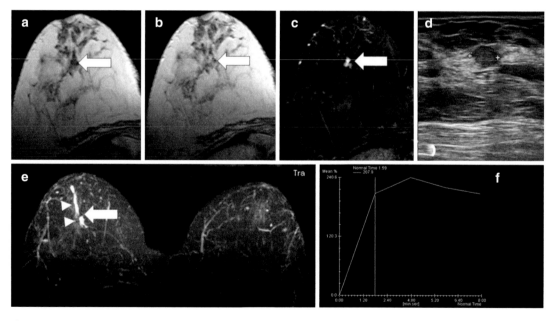

Fig. 15 Pathologic nipple discharge. A 52-year-old woman presented with single-duct bloody nipple discharge at the right breast. Mammography and first-look US (not shown) were negative. 1.5T breast MRI showed a small enhancing lesion in retroareolar region of the right breast: arrow in **a** (unenhanced T1-weighted image), **b** (first CE image obtained at about 2 min after injection of 0.1 mmol/kg of gadobenate dimeglumine), and **c** (subtracted image, i.e., **b** minus **a**). In **d**, second-look US shows the intraductal lesion (calipers). Partial MIP reconstructions from the T2-weighted STIR dataset (**e**) show the filling defect (arrows) in the dilated duct (arrowheads). The ROI-based dynamic behavior is shown to be a plateau (type 2) curve (**f**). Pathology of surgical specimen revealed an intraductal papilloma with stromal sclerosis

In fact, galactography is an invasive procedure that may cause discomfort and pain, feasible only when the duct discharge is demonstrated at the time of the study, with a rate of incompleteness or failure up to 15% and a low ability to distinguish between benign and malignant lesions. Ductoscopy provides a direct visualization of intraductal lesions, allowing for directed excision and facilitating targeted surgery, with a reported sensitivity of 94%; unfortunately, it is available in only a few centers and most clinicians are unfamiliar with its use (Panzironi et al. 2018).

The superiority of MRI compared to galactography has been demonstrated by a recent meta-analysis (Berger et al. 2017) including 921 patients from ten studies. MRI showed a significantly higher pooled sensitivity for any abnormality (92%) than galactography (69%); the pooled specificity was also significantly higher for MRI than for galactography (76% versus 39%). When considering the diagnostic performance for malignancy, MRI showed a 92% sensitivity and a 97% specificity.

11 Borderline (B3) Lesions at Mammography/US-Guided Needle Biopsy

B3 or *borderline lesions* encompass a heterogeneous spectrum of histological conditions whose subsequent management is challenging because they are pathologically defined as *lesions with uncertain potential for malignancy* (the term *high-risk lesions* is also used but should be avoided for the possible confusion between *high-risk lesions* and *high-risk women*) (Chapter "High Risk Lesions of the Breast: Diagnosis and Management"). The uncertainty is given by the possibility of an invasive cancer or a DCIS in the gland tissue nearby sampled under imaging guidance (Houssami et al. 2007; Sardanelli and Houssami 2008; Rageth et al. 2016). Taking into account different classifications, we can include a list of pathological entities among B3 lesion category: atypical ductal hyperplasia, flat epithelial atypia, lobular neoplasia (i.e., lobular carcinoma in situ and atypical lobular hyperplasia), papil-

lary lesions, benign phyllodes tumors, radial scars, mucocele-like lesions, and columnar cell lesions. They currently account for up to 9% of the results of needle biopsy under mammography/US (Londero et al. 2012) and their rate may be increased by the introduction of digital breast tomosynthesis. The range of malignancy rates associated with B3 lesions is variable, reported to be up to 25% (Lee et al. 2003) or also 33% (Houssami et al. 2007) in older series. Surgical excision still represents the standard of care in many countries although it is associated with the absence of cancer (invasive or DCIS) in more than 50% of cases.

The adoption of a more conserving approach has been proposed by a consensus conference (Rageth et al. 2016): first-line surgical excision for atypical ductal hyperplasia and phyllodes tumors; therapeutic excision by large-core vacuum-assisted biopsy with follow-up surveillance imaging for 5 years for flat epithelial atypia; lobular, papillary lesions; and radial scars. Other options are offered by subclassification into lesions with and without epithelial atypia, the former being associated with a lower rate of malignancy at surgical excision (Mayer et al. 2017).

Anyway, B3 lesions remain a clinical challenge for radiologists who should communicate the uncertainty of the pathology result of the needle sample they performed and for the multidisciplinary team as a whole. To date, few studies have investigated the role of MRI in the management of B3 lesions. A. Linda and coworkers (2008b) firstly reported on 76 B3 lesions: CE-MRI (interpreted using traditional morphologic/dynamic diagnostic criteria) showed an 89% sensitivity (8/9, with one false-negative grade 1 DCIS) and a 98% PPV. Pediconi and coworkers (2010) reported on 32 B3 lesions: BI-RADS-interpreted CE-MRI showed 88% sensitivity (7/8, with one false-negative 7 mm DCIS) and 96% NPV. Thereafter, Londero and coworkers (2012) evaluated 227 high-risk lesions at contrast-enhanced MRI considering them suspicious for malignancy if any contrast enhancement was detectable, without any consideration of size, shape, or dynamics (the same simple dichotomous criterion aimed at maximizing sensitivity, also adopted by Bennani-Baiti and coworkers (2017) for evaluating BI-RADS 4 microcalcifications). Of 155 contrast-enhancing lesions, 28 (18%) were upgraded to malignancy after surgical excision while of 72 non-contrast-enhancing lesions, only 2 (3%) were upgraded to malignancy after surgical excision, resulting in a 97% NPV, with both of the 2 false negatives being grade 1 DCIS.

Recently K. Tsuchiya and coworkers (2017) reported on 17 patients with ADH (15 from stereotactic biopsy, 2 from US-guided biopsy) who underwent 3T CE-MRI. Nine of 17 cases were upgraded to malignancy at final pathology. MRI sensitivity, specificity, positive predictive value, and negative predictive value resulted to be 100%, 88%, 90%, and 100%, respectively. At multivariate analysis, suspicious enhancement on MRI was the most significant predictor of malignancy. The authors concluded that patients with ADH without suspicious enhancement on CE-MRI might be followed with CE-MRI rather than undergoing surgical excision.

Although the evidence is still limited, CE-MRI dichotomous reading (enhancement versus no enhancement—Fig. 16) has a potential for avoiding surgery in a high proportion of B3 cases (of course, enhancing lesions that turn out to be B3 lesions at MRI-guided needle biopsy must undergo surgical excision because of their enhancement). Based on the cautious assumption of only 6% of B3 lesions among breast needle biopsy results, we estimated that using MRI in this setting could avoid approximately 10,000 breast surgical intervention for benign conditions in the USA and 15,000 in Europe (Londero et al. 2012).

This perspective needs to be investigated by large, prospective multicenter studies, taking into particular consideration the necessity to reduce inter-reader variability in the pathologic classification of these lesions, specifically for the crucial differentiation between atypical ductal dysplasia and DCIS, which is one factor contributing to overdiagnosis and overtreatment (Colin et al. 2014; Elmore et al. 2015; Sardanelli et al. 2018b).

To note, B3 lesions found at MRI-guided biopsy are a different set of lesions: they *are* contrast enhancing. A multicenter study (Verheyden et al. 2016) reporting on 1509 cases showed that for atypical ductal hyperplasia ($n = 72$) and DCIS ($n = 118$) at MRI-guided biopsy, the rates of underestimation were 26% and 23%, respectively. Another multicenter study (Khoury et al. 2016) reported on 63 cases of lobular neoplasia and a total of 1665 MRI-guided core biopsy, with a 24% rate of underestimation.

12 Conclusions

Breast MRI is a well-established clinical tool. As is for every substantial medical innovation, a learning curve could be observed during the years not only for the direct users, i.e., breast radiologists, but also for referring physicians, especially surgeons. To obtain optimal results, breast MRI has to be performed with state-of-the-art equipment and protocols as well as interpreted according to standardized lexicons and diagnostic categories (i.e., ACR BI-RADS (D'Orsi et al. 2013)).

Indications for breast MRI are a slowly evolving matter, also because they depend not only on the radiologists' opinions but also on the acceptance by referring physicians, in obvious relation with the levels of evidence that the method has reached in the published literature. An interesting debate is still open, especially for preoperative MRI. A survey from 177 EUSOBI members (Clauser et al. 2018) (52% of them from academic centers) recently showed that preoperative staging is the indication mostly practiced (all responders agree on this indication, in particular in the case of invasive lobular histology). As frequently happens, clinical practice in real life has its own track that depends on a lot of factors, including social and economic aspects as well as accessibility to the technology.

We foresee a bright future for breast MRI, even though for several indications illustrated in this chapter there are emerging competitors, the most important among them being contrast-enhanced mammography and automated breast

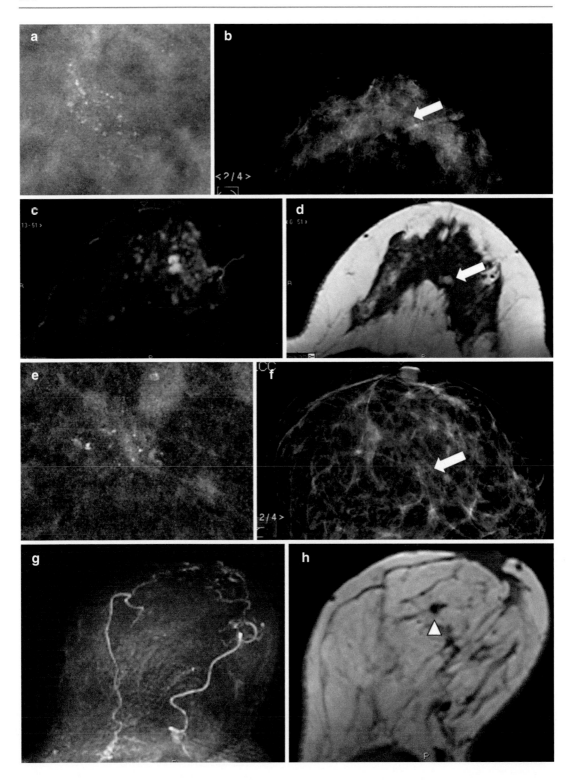

Fig. 16 Borderline (B3) lesions at mammography-guided needle biopsy. (**a–d**) A 48-year-old woman had a 9 mm cluster of punctate microcalcifications at the left breast as shown by an electronically magnified craniocaudal mammogram (**a**). In **b**, the left mammogram to be comparable with MRI (arrow pointing out the cluster). A vacuum-assisted biopsy under stereotactic guidance partially removed the cluster, resulting in the pathological diagnosis of atypical ductal hyperplasia. MRI (1.5T magnet, 0.1 mmol/kg of gadobenate dimeglumine) showed a 10-mm clumped enhancing lesion on the MIP of the first contrast-enhanced sequence (**c**), close to the hyperintensity of the residual post-biopsy hematoma visible on unenhanced T1-weighted image (arrowhead in **d**). Surgery revealed low-grade DCIS. (**e–h**) A 50-year-old woman had a 6 mm cluster of punctate microcalcifications at the left breast as shown by an electronically magnified craniocaudal mammogram (**e**). In **f**, the left mammogram to be comparable with MRI (arrow pointing out the cluster). A vacuum-assisted biopsy under stereotactic guidance partially removed the cluster resulting in the pathological diagnosis of atypical ductal hyperplasia; MRI (1.5T magnet, 0.1 mmol/kg of gadobenate dimeglumine) showed no enhancing lesions on the MIP of the first contrast-enhanced sequence (**g**). For completeness, the unenhanced T1-weighted image with the signal void artifact due to the localizing titanium clip placed after the biopsy (arrowhead in **h**) is shown. Pathology of surgical specimen confirmed atypical ductal hyperplasia

US. In particular, the former has already been shown in a multicenter study (Fallenberg et al. 2017) to provide information comparable to that given by MRI in the preoperative setting. Conversely, very preliminary results showed (Halshtok Neiman et al. 2016) a low agreement between automated breast US and MRI for screening BRCA1/2 mutation carriers, suggesting that its performance may be lower than that of MRI in this setting.

However, while the competitors are following MRI for BC diagnosis and staging, MRI is already on a new frontier, providing *in vivo* biomarkers for BC prognosis (Leithner et al. 2018). This will be the future competition, for which MRI is certainly in pole position. The application of artificial intelligence, especially of deep learning algorithms (Pesapane et al. 2018; Codari et al. 2019), to multiparametric breast MRI will probably play a crucial role. If breast MRI will be demonstrated to substantially contribute to the definition of therapy, all the hot discussions on preoperative MRI focused on surgical outcomes could be overcome.

References

Adrada BE, Miranda RN, Rauch GM et al (2014) Breast implant-associated anaplastic large cell lymphoma: sensitivity, specificity and findings of imaging studies in 44 patients. Breast Cancer Res Treat 147:1–14

Amarens H, Geuzinge MF, Bakker EAM et al (2021) Cost-effectiveness of magnetic resonance imaging screening for women with extremely dense breast tissue. JNCI: J Natl Cancer Inst 113:1476–1483. https://doi.org/10.1093/jnci/djab119

American College of Radiology (2003) Breast Imaging Reporting and Data System Atlas (BI-RADS Atlas), 4th edn. American College of Radiology, Reston, VA

American College of Radiology (2012) Appropriateness criteria on breast cancer screening. http://www.med.unc.edu/radiology/breastimaging/breast-density-law-files/american-college-of-radiology-acr. Accessed 12 Aug 2018

American College of Radiology (2018) Practice parameter for the performance of contrast-enhanced magnetic resonance imaging (MRI) of the breast. https://www.acr.org/-/media/ACR/Files/Practice-Parameters/mr-contrast-breast.pdf. Accessed 24 Sept 2018

American Society of Breast Surgeons (2018). http://www.choosingwisely.org/clinician-lists/breast-surgeons-mris-in-new-breast-cancer-patients/. Accessed 10 Jun 2018

American Society of Plastic Surgeons (2018). https://www.plasticsurgery.org/documents/News/Statistics/2017/plastic-surgery-statistics-full-report-2017.pdf. Accessed 17 Aug 2018

Bahl M, Pien IJ, Buretta KJ et al (2016) Can vascular patterns on preoperative magnetic resonance imaging help predict skin necrosis after nipple-sparing mastectomy? J Am Coll Surg 223:279–285

Bahl M, Gadd MA, Lehman CD (2017) Diagnostic utility of MRI after negative or inconclusive mammography for the evaluation of pathologic nipple discharge. AJR Am J Roentgenol 209:1404–1410

Ballesio L, Gigli S, Di Pastena F et al (2017) Magnetic resonance imaging tumor regression shrinkage patterns after neoadjuvant chemotherapy in patients with locally advanced breast cancer: correlation with tumor biological subtypes and pathological response after therapy. Tumour Biol 39:1010428317694540

Baltzer PA, Dietzel M, Vag T et al (2011) Clinical MR mammography: impact of hormonal status on background enhancement and diagnostic accuracy. Röfo 183:441–447

Baltzer P, Mann RM, Iima M et al (2020) Diffusion-weighted imaging of the breast-a consensus and mission statement from the EUSOBI International Breast Diffusion-Weighted Imaging working group. Eur Radiol 30:1436–1450

Barton SR, Smith IE, Kirby AM et al (2011) The role of ipsilateral breast radiotherapy in management of occult primary breast cancer presenting as axillary lymphadenopathy. Eur J Cancer 47:2099–2106

Baum F, Fischer U, Vosshenrich R, Grabbe E (2002) Classification of hypervascularized lesions in CE MR imaging of the breast. Eur Radiol 12:1087–1092

Belli P, Bufi E, Bonatesta A et al (2016) Unenhanced breast magnetic resonance imaging: detection of breast cancer. Eur Rev Med Pharmacol Sci 20:4220–4229

Bennani-Baiti B, Baltzer PA (2017) MR imaging for diagnosis of malignancy in mammographic microcalcifications: a systematic review and meta analysis. Radiology 283:692–701

Bennani-Baiti B, Bennani-Baiti N, Baltzer PA (2016) Diagnostic performance of breast magnetic resonance imaging in non-calcified equivocal breast findings: results from a systematic review and meta-analysis. PLoS One 11:e0160346

Bennani-Baiti B, Dietzel M, Baltzer PA (2017) MRI for the assessment of malignancy in BI-RADS 4 mammographic microcalcifications. PLoS One 12:e0188679

Berger N, Luparia A, Di Leo G et al (2017) Diagnostic performance of MRI versus galactography in women with pathologic nipple discharge: a systematic review and meta-analysis. AJR Am J Roentgenol 209:465–471

Bernardi D, Ciatto S, Pellegrini M, Valentini M, Houssami N (2012) EUSOMA criteria for performing preoperative MRI staging in candidates for breast conserving surgery: hype or helpful? Breast 21:406–408

Braman NM, Etesami M, Prasanna P et al (2017) Intratumoral and peritumoral radiomics for the pretreatment prediction of pathological complete response to neoadjuvant chemotherapy based on breast DCE-MRI. Breast Cancer Res 19:57. Erratum in: Breast Cancer Res 2017;19:80

Brennan ME, Houssami N, Lord S et al (2009) Magnetic resonance imaging screening of the contralateral breast in women with newly diagnosed breast cancer: systematic review and meta-analysis of incremental cancer detection and impact on surgical management. J Clin Oncol 27:5640–5649

Bucchi L, Belli P, Benelli E et al (2016) Recommendations for breast imaging follow-up of women with a previous history of breast cancer: position paper from the Italian Group for Mammography Screening (GISMa) and the Italian College of Breast Radiologists (ICBR) by SIRM. Radiol Med 121:891–896

Budhdeo S, Watkins J, Atun R, Williams C, Zeltner T, Maruthappu M (2015) Changes in government spending on healthcare and population mortality in the European Union, 1995–2010: a cross-sectional ecological study. J R Soc Med 108:490–498

Bufi E, Belli P, Costantini M et al (2015) Role of the apparent diffusion coefficient in the prediction of response to neoadjuvant chemotherapy in patients with locally advanced breast cancer. Clin Breast Cancer 15:370–380

Carbonaro LA, Tannaphai P, Trimboli RM et al (2012) Contrast-enhanced breast MRI: spatial displacement from prone to supine patient's position. Preliminary results. Eur J Radiol 81:e771–e774

Chan SE, Liao CY, Wang TY et al (2017) The diagnostic utility of preoperative breast magnetic resonance imaging (MRI) and/or intraoperative sub-nipple biopsy in nipple-sparing mastectomy. Eur J Surg Oncol 43:76–84

Charehbili A, Wasser MN, Smit VT et al (2014) Accuracy of MRI for treatment response assessment after taxane- and anthracycline-based neoadjuvant chemotherapy in HER2-negative breast cancer. Eur J Surg Oncol 40:1216–1221

Chen JH, Feig BA, Hsiang DJ et al (2009) Impact of MRI-evaluated neoadjuvant chemotherapy response on change of surgical recommendation in breast cancer. Ann Surg 249:448–454

Chiarelli AM, Prummel MV, Muradali D et al (2014) Effectiveness of screening with annual magnetic resonance imaging and mammography: results of the initial screen from the Ontario high risk breast screening program. J Clin Oncol 32:2224–2230

Cho N, Im SA, Cheon GJ et al (2018) Integrated 18F-FDG PET/MRI in breast cancer: early prediction of response to neoadjuvant chemotherapy. Eur J Nucl Med Mol Imaging 45:328–339

Choi BH, Choi N, Kim MY et al (2018) Usefulness of abbreviated breast MRI screening for women with a history of breast cancer surgery. Breast Cancer Res Treat 167:495–502

Chu W, Jin W, Liu D et al (2017) Diffusion-weighted imaging in identifying breast cancer pathological response to neoadjuvant chemotherapy: a meta-analysis. Oncotarget 9:7088–7100

Clauser P, Carbonaro LA, Pancot M et al (2015) Additional findings at preoperative breast MRI: the value of second-look digital breast tomosynthesis. Eur Radiol 25:2830–2839

Clauser P, Mann R, Athanasiou A (2018) A survey by the European Society of Breast Imaging on the utilisation of breast MRI in clinical practice. Eur Radiol 28:1909–1918

Codari M, Schiaffino S, Sardanelli F, Trimboli RM (2019) Artificial intelligence for breast MRI 2008–2018: a systematic mapping review. AJR Am J Roentgenol 212(2):280–292

Colin C, Foray N (2012) DNA damage induced by mammography in high family risk patients: only one single view in screening. Breast 21:409–410

Colin C, Devouassoux-Shisheboran M, Sardanelli F (2014) Is breast cancer overdiagnosis also nested in pathologic misclassification? Radiology 273:652–655

Colin C, Foray N, Di Leo G, Sardanelli F (2017) Radiation induced breast cancer risk in BRCA mutation carriers from low-dose radiological exposures: a systematic review. Radioprotection 52:231–240. https://doi.org/10.1051/radiopro/2017034

Corrigan-Curay J, Sacks L, Woodcock J (2018) Real-world evidence and real-world data for evaluating drug safety and effectiveness. JAMA. https://doi.org/10.1001/jama.2018.10136

Cox C, Holloway CM, Shaheta A et al (2013) What is the burden of axillary disease after neoadjuvant therapy in women with locally advanced breast cancer? Curr Oncol 20:111–117

D'Orsi C, Sickles E, Mendelson E, Morris E (2013) ACR BI-RADS® Atlas, Breast Imaging Reporting and Data System, 5th edn. American College of Radiology, Reston, VA

De Los Santos JF, Cantor A, Amos KD et al (2013) Magnetic resonance imaging as a predictor of pathologic response in patients treated with neoadjuvant systemic treatment for operable breast cancer. Translational Breast Cancer Research Consortium trial 017. Cancer 119:1776–1783

Dent R, Trudeau M, Pritchard KI et al (2007) Triple-negative breast cancer: clinical features and patterns of recurrence. Clin Cancer Res 13:4429–44234

Derias M, Subramanian A, Allan S, Shah E, Teraifi HE, Howlett D (2016) The role of magnetic resonance imaging in the investigation and management of invasive lobular carcinoma - a 3-year retrospective study in two district general hospitals. Breast J 22:384–389

Di Leo G, Trimboli RM, Benedek A et al (2015) MR imaging for selection of patients for partial breast irradiation: a systematic review and meta-analysis. Radiology 277:716–726

Dialani V, Chadashvili T, Slanetz PJ (2015) Role of imaging in neoadjuvant therapy for breast cancer. Ann Surg Oncol 22:1416–1424

Ding JR, Wang DN, Pan JL (2016) Apparent diffusion coefficient value of diffusion-weighted imaging for differential diagnosis of ductal carcinoma in situ and infiltrating ductal carcinoma. J Cancer Res Ther 12:744–750

Dongfeng H, Daqing M, Erhu J (2012) Dynamic breast magnetic resonance imaging: pretreatment prediction of tumor response to neoadjuvant chemotherapy. Clin Breast Cancer 12:94–101

Dorrius MD, Jansen-van der Weide MC et al (2011) Computer-aided detection in breast MRI: a systematic review and meta-analysis. Eur Radiol 21:1600–1608

Dorrius MD, Dijkstra H, Oudkerk M, Sijens PE (2014) Effect of b value and pre-admission of contrast on diagnostic accuracy of 1.5-T breast DWI: a systematic review and meta-analysis. Eur Radiol 24:2835–2847

Eisenhauer EA, Therasse P, Bogaerts J et al (2009) New response evaluation criteria in solid tumours: revised RECIST guideline (version 1.1). Eur J Cancer 45:228–247

Ellis RL (2009) Optimal timing of breast MRI examinations for premenopausal women who do not have a normal menstrual cycle. AJR Am J Roentgenol 193:1738–1740

Elmore JG, Longton GM, Carney PA et al (2015) Diagnostic concordance among pathologists interpreting breast biopsy specimens. JAMA 313:1122–1132

Elster AD (2018) Questions and answers in MRI. http://mriquestions.com/making-a-dw-image.html. Accessed 12 Aug 2018

Etxano J, Insausti LP, Elizalde A et al (2015) Analysis of the changes induced by bevacizumab using a high temporal resolution DCE-MRI as prognostic factors for response to further neoadjuvant chemotherapy. Acta Radiol 56:1300–1307

European Medicines Agency (2017) PRAC confirms restrictions on the use of linear gadolinium agents. http://www.ema.europa.eu/docs/cn_GB/document_library/Referrals_document/gadolinium_contrast_agents_31/Recommendation_provided_by_Pharmacovigilance_Risk_Assessment_Committee/WC500230928.pdf. Accessed 20 Aug 2017

Evans DG, Kesavan N, Lim Y et al, MARIBS Group (2014) MRI breast screening in high-risk women: cancer detection and survival analysis. Breast Cancer Res Treat 145:663–672

Evans A, Trimboli RM, et al, European Society of Breast Imaging (EUSOBI), with language review by Europa Donna–The European Breast Cancer Coalition (2018) Breast ultrasound: recommendations for information to women and referring physicians by the European Society of Breast Imaging. Insights Imaging. https://doi.org/10.1007/s13244-018-0636-z

Fakkert IE, Mourits MJ, Jansen L et al (2012) Breast cancer incidence after risk-reducing salpingo-oophorectomy in BRCA1 and BRCA2 mutation carriers. Cancer Prev Res (Phila) 5:1291–1297

Fallenberg EM, Schmitzberger FF, Amer H et al (2017) Contrast-enhanced spectral mammography vs. mammography and MRI - clinical performance in a multireader evaluation. Eur Radiol 27:2752–2764

Fan M, Wu G, Cheng H et al (2017) Radiomic analysis of DCE-MRI for prediction of response to neoadjuvant chemotherapy in breast cancer patients. Eur J Radiol 94:140–147

Fatayer H, Sharma N, Manuel D et al (2016) Serial MRI scans help in assessing early response to neoadjuvant chemotherapy and tailoring breast cancer treatment. Eur J Surg Oncol 42:965–972

Fausto A, Magaldi A, Babaei Paskeh B et al (2007) MR imaging and proton spectroscopy of the breast: how to select the images useful to convey the diagnostic message. Radiol Med 112:1060–1068

Fayanju OM, Jeffe DB, Margenthaler JA (2013) Occult primary breast cancer at a comprehensive cancer center. J Surg Res 185:684–689

Fischer U, Vosshenrich R, Keating D et al (1994) MR-guided biopsy of suspect breast lesions with a simple stereotaxic add-on-device for surface coils. Radiology 192:272–273

Fisher B, Anderson S, Bryant J et al (2002) Twenty-year follow-up of a randomized trial comparing total mastectomy, lumpectomy and lumpectomy plus irradiation for the treatment of invasive breast cancer. N Engl J Med 347:1233–1341

Fukuda T, Horii R, Gomi N et al (2016) Accuracy of magnetic resonance imaging for predicting pathological complete response of breast cancer after neoadjuvant chemotherapy: association with breast cancer subtype. Springerplus 5:152

Francesco S, Rubina MT, Nehmat H et al (2022) Magnetic resonance imaging before breast cancer surgery: results of an observational multicenter international prospective analysis (MIPA). Eur J Radiol 32:1611–1623. https://doi.org/10.1007/s00330-021-08240-x

Gao W, Guo N, Dong T (2018) Diffusion-weighted imaging in monitoring the pathological response to neoadjuvant chemotherapy in patients with breast cancer: a meta-analysis. World J Surg Oncol 16:145

Gervais MK, Maki E, Schiller DE, Crystal P, McCready DR (2017) Preoperative MRI of the breast and ipsilateral breast tumor recurrence: long-term follow up. J Surg Oncol 115:231–237

Giannini V, Mazzetti S, Marmo A et al (2017) A computer-aided diagnosis (CAD) scheme for pretreatment prediction of pathological response to neoadjuvant therapy using dynamic contrast-enhanced MRI texture features. Br J Radiol 90:20170269

Gonzalez V, Sandelin K, Karlsson A et al (2014) Preoperative MRI of the breast (POMB) influences primary treatment in breast cancer: a prospective, randomized, multicenter study. World J Surg 38:1685–1693

Green LA, Karow JA, Toman JE, Lostumbo A, Xie K (2018) Review of breast augmentation and reconstruction for the radiologist with emphasis on MRI. Clin Imaging 47:101–117. https://doi.org/10.1016/j.clinimag.2017.08.007

Grimm LJ, Soo MS, Yoon S et al (2015) Abbreviated screening protocol for breast MRI: a feasibility study. Acad Radiol 22:1157–1162

Gu YL, Pan SM, Ren J, Yang ZX, Jiang GQ (2017) Role of magnetic resonance imaging in detection of pathologic complete remission in breast cancer patients treated with neoadjuvant chemotherapy: a meta-analysis. Clin Breast Cancer 17:245–255

Gutierrez RL, Strigel RM, Partridge SC et al (2012) Dynamic breast MRI: does lower temporal resolution negatively affect clinical kinetic analysis? AJR Am J Roentgenol 199:703–708

Ha SM, Chae EY, Cha JH, Kim HH, Shin HJ, Choi WJ (2018) Breast MR imaging before surgery: outcomes in patients with invasive lobular carcinoma by using propensity score matching. Radiology 287:771–777

Halshtok Neiman O, Erlich Z, Friedman E et al (2016) Automated breast volumetric sonography compared with magnetic resonance imaging in Jewish BRCA 1/2 mutation carriers. Isr Med Assoc J 18:609–612

Harms SE, Flamig DP, Hesley KL et al (1993) MR imaging of the breast with rotating delivery of excitation off resonance: clinical experience with pathologic correlation. Radiology 187:493–501

Harvey SC, Di Carlo PA, Lee B et al (2016) An abbreviated protocol for high-risk screening breast MRI saves time and resources. J Am Coll Radiol 13:374–380

He M, Tang LC, Yu KD et al (2012) Treatment outcomes and unfavorable prognostic factors in patients with occult breast cancer. Eur J Surg Oncol 38:1022–1028

Heacock L, Melsaether AN, Heller SL et al (2016) Evaluation of a known breast cancer using an abbreviated breast MRI protocol: correlation of imaging characteristics and pathology with lesion detection and conspicuity. Eur J Radiol 85.815–823

Hegenscheid K, Schmidt CO, Seipel R et al (2012) Contrast enhancement kinetics of normal breast parenchyma in dynamic MR mammography: effects of menopausal status oral contraceptives and postmenopausal hormone therapy. Eur Radiol 22:2633–2640

Heldahl MG, Bathen TF, Rydland J et al (2010) Prognostic value of pretreatment dynamic contrast-enhanced MR imaging in breast cancer patients receiving neoadjuvant chemotherapy: overall survival predicted from combined time course and volume analysis. Acta Radiol 51:604–612

Henderson TO, Amsterdam A, Bhatia S et al (2010) Systematic review: surveillance for breast cancer in women treated with chest radiation for childhood, adolescent or young adult cancer. Ann Intern Med 152:444–455; W144–W154

Hendrick RE (2010) Breast magnetic resonance imaging acquisition protocols. In: Hendrick RE (ed) Breast MRI. Fundamentals and technical aspects. Springer, New York, pp 135–171

Heywang SH, Hahn D, Schmidt H et al (1986) MR imaging of the breast using gadolinium-DTPA. J Comput Assist Tomogr 10:199–204

Heywang-Köbrunner S, Beck R (1996) Contrast-enhanced MRI of the breast. Springer, Berlin

Heywang-Köbrunner SH, Heinig A, Schaumlöffel U et al (1999) MR-guided percutaneous excisional and incisional biopsy of breast lesions. Eur Radiol 9:1656–1665

Heywang-Köbrunner SH, Sinnatamby R, Lebeau A et al, Consensus Group (2009) Interdisciplinary consensus on the uses and technique of MR-guided vacuum-assisted breast biopsy (VAB): results of a European consensus meeting. Eur J Radiol 72:289–294

Holland R, Veling SH, Mravunac M, Hendriks JH (1985) Histologic multifocality of Tis, T1-2 breast carcinomas. Implications for clinical trials of breast-conserving surgery. Cancer 56:979–990

Houssami N, Ciatto S (2010) Design-related bias in estimates of accuracy when comparing imaging tests: examples from breast imaging research. Eur Radiol 20:2061–2066

Houssami N, Solin LJ (2010) An appraisal of preoperative MRI in breast cancer: more effective staging of the breast or much ado about nothing? Maturitas 67:291–293

Houssami N, Ciatto S, Bilous M, Vezzosi V, Bianchi S (2007) Borderline breast core needle histology: predictive values for malignancy in lesions of uncertain malignant potential (B3). Br J Cancer 96:1253–1257

Houssami N, Ciatto S, Macaskill P et al (2008) Accuracy and surgical impact of magnetic resonance imaging in breast cancer staging: systematic review and meta-analysis in detection of multifocal and multicentric cancer. J Clin Oncol 26:3248–3258

Houssami N, Macaskill P, Marinovich ML et al (2010) Meta-analysis of the impact of surgical margins on local recurrence in women with early-stage invasive breast cancer treated with breast-conserving therapy. Eur J Cancer 46:3219–3232

Houssami N, Turner R, Morrow M (2013) Preoperative magnetic resonance imaging in breast cancer: meta-analysis of surgical outcomes. Ann Surg 257:249–255

Houssami N, Turner R, Macaskill P et al (2014) An individual person data meta-analysis of preoperative magnetic resonance imaging and breast cancer recurrence. J Clin Oncol 32:392–401

Houssami N, Turner RM, Morrow M (2017) Meta-analysis of pre-operative magnetic resonance imaging (MRI) and surgical treatment for breast cancer. Breast Cancer Res Treat 165:273–283

Hylton NM (2005) Breast magnetic resonance imaging techniques. In: Morris E, Liberman L (eds) Breast MRI. Diagnosis and intervention. Springer, New York, pp 7–14

Iacconi C, Galman L, Zheng J et al (2016) Multicentric cancer detected at breast MR imaging and not at mammography: important or not? Radiology 279:378–384

IBIS Breast Cancer Risk Evaluation Tool (2018). http://www.ems-trials.org/riskevaluator/. Accessed 12 Aug 2018

Jatoi I, Benson JR (2013) The case against routine preoperative breast MRI. Future Oncol 9:347–353

Kaiser WA (1989) Magnetic resonance tomography of the breast. The results of 253 examinations. Dtsch Med Wochenschr 114:1351–1357

Kaiser WA (1993) Optimum procedure for the MRM examination. In: Kaiser WA (ed) MR mammography (MRM). Springer, Berlin, pp 29–35

Kaiser WA (1994) False-positive results in dynamic MR mammography. Causes, frequency and methods to avoid. Magn Reson Imaging Clin N Am 2: 539–555

Kaiser WA (2008) Signs in MR-mammography. Springer, Berlin

Kanal E (2017) Gadolinium-based contrast agents: the plot thickens. Radiology 285:340–342

Kazama T, Kuroki Y, Kikuchi M et al (2012) Diffusion-weighted MRI as an adjunct to mammography in women under 50 years of age: an initial study. J Magn Reson Imaging 36:139–144

Khoury T, Kumar PR, Li Z et al (2016) Lobular neoplasia detected in MRI-guided core biopsy carries a high risk

for upgrade: a study of 63 cases from four different institutions. Mod Pathol 29:25–33

Kim YS, Chang JM, Moon HG et al (2016) Residual mammographic microcalcifications and enhancing lesions on MRI after neoadjuvant systemic chemotherapy for locally advanced breast cancer: correlation with histopathologic residual tumor size. Ann Surg Oncol 23:1135–1142

Kim SY, Cho N, Park IA et al (2018) Dynamic contrast-enhanced breast MRI for evaluating residual tumor size after neoadjuvant chemotherapy. Radiology 289:327–334. https://doi.org/10.1148/radiol.2018172868

Koolen BB, Pengel KE, Wesseling J et al (2013) FDG PET/CT during neoadjuvant chemotherapy may predict response in ER-positive/HER2-negative and triple negative, but not in HER2-positive breast cancer. Breast 22:691–697

Krammer J, Price ER, Jochelson MS et al (2017) Breast MR imaging for the assessment of residual disease following initial surgery for breast cancer with positive margins. Eur Radiol 27:4812–4818

Kriege M, Brekelmans CT, Boetes C et al, Magnetic Resonance Imaging Screening Study Group (2004) Efficacy of MRI and mammography for breast-cancer screening in women with a familial or genetic predisposition. N Engl J Med 351:427–437

Kuhl C (2007) The current status of breast MR imaging. Part I. Choice of technique, image interpretation, diagnostic accuracy and transfer to clinical practice. Radiology 244:356–378

Kuhl CK, Mielcareck P, Klaschik S et al (1999) Dynamic breast MR imaging: are signal intensity time course data useful for differential diagnosis of enhancing lesions? Radiology 211:101–110

Kuhl C, Weigel S, Schrading S et al (2010) Prospective multicenter cohort study to refine management recommendations for women at elevated familial risk of breast cancer: the EVA trial. J Clin Oncol 28:1450–1457

Kuhl CK, Schrading S, Strobel K et al (2014) Abbreviated breast magnetic resonance imaging (MRI): first post-contrast subtracted images and maximum-intensity projection-a novel approach to breast cancer screening with MRI. J Clin Oncol 32:2304–2310

Kurniawan ED, Wong MH, Windle I et al (2008) Predictors of surgical margin status in breast-conserving surgery within a breast screening program. Ann Surg Oncol 15:2542–2549

Lauby-Secretan B, Scoccianti C, Loomis D et al, International Agency for Research on Cancer Handbook Working Group (2015) Breast-cancer screening—viewpoint of the IARC Working Group. N Engl J Med 372:2353–3258

Leach MO, Boggis CR, Dixon AK et al (2005) Screening with magnetic resonance imaging and mammography of a UK population at high familial risk of breast cancer: a prospective multicentre cohort study (MARIBS). Lancet 365:1769–1778

Lee AHS, Denley HE, Pinder SE et al, for the Nottingham Breast Team (2003) Excision biopsy findings of patients with breast needle core biopsies reported as suspicious of malignancy (B4) or lesion of uncertain malignant potential (B3). Histopathology 42:331–336

Lee J, Tanaka E, Eby PR et al (2017a) Preoperative breast MRI: surgeons' patient selection patterns and potential bias in outcomes analyses. AJR Am J Roentgenol 208:923–932

Lee SJ, Trikha S, Moy L et al (2017b) ACR Appropriateness criteria. Evaluation of nipple discharge. J Am Coll Radiol 14(5S):S138–S153

Lee J, Kim SH, Kang BJ (2018) Pretreatment prediction of pathologic complete response to neoadjuvant chemotherapy in breast cancer: perfusion metrics of dynamic contrast enhanced MRI. Sci Rep 8:9490

Lehman CD, Gatsonis C, Kuhl CK et al (2007) MRI evaluation of the contralateral breast in women with recently diagnosed breast cancer. N Engl J Med 356:1295–1303

Leithner D, Wengert GJ, Helbich TH et al (2018) Clinical role of breast MRI now and going forward. Clin Radiol 73:700–714

Li H, Yao L, Jin P et al (2018) MRI and PET/CT for evaluation of the pathological response to neoadjuvant chemotherapy in breast cancer: a systematic review and meta-analysis. Breast 40:106–115

Linda A, Zuiani C, Londero V, Bazzocchi M (2008a) Outcome of initially only magnetic resonance mammography-detected findings with and without correlate at second-look sonography: distribution according to patient history of breast cancer and lesion size. Breast 17:51–57

Linda A, Zuiani C, Bazzocchi M, Furlan A, Londero V (2008b) Borderline breast lesions diagnosed at core needle biopsy: can magnetic resonance mammography rule out associated malignancy? Preliminary results based on 79 surgically excised lesions. Breast 17:125–131

Liu Q, Wang C, Li P, Liu J, Huang G, Song S (2016) The role of (18)F-FDG PET/CT and MRI in assessing pathological complete response to neoadjuvant chemotherapy in patients with breast cancer: a systematic review and meta-analysis. Biomed Res Int 2016:3746232. Erratum in: Biomed Res Int 2016:1235429

Lo WC, Li W, Jones EF, Newitt DC et al (2016) Effect of imaging parameter thresholds on MRI prediction of neoadjuvant chemotherapy response in breast cancer subtypes. PLoS One 11:e0142047

Lo G, Scaranelo AM, Aboras H et al (2017) Evaluation of the utility of screening mammography for high-risk women undergoing screening breast MR imaging. Radiology 285:36–43

Lobbes MB, Vriens IJ, van Bommel AC et al (2017) Breast MRI increases the number of mastectomies for ductal cancers, but decreases them for lobular cancers. Breast Cancer Res Treat 162:353–364

Londero V, Zuiani C, Linda A, Girometti R, Bazzocchi M, Sardanelli F (2012) High-risk breast lesions at imaging-guided needle biopsy: usefulness of MRI for treatment decision. AJR Am J Roentgenol 199:W240–W250

Macedo FI, Eid JJ, Flynn J, Jacobs MJ, Mittal VK (2016) Optimal surgical management for occult breast carcinoma: a meta-analysis. Ann Surg Oncol 23:1838–1844

Machida Y, Shimauchi A, Kanemaki Y et al (2017) Feasibility and potential limitations of abbreviated breast MRI: an observer study using an enriched cohort. Breast Cancer 24:411–419

Maijers MC, Niessen FB, Veldhuizen JF, Ritt MJ, Manoliu RA (2014) MRI screening for silicone breast implant rupture: accuracy, inter- and intraobserver variability using explantation results as reference standard. Eur Radiol 24:1167–1175

Malya FU, Kadioglu H, Bektasoglu HK et al (2018) The role of PET and MRI in evaluating the feasibility of skin-sparing mastectomy following neoadjuvant therapy. J Int Med Res 46:626–636

Mango VL, Morris EA, Dershaw D et al (2015) Abbreviated protocol for breast MRI: are multiple sequences needed for cancer detection? Eur J Radiol 84:65–70

Mann RM, Boetes C (2010) MRI for breast conservation surgery. Lancet 375:2213

Mann RM, Kuhl CK, Kinkel K, Boetes C (2008) Breast MRI: guidelines from the European Society of Breast Imaging. Eur Radiol 18:1307–1318

Mann RM, Loo CE, Wobbes T et al (2010) The impact of preoperative breast MRI on the re-excision rate in invasive lobular carcinoma of the breast. Breast Cancer Res Treat 119:415–422

Mann RM, Balleyguier C, Baltzer PA et al (2015) Breast MRI: EUSOBI recommendations for women's information. Eur Radiol 25:3669–3678

Marije F, Bakker SV, de Lange RM, et al (2019) Supplemental MRI screening for women with extremely dense breast tissue. New Eng J Med 381:2091–2102. https://doi.org/10.1056/NEJMoa1903986

Marinovich ML, Sardanelli F, Ciatto S et al (2012) Early prediction of pathologic response to neoadjuvant therapy in breast cancer: systematic review of the accuracy of MRI. Breast 21:669–677

Marinovich ML, Houssami N, Macaskill P et al (2013a) Meta-analysis of magnetic resonance imaging in detecting residual breast cancer after neoadjuvant therapy. J Natl Cancer Inst 105:321–333

Marinovich ML, Macaskill P, Irwig L et al (2013b) Meta-analysis of agreement between MRI and pathologic breast tumour size after neoadjuvant chemotherapy. Br J Cancer 109:1528–1536

Marinovich ML, Macaskill P, Irwig L et al (2015) Agreement between MRI and pathologic breast tumor size after neoadjuvant chemotherapy and comparison with alternative tests: individual patient data meta-analysis. BMC Cancer 15:662

Mariscotti G, Belli P, Bernardi D et al (2016) Mammography and MRI for screening women who underwent chest radiation therapy (lymphoma survivors): recommendations for surveillance from the Italian College of Breast Radiologists by SIRM. Radiol Med 121:834–837

Mariscotti G, Durando M, Houssami N et al (2018) Preoperative MRI evaluation of lesion-nipple distance in breast cancer patients: thresholds for predicting occult nipple-areola complex involvement. Clin Radiol 738:735–743

Mayer S, Kayser G, Rücker G et al (2017) Absence of epithelial atypia in B3-lesions of the breast is associated with decreased risk for malignancy. Breast 31:144–149

McCartan DP, Zabor EC, Morrow M, Van Zee KJ, El-Tamer MB (2017) Oncologic outcomes after treatment for MRI occult breast cancer (pT0N+). Ann Surg Oncol 24:3141–3147

McDonald ES, Hammersley JA, Chou SH et al (2016) Performance of DWI as a rapid unenhanced technique for detecting mammographically occult breast cancer in elevated-risk women with dense breasts. AJR Am J Roentgenol 207:205–216

McGuire KP, Toro-Burguete J, Dang H et al (2011) MRI staging after neoadjuvant chemotherapy for breast cancer: does tumor biology affect accuracy? Ann Surg Oncol 18:3149–3154

McGuire KP, Hwang ES, Cantor A et al (2015) Surgical patterns of care in patients with invasive breast cancer treated with neoadjuvant systemic therapy and breast magnetic resonance imaging: results of a secondary analysis of TBCRC 017. Ann Surg Oncol 22:75–81

Melsaether A, Gudi A (2014) Breast magnetic resonance imaging performance: safety, techniques, and updates on diffusion-weighted imaging and magnetic resonance spectroscopy. Top Magn Reson Imaging 23:373–384

Miki Y, Swensen J, Shattuck-Eidens D et al (1994) A strong candidate for the breast and ovarian cancer susceptibility gene BRCA1. Science 266:66–71

Monticciolo DL, Newell MS, Moy L, Niell B, Monsees B, Sickles EA (2018) Breast cancer screening in women at higher-than-average risk: recommendations from the ACR. J Am Coll Radiol 15:408–414

Moon HG, Han W, Ahn SK et al (2013) Breast cancer molecular phenotype and the use of HER2-targeted agents influence the accuracy of breast MRI after neoadjuvant chemotherapy. Ann Surg 257:133–137

Morrogh M, Morris EA, Liberman L et al (2008) MRI identifies otherwise occult disease in select patients with Paget disease of the nipple. J Am Coll Surg 206:316–321

Morrow M, Harris JR (2009) More mastectomies: is this what patients really want? J Clin Oncol 27:4038–4040

National Institute for Clinical Excellence (2013) Breast cancer risk category. https://www.nice.org.uk. Accessed 18 Jan 2018

Newitt DC, Tan ET, Wilmes LJ et al (2015) Gradient nonlinearity correction to improve apparent diffusion coefficient accuracy and standardization in the ACRIN 6698 breast cancer trial. J Magn Reson Imaging 42:908–919

Obdeijn IM, Winter-Warnars GA, Mann RM et al (2014) Should we screen BRCA1 mutation carriers only with MRI? A multicenter study. Breast Cancer Res Treat 144:577–582

Ogston KN, Miller ID, Payne S et al (2003) A new histological grading system to assess response of breast cancers to primary chemotherapy: prognostic significance and survival. Breast 12:320–327

Oldrini G, Derraz I, Salleron J, Marchal F, Henrot P (2018) Impact of an abbreviated protocol for breast MRI in diagnostic accuracy. Diagn Interv Radiol 24:12–16

Onega T, Zhu W, Weiss JE (2018) Preoperative breast MRI and mortality in older women with breast cancer. Breast Cancer Res Treat 170:149–157

Oxford Centre for Evidence-based Medicine (2009) Levels of Evidence. https://www.cebm.net/2009/06/oxford-centre-evidence-based-medicine-levels-evidence-march-2009/. Accessed 16 Aug 2018

Panzironi G, Pediconi F, Sardanelli F (2018) Nipple discharge: the state of the art. Br J Radiol Open 1(1):20180016

Park SH, Moon WK, Cho N et al (2010) Diffusion-weighted MR imaging: pretreatment prediction of response to neoadjuvant chemotherapy in patients with breast cancer. Radiology 257(1):56–63

Park S, Yoon JH, Sohn J et al (2016) Magnetic resonance imaging after completion of neoadjuvant chemotherapy can accurately discriminate between no residual carcinoma and residual ductal carcinoma in situ in patients with triple-negative breast cancer. PLoS One 11:e0149347

Parker A, Schroen AT, Brenin DR (2013) MRI utilization in newly diagnosed breast cancer: a survey of practicing surgeons. Ann Surg Oncol 20:2600–2606

Pediconi F, Padula S, Dominelli V et al (2010) Role of breast MR imaging for predicting malignancy of histologically borderline lesions diagnosed at core needle biopsy: prospective evaluation. Radiology 257:653–666

Pesapane F, Codari M, Sardanelli F (2018) Artificial intelligence in medical imaging: threat or opportunity? Radiologists again at the forefront of innovation in medicine. Eur Radiol Exp 2:35. https://doi.org/10.1186/s41747-018-0061-6

Peter P, Dhillon R, Bose S, Bourke A (2016) MRI screening-detected breast lesions in high-risk young women: the value of targeted second-look ultrasound and imaging-guided biopsy. Clin Radiol 71:1037–1043

Peters NH, van Esser S, van den Bosch MA et al (2011) Preoperative MRI and surgical management in patients with nonpalpable breast cancer: the MONET - randomised controlled trial. Eur J Cancer 47:879–886

Phi XA, Houssami N, Obdeijn IM et al (2015) Magnetic resonance imaging improves breast screening sensitivity in BRCA mutation carriers age $\geq$ 50 years: evidence from an individual patient data meta-analysis. J Clin Oncol 33:349–356

Phi XA, Saadatmand S, De Bock GH et al (2016) Contribution of mammography to MRI screening in BRCA mutation carriers by BRCA status and age: individual patient data meta-analysis. Br J Cancer 114:631–637

Phi XA, Houssami N, Hooning MJ et al (2017) Accuracy of screening women at familial risk of breast cancer without a known gene mutation: individual patient data meta-analysis. Eur J Cancer 85:31–38

Plana MN, Carreira C, Muriel A et al (2012) Magnetic resonance imaging in the preoperative assessment of patients with primary breast cancer: systematic review of diagnostic accuracy and meta-analysis. Eur Radiol 22:26–38

Podo F, Santoro F, Di Leo G et al (2016) Triple-negative versus non-triple-negative breast cancers in high-risk women: phenotype features and survival from the HIBCRIT-1 MRI-including screening study. Clin Cancer Res 22:895–904

Rageth CJ, O'Flynn EA, Comstock C et al (2016) First international consensus conference on lesions of uncertain malignant potential in the breast (B3 lesions). Breast Cancer Res Treat 159:203–213

Richard R, Thomassin I, Chapellier M et al (2013) Diffusion-weighted MRI in pretreatment prediction of response to neoadjuvant chemotherapy in patients with breast cancer. Eur Radiol 23:2420–2431

Riedl CC, Luft N, Bernhart C et al (2015) Triple-modality screening trial for familial breast cancer underlines the importance of magnetic resonance imaging and questions the role of mammography and ultrasound regardless of patient mutation status, age and breast density. J Clin Oncol 33:1128–1135

Ritse M, Mann A, Athanasiou PAT et al (2022) Kuhl breast cancer screening in women with extremely dense breasts recommendations of the European Society of Breast Imaging (EUSOBI). Eur J Radiol. https://doi.org/10.1007/s00330-022-08617-6

Saadatmand S, Bretveld R, Siesling S, Tilanus-Linthorst MM (2015a) Influence of tumour stage at breast cancer detection on survival in modern times: population based study in 173,797 patients. BMJ 351:h4901

Saadatmand S, Obdeijn IM, Rutgers EJ et al (2015b) Survival benefit in women with BRCA1 mutation or familial risk in the MRI screening study (MRISC). Int J Cancer 137:1729–1738

Sackett DL, Rosenberg WM, Gray JA, Haynes RB, Richardson WS (1996) Evidence based medicine: what it is and what it isn't. BMJ 312:71–72

Sakakibara M, Nagashima T, Sangai T et al (2008) Breast-conserving surgery using projection and reproduction techniques of surgical-position breast MRI in patients with ductal carcinoma in situ of the breast. J Am Coll Surg 207:62–68

Santamaría G, Bargalló X, Fernández PL et al (2017) Neoadjuvant systemic therapy in breast cancer: association of contrast-enhanced MR imaging findings, diffusion-weighted imaging findings and tumor subtype with tumor response. Radiology 283: 663–672

Santoro F, Podo F, Sardanelli F (2014) MRI screening of women with hereditary predisposition to breast cancer: diagnostic performance and survival analysis. Breast Cancer Res Treat 147:685–687

Sardanelli F (2010a) Overview of the role of pre-operative breast MRI in the absence of evidence on patient outcomes. Breast 19:3–6

Sardanelli F (2010b) Additional findings at preoperative MRI: a simple golden rule for a complex problem? Breast Cancer Res Treat 124:717–721

Sardanelli F (2013) Considerations on the application of EUSOMA criteria for preoperative MRI. Breast 22:368–369

Sardanelli F, Di Leo G (2009a) Diagnostic performance. In: Sardanelli F, Di Leo G (eds) Biostatistics for radiologist. Springer, Milan, pp 19–40

Sardanelli F, Di Leo G (2009b) Study design, systematic reviews and levels of evidence. In: Sardanelli F, Di Leo G (eds) Biostatistics for radiologists. Springer, Milan, pp 141–164

Sardanelli F, Houssami N (2008) Evaluation of lesions of uncertain malignant potential (B3) at core needle biopsy using magnetic resonance imaging: a new approach warrants prospective studies. Breast 17:117–119

Sardanelli F, Trimboli RM (2012) Preoperative MRI: did randomized trials conclude the debate? Eur J Radiol 81(Suppl 1):S135–S1366

Sardanelli F, Fausto A, Iozzelli A, Rescinito G, Calabrese M (2004a) Dynamic breast magnetic resonance imaging. Effect of changing the region of interest on early enhancement using 2D and 3D techniques. J Comput Assist Tomogr 28:642–646

Sardanelli F, Giuseppetti GM, Panizza P et al (2004b) Sensitivity of MRI versus mammography for detecting foci of multifocal, multicentric breast cancer in Fatty and dense breasts using the whole-breast pathologic examination as a gold standard. AJR Am J Roentgenol 183:1149–1157

Sardanelli F, Podo F, D'Agnolo G et al (2007) Multicenter comparative multimodality surveillance of women at genetic-familial high risk for breast cancer (HIBCRIT study): interim results. Radiology 242:698–715

Sardanelli F, Boetes C, Borisch B et al (2010) Magnetic resonance imaging of the breast: recommendations from the EUSOMA working group. Eur J Cancer 46:1296–1316

Sardanelli F, Podo F, Santoro F et al, HIBCRIT-1 Study (2011) Multicenter surveillance of women at high genetic breast cancer risk using mammography, ultrasonography and contrast-enhanced magnetic resonance imaging (the high breast cancer risk Italian 1 study): final results. Invest Radiol 46:94–105

Sardanelli F, Esseridou A, Del Sole A, Sconfienza LM (2012) Response to treatment: the role of imaging. In: Aglietta M, Regge D (eds) Imaging tumor response to treatment. Springer, Milan, pp 15–37

Sardanelli F, Carbonaro LA, Montemezzi S, Cavedon C, Trimboli RM (2016a) Clinical breast MR using MRS or DWI: who is the winner? Front Oncol 6:217

Sardanelli F, Newstead GM, Putz B et al (2016b) Gadobutrol-enhanced magnetic resonance imaging of the breast in the preoperative setting: results of 2 prospective international multicenter Phase III studies. Invest Radiol 51:454–461

Sardanelli F, Alì M, Hunink MG, Houssami N, Sconfienza LM, Di Leo G (2018a) To share or not to share? Expected pros and cons of data sharing in radiological research. Eur Radiol 28:2328–2335

Sardanelli F, Trimboli RM, Tot T (2018b) Expert review of breast pathology in borderline lesions: a chance to reduce overdiagnosis and overtreatment? JAMA Oncol. https://doi.org/10.1001/jamaoncol.2018.1953

Sardanelli F, Trimboli RM, Houssami N et al (2020) Solving the preoperative breast MRI conundrum: design and protocol of the MIPA study. Eur Radiol 30(10):5427–5436

Saslow D, Boetes C, Burke W et al, American Cancer Society Breast Cancer Advisory Group (2007) American Cancer Society guidelines for breast screening with MRI as an adjunct to mammography. CA Cancer J Clin 57(2):75–89

Schaefgen B, Mati M, Sinn HP et al (2016) Can routine imaging after neoadjuvant chemotherapy in breast cancer predict pathologic complete response? Ann Surg Oncol 23:789–795

Schiaffino S, Carbonaro LA, Clauser P et al (2018) Side of contrast injection and breast size correlate with motion artifacts on breast MRI. ISMRM-SBI-EUSOBI workshop on breast MRI: advancing the state of the art Las Vegas, NV, USA, 10–13 Sept 2018. https://www.ismrm.org/workshops/2018/Breast/. Accessed 24 Sept 2018

Schmitz AMT, Teixeira SC, Pengel KE et al (2017) Monitoring tumor response to neoadjuvant chemotherapy using MRI and 18F-FDG PET/CT in breast cancer subtypes. PLoS One 12:e0176782

Schrading S, Distelmaier M, Dirrichs T et al (2015) Digital breast tomosynthesis-guided vacuum-assisted breast biopsy: initial experiences and comparison with prone stereotactic vacuum-assisted biopsy. Radiology 274:654–662

Seely JM, Lamb L, Malik N et al (2016) The yield of preoperative breast MRI in patients according to breast tissue density. Eur Radiol 26:3280–3289

Seiler SJ, Sharma PB, Hayes JC et al (2017) Multimodality imaging-based evaluation of single-lumen silicone breast implants for rupture. Radiographics 37: 366–382

Semiglazov V (2015) RECIST for response (clinical and imaging) in neoadjuvant clinical trials in operable breast cancer. J Natl Cancer Inst Monogr 2015(51):21–23

Shi RY, Yao QY, Wu LM, Xu JR (2018) Breast lesions: diagnosis using diffusion weighted imaging at 1.5T and 3.0T – systematic review and meta-analysis. Clin Breast Cancer 18:e305–e320

Slanetz PJ, Moy L, Baron P et al (2017) ACR Appropriateness Criteria® monitoring response to neoadjuvant systemic therapy for breast cancer. J Am Coll Radiol 14:S462–S475

Solin LJ (2010) Counterview: Pre-operative breast MRI (magnetic resonance imaging) is not recommended for all patients with newly diagnosed breast cancer. Breast 19:7–9

Song JW, Kim HM, Bellfi LT, Chung KC (2011) The effect of study design biases on the diagnostic accuracy of magnetic resonance imaging for detecting silicone breast implant ruptures: a meta-analysis. Plast Reconstr Surg 127:1029–1044

Spick C, Baltzer PA (2014) Diagnostic utility of second-look US for breast lesions identified at MR imaging: systematic review and meta-analysis. Radiology 273:401–409

Spick C, Bickel H, Pinker K et al (2016a) Diffusion-weighted MRI of breast lesions: a prospective clinical investigation of the quantitative imaging biomarker characteristics of reproducibility, repeatability and diagnostic accuracy. NMR Biomed 29:1445–1453

Spick C, Schernthaner M, Pinker K et al (2016b) MR-guided vacuum-assisted breast biopsy of MRI-only lesions: a single center experience. Eur Radiol 26:3908–3916

Sung JS, Li J, Da Costa G et al (2014) Preoperative breast MRI for early-stage breast cancer: effect on surgical and long-term outcomes. AJR Am J Roentgenol 202:1376–1382

Tannaphai P, Trimboli RM, Carbonaro LA et al (2012) Washout of mass-like benign breast lesions at dynamic magnetic resonance imaging. J Comput Assist Tomogr 36:301–330

Teruel JR, Heldahl MG, Goa PE et al (2014) Dynamic contrast-enhanced MRI texture analysis for pretreatment prediction of clinical and pathological response to neoadjuvant chemotherapy in patients with locally advanced breast cancer. NMR Biomed 27:887–896

The Council of the European Union (2003) Council recommendation of 2 December 2003 on cancer screening (2003/878/EC). https://ec.europa.eu/jrc/sites/jrcsh/files/2_December_2003%20cancer%20screening.pdf. Accessed 16 Aug 2018

Trimboli RM, Verardi N, Cartia F, Carbonaro LA, Sardanelli F (2014) Breast cancer detection using double reading of unenhanced MRI including T1-weighted, T2-weighted STIR and diffusion-weighted imaging: a proof of concept study. AJR Am J Roentgenol 203:674–681

Tsuchiya K, Mori N, Schacht DV et al (2017) Value of breast MRI for patients with a biopsy showing atypical ductal hyperplasia (ADH). J Magn Reson Imaging 46:1738–1747

Turnbull L, Brown S, Harvey I et al (2010) Comparative effectiveness of MRI in breast cancer (COMICE) trial: a randomized controlled trial. Lancet 375:563–571

Tyrer J, Duffy SW, Cuzick J (2004) A breast cancer prediction model incorporating familial and personal risk factors. Stat Med 23:1111–1130

U.S. Food and Drug Administration (2017) Medical devices: silicone gel-filled breast implants. https://www.fda.gov/MedicalDevices/ProductsandMedicalProcedures/ImplantsandProsthetics/BreastImplants/ucm063871.htm. Accessed 17 Aug 2018

Um E, Kang JW, Lee S et al (2018) Comparing accuracy of mammography and magnetic resonance imaging for residual calcified lesions in breast cancer patients undergoing neoadjuvant systemic therapy. Clin Breast Cancer 18(5):e1087–e1091

Verheyden C, Pages-Bouic E, Balleyguier C et al (2016) Underestimation rate at MR imaging-guided vacuum-assisted breast biopsy: a multi-institutional retrospective study of 1,509 breast biopsies. Radiology 281:708–719

Veronesi U, Cascinelli N, Mariani L et al (2002) Twenty-year follow-up of a randomized study comparing breast-conserving surgery with radical mastectomy for early breast cancer. N Engl J Med 347: 1227–1232

Vriens BE, de Vries B, Lobbes MB et al, INTENS Study Group (2016) Ultrasound is at least as good as magnetic resonance imaging in predicting tumour size post-neoadjuvant chemotherapy in breast cancer. Eur J Cancer 52:67–76

Wang SY, Long JB, Killelea BK et al (2018) Associations of preoperative breast magnetic resonance imaging with subsequent mastectomy and breast cancer mortality. Breast Cancer Res Treat 172(2):453–461

Warner E, Plewes DB, Hill KA et al (2004) Surveillance of BRCA1 and BRCA2 mutation carriers with magnetic resonance imaging, ultrasound, mammography, and clinical breast examination. JAMA 292:1317–1325

Wooster R, Bignell G, Lancaster J et al (1995) Identification of the breast cancer susceptibility gene BRCA2. Nature 378:789–792

Wu LM, Hu JN, Gu HY et al (2012) Can diffusion-weighted MR imaging and contrast-enhanced MR imaging precisely evaluate and predict pathological response to neoadjuvant chemotherapy in patients with breast cancer? Breast Cancer Res Treat 135:17–28

Wunderle M, Gass P, Häberle L et al (2018) BRCA mutations and their influence on pathological complete response and prognosis in a clinical cohort of neoadjuvantly treated breast cancer patients. Breast Cancer Res Treat 171:85–94

Yamada T, Kanemaki Y, Okamoto S, Nakajima Y (2018) Comparison of detectability of breast cancer by abbreviated breast MRI based on diffusion-weighted images and postcontrast MRI. Jpn J Radiol 36:331–339

Yılmaz E, Sarı O, Yılmaz A et al (2018) Diffusion-weighted imaging for the discrimination of benign and malignant breast masses; utility of ADC and relative ADC. J Belg Soc Radiol 102:24

Zhang L, Tang M, Min Z (2016) Accuracy of combined dynamic contrast-enhanced magnetic resonance imaging and diffusion-weighted imaging for breast cancer detection: a meta-analysis. Acta Radiol 57:651–660

Abbreviated Breast MRI: Short and Sweet?

Michelle Zhang, Victoria L. Mango, and Elizabeth Morris

Contents

1   **Introduction** 216

2   **Abbreviated Breast MRI** 216
    2.1   How? 216
    2.2   Why? 219
    2.3   Who? 222
    2.4   What? 222
    2.5   Limitations 224
    2.6   Future Directions 226

3   **Conclusion** 227

References 228

Abstract

Abbreviated breast magnetic resonance imaging (MRI) is a novel emerging tool for breast cancer screening. This chapter explores the commonly used abbreviated breast MRI protocols, its differences with conventional currently more widely used diagnostic breast MRI, its advantages over the current screening tools, the desired target screening population, its limitations and disadvantages, and its future directions. Abbreviated breast MRI is a potential game changer for the future of breast cancer screening, with comparable test performances as the standard conventional diagnostic MRI with high sensitivity for breast cancer detection; however, it is not without challenges (such as cost, gadolinium contrast injection, and accessibility). Its differences with the conventional diagnostic MRI, such as decreased scanning and radiologist interpretation time, make it much more attractive as a screening tool for a larger patient population.

M. Zhang (✉)
Department of Radiology, McGill University Health Center, Montreal, QC, Canada
e-mail: michelle.zhang@mail.mcgill.ca

V. L. Mango
Department of Radiology, Memorial Sloan Kettering Cancer Center, New York, NY, USA
e-mail: Mangov@mskcc.org

E. Morris
Department of Radiology, UC Davis Health, Sacramento, CA, USA
e-mail: eamorris@ucdavis.edu

© Springer Nature Switzerland AG 2022
M. Fuchsjäger et al. (eds.), *Breast Imaging*, Medical Radiology Diagnostic Imaging,
https://doi.org/10.1007/978-3-030-94918-1_10

1 Introduction

Breast magnetic resonance imaging (MRI) is currently the most sensitive imaging tool for breast cancer detection (DeMartini and Lehman 2008; DeMartini et al. 2008; Zakhireh et al. 2008). Though mammography is the standard of care for breast cancer screening in most countries, MRI demonstrates comparatively better sensitivity, especially in women with dense breast tissue and those at higher risk for breast cancer (Morrow et al. 2011; Melnikow et al. 2016; Warner et al. 2008). In fact, supplemental MRI after a normal mammogram reportedly detects an additional 3.5–26.8 breast cancers per 1000 examinations (Melnikow et al. 2016). Although MRI is an attractive alternative, using it as a routine widespread screening tool is limited by higher cost, relatively long scan times, and higher false-positive rates.

The role of MRI as a screening tool has significantly increased over the past decade. The current guidelines from the American Cancer Society recommend annual MRI screening for high-risk women such as those with BRCA mutations, lifetime breast cancer risk of more than 20%, certain genetic mutation carriers (i.e., Li-Fraumeni and Cowden syndromes), and prior chest radiation between the ages of 10 and 30 years (Saslow et al. 2007). Similar guidelines have also been adopted by other organizations such as the American College of Radiology, the Society of Breast Imaging, and the European Society of Breast Imaging (Lee et al. 2010; Mainiero et al. 2016; Mann et al. 2008).

Currently, regular diagnostic breast MRI takes approximately 20–40 min of scan time, and the routine protocol generates thousands of images for interpretation. These limitations can be addressed by an abbreviated MRI protocol, more tailored towards screening purposes, which is gaining popularity within the breast imaging community.

2 Abbreviated Breast MRI

2.1 How?

Multiple abbreviated MRI protocols have been proposed, and the fundamental backbone sequence of these protocols is the dynamic contrast-enhanced (DCE) sequence (Chhor and Mercado 2017). The DCE sequence is the optimal sequence to provide both morphology and contrast uptake characteristics, which are essential to differentiate between malignant and benign lesions (Szabo et al. 2003; Kinkel et al. 2000; Kuhl et al. 1999a) (Figs. 1 and 2). In order to assess lesion enhancement characteristics, the minimally required sequences include an unenhanced T1-weighted sequence and a contrast-enhanced T1-weighted sequence (obtained usually 80–100 s after gadolinium injection) without fat saturation (Chhor and Mercado 2017) (Fig. 3a, b). Using these fundamental sequences, subtraction and maximum-intensity projection (MIP) images can then be generated to improve diagnostic yield without increasing scan time (Fig. 3c, d).

Additional proposed sequences include T2-weighted images (such as short tau inversion recovery (STIR)) and more delayed DCE images (obtained 3 min after gadolinium injection) (Moschetta et al. 2016; Heacock et al. 2016) (Figs. 4 and 5). The rationale to include T2-weighted sequences is to acquire additional morphological information beyond margins and enhancement pattern obtained from DCE images. Circumscribed lesions with high T2 signal intensity are more likely to be a benign lesion such as fibroadenoma, and the additional T2 sequences could also increase lesion conspicuity (Heacock et al. 2016; Santamaria et al. 2010; Kuhl et al. 1999b) (Figs. 2 and 6). However, this significantly increases the total scan time. For example, the abbreviated protocols proposed by Kuhl et al. and Harvey et al. (which do not include T2-weighted sequences) average 3 min and 4.4 min to acquire, respectively, in contrast with the protocols by Grimm et al. and Moschetta et al. (which include at least one T2-weighted sequence), with average 11–13 min and 12 min, respectively, to acquire (Chhor and Mercado 2017; Moschetta et al. 2016; Grimm et al. 2015; Harvey et al. 2016; Kuhl et al. 2014). The usage of more delayed DCE images rather than the first was hypothesized to maximize assessment of the lesion's internal architecture and morphology characteristics (Kuhl et al. 1999a). However, Moschetta et al. utilized an abbreviated MRI protocol with

Fig. 1 Forty-seven-year-old female with right-breast biopsy-proven invasive ductal carcinoma. (**a**) MIP, (**b**) post-contrast T1, and (**c**) subtraction images showing right-breast irregularly enhancing mass. (**d**) Corresponding MLO mammogram does not easily show the mass, obscured by the heterogeneously dense breast tissue

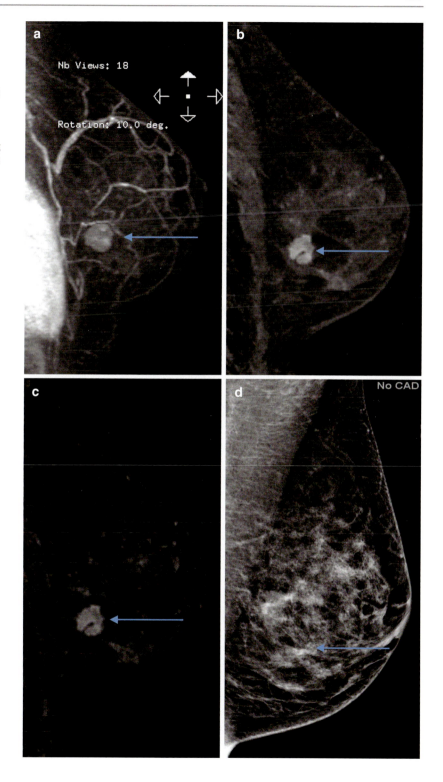

T2-weighted sequences and the third DCE images, but it did not yield better test performance with reported sensitivity of 89% and specificity of 91%, comparable to reported sensitivity of 96–100% and specificity of 94.3% by other authors using only first post-contrast DCE without T2 or more delayed DCE images (Moschetta et al. 2016).

Fig. 2 Left-breast intramammary lymph node. (**a**) MIP demonstrating a reniform-shaped mass in the upper outer quadrant adjacent to a coursing vessel, consistent with an intramammary lymph node. (**b**) STIR sequence demonstrating the lesion to be very T2 bright, more suggestive of a benign etiology, (**c**) T1 post-contrast and (**d**) subtraction image demonstrating the intramammary lymph node

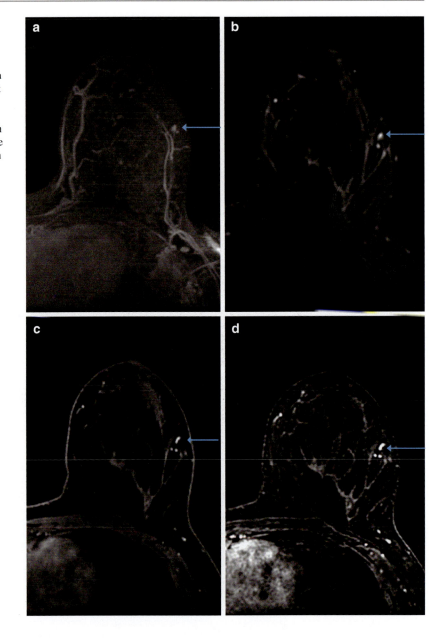

In addition, an abbreviated protocol with only interpretation of the post-contrast MIP images has also been proposed (Kuhl et al. 2014; Mango et al. 2015). The MIP image is the projection of the voxel with the highest signal throughout a 3D volume onto a 2D image (Cody 2002) (Fig. 7). It gives a good overview of the enhancement of the whole breast, yielding an image similar to a 2D mammogram but without lesion obscuration by the overlapping fibroglandular tissue.

By comparison, the standard full diagnostic breast MRI protocol, though variable by institutional practices, routinely includes a water-sensitive sequence (T2/STIR), multiple DCE sequences at different times following contrast bolus injection, multiplanar post-contrast acqui-

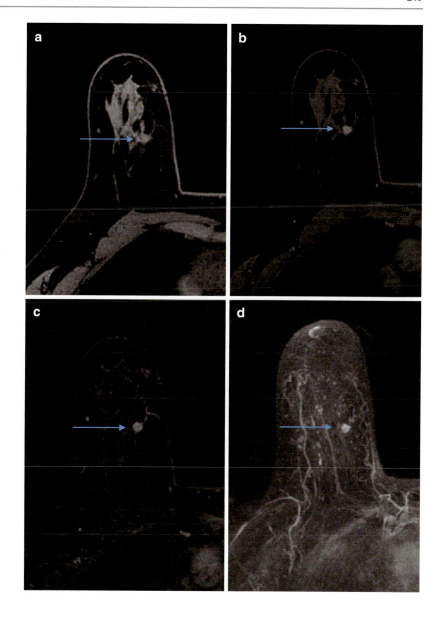

Fig. 3 Forty-seven-year-old female with right-breast biopsy-proven invasive ductal carcinoma. (**a**) Pre-contrast T1 image where the mass is not easily distinguishable from fibroglandular tissue without contrast. (**b**) Post-contrast DCE image easily demonstrating the enhancing irregularly shaped mass, biopsy proven to be cancer. (**c**) Subtraction image demonstrating increased conspicuity of the lesion. (**d**) MIP image demonstrating the malignant mass

sitions, and a pre-contrast T1 sequence (Chhor and Mercado 2017). The abbreviated MRI protocol puts emphasis on the DCE sequences, which are usually acquired only in one plane to shorten scanning time (Moschetta et al. 2016; Heacock et al. 2016; Grimm et al. 2015; Harvey et al. 2016; Kuhl et al. 2014; Mango et al. 2015). Given that abbreviated MRI sequences are the same as the ones used in the diagnostic routine protocols, the abbreviated protocol could be performed on any MRI scanner that is already currently being used for breast MRI, without the need for any additional software or hardware upgrade.

2.2 Why?

Abbreviated breast MRI addresses many of the limitations of breast MRI when used as a screening rather than a supplementary tool. The main

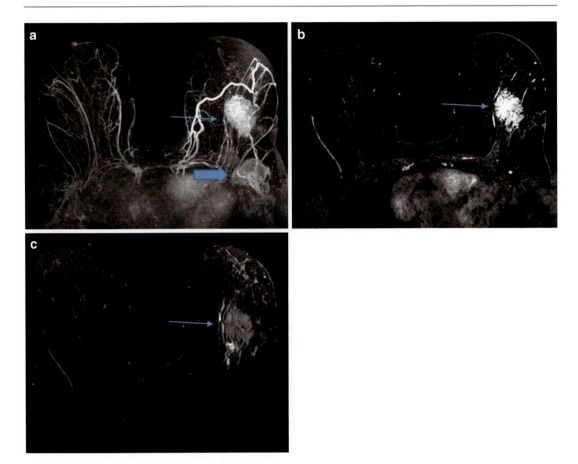

Fig. 4 Sixty-three-year-old female with left-breast biopsy-proven invasive ductal carcinoma and left axillary metastasis. (**a**) MIP and (**b**) post-contrast T1 images demonstrating left breast cancer (thin arrow) with left axillary metastatic adenopathy (thick arrow). (**c**) STIR image showing T2 intermediate signal of the tumor (in contrast with the T2 bright signal of the enhancing benign lesions in Figs. 2 and 5)

advantage is the reduced scan time. The average scan time for full diagnostic protocol ranges from 20 to 40 min, which can be reduced to 3–15 min for the abbreviated protocol (Chhor and Mercado 2017). Given that MRI may be less well tolerated by the patient, reduced time is highly important to consider given WHO criteria that screening tests be acceptable to the population (World Health Organization 2017). Reduced time increases the number of patients that could potentially be scanned and increases patient acceptance of a regularly occurring test (e.g., decreased test time and decreased discomfort). In the USA, 65% of all women over 40 years old reported having had a mammogram in the last 2 years (Huzarski et al. 2017). For MRI to be potentially offered to such a potential large target population, scan times of 3 min could be an acceptable alternative to the current usage of screening mammography. However, the need for intravenous contrast injection in both the full and abbreviated protocols may limit patients' acceptance of the exam.

Not only does the protocol take less time to acquire, but abbreviated MRI is also faster to interpret. Kuhl et al. reported abbreviated protocol average reading time of 28 s, and merely 3 s for the MIP-only protocol (Kuhl et al. 2014). The MIP-only image is also very similar to reading a mammogram and eliminates the need to scroll through multiple sets of images which can be time consuming (Fig. 8). These findings are corroborated by other similar studies by Harvey et al. and Moschetta et al., who found reading

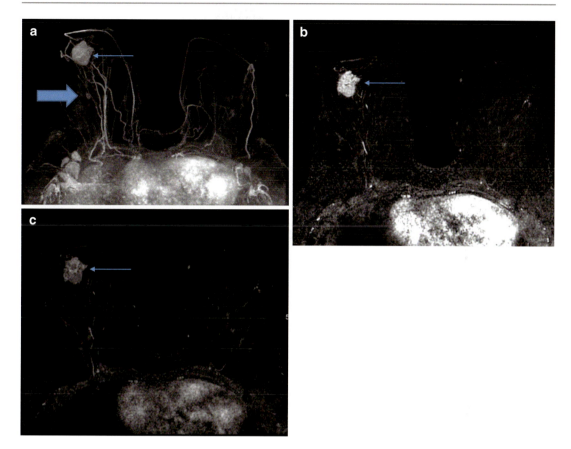

Fig. 5 Forty-year-old women with right-breast biopsy-proven invasive ductal carcinoma and fibroadenoma. (**a**) MIP image showing right-breast anterior cancer (thin arrow) and posterior fibroadenoma (thick arrow). (**b**) First post-contrast subtraction T1 image showing heterogeneously enhancing irregularly shaped cancer. (**c**) Third post-contrast subtraction T1 image showing tumor enhancement washout (3 min post-contrast injection)

times of 360–385 s for the full diagnostic protocol reduced to 93–120 s for the abbreviated protocol (Moschetta et al. 2016; Harvey et al. 2016). However, one study by Grimm et al. showed no substantial difference in reading times when comparing the full to the abbreviated protocol (Grimm et al. 2015). Possible explanations for this discrepancy may be that the additional sequences in the full diagnostic protocol (non fat-saturated T1 and additional post-contrast images) are not routinely relied upon and the radiologists took longer to look at the abbreviated images because of the unfamiliarity and the lack of other confirmatory sequences.

It is worth noting however that most of the current literature on abbreviated breast MRI involves interpretation by experienced fellowship-trained breast radiologists, and thus the reported test performance may not be transferable to community-based general radiologists (Moschetta et al. 2016; Heacock et al. 2016; Kuhl et al. 1999b; Grimm et al. 2015; Harvey et al. 2016; Mango et al. 2015). In addition, the amount of time saved interpreting an abbreviated protocol may not be as significant among radiologists less familiar with abbreviated MRIs. There may be a learning curve for radiologists comparable to that experienced by radiologists during the initial institution of widespread digital mammography screening.

Reduced scanner time and radiologist interpretation time could also translate into reduced exam costs and overall improved cost-effectiveness, an important consideration for widespread availability of any screening test.

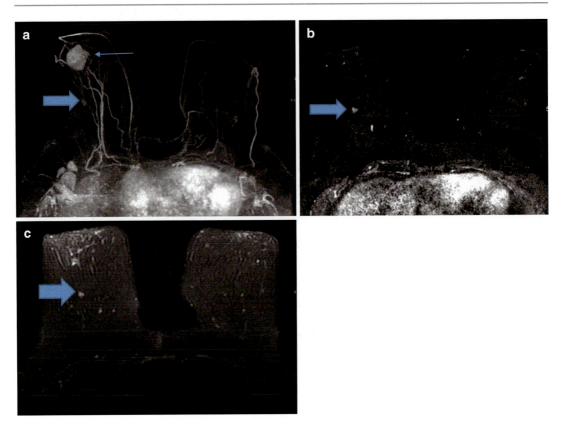

Fig. 6 Same patient as in Fig. 5. (**a**) MIP and (**b**) T1 post-contrast subtraction image demonstrating anterior invasive ductal carcinoma (thin arrow) and posterior fibroadenoma (thick arrow). (**c**) STIR image showing T2 bright signal of the benign lesion (in contrast to the T2 intermediate signal of the malignant lesion seen in Fig. 4)

2.3 Who?

Though the current guidelines by multiple organizations and societies recommend screening MRI in only high-risk patients, there remains a growing need for better cancer detection in patients who are at intermediate risk and those with high breast density (Melnikow et al. 2016; Huzarski et al. 2017; Berg et al. 2012) (Figs. 7 and 9). With the recent advent of the "breast density laws" in the USA, the physician is required to notify the patient of "dense breasts" (ACR BIRADS category C/D of heterogeneously dense or extremely dense breasts), leading to consideration of the need for supplemental screening by both physicians and patients (Freer et al. 2015; D'Orsi et al. 2013). Currently, there is no consensus on which supplemental screening modalities to utilize in these patients based on breast density, but abbreviated MRI, could be an attractive option. Higher breast density is associated with a higher risk of breast cancer, and mammographically occult cancers can be obscured by high breast density and instead be detected on MRI (Boyd et al. 2010; McCormack and dos Santos 2006; Chen et al. 2017) (Fig. 7). MRI is currently the most sensitive tool, and studies have suggested that this higher sensitivity persists even in patients with higher breast density (Melnikow et al. 2016; Riedl et al. 2015).

2.4 What?

Cancer detection rate and test accuracy are not significantly different between the full diagnostic and the abbreviated protocols. Abbreviated MRI has a reported sensitivity of

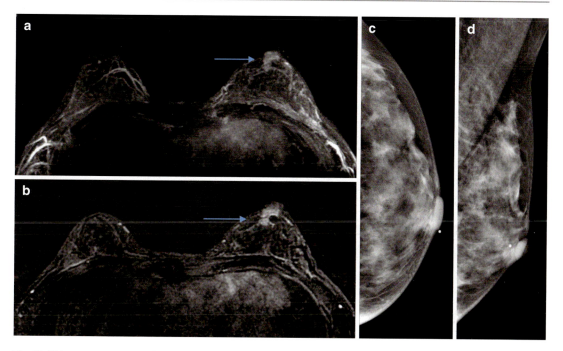

Fig. 7 Thirty-seven-year-old female with left retroareolar biopsy-proven invasive ductal carcinoma. (**a**) MIP and (**b**) T1 post-contrast subtraction images showing enhancing retroareolar cancer with internal susceptibility artifact from the biopsy marker. (**c**) Left-breast CC and (**d**) MLO views showing that the cancer is occult, hidden by the fibroglandular tissue

86–100% and specificity of 52–94% compared with full diagnostic MRI sensitivity (in the same studies) of 92–100% and 52–94% (Chhor and Mercado 2017). Studies on abbreviated MRI included both those for screening purposes and those with biopsy-proven carcinoma (Chhor and Mercado 2017; Ko and Morris 2019; Leithner et al. 2019). Mango et al. demonstrated that all 100 out of 100 biopsy-proven unicentric breast cancers were detected on abbreviated MRI protocol by at least one reader (Mango et al. 2015). Breast MRI is the most sensitive tool for breast cancer detection, outperforming conventional mammography, tomosynthesis, and ultrasound, and its higher sensitivity and higher breast cancer detection rates are conferred to abbreviated protocols. In fact, abbreviated MRI protocol had demonstrated very similar BI-RADS assessments as compared to standard full MRI protocol, with only differences in BI-RADS reporting in a small number (3.4%) of cases (Panigrahi et al. 2017). Additionally, a recent study by Weinstein et al. demonstrated that abbreviated breast MRI increased breast cancer detection rate by 27.4/1000 patients in women with dense breast after negative screening tomosynthesis (Weinstein et al. 2020).

In terms of the most useful sequences, the first post-contrast DCE sequence carried a sensitivity of 96–100% and specificity of 94%, without significant difference when comparing non-subtracted to subtracted DCE images (Kuhl et al. 1999b; Mango et al. 2015). The addition of a second post-contrast DCE sequence also did not improve the test performance (Grimm et al. 2015). When looking at an even more abbreviated MIP-only image, both the sensitivity and specificity slightly dropped, yielding 91–93% and 99.7%, respectively (Kuhl et al. 2014; Mango et al. 2015) (Fig. 10). The addition of a T2-weighted sequence also did not affect cancer detection rate, but increased lesion conspicuity (Moschetta et al. 2016; Heacock et al. 2016).

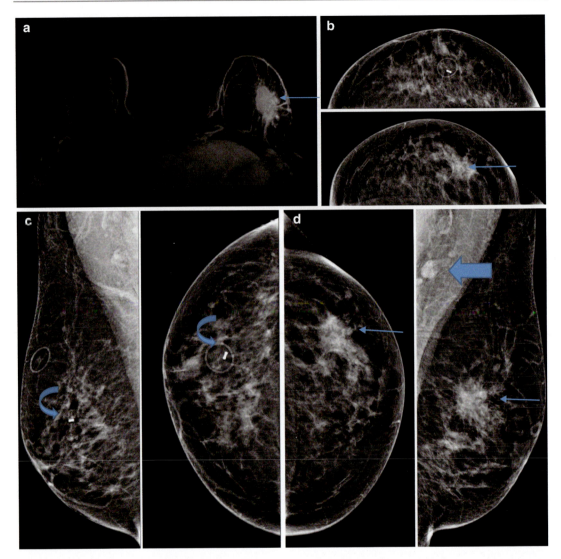

Fig. 8 Sixty-year-old female with left-breast invasive ductal carcinoma (thin arrow) and left axillary metastatic adenopathy (thick arrow). (**a**) MRI MIP is similar to reading (**b**) the mammographic CC views displayed in a similar orientation to the MIP image. (**c**) MLO and CC mammographic views of the right and (**d**) left breast in the same patient for comparison demonstrating a high-density spiculated mass in the left upper outer quadrant corresponding to the cancer. There is an incidental right-breast biopsy marker from a remote benign biopsy (curved arrow)

2.5 Limitations

The abbreviated MRI protocol's negative predictive value (98.0–100%) and positive predictive value (24.4–64%) are not significantly different from those of the full diagnostic protocol (Kuhl et al. 1999b; Mango et al. 2015). However, one of the main objections for widespread use of breast MRI is its high rate of false-positive results, which leads to additional imaging and biopsies and remains a problem for abbreviated MRIs with low positive predictive value (Morrow et al. 2011; Kuhl et al. 2014; Mango et al. 2015). By omitting additional post-contrast sequences in the abbreviated protocol as compared to the multiple post-contrast sequences on the conventional

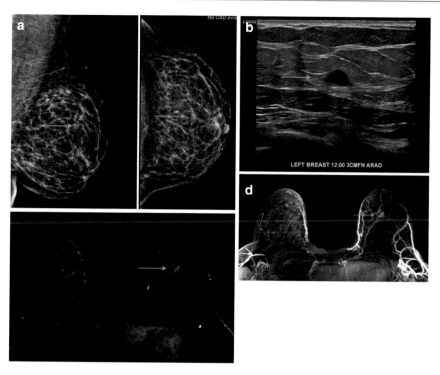

Fig. 9 Thirty-three-year-old female with first-degree family history of breast cancer and biopsy-proven triple-negative left-breast cancer. (**a**) MLO and CC views demonstrate a 12:00 well-circumscribed low-density oval mass (benign features), and (**b**) corresponding US demonstrates what was initially thought to represent a benign complicated cyst. (**c**) However, T1 post-contrast subtraction and (**d**) MIP images demonstrate a slightly irregularly shaped enhancing, which does not fit with a complicated benign cyst. This mass was then investigated further after the MRI and biopsied, yielding triple-negative breast cancer

MRI, there may be improvement of the positive predictive value, as seen in a study by Weinstein et al. (2020). This could be attributed to the fact that cancers tend to enhance early (seen in the first post-contrast sequence) and some benign lesions may be omitted on the abbreviated protocol as they enhance progressively and are usually seen on later sequences. This however requires further investigation and validation. In addition, known limitations of the full MRI protocol are also seen with abbreviated MRI protocols such as the possibility of missing non-enhancing DCIS, easily seen on mammogram as calcifications, but occult on MRI (Bazzocchi et al. 2006) (Fig. 11). However, cancers missed by MRI are usually less aggressive (Ko and Morris 2019).

The feasibility of offering an MRI screening program to a larger population may also be difficult to achieve in regions with less available resources and less access to MRI. Though abbreviated MRI is potentially less costly than a full MRI protocol, it is still currently more expensive than a routine mammogram. Further cost-benefit analysis taking into account lives and years saved secondary to increased cancer detection rate of MRI as compared to mammogram would be useful to help elucidate the best role for its future use. At this time, most of the published prospective MRI screening trials are performed using diagnostic MRI protocols and not abbreviated protocols, which may be more suited for screening purposes, and more research in this area is underway (Panigrahi et al. 2017; Strahle et al. 2017).

Furthermore, MRI screening, whether abbreviated or full protocol, requires the administration of gadolinium contrast agent. Gadolinium carries the risk of nephrogenic systemic fibrosis in those with severe renal dysfunction, though the risk is minimal (ACR Committee on Drugs and

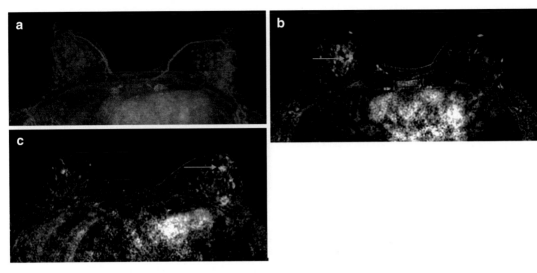

Fig. 10 Fifty-four-year-old female with bilateral biopsy-proven invasive ductal carcinoma, with false-negative MIP and detectable only on the diagnostic MRI images. (**a**) The bilateral breast cancers do not stand out on the MIP image due to marked background parenchymal enhancement. (**b**) However, the diagnostic T1 post-contrast subtraction images demonstrate right (thin arrow) and (**c**) left (thick arrow) subcentimeter irregularly shaped masses, subsequently biopsied, yielding bilateral breast cancer

Contrast Media 2016). By the same token, screening of patients for renal disease and additional testing for renal function may be an additional burden and cost to the health-care system. The recently discovered association of gadolinium deposition in neuronal tissue after repeated exposures, even in the setting of normal renal function, may also give reason for concern (McDonald et al. 2015; Stojanov et al. 2016a). However currently, this finding is not associated with any reported clinical symptoms or adverse health effects though its significance still remains unclear (Stojanov et al. 2016b). Given that the abbreviated breast MRI could potentially be performed annually for breast cancer screening, the effects of long-term regular gadolinium exposure should be an important consideration, especially since the target population includes mostly healthy individuals.

2.6 Future Directions

New and ultrafast sequences such as time-resolved angiography with stochastic trajectory (TWIST) sequence used by Mann et al. can allow optimal evaluation of the initial uptake kinetic curve for differentiating between benign and malignant lesions (Mann et al. 2014). This could potentially help improve breast MRI positive predictive value and false-positive rates while at the same time reducing scanning time as the delayed post-contrast sequences may no longer be needed (Mann et al. 2014; Platel et al. 2014).

In addition, breast MRI protocols without contrast, using T1 GRE, T2 STIR, and echo-planar DWI sequences, have also been investigated, showing cancer detection sensitivity of 76–78% and specificity of 90% (Trimboli et al. 2014) (Fig. 12). This could also be a promising future direction, given the attractiveness of a non-contrast scan, removing the potential gadolinium-associated risks.

Multiple studies are underway to better define the role of screening MRI. The recently published prospective ECOG-ACRIN EA1141 trial led by Comstock et al. comparing abbreviated breast MRI with digital tomosynthesis in screening women with dense breasts demonstrated an increased cancer detection rate with abbreviated MRI protocol with better sensitivity and specificity (U.S. National Institutes of

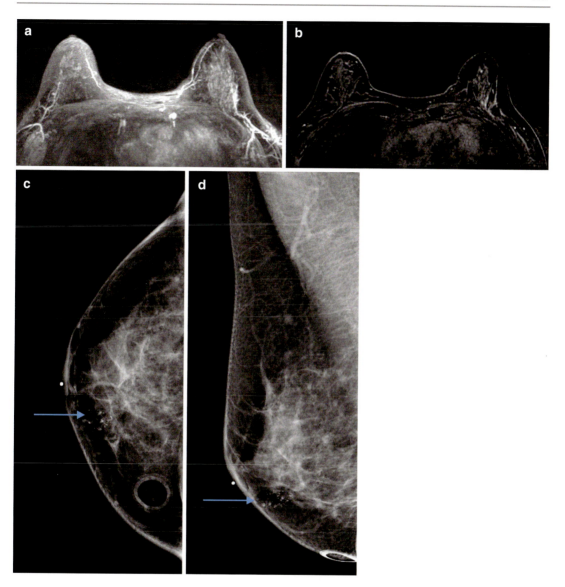

Fig. 11 Forty-five-year-old female with right-breast biopsy-proven DCIS seen as calcifications on mammograms but occult on MRI. (**a**) MIP and (**b**) T1 post-contrast subtraction images do not show abnormality other than moderate background enhancement. (**c**) However, there are fine pleomorphic suspicious calcifications on the CC and (**d**) MLO views, biopsied under stereotactic guidance to be intermediate- to high-grade DCIS

Health 2017; Comstock et al. 2020). Another ongoing prospective multicenter trial using abbreviated MRI is also underway in Korea to evaluate the breast cancer detection rate in high-risk women with a history of breast cancer who underwent BRCA mutation testing (but showing uninformative negative result or a variant of unknown significance) by comparing abbreviated MRI or ultrasound in addition to digital annual mammogram (US National Library of Medicine 2020).

3 Conclusion

Abbreviated MRI has similar test performance as the standard breast MRI full protocol, with less scanner time and reduced interpretation time. The

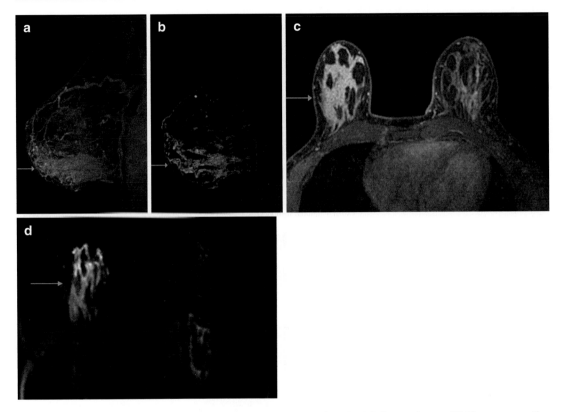

Fig. 12 Patient with biopsy-proven right inferior breast invasive lobular carcinoma. (**a**) MIP, (**b**) sagittal T1 post-contrast subtraction, (**c**) and axial T1 post-contrast images demonstrate extensive non-mass enhancement in the inferior right breast, corresponding to the site of biopsy-proven invasive lobular carcinoma. (**d**) The corresponding DWI image shows increased signal intensity at the site of tumor. But also note that the DWI image is prone to motion artifacts that are not seen on the other sequences

backbone of the abbreviated protocol includes the first post-contrast DCE and MIP sequences. This could be an attractive potential screening tool, especially in patients with intermediate risk and those with dense breasts, and has been described in the radiology literature as a "wave of the future for breast cancer screening" (Chhor and Mercado 2017). Current ongoing prospective trials will hopefully provide guidance on how best to incorporate supplemental screening modalities into routine clinical practice to best benefit patient care.

References

ACR Committee on Drugs and Contrast Media (2016) ACR manual on contrast media. Version 10.2

Bazzocchi M, Zuiani C, Panizza P, Del Frate C, Soldano F, Isola M et al (2006) Contrast-enhanced breast MRI in patients with suspicious microcalcifications on mammography: results of a multicenter trial. AJR Am J Roentgenol 186(6):1723–1732

Berg WA, Zhang Z, Lehrer D, Jong RA, Pisano ED, Barr RG et al (2012) Detection of breast cancer with addition of annual screening ultrasound or a single screening MRI to mammography in women with elevated breast cancer risk. JAMA 307(13):1394–1404

Boyd NF, Martin LJ, Bronskill M, Yaffe MJ, Duric N, Minkin S (2010) Breast tissue composition and susceptibility to breast cancer. J Natl Cancer Inst 102(16):1224–1237

Chen SQ, Huang M, Shen YY, Liu CL, Xu CX (2017) Abbreviated MRI protocols for detecting breast cancer in women with dense breasts. Korean J Radiol 18(3):470–475

Chhor CM, Mercado CL (2017) Abbreviated MRI protocols: wave of the future for breast cancer screening. AJR Am J Roentgenol 208(2):284–289

Cody DD (2002) AAPM/RSNA physics tutorial for residents: topics in CT. Image processing in CT. Radiographics 22(5):1255–1268

Comstock CE, Gatsonis C, Newstead GM, Snyder BS, Gareen IF, Bergin JT et al (2020) Comparison of abbreviated breast MRI vs digital breast tomosynthesis for breast cancer detection among women with dense breasts undergoing screening. JAMA 323(8):746–756

D'Orsi CJ, Sickles EA, Mendelson EB, Morris EA et al (2013) ACR BI-RADS® Atlas, breast imaging reporting and data system. American College of Radiology, Reston, VA

DeMartini W, Lehman C (2008) A review of current evidence-based clinical applications for breast magnetic resonance imaging. Top Magn Reson Imaging 19(3):143–150

DeMartini W, Lehman C, Partridge S (2008) Breast MRI for cancer detection and characterization: a review of evidence-based clinical applications. Acad Radiol 15(4):408–416

Freer PE, Slanetz PJ, Haas JS, Tung NM, Hughes KS, Armstrong K et al (2015) Breast cancer screening in the era of density notification legislation: summary of 2014 Massachusetts experience and suggestion of an evidence-based management algorithm by multidisciplinary expert panel. Breast Cancer Res Treat 153(2):455–464

Grimm LJ, Soo MS, Yoon S, Kim C, Ghate SV, Johnson KS (2015) Abbreviated screening protocol for breast MRI: a feasibility study. Acad Radiol 22(9):1157–1162

Harvey SC, Di Carlo PA, Lee B, Obadina E, Sippo D, Mullen L (2016) An abbreviated protocol for high-risk screening breast MRI saves time and resources. J Am Coll Radiol 13(11s):R74–R80

Heacock L, Melsaether AN, Heller SL, Gao Y, Pysarenko KM, Babb JS et al (2016) Evaluation of a known breast cancer using an abbreviated breast MRI protocol: correlation of imaging characteristics and pathology with lesion detection and conspicuity. Eur J Radiol 85(4):815–823

Huzarski T, Gorecka-Szyld B, Huzarska J, Psut-Muszynska G, Wilk G, Sibilski R et al (2017) Screening with magnetic resonance imaging, mammography and ultrasound in women at average and intermediate risk of breast cancer. Hered Cancer Clin Pract 15:4

Kinkel K, Helbich TH, Esserman LJ, Barclay J, Schwerin EH, Sickles EA et al (2000) Dynamic high-spatial-resolution MR imaging of suspicious breast lesions: diagnostic criteria and interobserver variability. AJR Am J Roentgenol 175(1):35–43

Ko ES, Morris EA (2019) Abbreviated magnetic resonance imaging for breast cancer screening: concept, early results, and considerations. Korean J Radiol 20(4):533–541

Kuhl CK, Mielcareck P, Klaschik S, Leutner C, Wardelmann E, Gieseke J et al (1999a) Dynamic breast MR imaging: are signal intensity time course data useful for differential diagnosis of enhancing lesions? Radiology 211(1):101–110

Kuhl CK, Klaschik S, Mielcarek P, Gieseke J, Wardelmann E, Schild HH (1999b) Do T2-weighted pulse sequences help with the differential diagnosis of enhancing lesions in dynamic breast MRI? J Magn Reson Imaging 9(2):187–196

Kuhl CK, Schrading S, Strobel K, Schild HH, Hilgers RD, Bieling HB (2014) Abbreviated breast magnetic resonance imaging (MRI): first postcontrast subtracted images and maximum-intensity projection-a novel approach to breast cancer screening with MRI. J Clin Oncol 32(22):2304–2310

Lee CH, Dershaw DD, Kopans D, Evans P, Monsees B, Monticciolo D et al (2010) Breast cancer screening with imaging: recommendations from the Society of Breast Imaging and the ACR on the use of mammography, breast MRI, breast ultrasound, and other technologies for the detection of clinically occult breast cancer. J Am Coll Radiol 7(1):18–27

Leithner D, Moy L, Morris EA, Marino MA, Helbich TH, Pinker K (2019) Abbreviated MRI of the breast: does it provide value? J Magn Reson Imaging 49(7): e85–e100

Mainiero MB, Lourenco A, Mahoney MC, Newell MS, Bailey L, Barke LD et al (2016) ACR appropriateness criteria breast cancer screening. J Am Coll Radiol 13(11s):R45–R49

Mango VL, Morris EA, David Dershaw D, Abramson A, Fry C, Moskowitz CS et al (2015) Abbreviated protocol for breast MRI: are multiple sequences needed for cancer detection? Eur J Radiol 84(1):65–70

Mann RM, Kuhl CK, Kinkel K, Boetes C (2008) Breast MRI: guidelines from the European Society of Breast Imaging. Eur Radiol 18(7):1307–1318

Mann RM, Mus RD, van Zelst J, Geppert C, Karssemeijer N, Platel B (2014) A novel approach to contrast-enhanced breast magnetic resonance imaging for screening: high-resolution ultrafast dynamic imaging. Invest Radiol 49(9):579–585

McCormack VA, dos Santos Silva I (2006) Breast density and parenchymal patterns as markers of breast cancer risk: a meta-analysis. Cancer Epidemiol Biomarkers Prev 15(6):1159–1169

McDonald RJ, McDonald JS, Kallmes DF, Jentoft ME, Murray DL, Thielen KR et al (2015) Intracranial gadolinium deposition after contrast-enhanced MR imaging. Radiology 275(3):772–782

Melnikow J, Fenton JJ, Whitlock EP, Miglioretti DL, Weyrich MS, Thompson JH et al (2016) Supplemental screening for breast cancer in women with dense breasts: a systematic review for the U.S. Preventive Services Task Force. Ann Intern Med 164(4):268–278

Morrow M, Waters J, Morris E (2011) MRI for breast cancer screening, diagnosis, and treatment. Lancet 378(9805):1804–1811

Moschetta M, Telegrafo M, Rella L, Stabile Ianora AA, Angelelli G (2016) Abbreviated combined MR protocol: a new faster strategy for characterizing breast lesions. Clin Breast Cancer 16(3):207–211

Panigrahi B, Mullen L, Falomo E, Panigrahi B, Harvey S (2017) An abbreviated protocol for high-risk screening breast magnetic resonance imaging: impact on performance metrics and BI-RADS assessment. Acad Radiol 24(9):1132–1138

Platel B, Mus R, Welte T, Karssemeijer N, Mann R (2014) Automated characterization of breast lesions imaged with an ultrafast DCE-MR protocol. IEEE Trans Med Imaging 33(2):225–232

Riedl CC, Luft N, Bernhart C, Weber M, Bernathova M, Tea MK et al (2015) Triple-modality screening trial for familial breast cancer underlines the importance of magnetic resonance imaging and questions the role of mammography and ultrasound regardless of patient mutation status, age, and breast density. J Clin Oncol 33(10):1128–1135

Santamaria G, Velasco M, Bargallo X, Caparros X, Farrus B, Luis Fernandez P (2010) Radiologic and pathologic findings in breast tumors with high signal intensity on T2-weighted MR images. Radiographics 30(2):533–548

Saslow D, Boetes C, Burke W, Harms S, Leach MO, Lehman CD et al (2007) American Cancer Society guidelines for breast screening with MRI as an adjunct to mammography. CA Cancer J Clin 57(2):75–89

Stojanov DA, Aracki-Trenkic A, Vojinovic S, Benedeto-Stojanov D, Ljubisavljevic S (2016a) Increasing signal intensity within the dentate nucleus and globus pallidus on unenhanced T1W magnetic resonance images in patients with relapsing-remitting multiple sclerosis: correlation with cumulative dose of a macrocyclic gadolinium-based contrast agent, gadobutrol. Eur Radiol 26(3):807–815

Stojanov D, Aracki-Trenkic A, Benedeto-Stojanov D (2016b) Gadolinium deposition within the dentate nucleus and globus pallidus after repeated administrations of gadolinium-based contrast agents-current status. Neuroradiology 58(5):433–441

Strahle DA, Pathak DR, Sierra A, Saha S, Strahle C, Devisetty K (2017) Systematic development of an abbreviated protocol for screening breast magnetic resonance imaging. Breast Cancer Res Treat 162(2):283–295

Szabo BK, Aspelin P, Wiberg MK, Bone B (2003) Dynamic MR imaging of the breast. Analysis of kinetic and morphologic diagnostic criteria. Acta Radiol 44(4):379–386

Trimboli RM, Verardi N, Cartia F, Carbonaro LA, Sardanelli F (2014) Breast cancer detection using double reading of unenhanced MRI including T1-weighted, T2-weighted STIR, and diffusion-weighted imaging: a proof of concept study. AJR Am J Roentgenol 203(3):674–681

U.S. National Institutes of Health (2017) Abbreviated breast MRI and digital tomosynthesis mammography in screening women with dense breasts. https://clinicaltrials.gov/ct2/show/NCT02933489

US National Library of Medicine (2020) Abbreviated breast MRI for second breast cancer detection in women with BRCA mutation testing. https://clinicaltrials.gov/ct2/show/NCT03475979

Warner E, Messersmith H, Causer P, Eisen A, Shumak R, Plewes D (2008) Systematic review: using magnetic resonance imaging to screen women at high risk for breast cancer. Ann Intern Med 148(9):671–679

Weinstein SP, Korhonen K, Cirelli C, Schnall MD, McDonald ES, Pantel AR et al (2020) Abbreviated breast magnetic resonance imaging for supplemental screening of women with dense breasts and average risk. J Clin Oncol 38(33):3874–3882

World Health Organization (2017) Screening for various cancers 2017. http://who.int/cancer/detection/variouscancer/en/

Zakhireh J, Gomez R, Esserman L (2008) Converting evidence to practice: a guide for the clinical application of MRI for the screening and management of breast cancer. Eur J Cancer 44(18):2742–2752

Breast MRI: Multiparametric and Advanced Techniques

Maria Adele Marino, Daly Avendano, Thomas Helbich, and Katja Pinker

Contents

1　Introduction 232

2　State of the Art of Breast MRI 232

3　Advanced Techniques 237
　3.1　Advanced DWI Approaches 237
　3.2　MR Spectroscopy 238
　3.3　Emerging Techniques 239

4　Screening MRI: Abbreviated MRI Protocols and Non-contrast mpMRI 243

5　Breast MRI Radiomics and Radiogenomics 244

6　Conclusions 249

References 249

M. A. Marino
Department of Biomedical Sciences and Morphologic and Functional Imaging, University of Messina, Messina, Italy

D. Avendano
School of medicine and health science, Tecnologico de Monterrey, Monterrey, México

T. Helbich
Division of Molecular and Gender Imaging, Department of Biomedical Imaging and Image-Guided Therapy, Medical University of Vienna, Vienna, Austria
e-mail: thomas.helbich@meduniwien.ac.at

K. Pinker (⊠)
Breast Imaging Service, Department of Radiology, Memorial Sloan Kettering Cancer Center, New York, NY, USA
e-mail: pinkerdk@mskcc.org

Abstract

Magnetic resonance imaging (MRI) is an essential tool in breast imaging with a high diagnostic accuracy for breast cancer diagnosis and several other established indications. The diagnostic value of breast MRI is based on its ability to provide not only morphological but also functional and metabolic information that can be used for both the detection and characterization of breast tumors. The combined application of different MRI parameters is defined as multiparametric MRI (mpMRI). There is conclusive data that mpMRI is superior to single-parametric MRI of the breast as it may simultaneously provide a multitude of

© Springer Nature Switzerland AG 2022
M. Fuchsjäger et al. (eds.), *Breast Imaging*, Medical Radiology Diagnostic Imaging,
https://doi.org/10.1007/978-3-030-94918-1_11

information, such as neo-angiogenesis, cellularity, tumor microenvironment, metabolite concentration, receptor status, tissue pH, and oxygenation, that can be used for an improved lesion evaluation. mpMRI can be performed at 1.5T, 3T, and event at 7T field strengths, although for research use only, using different combinations of MRI parameters. This review provides a comprehensive overview on the current clinical applications and emerging techniques of mpMRI of the breast. We will discuss the role of mpMRI for diagnosis, prognosis, response assessment, and screening of high-risk population and provide an outlook on the use of radiomics in this context.

1 Introduction

Breast cancer is the leading cause of cancer-related death among women worldwide, with variable incidence and mortality rates (Torre et al. 2016). Breast magnetic resonance imaging (MRI) is recognized as the most sensitive imaging method for the detection of breast cancer, especially those occult at conventional imaging (Riedl et al. 2015; Kuhl 2007a; Kuhl et al. 2006). Established recommendations for breast MRI are the evaluation of breast implants, preoperative staging, monitoring of neoadjuvant chemotherapy, differentiation between scar and recurrence, and patients with cancer of unknown primary origin (Mann et al. 2015; Sardanelli et al. 2010). Furthermore, its application in the screening setting for women at high (>20%) and intermediate lifetime (10–20%) risk has steadily increased in the past decade, facilitating earlier cancer detection and reducing interval cancers in this population (Leithner et al. 2018; Monticciolo et al. 2018).

The combination of multiple techniques, such as dynamic contrast-enhanced (DCE) MRI and T2-weighted and diffusion-weighted imaging (DWI) within the same examination, is called multiparametric MRI (mpMRI) and has been proven to increase the specificity of breast MRI

(Pinker et al. 2013, 2014a). Advanced functional techniques such as proton spectroscopy (MRS), sodium imaging (^{23}Na-MRI), phosphorus MRS (^{31}P MRS), chemical exchange saturation transfer (CEST) imaging, blood oxygen level-dependent (BOLD), and hyperpolarized MRI are currently being investigated for their clinical value and potential integration in multiparametric MRI protocols. Further, radiogenomics is an emerging area of research in breast imaging and is currently almost exclusively dominated by MRI (Grimm 2016).

This chapter provides a comprehensive overview of the current clinical applications and emerging techniques for mpMRI of the breast. We will discuss the role of mpMRI for diagnosis, prognosis, response assessment, and screening of high-risk population and provide an outlook of the use of radiomics in this context.

2 State of the Art of Breast MRI

Nowadays, a state-of-the-art breast MRI protocol is a comprehensive combination of different morphologic and functional MRI sequences, which is defined as multiparametric MRI (Kuhl et al. 2006; Baltzer et al. 2009, 2012; Marino et al. 2018a). In the clinical setting, a typical mpMRI protocol includes a three-place localizer sequence, a T2-weighted or short TI inversion recovery (STIR) sequence, a T1-weighted pre-contrast sequence, or three or more T1-weighted post-contrast sequences. Sequences are performed with or without fat saturation, while post-processing usually includes subtraction and maximum-intensity projection (MIP) images (Leithner et al. 2018).

Each individual MRI sequence contained in a mpMRI protocol interrogates different characteristics of breast tumor as detailed below, and with the combined information an improved diagnosis and characterization of breast tumors are facilitated.

- *DCE-MRI* is the most sensitive method for the detection of breast cancer, with a negative predictive value of up to 99% and a variable specificity, reported between 47% and 97% (Kuhl 2007a, b, c; Sardanelli et al. 2010; Helbich 2000; Pinker et al. 2009). Several studies have also demonstrated increased sensitivity and specificity in breast imaging at 3T (Pinker et al. 2009; Lourenco et al. 2014; Pinker-Domenig et al. 2012) and at ultrahigh field strength (Gruber et al. 2014), which can be translated into even higher temporal and spatial resolution imaging (van de Bank et al. 2013; Korteweg et al. 2011) or functional and metabolic imaging (Pinker et al. 2014a; Gruber et al. 2014; Klomp et al. 2011). DCE-MRI allows the simultaneous assessment of both tumor morphology and neo-angiogenesis, information that is necessary for the evaluation of breast lesions (Mann et al. 2015; Sardanelli et al. 2010; Spick et al. 2015; For the European Society of Breast Imaging (EUSOBI) et al. 2012; Kaiser et al. 2015a; Pinker et al. 2018a). The dynamic phases allow the assessment of different kinetic curves of a lesion (Rahbar and Partridge 2016): a slow, continuous enhancement curve (type I) is attributed to a benign lesion; a medium or strong enhancement followed by a plateau or persistent enhancement (type II) is indicative of either a benign or a malignant lesion; and a fast initial enhancement and washout (type III) are typically seen in malignancies, due to increased vascular permeability, density, and interstitial fluid (Helbich 2000) (Figs. 1 and 2). There is a considerable overlap of semiquantitative kinetic curve types among benign and malignant lesions since the rate of contrast agent uptake and washout depends on several factors, such as perfusion, capillary permeability, blood volume, contrast media distribution volume, and other aspects of local anatomy and physiology (Malich et al. 2005; Kaiser and Zeitler 1989; Kaiser 2007; Fischer et al. 2005; Berg et al. 2004; Kuhl et al. 1999). Quantitative evaluation of contrast enhancement kinetics through pharmacokinetic modeling enables the quantification of the contrast agent exchange between the intravascular and the interstitial space, providing measures of tumor blood flow, microvasculature, and capillary permeability. The Tofts two-compartment model (Tofts and Kermode 1991; Tofts et al. 1995) is the most commonly used approach and measures the exchange between the breast tissue plasma and the plasma space through different metrics such as Ktrans and Kep. Ktrans (min^{-1}) is the volume transfer constant and reflects the rate of transfer of contrast agent from the plasma to the tissue. Kep (min^{-1}) is

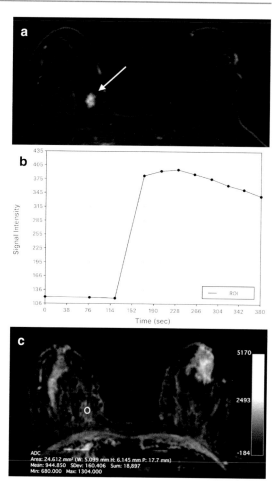

Fig. 1 Invasive ductal carcinoma G2 medially in the right breast in a 54-year-old woman: (**a**) DCE-MRI subtracted imaging shows an irregular mass with spiculated margins. The kinetic curve represented in (**b**) demonstrates a fast wash-in in the early phase with a rapid washout in the delayed phase. The malignant morphology and kinetic are corroborated by (**c**) decreased ADC values on DWI (0.944 × 10^{-3} mm^2/s). *DCE* dynamic contrast-enhanced, *MRI* magnetic resonance imaging, *DWI* diffusion-weighted imaging, *ADC* apparent diffusion coefficient

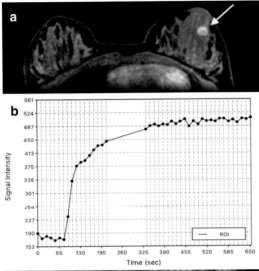

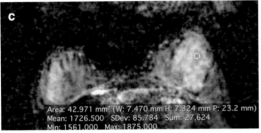

Fig. 2 Fibroadenoma in a 20-year-old woman in the retroareolar region of the left breast. (**a**) DCE-MRI shows the round circumscribed mass with (**b**) an initial moderate/persistent homogeneous contrast enhancement. (**c**) On DWI, the ADC values (1.762×10^{-3} mm^2/s) are above the threshold for malignancy, thus allowing an accurate classification as a benign finding. *DCE* dynamic contrast-enhanced, *MRI* magnetic resonance imaging, *DWI* diffusion-weighted imaging, *ADC* apparent diffusion coefficient

the transfer rate constant and reflects the reflux of contrast agent from the extravascular extracellular space to the plasma compartment. Different pharmacokinetic studies demonstrated that Ktrans and Kep have the potential to improve the discrimination of benign from malignant breast tumors and even between breast cancer subtypes. Huang et al. (2011) demonstrated that a potential cutoff could be used such that, in lesions with lower Ktrans values, biopsy could be obviated and thus false-positive MRI examinations could be decreased. Li et al. (2015) studied morphological and quantitative DCE-MRI for breast cancer diagnosis and found that Ktrans and Kep values were significantly higher in invasive ductal carcinoma and ductal carcinoma in situ (DCIS) than in borderline and benign lesions or healthy breast tissue. Pharmacokinetic MRI parameters have also been proven useful in patients who have undergone neoadjuvant chemotherapy for response assessment. Data from a recent meta-analysis from Marinovich et al. indicated that Ktrans is an early predictor of response and outperforms standard measures such as tumor size (Marinovich et al. 2013). Nevertheless, quantitative DCE-MRI with pharmacokinetic modeling remains challenging.

- *T2-weighted imaging* is usually performed as part of a standard full protocol because it increases the specificity of breast MRI, facilitating the recognition of important prognostic factors such as peritumoral edema (Uematsu 2015; Baltzer et al. 2011a; Kaiser et al. 2015b). Kaiser et al. (2017) demonstrated that the presence of peritumoral edema as a morphological sign in the T2-weighted images may be a strong prognostic indicator for lymphatic spread and cancerous infiltration of lymph nodes. It is also associated with the infiltration of the pectoral muscle, as well as high tumor grading. Furthermore, with the recent controversy about gadolinium-containing contrast agents and current recommendations to use gadolinium-based contrast agents only when essential diagnostic information cannot be obtained with unenhanced scans, there is an urgent need for non-contrast imaging methods for breast lesion detection and characterization. In this setting, T2-weighted imaging can serve as anatomic guidance for DWI (Baltzer et al. 2018).

- *DWI sequences with apparent diffusion coefficient (ADC)* mapping is an additional imaging biomarker and has shown diagnostic potential for an improved breast lesion characterization (Partridge et al. 2009; Kul et al. 2011) (Figs. 1 and 2). DWI provides additional functional information on tissue microstructure and cellularity that can be quantified by calculating the ADC values (Baltzer et al.

2009), thus providing valuable information for lesion characterization. In general, breast malignancies show lower ADC values compared with healthy breast tissue due to increased cell density in malignant tissue, which leads to compression of extracellular space and microstructural changes (Baltzer et al. 2009, 2010). Numerous studies investigated different ADC thresholds and b-values, with conflicting results (Marini et al. 2007; Thomassin-Naggara et al. 2013; Cho et al. 2015a). Bogner et al. (2009) found that a combined b-value protocol of 50 and 850 s/mm^2 yields a diagnostic accuracy of 96%, while in a recent meta-analysis including 26 studies, Dorrius et al. (2014) recommended the combination of $b = 0$ and 1000 s/mm^2 for the most accurate differentiation of benign and malignant lesions. Cutoff thresholds to rule out breast cancer have been proposed to potentially avoid unnecessary biopsy (Bogner et al. 2009, 2012; Tsushima et al. 2009; Costantini et al. 2010; Hatakenaka et al. 2008; Woodhams et al. 2005) and a threshold of 1300 for the ADC value is generally accepted now recommended in the consensus and mission statement by the European Society of Breast Imaging International DWI working group as the cutoff for the differentiation between benign (>1.4 × 10^{-3} mm^2/s) and malignant (<1.2 × 10^{-3} mm^2/s) breast lesions (Baltzer et al. 2020). DWI with ADC mapping can also be useful as a prognostic indicator. Martinicich et al. (2012) found that breast cancers characterized by high cellularity or a higher number of mitoses have lower ADC values. These results have been confirmed in triple-negative breast cancers, which are associated with higher ADC values compared with ER+ and HER2/neu-enriched tumors (Uematsu et al. 2009; Foulkes et al. 2010; Dogan et al. 2010; Kawashima 2011). In contrast, mucinous carcinoma usually presents ADC values similar to benign lesions, most likely due to the presence of both low cellularity and mucin-rich compartments (Woodhams et al. 2011). Bickel et al. evaluated the role of ADC with DWI at 3T for the differentiation of invasive breast cancer from DCIS, finding that ADC was a valuable tool for the assessment of breast cancer invasiveness (Bickel et al. 2015). DWI can also be used for monitoring the breast cancer response to treatment since ADC values are very sensitive to changes in tumor cellularity and necrosis. The cytotoxic effect of anticancer drugs would translate into an increase in ADC values which usually occurs earlier than lesion size changes or vascularity (Padhani et al. 2009; Pickles et al. 2006). Park et al. (2010) studied the potential of DWI for the prediction of response to neoadjuvant chemotherapy in breast cancer patients. Patients with a low pretreatment ADC tended to respond better to chemotherapy, and a cutoff of 1.17 × 10^{-3} mm^2/s could differentiate responders from nonresponders with a sensitivity of 94% and a specificity of 71%. Richards et al. (2013) found that pretreatment tumor ADC values differed between intrinsic subtypes and were predictive of pathologic response in triple-negative tumors. However, an international consensus has not been reached for the assessment of pre-chemotherapy ADC, and more data are warranted (Pickles et al. 2006; Woodhams et al. 2010; Sharma et al. 2009a; Iacconi et al. 2010) (Fig. 3).

mpMRI is nowadays an integral part of the diagnostic workup of breast tumors, as it has been shown to facilitate a significant increase in diagnostic accuracy and enable improved treatment planning and a reduction in unnecessary invasive procedures (Polanec et al. 2016; Loffroy et al. 2015; Kim et al. 2014; Gondo et al. 2014; Turkbey et al. 2013; Neto and Parente 2013). The clinical application of *mpMRI* enables an increase in the specificity of DCE-MRI, with the potential of reducing false-positive rates and unnecessary MRI-guided biopsies (Baltzer et al. 2010; Spick et al. 2014; Pinker et al. 2014b). Pinker et al. (2013) developed a reading scheme that adapted ADC thresholds to the assigned BI-RADS® classification. In that study, the sensitivity of the BI-RADS®-adapted reading was not significantly different from the high sensitivity of DCE-MRI ($p = 0.4$), whereas the specificity of the

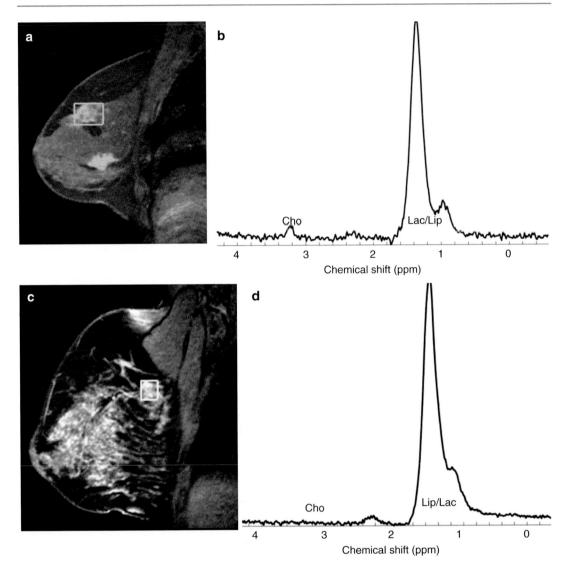

Fig. 3 Fibroadenoma and fibrocystic changes in a 40-year-old woman in the upper outer quadrant area of the right breast. (**a**) Sagittal fat-suppressed DCE-MRI shows the lesion within the MRS voxel of 1.1 cm^3 (white box). (**b**) PRESS spectrum (TR/TE = 2000/135 ms) shows no detectable Cho peak at 3.2 ppm. Multifocal invasive ductal carcinoma in a 56-year-old woman in the 9:00 and 12:00 axis of the right breast. (**c**) Sagittal fat-suppressed DCE-MRI shows the lesion within the MRS voxel of 9.4 cm^3 (white box). (**d**) PRESS spectrum (TR/TE = 2000/135 ms) shows a Cho peak at 3.2 ppm. *DCE* dynamic contrast-enhanced, *MRI* magnetic resonance imaging, *MRS* magnetic resonance spectroscopy, *Cho* choline, *Lac* lactate, *Lip* lipid

BI-RADS®-adapted reading was maximized to 89.4%, which was significantly higher compared with that of DCE-MRI ($p < 0.001$). The authors concluded that the BI-RADS®-adapted reading, which combined both DCE-MRI and DWI, improves diagnostic accuracy and is fast and easy to use in routine clinical practice. In a different approach, Baltzer et al. (2015) investigated the improvements in the specificity of breast MRI by integrating ADC values with DCE-MRI using a simple sum score. The additional integration of ADC scores achieved an improved specificity (92.4%) compared with DCE-MRI-only reading (specificity of 81.8%), with no false-negative results. Recently, the concept of multiparametric imaging has been extended to ultrahigh-field

MRI. mpMRI, combining high-resolution DCE-MRI and DWI at 7T, yielded a sensitivity and specificity of 100% and 88.2%, respectively, with an AUC of 0.941, which was significantly greater than that of DCE-MRI ($p = 0.003$) which had a sensitivity and specificity of 100% and 53.2%, respectively, with an AUC of 0.765, and greater than DWI, which had a sensitivity and specificity of 93.1% and 88.2%, respectively, with an AUC of 0.907 (Pinker et al. 2015). In that study, mpMRI of the breast at 7T accurately detected all cancers, reduced false positives from eight with DCE-MRI to two, and thus could have obviated unnecessary breast biopsies ($p = 0.031$).

3 Advanced Techniques

mpMRI allows the noninvasive visualization of different aspects of tumor biology and thus provides a deeper understanding of the hallmarks of cancer, which comprise sustaining proliferative signaling, evading growth suppressors, resisting cell death, enabling replicative immortality, inducing angiogenesis, and activating invasion and metastasis, on multiple levels (Hanahan and Weinberg 2000, 2011). New MRI parameters, such as advanced DWI approaches, proton MR spectroscopy, ^{23}Na MRI, ^{31}P MRS, ^{1}H-lipid MRS, CEST, BOLD, and hyperpolarized MRI, have been developed to further improve diagnosis, prognosis, and prediction of treatment response of breast tumors.

3.1 Advanced DWI Approaches

- *Intravoxel incoherent motion (IVIM)*: DWI is also sensitive to perfusion because the flow of blood in randomly oriented capillaries mimics a diffusion process through the IVIM effect (Le Bihan et al. 1988). Several studies have investigated IVIM in breast tumors, and preliminary data suggests that it can provide valuable information about both tissue microstructure and microvasculature that is beneficial for the diagnosis of breast cancer lesions (Cho et al. 2015b, c; Bokacheva et al. 2014; Iima et al. 2015; Liu et al. 2013).

- *Diffusion-weighted kurtosis (DKI)*: In living tissue, DWI is affected by Brownian incoherent motion and microperfusion or blood flow showing non-Gaussian phenomena (Jensen et al. 2005). The diffusion-weighted kurtosis (DKI) quantifies the deviation of tissue diffusion from a Gaussian pattern and has demonstrated a substantially higher sensitivity and specificity in cancer detection compared with ADC (Nogueira et al. 2014; Sun et al. 2015).

- *Diffusion tensor imaging (DTI)*: DTI is considered to be an extension of DWI, providing information about water motion in six or more directions and thus characterizing the motion of water (Baltzer et al. 2011b; Cakir et al. 2013) through two parameters: mean diffusivity (MD) and fractional anisotropy (FA). MD reflects the average anisotropy, whereas FA describes the degree of anisotropy (Cakir et al. 2013; Le Bihan et al. 2001). The diffusion of water molecules in the mammary glandular/ductal system is parallel to the walls of the ducts and lobules and leads to a restricted diffusion in the perpendicular directions, leading to an anisotropic diffusion (Eyal et al. 2012). Based on the histopathological data, most breast pathologies result in decreased structuring compared with healthy tissue. Therefore, any changes of this tissue structure by means of benign or malignant tumor growth should be reflected by changes in diffusion anisotropy detectable with DTI (Baltzer et al. 2011b; Cakir et al. 2013; Eyal et al. 2012). Partridge et al. (2010) investigated whether DTI measures of anisotropy in breast tumors are different from those in normal breast tissue and whether this could improve the discrimination between benign and malignant lesions. The authors demonstrated that diffusion anisotropy is significantly lower in breast cancers than in normal tissue, which may reflect alterations in tissue organization, but that it cannot reliably differentiate between benign and malignant lesions. Baltzer et al. (2011b) proved that DTI can visualize microanatomical differences between benign and malignant breast tumors, as well as normal breast parenchyma. However, FA did not have an incremental value compared with ADC. Although results for the diagnostic accuracy of FA are divergent (Partridge et al. 2009; Baltzer et al. 2011b; Cakir et al. 2013), it seems that DTI has the potential to serve not only as an adjunct method to DCE examination, but also as an alternative method when DCE imaging is contraindicated (Baltzer et al. 2011b; Eyal et al. 2012; Partridge et al. 2010).

3.2   MR Spectroscopy

- Proton magnetic resonance spectroscopy (^{1}H-MRS) is a noninvasive technique reflecting the chemical composition of a tissue by providing spatially localized signal spectra enabling the differentiation of various chemical compounds present in normal, benign, malignant, necrotic, or hypoxic region of interests (Marino et al. 2018a). Several studies have demonstrated that ^{1}H-MRS can improve diagnostic accuracy in breast cancer diagnosis based on the detection of choline (Cho) that is involved in cell membrane turnover (Rahbar and Partridge 2016; Baltzer and Dietzel 2013). However, in addition to Cho metabolites, water and other important lipids can be detected in breast lesions. Previous results in ex vivo human mammary tissue have reported that invasive ductal carcinomas contain a higher water/fat ratio compared with benign and normal tissue at 1.3 ppm (Sharma et al. 2009b; Thakur et al. 2006; Jagannathan et al. 1998). Several studies have explored the use of MRS at both 1.5 and 3T. The higher strength field offers approximately twice the signal-to-noise ratio (SNR) compared with a 1.5T system and allows metabolite peaks to be more widely separated. However, the number of required corrections for T1, T2, transmit, and receive efficiency to perform a quantitative spectroscopy analysis is increased at 3T (Vaughan et al. 2001; Hoult and Phil 2000; Bolan 2013). Moreover, from the clinical point of view although MRS at 3T is expected to perform better, no data in support of that have been found yet. In a recent systematic

review and meta-analysis, Baltzer and Dietzel (2013) examined 18 different studies with spectroscopic data acquired at both 1.5 and 3.0T field strength. The authors did not find any significant difference in diagnostic performance between the two systems. Therefore, both the currently available systems are suitable. Few studies have investigated the role of MRS at ultrahigh-field-strength scans (Korteweg et al. 2011; Klomp et al. 2011; Bolan et al. 2002, 2003, 2004; Haddadin et al. 2009). Korteweg et al. (2011) evaluated the feasibility of 7T breast MRI by determining the intrinsic sensitivity gain compared with 3T in healthy volunteers and explored the clinical application of 7T MRI in neoadjuvant chemotherapy patients. The authors found that more anatomic detail was depicted at 7T than at 3T, and in one case, a fat plane between the muscle and tumor was visible at 7T, but not at the clinically performed 3T examination, suggesting that there was no muscle invasion, which was confirmed by pathology. They therefore concluded that dedicated 7T breast MRI is technically feasible, can provide more SNR than at 3T, and has diagnostic potential. Several studies have demonstrated that ^{1}H-MRS can improve diagnostic accuracy in breast cancer diagnosis (Rahbar and Partridge 2016). In a recent meta-analysis of 19 studies, Baltzer and Dietzel (2013) evaluated the diagnostic performance and feasibility of ^{1}H-MRS for differentiating malignant from benign breast lesions. The pooled sensitivity and specificity of ^{1}H-MRS were 73% and 88%, respectively. ^{1}H-MRS seems to be limited in the diagnosis of early breast cancer and small breast tumors as well as in non-mass-enhancing lesions. Gruber et al. (2011) developed a high-spatial-resolution 3D ^{1}H-MRS protocol at 3T, designed to cover a large fraction of the breast in a clinically acceptable measurement time of 12–15 min with excellent data quality. In that study, with a Cho SNR threshold level of 2.6, 3D ^{1}H-MRS provided a sensitivity of 97% and a specificity of 84% in breast cancer diagnosis. ^{1}H-MRS might also be a valuable tool for the assessment of the response to neoadjuvant chemotherapy (Jagannathan et al. 2001; Danishad et al. 2010; Sharma et al. 2011). Meisamy et al. demonstrated that MRS of the breast was able to detect a change in Cho concentration from baseline (before receiving chemo) within 24 h of administration of the first dose of the regimen. This change had a statistically significant positive correlation with change in final size ($p = 0.001$) (Meisamy et al. 2005). In addition, Shin et al. showed that the tCho of tumors was higher in invasive versus in situ cancers and correlated this with several prognostic factors, including nuclear grade, histologic grade, and estrogen receptor status (Shin et al. 2012). Therefore, it can be expected that the addition of ^{1}H-MRSI of the breast will offer a substantial advantage over DCE-MRI of the breast alone in the prediction of response to neoadjuvant chemotherapy. In addition, tCho seems to be indicative not only of an increased proliferation, but also of a hallmark of imminent malignant transformation (Glunde et al. 2011; Aboagye and Bhujwalla 1999). Recently, Ramadan et al. (2015) demonstrated that, in BRCA-1 and BRCA-2 carriers, healthy breast tissue is likely to differ from each other as well as from non-mutation carriers with regard to levels of triglycerides, unsaturated fatty acids, and cholesterol in the absence of any other imaging findings. Further studies are warranted, but if these findings may be confirmed there might be relevant clinical implications for the screening of high-risk women.

- *Sodium (^{23}Na) MRI* has been introduced as a novel MRI parameter for the detection and therapy monitoring of breast cancer. ^{23}Na MRI provides information about the physiological and biochemical state of tissue with sodium concentration being an indicator of cellular metabolic integrity and ion hemostasis (Madelin and Regatte 2013; Ouwerkerk 2011). In normal cells, a low intracellular sodium concentration is maintained by the Na^+/K^+-ATPase pump, which actively pumps sodium out of the cell against a concentration gradient formed by the higher extracellular

sodium concentration. ^{23}Na MRI can detect increased sodium levels secondary to failure of the Na^+/K^+-ATPase pump due to the breakdown of cell membranes, as observed in malignancy. At field strengths of 1.5 and 3T, ^{23}Na MRI is technically limited due to the intrinsically low SNR, resulting long imaging times (approximately 20–30 min), and poor spatial resolution. Substantial improvements can be facilitated with dedicated MRI coils, higher static magnetic field strengths such as 7T, and optimized sequences, which shorten measurement times and improve the coverage and spatial resolution. Recently, Zaric et al. (2016) studied quantitative ^{23}Na MRI at 7T compared with DWI, demonstrating a good resolution and image quality in patients with breast tumors. They showed that discrimination of benign and malignant breast lesions ($p = 0.002$) with similar results to DWI ($p = 0.002$) is feasible.

- *Phosphorus spectroscopy (^{31}P MRS)* measures the bioenergetics of tissue and membrane phospholipid metabolism. The signals of phospholipid precursors and catabolites can be used as imaging biomarkers for tumor progression and response to therapy (Ackerstaff et al. 2003; Arias-Mendoza et al. 2006). It has been demonstrated in several in vitro and in vivo ^{31}P MRS studies that elevated levels of phosphocholine (PC)/phosphoethanolamine (PE) are detectable in several cancers. At 1.5 and 3T field strengths, ^{31}P MRS is restricted to relatively large and primarily superficial tumors. The application of ^{31}P MRS is significantly improved at 7T. In addition to a higher spectral resolution, 7T MRS provides a higher SNR that can be traded off for improving spatial resolution or shortening scan time.

3.3 Emerging Techniques

- *Chemical exchange saturation transfer (CEST)* imaging is a MRI parameter that enables visualization of chemical exchange processes between protons bound to solutes and surrounding bulk water molecules (Ward et al. 2000; Schmitt et al. 2012). It has been demonstrated that endogenous CEST can discriminate tumor from healthy breast tissue based on the information about protons associated with mobile proteins through the amide proton transfer (APT) effect, and it has also been implicated as a prognosticator of response to therapy. Dynamic CEST after the administration of glucose (glucoCEST) enables the evaluation of glycolysis. It was found that glucoCEST could noninvasively depict the kinetics of glycolysis, which is typically enhanced in malignant lesions. Initial data suggest that glucoCEST might be used as a substitute for PET/CT or PET/MRI in the clinical setting to detect tumors and metastases, distinguish between malignant and solid tumors, and monitor tumor response to therapy (Nasrallah et al. 2013; Rivlin et al. 2013). Amide, amine, and aliphatic CEST (aaaCEST) allows the differentiation of areas of apoptosis/necrosis from actively progressing cancer (Klomp et al. 2013).

- *Blood oxygen level-dependent (BOLD) MRI* depicts tissue hypoxia, which is typically associated with tumor progression, recurrence, treatment resistance, and metastasis. To date, tumor hypoxia is assessed on biopsy-derived tumor tissue samples, with the main limitations being the invasiveness, nonrepresentative sampling (the tumor can be quite heterogeneous, and biopsies can be nonrepresentative of the whole tumor), and necessity to perform multiple evaluations to follow changes in tumor oxygenation after treatment (Shin et al. 2012) These limitations highlight the importance of developing imaging biomarkers that can reliably detect tumor hypoxia for tumor grading and noninvasive monitoring spatio-longitudinally during treatment. Initial data suggest that BOLD MRI may be used as a simple, indirect, and noninvasive technique that yields hypoxia information on breast cancer (Stadlbauer et al. 2019) (Figs. 4 and 5) and can assess the response to neoadjuvant treat-

ment (Jiang et al. 2013). A recent study investigated the potential of quantitative BOLD MRI combined with vascular architectural for the characterization of breast cancers and showed that such a noninvasive synergistic assessment of tumor microenvironment (TME) hypoxia and induced neovascularization enables the noninvasive identification of aggressive breast cancer (Bennani-Baiti et al. 2020) (Fig. 6).

- *Hyperpolarized MRI (HP MRI)* is one of the most recent advances in molecular imaging, which allows a rapid, radiation-free, noninvasive investigation of tumor metabolism by exploiting exogenous contrast agents that have been "hyperpolarized." While in conventional MRI nuclear spins are polarized on the order of a few parts per million, in HP MRI, spins reach near-unity polarization, resulting in a substantially increased signal intensity (Ardenkjaer-Larsen et al. 2003; Brindle et al. 2011). HP MRI nuclear spins are polarized in an amorphous solid state at ~1.2 K through coupling of the nuclear spins with unpaired electrons that are added to the sample via an organic free radical. In addition to the distinction of cancerous and normal cells (Golman et al. 2006; Chen et al. 2007; Kurhanewicz et al. 2008), HP MRI using ^{13}C pyruvate has been demonstrated to have potential for the assessment of cancer progression (Albers et al. 2008; Zierhut et al. 2010). Recently, other novel probes for redox (^{13}C dehydroascorbate), necrosis (^{13}C fumarate), and glutamine metabolism (^{13}C glutamine) have been developed to interrogate other metabolic pathways, with promising results (Keshari et al. 2013). To date, there is no specific clinical application for HP MRI in breast cancer. Nevertheless, several preclinical and initial studies in cancer, including breast cancer (Asghar Butt et al. 2014), indicated that this technique may be applicable for the detection of breast cancer and assessment of treatment response in the future.

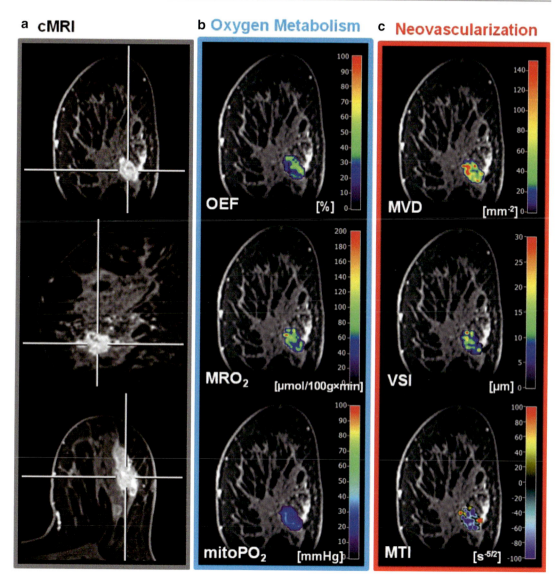

Fig. 4 Noninvasive synergistic assessment of neovascularization, oxygen metabolism, and hypoxia, respectively, in a 53-year-old patient with an invasive ductal carcinoma. Conventional MRI using DCE T1-weighted perfusion MR images in coronal, sagittal, and axial orientation (**a**, top-down) shows lesion size and position. The white line indicates the slice intersection. Imaging biomarker maps of OEF, MRO$_2$, and mitoPO$_2$ in coronal orientation (**b**, top-down) as well as of MVD, VSI, and MTI in coronal orientation (**c**, top-down) demonstrate intratumoral spatial heterogeneity. The invasive ductal carcinoma showed high MRO$_2$, low mitoPO$_2$, high MVD, and low (i.e., more pathologic) MTI. *MRI* magnetic resonance imaging, *DCE* dynamic contrast-enhanced, *OEF* oxygen extraction fraction, *MRO$_2$* metabolic rate of oxygen, *mitoPO$_2$* mitochondrial oxygen tension, *MVD* microvessel density, *VSI* vessel size index, *MTI* microvessel type indicator. (Reprinted under a Creative Commons license (https://creativecommons.org/licenses/by/4.0/) from Stadlbauer A, Zimmermann M, Bennani-Baiti B, Helbich TH, Baltzer P, Clauser P, Kapetas P, Bago-Horvath Z, Pinker K. Development of a Non-invasive Assessment of Hypoxia and Neovascularization with Magnetic Resonance Imaging in Benign and Malignant Breast Tumors: Initial Results. Mol Imaging Biol. 2019 Aug;21(4):758–770. https://doi.org/10.1007/s11307-018-1298-4 (Stadlbauer et al. 2019))

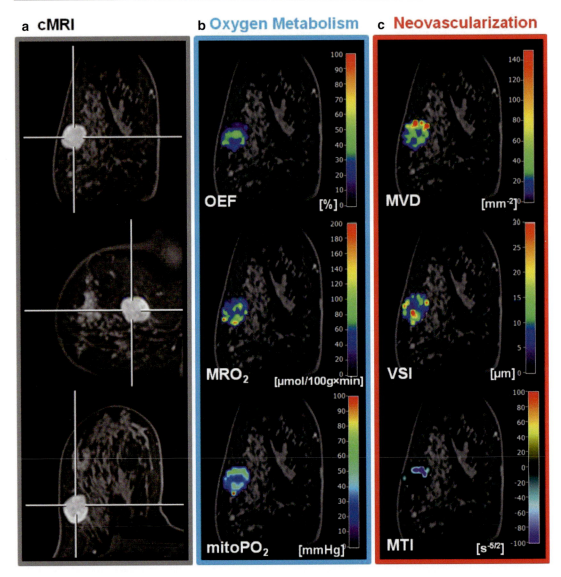

Fig. 5 Noninvasive synergistic assessment of neovascularization, oxygen metabolism, and hypoxia, respectively, in a 31-year-old patient with a benign fibroadenoma. Conventional MRI using DCE T1-weighted perfusion MR images in coronal, sagittal, and axial orientation (**a**, top-down) shows lesion size and position. The white line indicates the slice intersection. Imaging biomarker maps of OEF, MRO$_2$, and mitoPO$_2$ in coronal orientation (**b**, top-down) as well as of MVD, VSI, and MTI in coronal orientation (**c**, top-down) demonstrate intratumoral spatial heterogeneity with lower MRO$_2$, higher mitoPO$_2$, lower MVD, and higher MTI as compared to malignant tumors. *MRI* magnetic resonance imaging, *DCE* dynamic contrast-enhanced, *OEF* oxygen extraction fraction, *MRO$_2$* metabolic rate of oxygen, *mitoPO$_2$* mitochondrial oxygen tension, *MVD* microvessel density, *VSI* vessel size index, *MTI* microvessel type indicator. (Reprinted under a Creative Commons license (https://creativecommons.org/licenses/by/4.0/) from Stadlbauer A, Zimmermann M, Bennani-Baiti B, Helbich TH, Baltzer P, Clauser P, Kapetas P, Bago-Horvath Z, Pinker K. Development of a Non-invasive Assessment of Hypoxia and Neovascularization with Magnetic Resonance Imaging in Benign and Malignant Breast Tumors: Initial Results. Mol Imaging Biol. 2019 Aug;21(4):758-770. https://doi.org/10.1007/s11307-018-1298-4 (Stadlbauer et al. 2019))

4 Screening MRI: Abbreviated MRI Protocols and Non-contrast mpMRI

Randomized controlled trials have shown that mammographic screening in women at an average risk can reduce breast cancer mortality by up to 50% (Brenner 2002; Tabár et al. 2011; Feig 2014). In high-risk population, mammographic screening has shown several drawbacks inherent to this group of women, such as young age of the onset of the disease (Kerlikowske et al. 1993; Brekelmans et al. 2001; Huo et al. 2002; Tilanus-Linthorst et al. 2002; Adem et al. 2003; Komenaka et al. 2004), dense breast tissue (Mandelson et al. 2000; Kolb et al. 2002; Olsen et al. 2009), rapid tumor growth (Tilanus-Linthorst et al. 2005), atypical imaging features of breast cancers (Schrading and Kuhl 2008; Veltman et al. 2008; Marino et al. 2018b), and cumulative effect of radiation from yearly mammograms (Powell and Kachnic 2003; Jansen-van der Weide et al. 2010). In several prospective high-risk screening studies, MRI has widely proven its high sensitivity, outperforming other breast imaging techniques, such as mammography and/or ultrasound (Mann et al. 2008; Sardanelli et al. 2011). Therefore, international guidelines currently recommend annual MRI screening from age 25 years onward and additional mammography from age 30 years for women at high risk (Mann et al. 2015; Sardanelli et al. 2010; Expert Panel on Breast Imaging et al. 2017). Major criticisms of breast MRI screening are the high costs as a consequence of relatively long acquisition and interpretation times involved in a full diagnostic protocol. To overcome these limitations, Kuhl et al. (2014) in 2014 first introduced an abbreviated breast MRI protocol consisting of only one pre- and one post-contrast acquisition screening purpose. The authors proposed a 3-min acquisition time with a reading time of <30 s that achieved similar diagnostic accuracy compared with a full diagnostic protocol. Similar results have been obtained by other study groups who reproduced the abbreviated protocols for breast cancer screening (Kuhl et al. 2014; Mango et al. 2015; Grimm et al. 2015; Moschetta et al. 2016; Harvey et al. 2016). Mango et al. investigated the diagnostic value of an abbreviated protocol consisting of a pre-contrast T1-weighted sequence and an initial post-contrast T1-weighted sequence, both with fat saturation in cancers (Mango et al. 2015). Mean sensitivities of 93–96% for each sequence were reached, at a mean interpretation time of 44 s. The authors concluded that an abbreviated examination could translate into decreased cost and make breast MRI a more accessible modality. In a different approach, Mann et al. (2014) evaluated the use of ultrafast breast MRI with stochastic trajectory (TWIST) acquisitions ($0.9 \times 1 \times 2.5$ mm, temporal resolution, 4.3 s) as a screening tool. The authors found that ultrafast dynamic breast MRI allows detection of breast lesions and classification with high accuracy allowing substantial shortening of scan protocols and hence reducing imaging costs. Kuhl et al. investigated the utility of MRI as a supplemental screening tool in 2120 women at average breast cancer risk and found that MRI depicted 60 additional breast cancers, while 12 of 13 incident cancers were found with MRI alone (Kuhl et al. 2017). Despite such encouraging results, breast MRI is currently not implemented in the screening of women at average risk of breast cancer, with the limiting factor being its relatively high direct and indirect costs compared with conventional imaging (Cott Chubiz et al. 2013; Lowry et al. 2012).

Several authors have investigated abbreviated non-contrast protocols with different combinations of T1 weighted and/or T2 weighted with DWI, with encouraging results (Baltzer et al. 2018, 2010; Trimboli et al. 2014; McDonald et al. 2016; Shin et al. 2016; Yabuuchi et al. 2011; Bickelhaupt et al. 2016). Shin et al. investigated two abbreviated protocols—non-contrast high b-value DWI and T1-weighted imaging vs. a contrast-enhanced protocol including early DCE-MRI sequences. They showed that both abbreviated protocols achieved similar detection rates and diagnostic accuracy (Kuhl 2007a). Baltzer et al. compared a non-contrast DWI protocol with a full contrast-enhanced protocol with DCE-MRI and T2-weighted imaging protocol; both protocols achieved similar results with high diagnostic performance and inter-reader agreement (Monticciolo et al. 2018). Bickelhaupt et al. compared a non-contrast MRI protocol consisting of maximum-intensity projections from DWI with background suppression and unenhanced morphologic sequence with an abbreviated DCE-MRI protocol and a full diagnostic MRI protocol to predict the likelihood of malignancy in patients recalled from screening mammography. The non-contrast MRI protocol was able to exclude malignancy in these patients with a negative predictive value of 0.92 (Leithner et al. 2018). While these results are encouraging and highlight the potential of DWI as a promising MRI technique for non-contrast screening with MRI, a recent study comparing DCE-MRI, DWI as a stand-alone parameter for breast cancer detection, and mpMRI demonstrated that DCE-MRI remains the most sensitive protocol for breast cancer detection (Pinker et al. 2018a). A current limitation of DWI is that its sensitivity is limited in smaller lesions ≤ 12 mm and in lesions presenting as diffuse non-mass enhancement (NME) (Pinker et al. 2013). Nevertheless, research to improve the spatial resolution of DWI is ongoing, and it can be expected that further advances are possible to overcome its current limitations. In the meantime, as several studies have demonstrated that the mpMRI with DCE-MRI and DWI maximizes diagnostic accuracy, it seems that there is potential for the application of abbreviated MRI protocols with combined DCE-MRI and DWI in breast cancer screening.

5 Breast MRI Radiomics and Radiogenomics

Radiomics extracts information on phenotypic characteristics of the entire tumor in a noninvasive and cost-effective way by converting medical images into quantifiable data (Valdora et al. 2018; Gillies et al. 2016). Meanwhile, radiogenomics aims to correlate imaging characteristics (i.e., the imaging phenotype) with gene expression patterns, gene mutations, and other genome-related characteristics (Grimm 2016; Pinker et al. 2018b; Mazurowski et al. 2014). To date, radiomic and radiogenomics research in breast imaging has focused on DCE-MRI (Grimm 2016; Pinker et al. 2018b; Dong et al. 2018; Saha et al. 2018a, b), extracting morphologic and functional image features for determining individual gene signatures for the differentiation of molecular breast cancer subtypes as well as for correlation with recurrence scores (RS) (Sutton et al. 2015; Li et al. 2016a, b).

Different radiogenomic studies have shown encouraging results. Yamamoto et al. (2012) investigated ten patients undergoing preoperative DCE-MRI and global gene expression analysis. They presented a preliminary radiogenomic association map linking MRI phenotypes to underlying global gene expression patterns in breast cancer. High-level analysis identified 21 imaging traits globally correlated with 71% of the total

Fig. 6 Radiologic-histopathologic correlation: 58-year-old patient with an invasive ductal carcinoma (estrogen receptor (ER)/progesterone receptor (PR) positive and human epidermal growth receptor 2 (HER2) negative, ki-67 20%). (**a**) MRI biomarkers. (**b**) Contrast-enhanced T1 (CE-T1) image coronal. (**c**) CE-T1 image axial. (**d**) Vascular endothelial growth factor receptor 1 (FLT1), (**e**) Podoplanin. (**f**) Hypoxia-inducible factor 1-alpha (HIF-1alpha). (**g**) Carbonic anhydrase 9 (CA IX). (**h**) Vascular endothelial growth factor C (VEGF-C). HIF-1alpha is expressed ubiquitously, along with VEGF-C and FLT1 in the more solid areas of the tumor. This is matched by higher levels of mitoPO$_2$ values and OEF which are MRI biomarker for oxygen metabolism, especially in the tumor center. (Reprinted under a Creative Commons license (https://creativecommons.org/licenses/by/4.0/) from Bennani-Baiti B, Pinker K, Zimmermann M, Helbich TH, Baltzer PA, Clauser P, Kapetas P, Bago-Horvath Z, Stadlbauer A. Non-Invasive Assessment of Hypoxia and Neovascularization with MRI for Identification of Aggressive Breast Cancer. Cancers (Basel). 2020 Jul 24;12(8):E2024. https://doi.org/10.3390/cancers12082024 (Bennani-Baiti et al. 2020))

Breast MRI: Multiparametric and Advanced Techniques

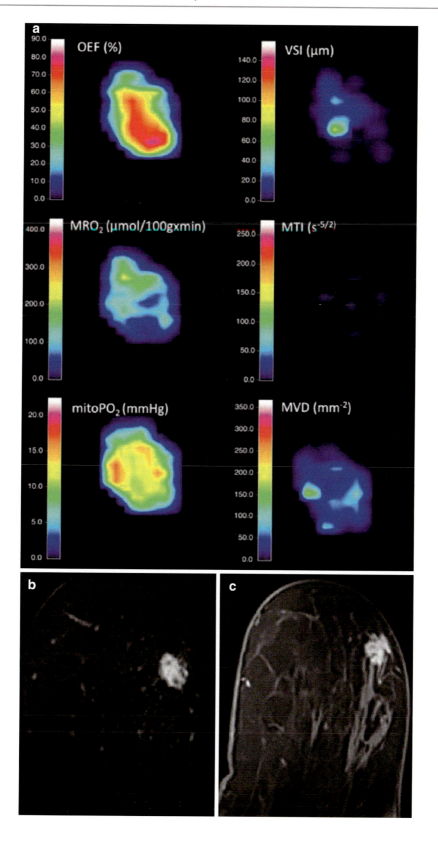

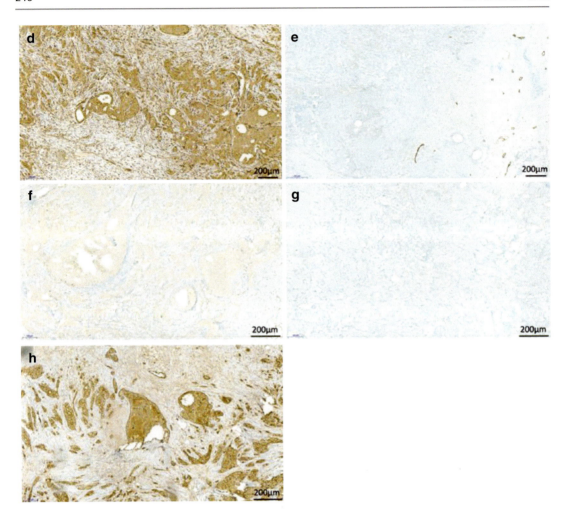

Fig. 6 (continued)

genes measured in patients with breast cancer ($p < 0.05$). Moreover, there were significant correlations between heterogeneous enhancement patterns and interferon breast cancer subtype ($p < 0.01$). In addition, 12 imaging traits significantly correlated with breast cancer gene sets, and 11 traits correlated with prognostic gene sets (false discovery rate <0.25, respectively). Mazurowski et al. (2014) performed radiogenomic analysis on a subset of 48 cases from The Cancer Genome Atlas database to investigate whether enhancement kinetics could predict the luminal B subtype. The authors found an increased ratio of tumor-to-background parenchymal enhancement in the luminal B subtype compared with other subtypes. MRI radiomics studies indicate that tumor enhancement kinetics reflect underlying tumor biology. Bhooshan et al. (2010, 2011) investigated breast MRI radiomics features for determining tumor invasiveness, achieving high accuracies of 83%. Yamaguchi et al. (2015) investigated the relationship between kinetic curve pattern and molecular subtypes, finding that HR+/HER2− and triple-negative (TN) breast cancer subtypes demonstrated less washout on the delayed phase of enhancement compared with HER2–luminal (HR+/HER2+) and HER2-positive (HR−/HER2+) subtypes. Blaschke and Abe (2015) reported that HER2-positive tumors have a more rapid initial enhancement compared with other molecular subtypes. Li et al. (2016b) observed faster contrast enhancement in estrogen receptor-negative, progesterone receptor-negative, and TN cancers relative to estrogen receptor-positive, progesterone receptor-positive, and non-TN cancers. In a recent study, Leithner et al. (2020) evaluated the performance of radiomics and artificial intelligence (AI) from mpMRI in 91 breast cancer patients for the assessment of breast cancer molecular subtypes. The authors found that radiomics and AI from multiparametric MRI may aid in the noninvasive differentiation of TN and luminal A breast cancers from other subtypes, with an overall median AUC of 0.8.

Different recurrence scores, such as Oncotype DX (Genomic Health, CA), MammaPrint (Agendia, CA), Mammostrat (Clarient Diagnostic Services, CA), and PAM50/Prosigna (NanoString, WA), have been studied in association with breast cancer MRI features. Ashraf et al. in two different studies presented a method for identifying intrinsic imaging phenotypes in breast cancer tumors and investigated their association with prognostic gene expression profiles (Ashraf et al. 2014). In this study, the authors retrospectively analyzed breast DCE-MRI in 56 women and found a moderate correlation between DCE-MR imaging features and RS. Four dominant imaging phenotypes were detected, with two including only low- and medium-risk tumors. Sutton et al. investigated the association between a validated, gene expression-based, aggressiveness assay, Oncotype DX RS, and morphological and texture-based image features extracted from breast MRI. In their cohort of 95 patients, they found that a model for invasive ductal carcinoma correlates with Oncotype DX RS, suggesting that image-based features could also predict the likelihood of recurrence and magnitude of chemotherapy benefit (Sutton et al. 2015). Li et al. assessed the relationships of computer-extracted breast MRI phenotypes with MammaPrint, Oncotype DX, and PAM50/Prosigna to evaluate the role of radiogenomics in the risk of breast cancer recurrence. In this study, there were significant associations between breast cancer MRI radiomics signatures and multigene assay recurrence scores, specifically MammaPrint, Oncotype DX, and PAM50/Prosigna risk of relapse based on the subtype (Li et al. 2016b) (Figs. 7 and 8).

Radiomics and radiogenomics aim to facilitate a deeper understanding of tumor biology and

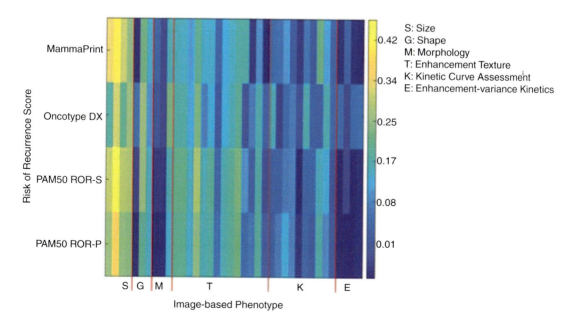

Fig. 7 Correlation heat map based on the univariate linear regression analysis between each individual MRI phenotype and the recurrence predictor models of MammaPrint, Oncotype DX, PAM50 ROR-S, and PAM50 ROR-P. In this color scale, yellow indicates higher correlation as compared with blue and the different gene assays served as the "reference standard" in this study. Some phenotypes correlate similarly (i.e., similar color on the color scale) across the risk estimate models, while others do not. (Reprinted with permission from: Li H, Zhu Y, Burnside ES, et al. Radiology 2016;281:382–391)

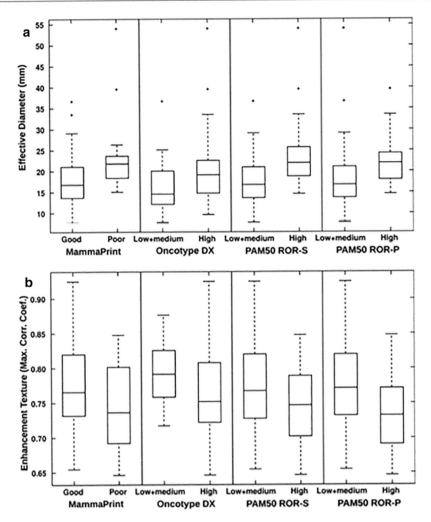

Fig. 8 Box-and-whisker plots show the relationship of the MRI-based phenotypes of (**a**) size (effective diameter), and (**b**) enhancement texture (maximum correlation coefficient) with the recurrence predictor models of MammaPrint, Oncotype DX, PAM50 ROR-S, and PAM50 ROR-P. A positive correlation between the selected MRI phenotypes of size (effective diameter) and negative correlation with enhancement texture (maximum correlation coefficient) and increasing levels of risk of recurrence for MammaPrint, Oncotype DX, PAM50 ROR-S, and PAM50 ROR-P were observed. A low value of this enhancement texture feature indicates a more heterogeneous enhancement pattern. (Reprinted with permission from Li H, Zhu Y, Burnside ES, et al. Radiology. 2016;281:382–391)

capture the intrinsic tumor heterogeneity. Ultimately, the overarching goal is to develop imaging biomarkers for outcome that incorporate both phenotypic and genotypic metrics. Due to the noninvasive nature of medical imaging and its ubiquitous use in clinical practice, this young field of research is rapidly evolving. The previously detailed initial results are encouraging that the overarching goal to provide meaningful imaging biomarkers that can be incorporated in clinical practice for precision medicine in breast cancer can be achieved. To date, radiomics and radiogenomics in breast imaging have focused mainly on DCE-MRI, molecular breast cancer subtypes, and recurrence scores. However, it is expected that other well-established and emerging breast imaging techniques such as DWI or multi-nuclei MR spectroscopy will emerge in the field of radiomics and radiogenomics. It has to be noted that to date radiomics and radiogenomics are still limited somewhat by the heterogeneity of datasets from different institutions and challenges in genetic testing. Therefore, larger prospective studies are warranted to define the future role of radiomics and radiogenomics in the clinical management of breast cancer.

6 Conclusions

DCE-MRI not only has become an essential method in breast imaging but is also undisputedly the most sensitive test for breast cancer detection outperforming conventional breast imaging. Due to its limitations in specificity, several other functional MRI parameters as an adjunct to DCE-MRI have been explored with excellent success. Currently, mpMRI comprises established (DCE-MRI, DWI, T2-weighted) parameters and can be performed at 1.5, 3, and 7T. Emerging MRI parameters, such as multi-nuclei spectroscopy, sodium imaging, CEST, BOLD, and hyperpolarized MRI, are being investigated and translated from the experimental to clinical. mpMRI allows for different combinations of interchangeable functional MRI parameters and thus can simultaneously assess a multitude of processes relevant for cancer development, progression, and response to treatment. In the clinical routine, mpMRI is mainly performed using DCE-MRI, T2 weighted, and DWI and has been shown to improve diagnostic accuracy and aid treatment decision-making. It has to be noted that the implementation of mpMRI is currently not uniform worldwide as the level of its integration is often dependent on the institution (academic vs. private practice), associated costs (e.g., specific coils, 7T), and each individual country's reimbursement policies. Abbreviated ultrafast MRI and non-contrast mpMRI protocols are being investigated to save costs and hence make breast cancer screening with MRI available not only to high-risk women. Moreover, with advances in medical imaging techniques and image analysis and the development of high-throughput methods to extract and correlate multiple imaging parameters with genomic data, the field of radiogenomics has emerged, aiming to correlate imaging phenotypes with genomic cancer characteristics to provide deeper insights in pathologic processes. In conclusion, mpMRI of the breast is a still-evolving field, and a paradigm shift establishing advanced morpho-functional imaging with MRI potentially coupled with radiogenomics is expected to further improve the diagnosis, prediction, and prognosis of breast cancer, ultimately realizing the goal of precision medicine.FundingFunding was provided in part by the 2020—Research and Innovation Framework Programme PHC-11-2015 Nr. 667211–2 and under grant agreement Nr. 688188.

References

Aboagye EO, Bhujwalla ZM (1999) Malignant transformation alters membrane choline phospholipid metabolism of human mammary epithelial cells. Cancer Res 59:80–84

Ackerstaff E, Glunde K, Bhujwalla ZM (2003) Choline phospholipid metabolism: a target in cancer cells? J Cell Biochem 90:525–533. https://doi.org/10.1002/jcb.10659

Adem C, Reynolds C, Soderberg CL et al (2003) Pathologic characteristics of breast parenchyma in patients with hereditary breast carcinoma, including BRCA1 and BRCA2 mutation carriers. Cancer 97:1–11. https://doi.org/10.1002/cncr.11048

Albers MJ, Bok R, Chen AP et al (2008) Hyperpolarized 13C lactate, pyruvate, and alanine: noninvasive biomarkers for prostate cancer detection and grading. Cancer Res 68:8607–8615. https://doi.org/10.1158/0008-5472.CAN-08-0749

Ardenkjaer-Larsen JH, Fridlund B, Gram A et al (2003) Increase in signal-to-noise ratio of >10,000 times in liquid-state NMR. Proc Natl Acad Sci U S A 100:10158–10163. https://doi.org/10.1073/pnas.1733835100

Arias-Mendoza F, Payne GS, Zakian KL et al (2006) In vivo 31P MR spectral patterns and reproducibility in cancer patients studied in a multi-institutional trial. NMR Biomed 19:504–512. https://doi.org/10.1002/nbm.1057

Asghar Butt S, Søgaard LV, Ardenkjaer-Larsen JH et al (2014) Monitoring mammary tumor progression and effect of tamoxifen treatment in MMTV-PymT using MRI and magnetic resonance spectroscopy with hyperpolarized [1-(13) C]pyruvate. Magn Reson Med. https://doi.org/10.1002/mrm.25095

Ashraf AB, Daye D, Gavenonis S et al (2014) Identification of intrinsic imaging phenotypes for breast cancer tumors: preliminary associations with gene expression profiles. Radiology 272:374–384. https://doi.org/10.1148/radiol.14131375

Baltzer PAT, Dietzel M (2013) Breast lesions: diagnosis by using proton MR spectroscopy at 1.5 and 3.0 T—systematic review and meta-analysis. Radiology 267:735–746. https://doi.org/10.1148/radiol.13121856

Baltzer PAT, Renz DM, Herrmann K-H et al (2009) Diffusion-weighted imaging (DWI) in MR mammography (MRM): clinical comparison of echo planar imaging (EPI) and half-Fourier single-shot turbo spin echo (HASTE) diffusion techniques. Eur Radiol 19:1612–1620. https://doi.org/10.1007/s00330-009-1326-5

Baltzer PAT, Benndorf M, Dietzel M et al (2010) Sensitivity and specificity of unenhanced MR mammography (DWI combined with T2-weighted TSE imaging, ueMRM) for the differentiation of mass lesions. Eur Radiol 20:1101–1110. https://doi.org/10.1007/s00330-009-1654-5

Baltzer PAT, Dietzel M, Kaiser WA (2011a) Nonmass lesions in magnetic resonance imaging of the breast: additional T2-weighted images improve diagnostic accuracy. J Comput Assist Tomogr 35:361–366. https://doi.org/10.1097/RCT.0b013e31821065c3

Baltzer PAT, Schäfer A, Dietzel M et al (2011b) Diffusion tensor magnetic resonance imaging of the breast: a pilot study. Eur Radiol 21:1–10. https://doi.org/10.1007/s00330-010-1901-9

Baltzer PAT, Dietzel M, Kaiser WA (2012) MR-spectroscopy at 1.5 tesla and 3 tesla. Useful? A systematic review and meta-analysis. Eur J Radiol 81(Suppl 1):S6–S9. https://doi.org/10.1016/S0720-048X(12)70003-7

Baltzer A, Dietzel M, Kaiser CG, Baltzer PA (2015) Combined reading of contrast enhanced and diffusion weighted magnetic resonance imaging by using a simple sum score. Eur Radiol. https://doi.org/10.1007/s00330-015-3886-x

Baltzer PAT, Bickel H, Spick C et al (2018) Potential of noncontrast magnetic resonance imaging with diffusion-weighted imaging in characterization of breast lesions: intraindividual comparison with dynamic contrast-enhanced magnetic resonance imaging. Invest Radiol 53:229–235. https://doi.org/10.1097/RLI.0000000000000433

Baltzer P, Mann RM, Iima M et al (2020) Diffusion-weighted imaging of the breast-a consensus and mission statement from the EUSOBI International Breast Diffusion-Weighted Imaging working group. Eur Radiol 30:1436–1450. https://doi.org/10.1007/s00330-019-06510-3

Bennani-Baiti B, Pinker K, Zimmermann M et al (2020) Non-invasive assessment of hypoxia and neovascularization with MRI for identification of aggressive breast cancer. Cancers (Basel) 12(8):2024. https://doi.org/10.3390/cancers12082024

Berg WA, Gutierrez L, NessAiver MS et al (2004) Diagnostic accuracy of mammography, clinical examination, US, and MR imaging in preoperative assessment of breast cancer. Radiology 233:830–849. https://doi.org/10.1148/radiol.2333031484

Bhooshan N, Giger ML, Jansen SA et al (2010) Cancerous breast lesions on dynamic contrast-enhanced MR images: computerized characterization for image-based prognostic markers. Radiology 254:680–690. https://doi.org/10.1148/radiol.09090838

Bhooshan N, Giger M, Edwards D et al (2011) Computerized three-class classification of MRI-based prognostic markers for breast cancer. Phys Med Biol 56:5995–6008. https://doi.org/10.1088/0031-9155/56/18/014

Bickel H, Pinker-Domenig K, Bogner W et al (2015) Quantitative apparent diffusion coefficient as a non-invasive imaging biomarker for the differentiation of invasive breast cancer and ductal carcinoma in situ. Invest Radiol 50:95–100. https://doi.org/10.1097/RLI.0000000000000104

Bickelhaupt S, Laun FB, Tesdorff J et al (2016) Fast and noninvasive characterization of suspicious lesions detected at breast cancer X-ray screening: capability of diffusion-weighted MR imaging with MIPs. Radiology 278:689–697. https://doi.org/10.1148/radiol.2015150425

Blaschke E, Abe H (2015) MRI phenotype of breast cancer: kinetic assessment for molecular subtypes. J Magn Reson Imaging 42:920–924. https://doi.org/10.1002/jmri.24884

Bogner W, Gruber S, Pinker K et al (2009) Diffusion-weighted MR for differentiation of breast lesions at 3.0 T: how does selection of diffusion protocols affect diagnosis? Radiology 253:341–351. https://doi.org/10.1148/radiol.2532081718

Bogner W, Pinker-Domenig K, Bickel H et al (2012) Readout-segmented echo-planar imaging improves the diagnostic performance of diffusion-weighted MR breast examinations at 3.0 T. Radiology 263:64–76. https://doi.org/10.1148/radiol.12111494

Bokacheva L, Kaplan JB, Giri DD et al (2014) Intravoxel incoherent motion diffusion-weighted MRI at 3.0 T differentiates malignant breast lesions from benign lesions and breast parenchyma. J Magn Reson Imaging 40:813–823. https://doi.org/10.1002/jmri.24462

Bolan PJ (2013) Magnetic resonance spectroscopy of the breast: current status. Magn Reson Imaging Clin N Am 21:625–639. https://doi.org/10.1016/j.mric.2013.04.008

Bolan PJ, DelaBarre L, Baker EH et al (2002) Eliminating spurious lipid sidebands in 1H MRS of breast lesions. Magn Reson Med 48:215–222. https://doi.org/10.1002/mrm.10224

Bolan PJ, Meisamy S, Baker EH et al (2003) In vivo quantification of choline compounds in the breast with 1H MR spectroscopy. Magn Reson Med 50:1134–1143. https://doi.org/10.1002/mrm.10654

Bolan PJ, Henry P-G, Baker EH et al (2004) Measurement and correction of respiration-induced B0 variations in breast 1H MRS at 4 Tesla. Magn Reson Med 52:1239–1245. https://doi.org/10.1002/mrm.20277

Brekelmans CT, Seynaeve C, Bartels CC et al (2001) Effectiveness of breast cancer surveillance in BRCA1/2 gene mutation carriers and women with high familial risk. J Clin Oncol 19:924–930. https://doi.org/10.1200/jco.2001.19.4.924

Brenner H (2002) Long-term survival rates of cancer patients achieved by the end of the 20th century: a period analysis. Lancet 360:1131–1135. https://doi.org/10.1016/S0140-6736(02)11199-8

Brindle KM, Bohndiek SE, Gallagher FA, Kettunen MI (2011) Tumor imaging using hyperpolarized 13C magnetic resonance spectroscopy. Magn Reson Med 66:505–519. https://doi.org/10.1002/mrm.22999

Cakir O, Arslan A, Inan N et al (2013) Comparison of the diagnostic performances of diffusion parameters in diffusion weighted imaging and diffusion tensor imaging of breast lesions. Eur J Radiol 82:e801–e806. https://doi.org/10.1016/j.ejrad.2013.09.001

Chen AP, Albers MJ, Cunningham CH et al (2007) Hyperpolarized C-13 spectroscopic imaging of the TRAMP mouse at 3T-initial experience. Magn Reson Med 58:1099–1106. https://doi.org/10.1002/mrm.21256

Cho GY, Moy L, Kim SG et al (2015a) Comparison of contrast enhancement and diffusion-weighted magnetic resonance imaging in healthy and cancerous breast tissue. Eur J Radiol 84:1888–1893. https://doi.org/10.1016/j.ejrad.2015.06.023

Cho GY, Moy L, Kim SG et al (2015b) Evaluation of breast cancer using intravoxel incoherent motion (IVIM) histogram analysis: comparison with malignant status, histological subtype, and molecular prognostic factors. Eur Radiol. https://doi.org/10.1007/s00330-015-4087-3

Cho GY, Moy L, Zhang JL et al (2015c) Comparison of fitting methods and b-value sampling strategies for intravoxel incoherent motion in breast cancer. Magn Reson Med 74:1077–1085. https://doi.org/10.1002/mrm.25484

Costantini M, Belli P, Rinaldi P et al (2010) Diffusion-weighted imaging in breast cancer: relationship between apparent diffusion coefficient and tumour aggressiveness. Clin Radiol 65:1005–1012. https://doi.org/10.1016/j.crad.2010.07.008

Cott Chubiz JE, Lee JM, Gilmore ME et al (2013) Cost-effectiveness of alternating magnetic resonance imaging and digital mammography screening in BRCA1 and BRCA2 gene mutation carriers. Cancer 119:1266–1276. https://doi.org/10.1002/cncr.27864

Danishad KKA, Sharma U, Sah RG et al (2010) Assessment of therapeutic response of locally advanced breast cancer (LABC) patients undergoing neoadjuvant chemotherapy (NACT) monitored using sequential magnetic resonance spectroscopic imaging (MRSI). NMR Biomed 23:233–241. https://doi.org/10.1002/nbm.1436

Dogan BE, Gonzalez-Angulo AM, Gilcrease M et al (2010) Multimodality imaging of triple receptor-negative tumors with mammography, ultrasound, and

MRI. AJR Am J Roentgenol 194:1160–1166. https://doi.org/10.2214/AJR.09.2355

Dong Y, Feng Q, Yang W et al (2018) Preoperative prediction of sentinel lymph node metastasis in breast cancer based on radiomics of T2-weighted fat-suppression and diffusion-weighted MRI. Eur Radiol 28:582–591. https://doi.org/10.1007/s00330-017-5005-7

Dorrius MD, Dijkstra H, Oudkerk M, Sijens PE (2014) Effect of b value and pre-admission of contrast on diagnostic accuracy of 1.5-T breast DWI: a systematic review and meta-analysis. Eur Radiol 24:2835–2847. https://doi.org/10.1007/s00330-014-3338-z

Expert Panel on Breast Imaging, Mainiero MB, Moy L et al (2017) ACR Appropriateness Criteria® breast cancer screening. J Am Coll Radiol 14:S383–S390. https://doi.org/10.1016/j.jacr.2017.08.044

Eyal E, Shapiro-Feinberg M, Furman-Haran E et al (2012) Parametric diffusion tensor imaging of the breast. Invest Radiol 47:284–291. https://doi.org/10.1097/RLI.0b013e3182438e5d

Feig SA (2014) Screening mammography benefit controversies: sorting the evidence. Radiol Clin North Am 52:455–480. https://doi.org/10.1016/j.rcl.2014.02.009

Fischer DR, Wurdinger S, Boettcher J et al (2005) Further signs in the evaluation of magnetic resonance mammography: a retrospective study. Invest Radiol 40:430–435

For the European Society of Breast Imaging (EUSOBI), Sardanelli F, Helbich TH (2012) Mammography: EUSOBI recommendations for women's information. Insights Imaging 3:7–10. https://doi.org/10.1007/s13244-011-0127-y

Foulkes WD, Smith IE, Reis-Filho JS (2010) Triple-negative breast cancer. N Engl J Med 363:1938–1948. https://doi.org/10.1056/NEJMra1001389

Gillies RJ, Kinahan PE, Hricak H (2016) Radiomics: images are more than pictures, they are data. Radiology 278:563–577. https://doi.org/10.1148/radiol.2015151169

Glunde K, Bhujwalla ZM, Ronen SM (2011) Choline metabolism in malignant transformation. Nat Rev Cancer 11:835–848. https://doi.org/10.1038/nrc3162

Golman K, Zandt RI, Lerche M et al (2006) Metabolic imaging by hyperpolarized 13C magnetic resonance imaging for in vivo tumor diagnosis. Cancer Res 66:10855–10860. https://doi.org/10.1158/0008-5472.CAN-06-2564

Gondo T, Hricak H, Sala E et al (2014) Multiparametric 3T MRI for the prediction of pathological downgrading after radical prostatectomy in patients with biopsy-proven Gleason score 3+4 prostate cancer. Eur Radiol 24:3161–3170. https://doi.org/10.1007/s00330-014-3367-7

Grimm LJ (2016) Breast MRI radiogenomics: current status and research implications. J Magn Reson Imaging 43:1269–1278. https://doi.org/10.1002/jmri.25116

Grimm LJ, Soo MS, Yoon S et al (2015) Abbreviated screening protocol for breast MRI: a feasibility study. Acad Radiol 22:1157–1162. https://doi.org/10.1016/j.acra.2015.06.004

Gruber S, Debski B-K, Pinker K et al (2011) Three-dimensional proton MR spectroscopic imaging at 3 T for the differentiation of benign and malignant breast lesions. Radiology 261:752–761. https://doi.org/10.1148/radiol.11102096

Gruber S, Pinker K, Zaric O et al (2014) Dynamic contrast-enhanced magnetic resonance imaging of breast tumors at 3 and 7 T: a comparison. Invest Radiol 49:354–362. https://doi.org/10.1097/RLI.0000000000000034

Haddadin IS, McIntosh A, Meisamy S et al (2009) Metabolite quantification and high-field MRS in breast cancer. NMR Biomed 22:65–76. https://doi.org/10.1002/nbm.1217

Hanahan D, Weinberg RA (2000) The hallmarks of cancer. Cell 100:57–70

Hanahan D, Weinberg RA (2011) Hallmarks of cancer: the next generation. Cell 144:646–674. https://doi.org/10.1016/j.cell.2011.02.013

Harvey SC, Di Carlo PA, Lee B et al (2016) An abbreviated protocol for high-risk screening breast MRI saves time and resources. J Am Coll Radiol 13:R74–R80. https://doi.org/10.1016/j.jacr.2016.09.031

Hatakenaka M, Soeda H, Yabuuchi H et al (2008) Apparent diffusion coefficients of breast tumors: clinical application. Magn Reson Med Sci 7:23–29

Helbich TH (2000) Contrast-enhanced magnetic resonance imaging of the breast. Eur J Radiol 34:208–219

Hoult DI, Phil D (2000) Sensitivity and power deposition in a high-field imaging experiment. J Magn Reson Imaging 12:46–67

Huang W, Tudorica LA, Li X et al (2011) Discrimination of benign and malignant breast lesions by using shutter-speed dynamic contrast-enhanced MR imaging. Radiology 261:394–403. https://doi.org/10.1148/radiol.11102413

Huo Z, Giger ML, Olopade OI et al (2002) Computerized analysis of digitized mammograms of BRCA1 and BRCA2 gene mutation carriers. Radiology 225:519–526. https://doi.org/10.1148/radiol.2252010845

Iacconi C, Giannelli M, Marini C et al (2010) The role of mean diffusivity (MD) as a predictive index of the response to chemotherapy in locally advanced breast cancer: a preliminary study. Eur Radiol 20:303–308. https://doi.org/10.1007/s00330-009-1550-z

Iima M, Yano K, Kataoka M et al (2015) Quantitative non-Gaussian diffusion and intravoxel incoherent motion magnetic resonance imaging: differentiation of malignant and benign breast lesions. Invest Radiol 50:205–211. https://doi.org/10.1097/RLI.0000000000000094

Jagannathan NR et al (1998) Volume localized in vivo proton MR spectroscopy of breast carcinoma: variation of water–fat ratio in patients receiving chemotherapy. NMR Biomed 11(8):414–422

Jagannathan NR, Kumar M, Seenu V et al (2001) Evaluation of total choline from in-vivo volume localized proton MR spectroscopy and its response to neoadjuvant chemotherapy in locally advanced breast cancer. Br J Cancer 84:1016–1022. https://doi.org/10.1054/bjoc.2000.1711

Jansen-van der Weide MC, Greuter MJW, Jansen L et al (2010) Exposure to low-dose radiation and the risk of breast cancer among women with a familial or genetic predisposition: a meta-analysis. Eur Radiol 20:2547–2556. https://doi.org/10.1007/s00330-010-1839-y

Jensen JH, Helpern JA, Ramani A et al (2005) Diffusional kurtosis imaging: the quantification of non-gaussian water diffusion by means of magnetic resonance imaging. Magn Reson Med 53:1432–1440. https://doi.org/10.1002/mrm.20508

Jiang L, Weatherall PT, McColl RW et al (2013) Blood oxygenation level-dependent (BOLD) contrast magnetic resonance imaging (MRI) for prediction of breast cancer chemotherapy response: a pilot study. J Magn Reson Imaging 37:1083–1092. https://org/10.1002/jmri.23891

Kaiser WA (2007) Breast magnetic resonance imaging: principles and techniques. Semin Roentgenol 42:228–235. https://doi.org/10.1053/j.ro.2007.07.003

Kaiser WA, Zeitler E (1989) MR imaging of the breast: fast imaging sequences with and without Gd-DTPA. Preliminary observations. Radiology 170:681–686. https://doi.org/10.1148/radiology.170.3.2916021

Kaiser CG, Reich C, Dietzel M et al (2015a) DCE-MRI of the breast in a stand-alone setting outside a complementary strategy - results of the TK-study. Eur Radiol 25:1793–1800. https://doi.org/10.1007/s00330-014-3580-4

Kaiser CG, Herold M, Baltzer PAT et al (2015b) Is "prepectoral edema" a morphologic sign for malignant breast tumors? Acad Radiol 22:684–689. https://doi.org/10.1016/j.acra.2015.01.009

Kaiser CG, Herold M, Krammer J et al (2017) Prognostic value of "prepectoral edema" in MR-mammography. Anticancer Res 37:1989–1995. https://doi.org/10.21873/anticanres.11542

Kawashima H (2011) Imaging findings of triple-negative breast cancer. Breast Cancer 18:145. https://doi.org/10.1007/s12282-010-0247-0

Kerlikowske K, Grady D, Barclay J et al (1993) Positive predictive value of screening mammography by age and family history of breast cancer. JAMA 270:2444–2450

Keshari KR, Sai V, Wang ZJ et al (2013) Hyperpolarized [1-13C]dehydroascorbate MR spectroscopy in a murine model of prostate cancer: comparison with 18F-FDG PET. J Nucl Med 54:922–928. https://doi.org/10.2967/jnumed.112.115402

Kim JH, Choi SH, Ryoo I et al (2014) Prognosis prediction of measurable enhancing lesion after completion of standard concomitant chemoradiotherapy and adjuvant temozolomide in glioblastoma patients: application of dynamic susceptibility contrast perfusion and diffusion-weighted imaging. PLoS One 9:e113587. https://doi.org/10.1371/journal.pone.0113587

Klomp DWJ, van de Bank BL, Raaijmakers A et al (2011) 31P MRSI and 1H MRS at 7 T: initial results in human breast cancer. NMR Biomed 24:1337–1342. https://doi.org/10.1002/nbm.1696

Klomp DWJ, Dula AN, Arlinghaus LR et al (2013) Amide proton transfer imaging of the human breast at 7T: development and reproducibility. NMR Biomed 26:1271–1277. https://doi.org/10.1002/nbm.2947

Kolb TM, Lichy J, Newhouse JH (2002) Comparison of the performance of screening mammography, physical examination, and breast US and evaluation of factors that influence them: an analysis of 27,825 patient evaluations. Radiology 225:165–175. https://doi.org/10.1148/radiol.2251011667

Komenaka IK, Ditkoff B-A, Joseph K-A et al (2004) The development of interval breast malignancies in patients with BRCA mutations. Cancer 100:2079–2083. https://doi.org/10.1002/cncr.20221

Korteweg MA, Veldhuis WB, Visser F et al (2011) Feasibility of 7 Tesla breast magnetic resonance imaging determination of intrinsic sensitivity and high-resolution magnetic resonance imaging, diffusion-weighted imaging, and (1)H-magnetic resonance spectroscopy of breast cancer patients receiving neoadjuvant therapy. Invest Radiol 46:370–376. https://doi.org/10.1097/RLI.0b013e31820df706

Kuhl CK (2007a) Current status of breast MR imaging. Part 2. Clinical applications. Radiology 244:672–691. https://doi.org/10.1148/radiol.2443051661

Kuhl C (2007b) The current status of breast MR imaging. Part I. Choice of technique, image interpretation, diagnostic accuracy, and transfer to clinical practice. Radiology 244:356–378. https://doi.org/10.1148/radiol.2442051620

Kuhl CK (2007c) Breast MR imaging at 3T. Magn Reson Imaging Clin N Am 15:315–320, vi. https://doi.org/10.1016/j.mric.2007.08.003

Kuhl CK, Mielcareck P, Klaschik S et al (1999) Dynamic breast MR imaging: are signal intensity time course data useful for differential diagnosis of enhancing lesions? Radiology 211:101–110. https://doi.org/10.1148/radiology.211.1.r99ap38101

Kuhl CK, Jost P, Morakkabati N et al (2006) Contrast-enhanced MR imaging of the breast at 3.0 and 1.5 T in the same patients: initial experience. Radiology 239:666–676. https://doi.org/10.1148/radiol.2392050509

Kuhl CK, Schrading S, Strobel K et al (2014) Abbreviated breast magnetic resonance imaging (MRI): first postcontrast subtracted images and maximum-intensity projection-a novel approach to breast cancer screening with MRI. J Clin Oncol 32:2304–2310. https://doi.org/10.1200/JCO.2013.52.5386

Kuhl CK, Strobel K, Bieling H et al (2017) Supplemental breast MR imaging screening of women with average risk of breast cancer. Radiology 283:361–370. https://doi.org/10.1148/radiol.2016161444

Kul S, Cansu A, Alhan E et al (2011) Contribution of diffusion-weighted imaging to dynamic contrast-enhanced MRI in the characterization of breast tumors. AJR Am J Roentgenol 196:210–217. https://doi.org/10.2214/AJR.10.4258

Kurhanewicz J, Bok R, Nelson SJ, Vigneron DB (2008) Current and potential applications of clinical 13C MR spectroscopy. J Nucl Med 49:341–344. https://doi.org/10.2967/jnumed.107.045112

Le Bihan D, Breton E, Lallemand D et al (1988) Separation of diffusion and perfusion in intravoxel incoherent motion MR imaging. Radiology 168:497–505. https://doi.org/10.1148/radiology.168.2.3393671

Le Bihan D, Mangin JF, Poupon C et al (2001) Diffusion tensor imaging: concepts and applications. J Magn Reson Imaging 13:534–546

Leithner D, Moy L, Morris EA et al (2018) Abbreviated MRI of the breast: does it provide value? J Magn Reson Imaging. https://doi.org/10.1002/jmri.26291

Leithner D, Mayerhoefer ME, Martinez DF et al (2020) Non-invasive assessment of breast cancer molecular subtypes with multiparametric magnetic resonance imaging radiomics. J Clin Med 9(6):1853. https://doi.org/10.3390/jcm9061853

Li L, Wang K, Sun X et al (2015) Parameters of dynamic contrast-enhanced MRI as imaging markers for angiogenesis and proliferation in human breast cancer. Med Sci Monit 21:376–382. https://doi.org/10.12659/MSM.892534

Li H, Zhu Y, Burnside ES et al (2016a) Quantitative MRI radiomics in the prediction of molecular classifications of breast cancer subtypes in the TCGA/TCIA data set. NPJ Breast Cancer 2:16012. https://doi.org/10.1038/npjbcancer.2016.12

Li H, Zhu Y, Burnside ES et al (2016b) MR imaging radiomics signatures for predicting the risk of breast cancer recurrence as given by research versions of MammaPrint, Oncotype DX, and PAM50 gene assays. Radiology 281:382–391. https://doi.org/10.1148/radiol.2016152110

Liu C, Liang C, Liu Z et al (2013) Intravoxel incoherent motion (IVIM) in evaluation of breast lesions: comparison with conventional DWI. Eur J Radiol 82:e782–e789. https://doi.org/10.1016/j.ejrad.2013.08.006

Loffroy R, Chevallier O, Moulin M et al (2015) Current role of multiparametric magnetic resonance imaging for prostate cancer. Quant Imaging Med Surg 5:754–764. https://doi.org/10.3978/j.issn.2223-4292.2015.10.08

Lourenco AP, Donegan L, Khalil H, Mainiero MB (2014) Improving outcomes of screening breast MRI with practice evolution: initial clinical experience with 3T compared to 1.5T. J Magn Reson Imaging 39:535–539. https://doi.org/10.1002/jmri.24198

Lowry KP, Lee JM, Kong CY et al (2012) Annual screening strategies in BRCA1 and BRCA2 gene mutation carriers: a comparative effectiveness analysis. Cancer 118:2021–2030

Madelin G, Regatte RR (2013) Biomedical applications of sodium MRI in vivo. J Magn Reson Imaging 38:511–529. https://doi.org/10.1002/jmri.24168

Malich A, Fischer DR, Wurdinger S et al (2005) Potential MRI interpretation model: differentiation of benign from malignant breast masses. AJR Am J Roentgenol 185:964–970. https://doi.org/10.2214/AJR.04.1073

Mandelson MT, Oestreicher N, Porter PL et al (2000) Breast density as a predictor of mammographic detection: comparison of interval- and screen-detected cancers. J Natl Cancer Inst 92:1081–1087

Mango VL, Morris EA, David Dershaw D et al (2015) Abbreviated protocol for breast MRI: are multiple sequences needed for cancer detection? Eur J Radiol 84:65–70. https://doi.org/10.1016/j.ejrad.2014.10.004

Mann RM, Kuhl CK, Kinkel K, Boetes C (2008) Breast MRI: guidelines from the European Society of Breast Imaging. Eur Radiol 18:1307–1318. https://doi.org/10.1007/s00330-008-0863-7

Mann RM, Mus RD, van Zelst J et al (2014) A novel approach to contrast-enhanced breast magnetic resonance imaging for screening: high-resolution ultrafast dynamic imaging. Invest Radiol 49:579–585. https://doi.org/10.1097/RLI.0000000000000057

Mann RM, Balleyguier C, Baltzer PA et al (2015) Breast MRI: EUSOBI recommendations for women's information. Eur Radiol. https://doi.org/10.1007/s00330-015-3807-z

Marini C, Iacconi C, Giannelli M et al (2007) Quantitative diffusion-weighted MR imaging in the differential diagnosis of breast lesion. Eur Radiol 17:2646–2655. https://doi.org/10.1007/s00330-007-0621-2

Marino MA, Helbich T, Baltzer P, Pinker-Domenig K (2018a) Multiparametric MRI of the breast: a review. J Magn Reson Imaging 47:301–315. https://doi.org/10.1002/jmri.25790

Marino MA, Riedl CC, Bernathova M et al (2018b) Imaging phenotypes in women at high risk for breast cancer on mammography, ultrasound, and magnetic resonance imaging using the fifth edition of the breast imaging reporting and data system. Eur J Radiol 106:150–159. https://doi.org/10.1016/j.ejrad.2018.07.026

Marinovich ML, Houssami N, Macaskill P et al (2013) Meta-analysis of magnetic resonance imaging in detecting residual breast cancer after neoadjuvant therapy. J Natl Cancer Inst 105:321–333. https://doi.org/10.1093/jnci/djs528

Martincich L, Deantoni V, Bertotto I et al (2012) Correlations between diffusion-weighted imaging and breast cancer biomarkers. Eur Radiol 22:1519–1528. https://doi.org/10.1007/s00330-012-2403-8

Mazurowski MA, Zhang J, Grimm LJ et al (2014) Radiogenomic analysis of breast cancer: luminal B molecular subtype is associated with enhancement dynamics at MR imaging. Radiology 273:365–372. https://doi.org/10.1148/radiol.14132641

McDonald ES, Hammersley JA, Chou S-HS et al (2016) Performance of DWI as a rapid unenhanced technique for detecting mammographically occult breast cancer in elevated-risk women with dense breasts. AJR Am J Roentgenol 207:205–216. https://doi.org/10.2214/AJR.15.15873

Meisamy S, Bolan PJ, Baker EH et al (2005) Adding in vivo quantitative 1H MR spectroscopy to improve diagnostic accuracy of breast MR imaging: preliminary results of observer performance study at 4.0 T. Radiology 236:465–475. https://doi.org/10.1148/radiol.2362040836

Monticciolo DL, Newell MS, Moy L et al (2018) Breast cancer screening in women at higher-than-average risk: recommendations from the ACR. J Am Coll Radiol 15:408–414. https://doi.org/10.1016/j.jacr.2017.11.034

Moschetta M, Telegrafo M, Rella L et al (2016) Abbreviated combined MR protocol: a new faster strategy for characterizing breast lesions. Clin Breast Cancer 16:207–211. https://doi.org/10.1016/j.clbc.2016.02.008

Nasrallah FA, Pagès G, Kuchel PW et al (2013) Imaging brain deoxyglucose uptake and metabolism by glucoCEST MRI. J Cereb Blood Flow Metab 33:1270–1278. https://doi.org/10.1038/jcbfm.2013.79

Neto JAO, Parente DB (2013) Multiparametric magnetic resonance imaging of the prostate. Magn Reson Imaging Clin N Am 21:409–426. https://doi.org/10.1016/j.mric.2013.01.004

Nogueira L, Brandão S, Matos E et al (2014) Application of the diffusion kurtosis model for the study of breast lesions. Eur Radiol 24:1197–1203. https://doi.org/10.1007/s00330-014-3146-5

Olsen AH, Bihrmann K, Jensen M-B et al (2009) Breast density and outcome of mammography screening: a cohort study. Br J Cancer 100:1205–1208. https://doi.org/10.1038/sj.bjc.6604989

Ouwerkerk R (2011) Sodium MRI. Methods Mol Biol 711:175–201. https://doi.org/10.1007/978-1-61737-992-5_8

Padhani AR, Liu G, Koh DM et al (2009) Diffusion-weighted magnetic resonance imaging as a cancer biomarker: consensus and recommendations. Neoplasia 11:102–125

Park SH, Moon WK, Cho N et al (2010) Diffusion-weighted MR imaging: pretreatment prediction of response to neoadjuvant chemotherapy in patients with breast cancer. Radiology 257:56–63. https://doi.org/10.1148/radiol.10092021

Partridge SC, DeMartini WB, Kurland BF et al (2009) Quantitative diffusion-weighted imaging as an adjunct to conventional breast MRI for improved positive predictive value. AJR Am J Roentgenol 193:1716–1722. https://doi.org/10.2214/AJR.08.2139

Partridge SC, Ziadloo A, Murthy R et al (2010) Diffusion tensor MRI: preliminary anisotropy measures and mapping of breast tumors. J Magn Reson Imaging 31:339–347. https://doi.org/10.1002/jmri.22045

Pickles MD, Gibbs P, Lowry M, Turnbull LW (2006) Diffusion changes precede size reduction in neoadjuvant treatment of breast cancer. Magn Reson Imaging 24:843–847, https://doi.org/10.1016/j.mri.2005.11.005

Pinker K, Grabner G, Bogner W et al (2009) A combined high temporal and high spatial resolution 3 Tesla MR imaging protocol for the assessment of breast lesions: initial results. Invest Radiol 44:553–558. https://doi.org/10.1097/RLI.0b013e3181b4c127

Pinker K, Bickel H, Helbich TH et al (2013) Combined contrast-enhanced magnetic resonance and diffusion-weighted imaging reading adapted to the "Breast

Imaging Reporting and Data System" for multiparametric 3-T imaging of breast lesions. Eur Radiol 23:1791–1802. https://doi.org/10.1007/s00330-013-2771-8

Pinker K, Bogner W, Baltzer P et al (2014a) Improved differentiation of benign and malignant breast tumors with multiparametric 18fluorodeoxyglucose positron emission tomography magnetic resonance imaging: a feasibility study. Clin Cancer Res 20:3540–3549. https://doi.org/10.1158/1078-0432.CCR-13-2810

Pinker K, Bogner W, Baltzer P et al (2014b) Improved diagnostic accuracy with multiparametric magnetic resonance imaging of the breast using dynamic contrast-enhanced magnetic resonance imaging, diffusion-weighted imaging, and 3-dimensional proton magnetic resonance spectroscopic imaging. Invest Radiol 49:421–430. https://doi.org/10.1097/RLI.0000000000000029

Pinker K, Baltzer P, Bogner W et al (2015) Multiparametric MR imaging with high-resolution dynamic contrast-enhanced and diffusion-weighted imaging at 7 T improves the assessment of breast tumors: a feasibility study. Radiology 276:360–370. https://doi.org/10.1148/radiol.15141905

Pinker K, Moy L, Sutton EJ et al (2018a) Diffusion-weighted imaging with apparent diffusion coefficient mapping for breast cancer detection as a stand-alone parameter: comparison with dynamic contrast-enhanced and multiparametric magnetic resonance imaging. Invest Radiol. https://doi.org/10.1097/RLI.0000000000000465

Pinker K, Shitano F, Sala E et al (2018b) Background, current role, and potential applications of radiogenomics. J Magn Reson Imaging 47:604–620. https://doi.org/10.1002/jmri.25870

Pinker-Domenig K, Bogner W, Gruber S et al (2012) High resolution MRI of the breast at 3 T: which BI-RADS® descriptors are most strongly associated with the diagnosis of breast cancer? Eur Radiol 22:322–330. https://doi.org/10.1007/s00330-011-2256-6

Polanec SH, Pinker-Domenig K, Brader P et al (2016) Multiparametric MRI of the prostate at 3 T: limited value of 3D (1)H-MR spectroscopy as a fourth parameter. World J Urol 34:649–656. https://doi.org/10.1007/s00345-015-1670-9

Powell SN, Kachnic LA (2003) Roles of BRCA1 and BRCA2 in homologous recombination, DNA replication fidelity and the cellular response to ionizing radiation. Oncogene 22:5784–5791. https://doi.org/10.1038/sj.onc.1206678

Rahbar H, Partridge SC (2016) Multiparametric MR imaging of breast cancer. Magn Reson Imaging Clin N Am 24:223–238. https://doi.org/10.1016/j.mric.2015.08.012

Ramadan S, Arm J, Silcock J et al (2015) Lipid and metabolite deregulation in the breast tissue of women carrying BRCA1 and BRCA2 genetic mutations. Radiology 275:675–682. https://doi.org/10.1148/radiol.15140967

Richard R, Thomassin I, Chapellier M et al (2013) Diffusion-weighted MRI in pretreatment prediction of response to neoadjuvant chemotherapy in patients with breast cancer. Eur Radiol 23:2420–2431. https://doi.org/10.1007/s00330-013-2850-x

Riedl CC, Luft N, Bernhart C et al (2015) Triple-modality screening trial for familial breast cancer underlines the importance of magnetic resonance imaging and questions the role of mammography and ultrasound regardless of patient mutation status, age, and breast density. J Clin Oncol 33:1128–1135. https://doi.org/10.1200/JCO.2014.56.8626

Rivlin M, Horev J, Tsarfaty I, Navon G (2013) Molecular imaging of tumors and metastases using chemical exchange saturation transfer (CEST) MRI. Sci Rep 3:3045. https://doi.org/10.1038/srep03045

Saha A, Harowicz MR, Mazurowski MA (2018a) Breast cancer MRI radiomics: an overview of algorithmic features and impact of inter-reader variability in annotating tumors. Med Phys. https://doi.org/10.1002/mp.12925

Saha A, Harowicz MR, Wang W, Mazurowski MA (2018b) A study of association of Oncotype DX recurrence score with DCE-MRI characteristics using multivariate machine learning models. J Cancer Res Clin Oncol 144:799–807. https://doi.org/10.1007/s00432-018-2595-7

Sardanelli F, Boetes C, Borisch B et al (2010) Magnetic resonance imaging of the breast: recommendations from the EUSOMA working group. Eur J Cancer 46:1296–1316. https://doi.org/10.1016/j.ejca.2010.02.015

Sardanelli F, Podo F, Santoro F et al (2011) Multicenter surveillance of women at high genetic breast cancer risk using mammography, ultrasonography, and contrast-enhanced magnetic resonance imaging (the high breast cancer risk Italian 1 study): final results. Invest Radiol 46:94–105. https://doi.org/10.1097/RLI.0b013e3181f3fcdf

Schmitt B, Trattnig S, Schlemmer H-P (2012) CEST-imaging: a new contrast in MR-mammography by means of chemical exchange saturation transfer. Eur J Radiol 81(Suppl 1):S144–S146. https://doi.org/10.1016/S0720-048X(12)70060-8

Schrading S, Kuhl CK (2008) Mammographic, US, and MR imaging phenotypes of familial breast cancer. Radiology 246:58–70. https://doi.org/10.1148/radiol.2461062173

Sharma U, Danishad KKA, Seenu V, Jagannathan NR (2009a) Longitudinal study of the assessment by MRI and diffusion-weighted imaging of tumor response in patients with locally advanced breast cancer undergoing neoadjuvant chemotherapy. NMR Biomed 22:104–113. https://doi.org/10.1002/nbm.1245

Sharma U, Kumar M, Sah RG, Jagannathan NR (2009b) Study of normal breast tissue by in vivo volume localized proton MR spectroscopy: variation of water-fat ratio in relation to the heterogeneity of the breast and the menstrual cycle. Magn Reson Imaging 27:785–791. https://doi.org/10.1016/j.mri.2009.01.004

Sharma U, Baek HM, Su MY, Jagannathan NR (2011) In vivo 1H MRS in the assessment of the therapeutic response of breast cancer patients. NMR Biomed 24:700–711. https://doi.org/10.1002/nbm.1654

Shin HJ, Baek H-M, Cha JH, Kim HH (2012) Evaluation of breast cancer using proton MR spectroscopy: total choline peak integral and signal-to-noise ratio as prognostic indicators. AJR Am J Roentgenol 198:W488–W497. https://doi.org/10.2214/AJR.11.7292

Shin HJ, Chae EY, Choi WJ et al (2016) Diagnostic performance of fused diffusion-weighted imaging using unenhanced or postcontrast T1-weighted MR imaging in patients with breast cancer. Medicine (Baltimore) 95:e3502. https://doi.org/10.1097/MD.0000000000003502

Spick C, Pinker-Domenig K, Rudas M et al (2014) MRI only lesions: application of diffusion-weighted imaging obviates unnecessary MR-guided breast biopsies. Eur Radiol 24:1204–1210. https://doi.org/10.1007/s00330-014-3153-6

Spick C, Szolar DHM, Preidler KW et al (2015) Breast MRI used as a problem-solving tool reliably excludes malignancy. Eur J Radiol 84:61–64. https://doi.org/10.1016/j.ejrad.2014.10.005

Stadlbauer A, Zimmermann M, Bennani-Baiti B et al (2019) Development of a non-invasive assessment of hypoxia and neovascularization with magnetic resonance imaging in benign and malignant breast tumors: initial results. Mol Imaging Biol 21(4):758–770

Sun K, Chen X, Chai W et al (2015) Breast cancer: diffusion kurtosis MR imaging-diagnostic accuracy and correlation with clinical-pathologic factors. Radiology 277:46–55. https://doi.org/10.1148/radiol.15141625

Sutton EJ, Oh JH, Dashevsky BZ et al (2015) Breast cancer subtype intertumor heterogeneity: MRI-based features predict results of a genomic assay. J Magn Reson Imaging 42:1398–1406. https://doi.org/10.1002/jmri.24890

Tabár L, Vitak B, Chen TH-H et al (2011) Swedish two-county trial: impact of mammographic screening on breast cancer mortality during 3 decades. Radiology 260:658–663. https://doi.org/10.1148/radiol.11110469

Thakur SB, Bartella L, Ishill NM et al (2006) Comparisons of water-to-fat ratios in malignant, benign breast lesions, and normal breast parenchyma: an in vivo proton MRS study. In: Proceedings of the International Society for Magnetic Resonance in Medicine, p 2874

Thomassin-Naggara I, De Bazelaire C, Chopier J et al (2013) Diffusion-weighted MR imaging of the breast: advantages and pitfalls. Eur J Radiol 82:435–443. https://doi.org/10.1016/j.ejrad.2012.03.002

Tilanus-Linthorst M, Verhoog L, Obdeijn I-M et al (2002) A BRCA1/2 mutation, high breast density and prominent pushing margins of a tumor independently contribute to a frequent false-negative mammography. Int J Cancer 102:91–95. https://doi.org/10.1002/ijc.10666

Tilanus-Linthorst MMA, Kriege M, Boetes C et al (2005) Hereditary breast cancer growth rates and its impact on screening policy. Eur J Cancer 41:1610–1617. https://doi.org/10.1016/j.ejca.2005.02.034

Tofts PS, Kermode AG (1991) Measurement of the blood-brain barrier permeability and leakage space using dynamic MR imaging. 1. Fundamental concepts. Magn Reson Med 17:357–367

Tofts PS, Berkowitz B, Schnall MD (1995) Quantitative analysis of dynamic Gd-DTPA enhancement in breast tumors using a permeability model. Magn Reson Med 33:564–568

Torre LA, Siegel RL, Ward EM, Jemal A (2016) Global cancer incidence and mortality rates and trends—an update. Cancer Epidemiol Biomarkers Prev 25:16–27. https://doi.org/10.1158/1055-9965.EPI-15-0578

Trimboli RM, Verardi N, Cartia F et al (2014) Breast cancer detection using double reading of unenhanced MRI including T1-weighted, T2-weighted STIR, and diffusion-weighted imaging: a proof of concept study. AJR Am J Roentgenol 203:674–681. https://doi.org/10.2214/AJR.13.11816

Tsushima Y, Takahashi-Taketomi A, Endo K (2009) Magnetic resonance (MR) differential diagnosis of breast tumors using apparent diffusion coefficient (ADC) on 1.5-T. J Magn Reson Imaging 30:249–255. https://doi.org/10.1002/jmri.21854

Turkbey B, Mani H, Aras O et al (2013) Prostate cancer: can multiparametric MR imaging help identify patients who are candidates for active surveillance? Radiology 268:144–152. https://doi.org/10.1148/radiol.13121325

Uematsu T (2015) Focal breast edema associated with malignancy on T2-weighted images of breast MRI: peritumoral edema, prepectoral edema, and subcutaneous edema. Breast Cancer 22:66–70. https://doi.org/10.1007/s12282-014-0572-9

Uematsu T, Kasami M, Yuen S (2009) Triple-negative breast cancer: correlation between MR imaging and pathologic findings. Radiology 250:638–647. https://doi.org/10.1148/radiol.2503081054

Valdora F, Houssami N, Rossi F et al (2018) Rapid review: radiomics and breast cancer. Breast Cancer Res Treat. https://doi.org/10.1007/s10549-018-4675-4

van de Bank BL, Voogt IJ, Italiaander M et al (2013) Ultra high spatial and temporal resolution breast imaging at 7T. NMR Biomed 26:367–375. https://doi.org/10.1002/nbm.2868

Vaughan JT, Garwood M, Collins CM et al (2001) 7T vs. 4T: RF power, homogeneity, and signal-to-noise comparison in head images. Magn Reson Med 46:24–30

Veltman J, Mann R, Kok T et al (2008) Breast tumor characteristics of BRCA1 and BRCA2 gene mutation carriers on MRI. Eur Radiol 18:931–938. https://doi.org/10.1007/s00330-008-0851-y

Ward KM, Aletras AH, Balaban RS (2000) A new class of contrast agents for MRI based on proton chemical exchange dependent saturation transfer (CEST). J Magn Reson 143:79–87. https://doi.org/10.1006/jmre.1999.1956

Woodhams R, Matsunaga K, Iwabuchi K et al (2005) Diffusion-weighted imaging of malignant breast tumors: the usefulness of apparent diffusion coefficient (ADC) value and ADC map for the detection of malignant breast tumors and evaluation of cancer extension. J Comput Assist Tomogr 29:644–649

Woodhams R, Kakita S, Hata H et al (2010) Identification of residual breast carcinoma following neoadjuvant chemotherapy: diffusion-weighted imaging—comparison with contrast-enhanced MR imaging and pathologic findings. Radiology 254:357–366. https://doi.org/10.1148/radiol.2542090405

Woodhams R, Ramadan S, Stanwell P et al (2011) Diffusion-weighted imaging of the breast: principles and clinical applications. Radiographics 31:1059–1084. https://doi.org/10.1148/rg.314105160

Yabuuchi H, Matsuo Y, Sunami S et al (2011) Detection of non-palpable breast cancer in asymptomatic women by using unenhanced diffusion-weighted and T2-weighted MR imaging: comparison with mammography and dynamic contrast-enhanced MR imaging. Eur Radiol 21:11–17. https://doi.org/10.1007/s00330-010-1890-8

Yamaguchi K, Abe H, Newstead GM et al (2015) Intratumoral heterogeneity of the distribution of kinetic parameters in breast cancer: comparison based on the molecular subtypes of invasive breast cancer. Breast Cancer 22:496–502. https://doi.org/10.1007/s12282-013-0512-0

Yamamoto S, Maki DD, Korn RL, Kuo MD (2012) Radiogenomic analysis of breast cancer using MRI: a preliminary study to define the landscape. AJR Am J Roentgenol 199:654–663. https://doi.org/10.2214/AJR.11.7824

Zaric O, Pinker K, Zbyn S et al (2016) Quantitative sodium MR imaging at 7 T: initial results and comparison with diffusion-weighted imaging in patients with breast tumors. Radiology 280(1):39–48. https://doi.org/10.1148/radiol.2016151304

Zierhut ML, Yen Y-F, Chen AP et al (2010) Kinetic modeling of hyperpolarized 13C1-pyruvate metabolism in normal rats and TRAMP mice. J Magn Reson 202:85–92. https://doi.org/10.1016/j.jmr.2009.10.003

MRI-Guided Breast Interventions

Karim Rebeiz and Elizabeth Morris

Contents

1   **Introduction** 260

2   **Breast MRI-Guided Biopsy** 260
    2.1   Indications 260
    2.2   Pre-procedure 260
    2.3   Procedure 264

3   **MRI-Guided Wire Localization** 267

4   **MRI-Guided Percutaneous Ablative Treatment** ... 268
    4.1   Radiofrequency Ablation (RFA) 268
    4.2   Laser Interstitial Thermal Therapy (LITT) 268
    4.3   Cryoablation (Pediconi et al. 2018; Gombos et al. 2015) 268
    4.4   High-Intensity Focused Ultrasound Ablation (HIFU) 269

5   **Conclusion** 269

References 269

Abstract

Magnetic resonance imaging (MRI) is an integral part of breast imaging due to its high sensitivity in identifying malignancy and high-risk lesions (0.88–0.92, 95% confidence interval) (Mcgrath et al., J Magn Reson Imaging 46(3):631–645, https://doi.org/10.1002/jmri.25738, 2017) and its comparability in positive predictive value to that of conventional imaging (15–30%). However, its specificity is lower (0.67–0.77, 95% confidence interval) (Mcgrath et al., J Magn Reson Imaging 46(3):631–645, https://doi.org/10.1002/jmri.25738, 2017; Myers et al., Clin Breast Cancer 15(2):143–152, https://doi.org/10.1016/j.clbc.2014.11.003, 2015) due to an overlap in imaging characteristics between benign and malignant lesions. Histologic sampling is therefore sometimes needed.

K. Rebeiz (✉)
Department of Radiology, Memorial Sloan Kettering Cancer Center, New York, NY, USA
e-mail: rebeizk@mskcc.org

E. Morris
Department of Radiology, UC Davis Health, Sacramento, CA, USA
e-mail: eamorris@ucdavis.edu

© Springer Nature Switzerland AG 2022
M. Fuchsjäger et al. (eds.), *Breast Imaging*, Medical Radiology Diagnostic Imaging,
https://doi.org/10.1007/978-3-030-94918-1_12

1 Introduction

Magnetic resonance imaging (MRI) is an integral part of breast imaging due to its high sensitivity in identifying malignancy and high-risk lesions (0.88–0.92, 95% confidence interval) (Mcgrath et al. 2017) and its comparability in positive predictive value to that of conventional imaging (15–30%). However, its specificity is lower (0.67–0.77, 95% confidence interval) (Mcgrath et al. 2017; Myers et al. 2015) due to an overlap in imaging characteristics between benign and malignant lesions. Histologic sampling is therefore sometimes needed.

Often, suspicious lesions on MRI cannot be found on ultrasound and mammogram, the cheaper and more readily available modalities. Ultrasound correlates are found and biopsied in only half of the cases, usually a mass >10 mm, a lesion categorized as BI-RADS 5 or located in the axilla (Gombos et al. 2015; Meissnitzer et al. 2009; Abe et al. 2010). In addition, non-mass enhancement only at times is correlated to an overlooked area of microcalcifications on mammogram (Mcgrath et al. 2017; Papalouka et al. 2018). Moreover, in a recent study conducted by Lee et al. (2018) with percutaneous sampling of presumed ultrasound correlates to suspicious lesions identified by MRI, the correlate was only accurate in 26% of cases, and 10% of these discordant cases ultimately revealed malignancy (Lee et al. 2018). This chapter focuses on detailing the technique and approach to MRI-guided breast interventions, specifically biopsies, but also wire localization and cancer ablation treatment options.

2 Breast MRI-Guided Biopsy

2.1 Indications

A suspicious mass, unique focus, non-mass enhancement on MRI not reliably identified on mammogram or ultrasound is an indication for MRI-guided biopsy (Papalouka et al. 2018).

Once a lesion is detected on MRI, it is imperative to correlate with mammography and perform targeted focal ultrasound. Suspicious non-mass enhancement usually does not have a correlate on ultrasound.

A sonographic correlate is more likely to be found when the lesion is larger than 10 mm, categorized as BI-RADS 5, or located within the axilla, rendering it more accessible with ultrasound (Mcgrath et al. 2017).

If the lesion is identified on focal ultrasound, an ultrasound-guided biopsy will be performed as it provides improved operator flexibility and patient comfort.

2.2 Pre-procedure

2.2.1 Patient Preparation, Counseling, and Consent

Patients should be interviewed, and medical records assessed prior to the MRI-guided biopsy to ensure success and appropriateness. Anxiety, allergies, coagulopathies, medications, presence of MRI-incompatible implanted device, status of pregnancy and lactation, and renal disease are key points to take into account.

Patient anxiety and motion artifacts can lead to repositioning, prolonged procedure time, and procedure termination (Mcgrath et al. 2017; Bhole and Neuschler 2015; Santiago et al. 2018; Gombos et al. 2015). To improve the success of the procedure, the procedure is discussed with the patient in detail. Anxiolytics such as lorazepam 1 mg tablets, 1–2 h before the MRI-guided biopsy appointment, can be prescribed for anxious or claustrophobic patients who cannot tolerate the scan. A second tablet can be administered if the patient is still anxious immediately before going into the scanner.

In patients with allergy to gadolinium or lidocaine (Mcgrath et al. 2017; Bhole and Neuschler 2015; Santiago et al. 2018), premedication can be performed with methylprednisolone 32 mg PO administered at 12 h and 2 h before contrast and diphenhydramine 50 mg PO/IV/IM 1 h before contrast injection.

Bleeding disorders and anticoagulant medication are associated with increased risk of hematoma and bruising. For patients on warfarin, vacuum-assisted biopsy can be performed if INR is within the therapeutic range (Somerville et al. 2008; British Society of Radiology n.d.). For patients at high or intermediate risk of thromboembolic events where stopping anticoagulation is preferred, supervised bridge therapy with short-acting injectable blood thinners may be considered. Antiplatelets such as aspirin and clopidogrel do not need to be discontinued (Santiago et al. 2018).

The patient should be evaluated for pregnancy. MRI-guided procedures are not deemed appropriate in pregnancy due to the need of IV contrast administration (Expert Panel on Breast Imaging 2018; Vashi et al. 2013). Gadolinium contrast-enhanced MRI scans at any time during pregnancy may be associated with an increased risk of a broad set of disorders, including rheumatological, inflammatory, or skin conditions, and, possibly, with stillbirth and neonatal death (Ray et al. 2016).

MRI-guided breast biopsy is not contraindicated in lactating women (Expert Panel on Breast Imaging 2018; Vashi et al. 2013). There is a slightly increased risk of bleeding and infection due to the increased breast vascularization and ductal dilatation associated with pregnancy and lactation (Expert Panel on Breast Imaging 2018; Vashi et al. 2013). There is a small risk of milk fistula formation (Expert Panel on Breast Imaging 2018; Vashi et al. 2013). After the biopsy, blood and lidocaine may be present in the breast milk. Pumping and discarding milk from the affected breast for up to 12–24 h may be performed (Vashi et al. 2013).

Presence of renal disease with a GFR rate <30 mL/min/1.73 m^2 may be a contraindication for gadolinium-based contrast administration due to an increased risk of nephrogenic systemic fibrosis (Expert Panel on Urologic Imaging 2021). This is especially true with linear nonionic or older linear ionic gadolinium-based contrast agents (Khawaja et al. 2015).

At the time of interview, the patient is asked about implanted devices. Presence of non-MRI-safe devices such as metallic implants, aneurysm clips, or MR-incompatible pacemakers is a contraindication to MRI.

The procedure, risks, benefits, and alternatives are discussed with the patient. Risks and complication rates are low. The patient must be instructed to avoid driving on the day of the procedure and be accompanied. Infection, pain, bruising, bleeding, possible injury to adjacent structures, and possibility of scarring are discussed with the patient (Santiago et al. 2018). In addition, the biopsy-marking clip purpose and placement and post-biopsy mammograms are discussed (Mcgrath et al. 2017; Bhole and Neuschler 2015). Lastly, the radiologist should discuss the possibility of termination of the procedure, should the target not be visualized with contrast administration.

After assessing relevant medical records, interviewing the patient, discussing the procedure with the patient, and properly identifying the patient and the site of biopsy, the consent is signed.

The procedure and potential risks should be discussed while avoiding the use of complex medical jargon. For example, the following can be used: "Your radiologist has recommended that you have an MRI-guided breast biopsy to take samples of tissue from your breast and examine them for cancer. You will first have an MRI done to find the exact area of your breast to biopsy. An MRI is a test that uses strong magnetic fields and injected contrast to take pictures of the inside of your body. Once the area to biopsy is found, your radiologist will insert a thin needle into your breast and remove a sample of tissue or cells. The sample is then checked for cancer. A tiny clip will be placed for reference. After your biopsy, you will have a mammogram" (MRI-guided breast biopsy n.d.).

2.2.2 Equipment

A magnet strength of 1.5T or higher is recommended. A phased array dedicated breast coil, which has open access to the lateral and/or medial aspect of the breasts, is used (Papalouka et al. 2018).

A vacuum-assisted device is utilized to maximize the volume of tissue and ensure adequate sample size. The vacuum console itself is not MRI compatible, only the foot pedal and biopsy driver can be brought into the MRI suite (Bhole and Neuschler 2015). A grid is used with a pillar and post system for localization. The grid is a plastic panel made of uniformly spaced square openings, which will receive the needle guide and allow access to the breast (Fig. 1a, b). The pillar and positioning device has medial and lateral compression plates, a needle guide (Fig. 1c, d) for placing the fiducial marker, and a needle sleeve (Taneja et al. 2010). A T1 hyperintense fiducial or vitamin E marker (black arrows in Fig. 1a, b) is placed within one of the grid's openings and acts as a reference to determine the optimal position for the needle guide and the needle entry site (Mcgrath et al. 2017; Santiago et al. 2018; Gombos et al. 2015).

The MRI-guided biopsy kit consists of a coaxial system that is MR compatible (Fig. 2). The outer component consists of a plastic introducer sheath with depth gradation, and a small surrounding mobile depth marker. The inner component is a metallic, sharp, introducer stylet, which can be interchanged with a plastic obturator (Mcgrath et al. 2017; Bhole and Neuschler 2015; Santiago et al. 2018). The biopsy needle gauge and size will depend on the tissue, lesion size, and depth. In general, a beveled-tip large 9–14 G needle is used (Bhole and Neuschler 2015; Gombos et al. 2015; Ghate et al. 2006; Orel et al. 2006; Meeuwis et al. 2012; Papalouka et al. 2018).

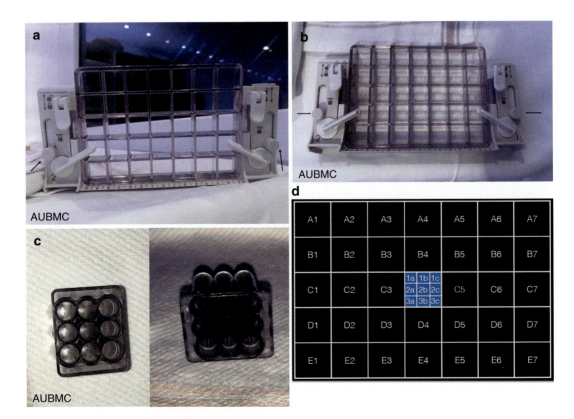

Fig. 1 (**a, b**) Grid with uniformly spaced square openings and two fiducial markers (black arrows) as well as a needle guide (**c**). The needle guide is made of multiple short tunnels. It fits into a predetermined square in the grid (**d**), and the coaxial system fits into one of the tunnels in the needle guide allowing accurate direct targeting of the lesion. (**d**) Schematic representation of the needle guide within the grid

MRI-Guided Breast Interventions

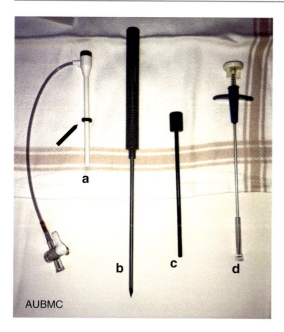

Fig. 2 MRI-guided breast biopsy kit: (**a**) plastic introducer sheath with mobile depth marker (black arrow); (**b**) metallic sharp introducer stylet; (**c**) plastic obturator; (**d**) clip marker

2.2.3 Imaging Protocol

The adapted sequences may vary between institutions, but the common goal is to minimize the image acquisition and procedure time without compromising lesion visualization and image quality (Santiago et al. 2018; Gombos et al. 2015). The most commonly used protocol includes an initial triplane localizer sequence followed by pre-contrast fat-saturated T1W images in the sagittal plane. These initial images help ensure the area with the target lesion, the grid, and fiducial markers are all included in the field of view. Dynamic post-contrast fat saturation T1W images with subtractions are then performed. A gadolinium-based contrast agent (GBCAs) is administered intravenously as a bolus with standard dosing by weight of 0.1 mmol/kg followed by a saline flush of at least 10 mL (American College of Radiology 2016). If a single post-contrast scan is acquired, the scan time should not extend beyond 4 min after bolus injection (American College of Radiology 2016). Slice thickness of 3 mm or less is preferred (Gombos et al. 2015). CAD localization software is optional, but knowledge of manual calculation of the index lesion is essential.

	LOC	Sagittal T1 pre	Sagittal T1 post
Generic sequence name	3-PLANE	VIBRANT	VIBRANT
Plane		Sagittal	Sagittal
Options		ASSET	ASSET
Field of view (cm)	48	22–24	22–24
Slice thickness (mm)	12	3	3
Gap (mm)	0	0	0
Saturation pulse		FAT	FAT
TE1/TE2	80	4.2	4.2
TR			
Flip angle		10	10
Bandwidth (kHz)	83	83.3	83.3
ETL			
NEX		1	1
Phase encoding steps	128	320	320
Frequency steps	128	320	320
Frequency direction			A/P
Comments		ISOTROPIC	ISOTROPIC

2.3 Procedure

2.3.1 Planning

Prior diagnostic MR images are reviewed to assess the location of the target lesion including the lesion depth and distance from the nipple and midline in all three planes. These parameters dictate the side and approach of the biopsy. Anatomical landmarks aid in localizing the lesion during the pre-contrast biopsy images (Mcgrath et al. 2017). In addition, prior mammograms are assessed for biopsy clips in order to choose a different clip shape for the upcoming procedure.

It is important that, when sampling more than one lesion, the most suspicious lesion should be biopsied first. Planning for multiple biopsies should be done beforehand (Mcgrath et al. 2017; Santiago et al. 2018).

2.3.2 Positioning (Fig. 3a, b)

The patient lies in the prone position, and the targeted breast is compressed to provide immobility and reproducibility of prior diagnostic imaging. The breast is adequately compressed to stabilize the breast and the needle (Mcgrath et al. 2017; Bhole and Neuschler 2015; Santiago et al. 2018; Gombos et al. 2015). Excessive compression will lead to decreased blood and contrast flow to the lesion. Too little or loose compression will increase the risk of ill-positioned needle and skin tenting.

The positioning of the patient's arms must take into consideration the target lesion depth and subjacent tissues (Mcgrath et al. 2017; Santiago et al. 2018). If the lesion is posterior, the arms are set down alongside the body. This will help relax the pectoralis muscle and allow more tissue to fall dependently into the coil (Mcgrath et al. 2017).

If the lesion is too close to the pectoralis muscle, the arms can be positioned over the head to lift the muscle out of the grid and keep the breast parenchyma behind. This allows greater separation of the lesion from the muscle and makes it more accessible (Mcgrath et al. 2017).

If the lesion is anterior or periareolar, the distance from the nipple is evaluated to estimate whether the lesion will be included within the positioning device before image acquisition (Bhole and Neuschler 2015).

The breast can be approached from the lateral or the medial side, whichever allows the shortest distance from the skin to the index lesion. The grid is placed on the side of the predicted approach, and the marker is placed on the skin (vitamin E vs. fiducial). The skin should be marked where the marker is set.

2.3.3 Imaging

After the pre-contrast images are acquired, comparison with prior diagnostic MR images is performed, and positioning is readjusted accordingly. The breast fibroglandular/fat interface can be used as the landmark to deduce the location of the lesion on the precontract images. Gadolinium-based contrast is then administered, and images are acquired within the first 2 min (Fig. 4a–c).

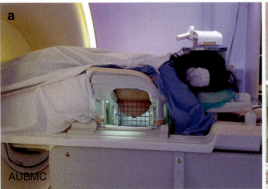
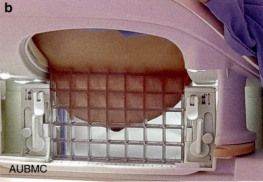

Fig. 3 (**a**, **b**) Patient lying prone with the targeted breast compressed against the grid

MRI-Guided Breast Interventions

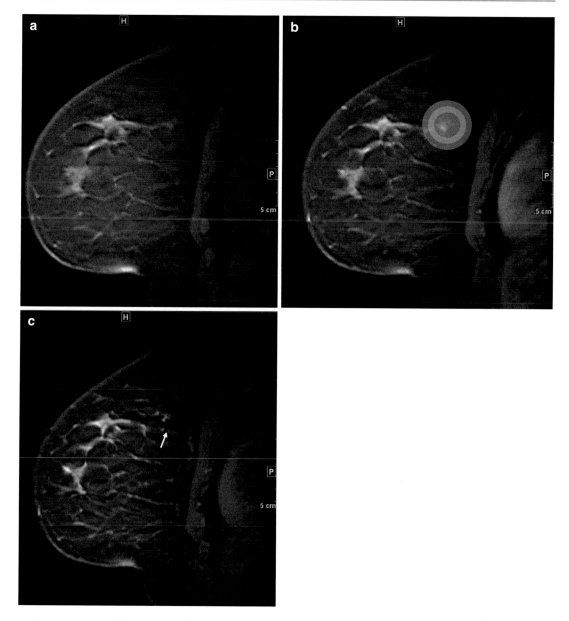

Fig. 4 Pre-contrast (**a**), post-contrast (**b**), and post-biopsy sagittal T1-weighted images of the breast. (**b**) Demonstrates a focus of enhancement (yellow border circle) corresponding to the target lesion with post-biopsy changes (white arrow, **c**)

2.3.4 Localization

After the enhancing lesion is visualized, the biopsy entry point is calculated using the CAD or the manual approach. The X and Y axes indicate the needle entry site, and Z-axis indicates the lesion depth. Either a manual approach or a digital technique can be used.

For the manual approach, the operator scrolls from the lesion to the skin surface (identified by visualization of the grid and fiducial marker). This will determine the number of slices/depth (Z-axis) and the appropriate grid square and needle guide tunnel to enter the skin (X- and Y-axis) (Mcgrath et al. 2017).

The number of slices from the skin to the lesion is then multiplied by the slice thickness of acquisition (3 mm in our institution). For example, a lesion that is 7 slices away from the fiducial marker would be 2.1 cm deep. Some setups require an additional 2 cm to be added to the calculated depth to account for the length of the tunneled needle guide (Mcgrath et al. 2017; Bhole and Neuschler 2015).

For the digital technique, the fiducial serves as a reference, and the lesion is marked on a dedicated software which then calculates the entry point (X and Y) as well as depth (Z) (Mcgrath et al. 2017; Santiago et al. 2018).

If the patient is oriented headfirst in the MRI scanner, the chest wall is at the 12 o'clock position, the nipple is at the 6 o'clock, and the orientation of the head is at the 3 o'clock (Bhole and Neuschler 2015).

If the target lesion is not visualized, the equipment including coil or contrast injection pump should first be checked for failure. The patient should also be examined for contrast extravasation. If this initial evaluation is unrevealing, breast compression should be lessened and delayed and subtracted images obtained. Both axial and sagittal views should be obtained.

If the lesion is still not visualized, the ACR recommends short-term MRI follow-up in 3–6 months (Mcgrath et al. 2017). In a study by Niell et al. where 445 lesions were biopsied, 13% of the procedures were aborted due to non-visualization of biopsy target. In their population, 10% of these patients who were followed ultimately were diagnosed with a malignancy (Niell et al. 2014). In another study by Pinnamaneni et al., the malignancy rate in an aborted biopsy due to non-visualization was much lower, at 1.9% (Pinnamaneni et al. 2018). Lastly, in a third retrospective trial by Brennan et al., with 907 patients, 8% of biopsies were aborted due to non-visualization, and the cancer detection rate in this population was similar at 2% (Brennan et al. 2011).

2.3.5 Biopsy

The vacuum-assisted breast biopsy (VABB) device must be flushed ahead of the procedure to ensure the elimination of air bubbles which would otherwise produce susceptibility artifact (Mcgrath et al. 2017; Bhole and Neuschler 2015). The skin is then marked

and cleansed with betadine or chlorhexidine at the predetermined entry site. Afterwards, superficial and deep local anesthesia is injected, ensuring that a wheel is performed and adequate time is given for the anesthesia to take effect. A superficial skin incision is sometimes needed. The introducer stylet is then inserted into the plastic introducer sheath and advanced through the skin using the "push and twist" technique until the correct predetermined depth is reached as indicated by the stopper on the plastic introducer sheath (Fig. 5a) (Mcgrath et al. 2017; Bhole and Neuschler 2015). The "push and twist" technique decreases the risk of "skin tenting" and the "snowplow effect." "Snowplowing" occurs when the breast tissue and the target lesion are pushed away from the needle tip as the needle advances deeper (Mcgrath et al. 2017). This effect is worse with dense breast and suboptimal compression.

The cutting stylet is then replaced with the plastic obturator (Fig. 5b). T1-weighted sequences are then reacquired to ensure that the introducer/obturator tip is subjacent to the lesion, ideally within the center of a large lesion or proximal margin of a small lesion. Once the target position has been confirmed, the plastic obturator is replaced by the biopsy device (Fig. 5c), and sampling can be performed (Santiago et al. 2018).

2.3.6 Sampling

In general, 12 samples about the clockface or directed in the region of the lesion usually suffices for proper histological analysis (Bhole and Neuschler 2015). Placing the tip in or too close to a small lesion may result in biopsy firing beyond the lesion and the sampling notch incompletely covering the target site. This is less of a concern for larger lesions. Once all samples have been obtained, post-biopsy images are obtained to confirm adequate sampling of the target lesion. The biopsy site is then irrigated and suctioned to minimize the risk of post-biopsy hematoma (Mcgrath et al. 2017). A biopsy clip of unique shape is placed to avoid confusion with prior clips (Fig. 5d).

2.3.7 Post-biopsy Care

As soon as the biopsy system is removed, compression is administered to minimize hematoma formation and bleeding. It should be applied for 10–15 min. A post-biopsy mammogram confirms

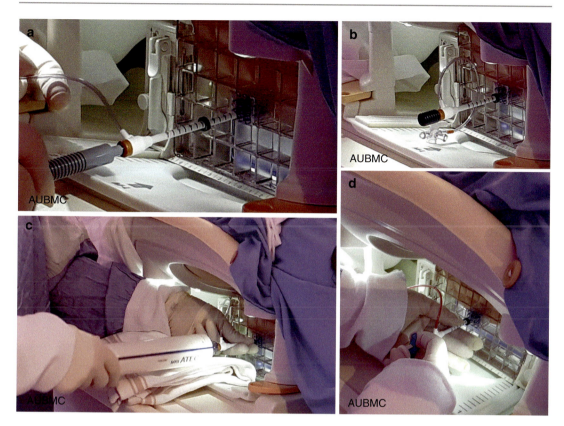

Fig. 5 The metallic cutting stylet (**a**) is first mounted into the sheath, and the entire coaxial system is introduced into the predetermined tunnel of the needle guide. Once the appropriate depth is reached, the cutting stylet is exchanged for the obturator (**b**). The sample is then obtained using a VAB device (**c**). After the biopsy, repeat imaging is performed to ensure adequate sampling of the target lesion, and a clip marker (**d**) is deployed

deployment and position of biopsy clip. If a hematoma has formed and the patient does not have a supportive bra, an ACE bandage can be considered (Bhole and Neuschler 2015). If bleeding does not stop, additional compression and epinephrine injection usually suffice. Sometimes, the hematoma may be aspirated with a large-gauge needle or small catheter.

2.3.8 Assessment of Sampling Accuracy and Technical Limitations

Imaging evaluation of the biopsied region by MRI guidance is limited by several factors (Mcgrath et al. 2017; Bhole and Neuschler 2015; Santiago et al. 2018).

When compared to ultrasound-guided biopsy, real-time visual confirmation of the needle targeting the lesion is not possible. Moreover, in post images, the contrast will be washed out, and additionally blood, air, and biopsy clip susceptibility further obscure the biopsied region (Mcgrath et al. 2017). As such, 7–9% of MRI-guided biopsies result in discordant imaging-pathologic results, requiring repeat biopsy (Mcgrath et al. 2017).

3 MRI-Guided Wire Localization

Similar to mammography guide wire localization, MRI guidance is performed to evaluate the disease extent in the preoperative setting. Patient preparation, risks, and procedural planning are similar to the MRI-guided biopsy. After identifying the lesion, a hollow needle with a loaded MRI-compatible wire is placed at the targeted depth. When the position is established, the wire is deployed into the lesion (Mcgrath et al. 2017; Santiago et al. 2018).

4 MRI-Guided Percutaneous Ablative Treatment

Local regional treatment of breast cancer is evolving. Previously, mastectomy, either radical or modified radical, was the mainstay of the treatment of breast cancer. Although this remains appropriate for some patients, breast conservation has become the method of choice in many patients in achieving both optimal cosmetic results and minimal rates of in-breast recurrences after treatment. In the exploration of less invasive techniques, imaging-guided ablation treatments are a promising emerging alternative to surgical resection in select cases with fewer complications, better cosmetic outcome, and less patient discomfort. A potential usage can be considered for the control of local tumor growth, as palliative therapy or in patients who are poor surgical candidates (Pediconi et al. 2018) (Chapter "Minimal Invasive Therapy").

The purpose of these procedures is to achieve irreversible cell damage while sparing the overlying and surrounding tissues (Gombos et al. 2015). Both ultrasound and MRI can be used, with MRI best equipped to include the extent of disease and monitor the ablation progress (Pediconi et al. 2018; Gombos et al. 2015). The most commonly used and studied techniques are the minimally invasive radiofrequency ablation (RFA), laser-induced thermal therapy (LITT), cryoablation therapy, and noninvasive high-intensity focused ultrasound (HIFU) ablation. RFA, LITT, and HIFU rely on hyperthermic ablation, while cryoablation uses freezing temperatures (Pediconi et al. 2018; Gombos et al. 2015). At this time, surgery remains the mainstay of treatment. MRI-guided ablative procedures are currently only used in clinical trials and specific institutions.

4.1 Radiofrequency Ablation (RFA)

Performed under ultrasound or MRI guidance, this procedure relies on high-frequency alternating current being delivered via needle electrodes. The needle is introduced at the target lesion, and the increase in temperature results in cellular damage and coagulation necrosis (Pediconi et al. 2018; Gombos et al. 2015). Ultrasound-guided RFA faces many technical limitations resulting from the hyperechogenicity of the heated breast tissue and shadowing artifact from gas bubbles formed during ablation. These issues can be overcome with the use of MRI instead. Studies demonstrated a reliable correlation between tumor ablation volume on MRI images and histopathologic analysis (Pediconi et al. 2018; Vilar et al. 2012).

On post-ablation contrast-enhanced MRI, the viable residual tumor appears as an irregular or nodular enhancement at the ablation margin, and necrosis correlates with non-perfused tissue or fluid collection surrounded by an enhancing rim of reactive hyperemia. Skin burn and injury to the pectoralis muscle are the most common complications and described in up to 5% of cases (Pediconi et al. 2018; Vilar et al. 2012).

4.2 Laser Interstitial Thermal Therapy (LITT)

LITT relies on MRI-compatible cooled optic fibers percutaneously inserted into the target lesion to deliver laser-generated ablative heat and tissue necrosis. Target tissue temperature reaches 60 °C for up to 20 min. This results in a centrally necrotic cavity surrounded by pale tissue and an external hemorrhagic rim (Pediconi et al. 2018; Gombos et al. 2015). The optic fibers used in LITT can be placed through the outer cannula of a breast biopsy needle, allowing it to be directly performed following a breast biopsy. Potential complications include skin burn and gaseous rupture of the tumor.

Some institutions have successfully applied LITT for the treatment of benign fibroadenomas (Gombos et al. 2015; Lai et al. 1999; Harms et al. 1999).

4.3 Cryoablation (Pediconi et al. 2018; Gombos et al. 2015)

In contrast to RFA and LITT, cryoablation uses hypothermia. Tissue ablation is achieved through rapid decrease in temperature (from −187 to −70 °C) using the Joule-Thomson effect with argon gas needle probes or cooled liquid nitrogen probes. Tissue freezing leads to rapid formation of intra- and extracellular ice crystals that lead to mechanical damage and disruption of the microcirculation. In a study by Roubidoux et al., 78% of treated patients had no residual disease following resection and histopathologic examination (Pediconi et al. 2018). Another study conducted by Morin et al. (Gombos et al. 2015; Morin et al. 2004) found that almost 50% of treated tumors achieved total ablation on surgical excision specimens performed 4 weeks following the ablation. The targeted zone for cryoablation must be larger than the lesion size. The ice ball will appear as a signal void on MRI due to T2*-shortening effect. Post-therapy local swelling and ecchymosis are common and resolve within 2–3 weeks. A palpable lump resolves slowly over time.

4.4 High-Intensity Focused Ultrasound Ablation (HIFU)

HIFU ablation is a noninvasive external transducer that generates sonic waves. The piezoelectric transducer located inside the MRI table generates an ultrasound beam (1.5 MHz) that is focused on the target lesion, which can be up to 20 cm deep. The target area is subjected to a rapid elevation in temperature (56–90 °C for 10–20 s), resulting in coagulative necrosis (Pediconi et al. 2018; Gombos et al. 2015). In addition, gas bubbles are created by the ultrasound property of compression and rarefaction of the tissue also known as mechanical cavitation mechanism. Those microbubbles are compressed and expanded by the ultrasound wave and cause cell damage, thus increasing the overall ablation efficiency (Gombos et al. 2015). On imaging, the ablated region will appear as a sharp circumscribed, elliptical lesion with a volume of 50–300 mm.

5 Conclusion

The role of MRI-guided interventions in the field of breast imaging has become strongly established over the past few years. Adequate in-depth knowledge, understanding, and training in MRI-guided breast biopsy procedure are of utmost importance for every breast radiologist in order to ensure satisfactory and diagnostic sampling and treatment as appropriate of all suspicious lesions that are mammographically and sonographically occult.

References

Abe H et al (2010) MR-directed ("second-look") ultrasound examination for breast lesions detected initially on MRI: MR and sonographic findings. AJR Am J Roentgenol 194(2):370–377

American College of Radiology (2016) ACR Practice parameter for the performance of Magnetic Resonance; Image-guided breast interventional procedures. https://www.acr.org/-/media/ACR/Files/Practice-Parameters/MR-Guided-Breast.pdf

Bhole S, Neuschler E (2015) MRI-guided breast interventions. Appl Radiol 44(10):7–13

Brennan SB, Sung JS, Dershaw DD, Liberman L, Morris EA (2011) Cancellation of MR imaging-guided breast biopsy due to lesion nonvisualization: frequency and follow-up. Radiology 261(1):92–99. https://doi.org/10.1148/radiol.11100720

British Society of Radiology (n.d.) Guidelines for performing breast and axillary biopsies in patients on anticoagulant and anti-platelet therapy

Expert Panel on Breast Imaging et al (2018) ACR Appropriateness Criteria for breast imaging of pregnant and lactating women. J Am Coll Radiol 15(11S):S263–S275

Expert Panel on Urologic Imaging et al (2021) ACR Appropriateness Criteria® renal failure. J Am Coll Radiol 18(5S):S174–S188

Ghate SV, Rosen EL, Soo MC, Baker JA (2006) MRI-guided vacuum-assisted breast biopsy with a handheld portable biopsy system. AJR Am J Roentgenol 186(6). https://doi.org/10.2214/AJR.05.0551

Gombos EC, Jagadeesan J, Richman DM, Kacher DF (2015) MR guided breast interventions: role in biopsy targeting and lumpectomies. Magn Reson Imaging Clin N Am 23(4):547–561. https://doi.org/10.1016/j.mric.2015.05.004

Harms S et al (1999) MRI directed interstitial thermal ablation of breast fibroadenomas. Wiley, Hoboken, NJ

Khawaja AZ, Cassidy DB, Shakarchi JA, Mcgrogan DG, Inston NG, Jones RG (2015) Revisiting the risks of MRI with gadolinium based contrast agents—review of literature and guidelines. Insights Imaging 6(5):553–558. https://doi.org/10.1007/s13244-015-0420-2

Lai LM et al (1999) Interstitial laser photocoagulation for fibroadenomas of the breast. Breast 8(2):89–94

Lee AY, Nguyen VT, Arasu VA, Greenwood HI, Ray KM, Joe BN, Price ER (2018) Sonographic-MRI correlation after percutaneous sampling of targeted breast ultrasound lesions: initial experiences with limited-sequence unenhanced MRI for postprocedural clip localization. AJR Am J Roentgenol 210(4):927–934

Mcgrath AL, Price ER, Eby PR, Rahbar H (2017) MRI-guided breast interventions. J Magn Reson Imaging 46(3):631–645. https://doi.org/10.1002/jmri.25738

Meeuwis C, Veltman J, van Hall HN, Mus RDM, Boetes C, Barentsz JO, Mann RM (2012) MR-guided breast biopsy at 3T: diagnostic yield of large core needle biopsy compared with vacuum-assisted biopsy. Eur Radiol 22(2):341–349. https://doi.org/10.1007/s00330-011-2272-6

Meissnitzer M et al (2009) Targeted ultrasound of the breast in women with abnormal MRI findings for whom biopsy has been recommended. AJR Am J Roentgenol 193(4):1025–1029

Morin J et al (2004) Magnetic resonance-guided percutaneous cryosurgery of breast carcinoma: technique and early clinical results. Can J Surg 47(5):347–351

MRI-guided breast biopsy. mskcc.org. https://www.mskcc.org/cancer-care/patient-education/mri-guided-breast-biopsy

Myers KS, Kamel IR, Macura KJ (2015) MRI-guided breast biopsy: outcomes and effect on patient management. Clin Breast Cancer 15(2):143–152. https://doi.org/10.1016/j.clbc.2014.11.003

Niell BL, Lee JM, Johansen C, Halpern EF, Rafferty EA (2014) Patient outcomes in canceled MRI-guided breast biopsies. AJR Am J Roentgenol 202(1):223–228. https://doi.org/10.2214/ajr.12.10228

Orel SG, Rosen M, Mies C, Schnall MD (2006) MR imaging-guided 9-gauge vacuum-assisted core-needle breast biopsy: initial experience. Radiology 238(1):54–61. Epub 2005 Nov 22

Papalouka V, Kilburn-Toppin F, Gaskarth M, Gilbert F (2018) MRI-guided breast biopsy: a review of technique, indications, and radiological–pathological correlations. Clin Radiol 73(10):908.e17–908.e25

Pediconi F, Marzocca F, Marincola BC, Napoli A (2018) MRI-guided treatment in the breast. J Magn Reson Imaging. https://doi.org/10.1002/jmri.26282

Pinnamaneni N, Moy L, Gao Y, Melsaether AN, Babb JS, Toth HK, Heller SL (2018) Canceled MRI-guided breast biopsies due to nonvisualization. Acad Radiol 25(9):1101–1110. https://doi.org/10.1016/j.acra.2018.01.016

Ray JG, Vermeulen MJ, Bharatha A, Montanera WJ, Park AL (2016) Association between MRI exposure during pregnancy and fetal and childhood. JAMA 316(9):952–961

Santiago L, Candelaria RP, Huang ML (2018) MR imaging-guided breast interventions. Magn Reson Imaging Clin N Am 26(2):235–246. https://doi.org/10.1016/j.mric.2017.12.002

Somerville P, Seifert PJ, Destounis SV, Murphy PF, Young W (2008) Anticoagulation and bleeding risk after core needle biopsy. AJR Am J Roentgenol 191(4):1194–1197

Taneja S, Jena A, Kumar K, Mehta A (2010) Technical note: MRI-guided breast biopsy - our preliminary experience. Indian J Radiol Imaging 20(3):218. https://doi.org/10.4103/0971-3026.69362

Vashi R, Hooley R, Butler R, Geisel J, Philpotts L (2013) Breast imaging of the pregnant and lactating patient: imaging modalities and pregnancy-associated breast cancer. AJR Am J Roentgenol 200(2):321–328

Vilar VS, Goldman SM, Ricci MD et al (2012) Analysis by MRI of residual tumor after radiofrequency ablation for early-stage breast cancer. Am J Roentgenol 198:W285–W291

Imaging the Axilla

Fleur Kilburn-Toppin

Contents

1 Indications for Axillary Imaging and Clinical Relevance 272

2 Anatomy and Ultrasound Examination Technique 272

3 US Features of Morphologically Normal and Abnormal Lymph Nodes 274

4 US-Guided Biopsy Technique of Axillary Lymph Nodes 276

5 Clinical Utility of Axillary US 277

6 Neoadjuvant Chemotherapy and Imaging of Axillary Lymph Nodes 280

7 Multimodality Imaging of Axillary Lymph Nodes 281

8 Summary 283

References 283

Abstract

The presence of axillary lymph node metastases remains one of the most important prognostic factors in breast cancer. Axillary ultrasound is used routinely in clinical practice, with both morphological features and cortical thickness prompting selective needle biopsy of lymph nodes. Ultrasound and axillary core needle biopsy have a positive impact on the management of patients with breast

cancer, as preoperative identification of axillary metastases allows the patient to proceed directly to full axillary lymph node dissection, avoiding unnecessary sentinel lymph node biopsy. The performance characteristics of axillary US vary widely in the literature, and its clinical utility has been called into question with the advent of the American College of Surgeons Oncology Group Z0011 trial. Subsequently, focus has been on imaging to improve discrimination between limited and advanced nodal disease as well as improved targeting of the sentinel lymph node. The timing of sentinel lymph node biopsy and the use of imaging in the setting of neoadjuvant chemotherapy have also been a subject of much debate. While US is the most widely used

F. Kilburn-Toppin (✉)
Cambridge University NHS Foundation Trust,
Cambridge, UK
e-mail: fk224@cam.ac.uk

© Springer Nature Switzerland AG 2022
M. Fuchsjäger et al. (eds.), *Breast Imaging*, Medical Radiology Diagnostic Imaging,
https://doi.org/10.1007/978-3-030-94918-1_13

technique for axillary assessment, multimodality imaging techniques including MRI and PET-CT have been investigated to provide nodal staging information.

1 Indications for Axillary Imaging and Clinical Relevance

The presence of axillary node metastases remains one of the most important prognostic factors in breast cancer, and for determining the need for systemic chemotherapy and radiation therapy (Kleer and Sabel 2010). Approximately 30–40% of newly diagnosed breast cancer patients will have nodal metastases (Siesling et al. 2003). The AJCC TNM staging system (eighth edition) includes both clinical and pathological staging (Amin et al. 2017). Clinical nodal staging is based on the findings on both clinical examination and imaging, while pathological nodal staging is defined according to node assessment at sentinel lymph node (SLN) surgery or complete axillary lymph node dissection (ALND). Clinically detected nodes are defined as nodes that have suspicious characteristics on clinical examination or imaging. Pathologic lymph node staging is dependent on the size of the metastasis, the total number of positive nodes, and the anatomic location of the involved nodes. The pathologic node staging criteria are based on the number of nodes identified histologically as containing metastases. One to three positive nodes are considered pN1, four to nine positive nodes are considered pN2, and ten or more positive nodes are considered pN3.

Historically, ALND has been used for the evaluation and treatment of axillary metastases (Banerjee et al. 2004; Benson et al. 2007). However, ALND is associated with noteworthy morbidity, including postoperative seroma, paresthesia, and lymphoedema (Fleissig et al. 2005; Lucci et al. 2007; Ahmed et al. 2008; Liu et al. 2009). Subsequently, sentinel lymph node biopsy (SLNB), involving intramammary injection of a radiolabeled colloid (Tc-99 sulfur colloid) with or without the addition of a blue dye (lymphazurin or methylene blue) followed by an open surgical biopsy of axillary nodes demonstrating radioactive or blue dye uptake, emerged as a safe and accurate minimally invasive alternative for clinically node-negative patients. SLNB was shown to have a low false-negative rate, high negative predictive value, and importantly considerably less morbidity (Veronesi et al. 2003). In 2005, a panel from the American Society of Clinical Oncology (ASCO) published guidelines recommending SLNB as an initial alternative for ALND with early-stage breast cancer, and only patients who were detected as lymph node positive at SLNB required complete axillary dissection (Lyman et al. 2005).

The benefit of preoperative identification of axillary metastases means that the patient, if node positive, can proceed directly to ALND at the time of tumor excision, thereby sparing a second operation and general anesthetic, as well as the small risk of complications from SLNB.

While multiple imaging modalities have been used to determine axillary status preoperatively (Hyun et al. 2016), it is only axillary ultrasound with selective needle biopsy of morphologically abnormal nodes which is used routinely in clinical practice (NICE 2009; ACBS 2011), given its relatively high sensitivity and specificity compared to physical examination of the axilla as well as its ease of use. The strategy for identifying axillary metastases with US prior to surgery varies among countries and institutions, ranging from imaging only patients with suspicious clinical findings of the axilla to specific protocols imaging patients with invasive tumors larger than a certain size. It is routine practice in the UK to perform axillary US in all patients with suspected breast cancer on initial imaging (NICE 2009).

2 Anatomy and Ultrasound Examination Technique

Axillary ultrasound should be performed using a high-resolution, linear array, high-frequency transducer of at least 10 MHz, with the frequency suitably adjusted based on patient body habitus and imaging findings. The patient should lie in a supine oblique position, with their hand held behind their head and with the arm abducted and externally rotated. Nodes should be imaged in orthogonal planes with grayscale US. If color Doppler US is used, it is recommended to use low-wall filter settings and low-velocity settings to detect abnormal cortical blood flow (Dialani et al. 2015).

Anatomically, the axilla has a three-dimensional shape resembling a pyramid, with borders consisting of four sides, and a base with an opening at the apex. The size and shape of the axilla varies with arm abduction, and it contains structures including the axillary artery and vein, brachial plexus, and axillary lymph nodes. The axilla is divided into three levels by the pectoralis minor muscle. Level I is bounded by the axillary vessels and the lateral border of pectoralis minor, with level I lymph nodes lying lateral and inferior to pectoralis minor (Fig. 1). Lymph nodes lying beneath pectoralis minor are classified as level II, and those deep and medial to the medial border of pectoralis minor are level III (infraclavicular). Drainage generally proceeds in a stepwise fashion from level I to II to III, and finally into the thorax (Moore 1985). Nodal metastases to level III carry a worse prognosis than metastases to level I and level II axillary nodes. Metastases to the internal mammary nodes usually occur after a tumor has metastasized to the axilla, although isolated metastases to the internal mammary nodes occur in up to 5% of breast cancers and often come from deep or medially situated lesions. The presence of internal mammary node metastases does have prognostic significance and carries a small risk of local recurrence (Chen et al. 2010).

A set routine is recommended when performing ultrasound of the axilla so that lymph nodes are not overlooked (Britton et al. 2009a, b). A thorough examination of level I should be performed, with emphasis placed on scanning inferiorly through the axillary tail, with the reason being the majority of sentinel lymph nodes lying low in the axilla at a distance from the axillary vessels, with more than three-quarters of the SLNs being the lowest identifiable node (Britton

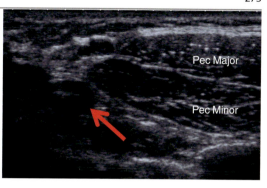

Fig. 1 US of level 1 lymph node (arrow) lying lateral to pectoralis minor

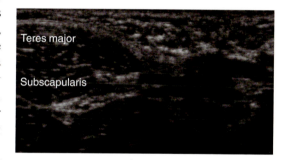

Fig. 2 US of the lateral border of the axilla demonstrating teres major and subscapularis muscles

et al. 2010). High rates of ultrasound targeting of the SLN have been demonstrated by tightly focused US technique examining the axilla 2 cm above to 3 cm below the lowest axillary hair follicles (Nathanson et al. 2007). The examination should start in the axillary tail with the probe moved cranially along the lateral border of the pectoralis muscles to the level of the axillary vessels. Then further similar sweeps can be performed moving further laterally until teres major and subscapularis muscles are seen at the lateral edge (Fig. 2). The lateral thoracic and thoracodorsal arteries may be seen along each margin, although lymph nodes are often found in isolation within the axillary fat (Fig. 3). Occasionally, the hilar vessels to a particular node can be seen and traced back to their artery of origin. Only if morphologically abnormal nodes are seen in level I should level II and III be scanned to determine the likely extent of lymph node involvement. This practice varies between institutions, with some centers advocating examination of

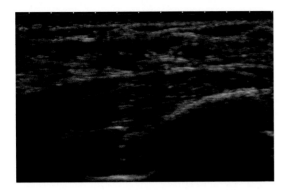

Fig. 3 US of normal lymph node lying in axillary fat

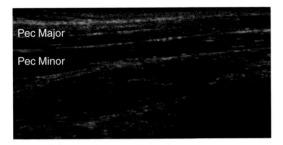

Fig. 4 US appearances of level II of the axilla demonstrating pectoralis major and minor muscles

level II, the fat behind pectoralis minor muscle, in patients whose cancer is located superiorly in the breast and where lymph node spread may bypass level I (Fig. 4). Some institutions also scan the supraclavicular area and along the margin of the sternum, following the course of the internal mammary artery if abnormal nodes are found in level I.

3 US Features of Morphologically Normal and Abnormal Lymph Nodes

The normal axillary lymph node should be oval with a smooth, well-defined margin and a uniformly thin hypoechoic cortex. The echogenic hilum should comprise most of the lymph node (Fig. 5). US findings which should prompt lymph node biopsy due to suspicion of metastatic involvement include both morphological features and cortical thickness. Overall size of the node has been shown to have a very poor diagnostic accuracy for predicting metastasis; however, in some centers, the ratio of longitudinal length to transverse length of <2 is used as a criterion for biopsy (Feu et al. 1997). When considering the morphological appearances of abnormal lymph nodes, it is helpful to consider the fashion in which metastatic deposits spread to the lymph nodes. One model suggests that tumor cells enter the lymph nodes through afferent lymphatics and are deposited in the subcapsular sinusoids, proliferating in the medullary sinusoids and then into the efferent lymphatics. As deposits spread in the nodal parenchyma, they replace the normal nodal architecture as they proliferate (Ching et al. 2010). As the metastatic deposits get bigger, they can obliterate the normal histological features of large parts of the node, and then eventually replace the entire lymph node. Finally, extra-nodal spread of the tumor into the adjacent axillary fat can occur, and the node is ultimately replaced by an irregular mass.

It is not surprising therefore that diffuse cortical thickening and eccentric cortical thickening, or a focal cortical budge, are considered the earliest detectable changes (Figs. 6 and 7). It is important to note that normal lymph nodes often have a lobulated shape because of concurrent constrictions and bulges of both the cortex and fatty hilum. A true abnormal cortical bulge is seen as focal thickening of the cortex that does not follow the margin of the echogenic hilum and should be distinctly hypoechoic (Fig. 8). Findings seen in cases with more advanced nodal involvement, such as effacement of the fatty hilum or a rounded hypoechoic mass, have a higher positive predictive value in patients with invasive breast cancer (Fig. 9). Replacement of the entire node by an ill-defined mass is highly suspicious for malignant involvement (Fig. 10). Color Doppler may also be useful in the assessment of abnormal lymph nodes, with metastatic deposits leading to distortion of the intranodal angioarchitecture and engorgement of the peripheral vascularity. This is hypothesized to result in non-hilar blood flow demonstrated at color Doppler as peripheral vascular flow at the cortex of the node with no detectable connection to the hilum. Various authors have published odds ratios for biopsy cri-

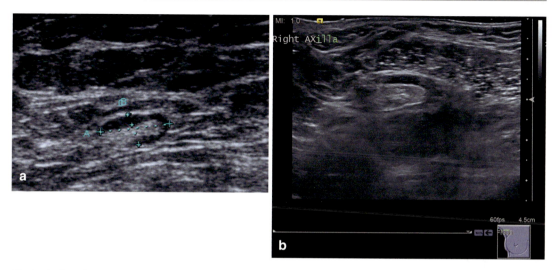

Fig. 5 (a, b) US appearances of morphologically normal lymph nodes with a uniform smooth hypoechoic cortex and fatty hilum

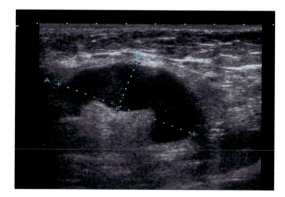

Fig. 6 Diffuse cortical thickening in a metastatic axillary lymph node

teria (Britton et al. 2009a, b; Abe et al. 2009; Mainiero et al. 2010), but it is important to note that these are not pathognomonic of malignancy and biopsy confirmation is required.

Diffuse cortical thickening can also be seen with metastatic involvement of nodes; however, this finding is nonspecific and is often associated with reactive nodes (Fig. 11). There is a significant correlation between increasing cortical thickness of nodes and presence of malignancy, and investigators have suggested multiple cutoff values for cortical thickness, with inevitable trade-off in sensitivity and specificity (Bedi et al. 2008; Choi et al. 2009; Saffar et al. 2015). Work done by Duerloo demonstrated that a diffusely thickened cortex of 4 mm or greater was 80% sensitive and 80% specific for malignancy, but if the cutoff was lowered to 2 mm, sensitivity increased to 95% but specificity dropped to 44% (Deurloo et al. 2003). Submitting of a greater proportion of patients to biopsy to see if this improves sensitivity was performed by Britton et al., with 87% of patients undergoing lymph node biopsy resulting in only a modest increment in sensitivity to 53% but with a substantial increase in biopsies. All centers will use their own cutoff criteria, but consideration should be given to the fact that the highest needle biopsy sensitivities will be achieved in patient groups with high likelihood of metastatic disease. Patients who present with a palpable lump, multifocal or multicentric malignancy, central cancers, and cancers >20 mm are more likely to have axillary nodal involvement than asymptomatic screen-detected patients with small <20 mm tumors.

Other techniques such as US elastography have shown potential for preoperative axillary staging in breast cancer (Taylor et al. 2011; Wojcinski et al. 2012), with significantly harder cortex seen in metastatic lymph nodes. The highest sensitivity and specificity of 73% and 99.3%, respectively, in these studies were achieved with a combination of conventional US and elastogra-

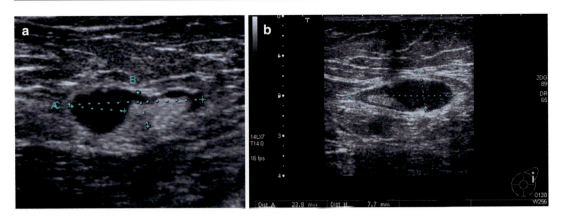

Fig. 7 (**a**, **b**) US appearances of a focal cortical bulge in metastatic axillary lymph nodes

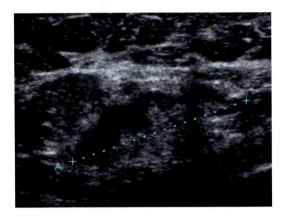

Fig. 8 Multiple cortical bulges in a metastatic axillary lymph node

phy, suggesting that elastography may be a useful adjunct to conventional US to improve diagnostic performance.

4 US-Guided Biopsy Technique of Axillary Lymph Nodes

If US evaluation of the axilla reveals a suspicious finding, percutaneous procedures including ultrasound-guided fine needle aspiration (FNA) or ultrasound-guided core needle biopsy (CNB) should be performed to substantiate clinical decision-making. FNA is preferred by some centers, usually using a 22–25 G needle with three passes and with aspirates sent to cytology. However, FNA is operator dependent, requires access to reliable cytology, and has a relatively high false-negative rate of 12–23% (Krishnamurthy et al. 2002). CNB is now widely used as an alternative because it has been shown in several studies to be more sensitive than FNA (90–94%), with no reported false positives and equivalent low rate of morbidity, with multiple studies reporting no significant complications (Rautiainen et al. 2013). The latter is of importance as concerns have been raised regarding vascular or nerve damage with CNB. Although most SLNs are located low in the axilla in axillary fat, for those that are located near axillary vessels potential complications can be avoided by continuous US monitoring, clear operator understanding of axillary anatomy, and operator experience (Fig. 12). Furthermore, most spring-loaded biopsy devices offer the option of a "no-throw" technique, with an open bowl advanced through the lymph node and a cutting cannula then released over the open bowl, which may be desirable in situations with vessels located nearby to the targeted lymph node. Either FNA or CNB of the axilla provides good accuracy in this clinical context, and it may be more relevant to consider each center's expertise in breast cytology or core needle histology in deciding on the type of percutaneous procedure to perform.

Imaging the Axilla

Fig. 9 Enlarged metastatic lymph node with absent fatty hilum

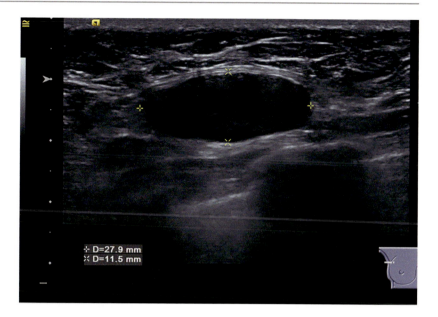

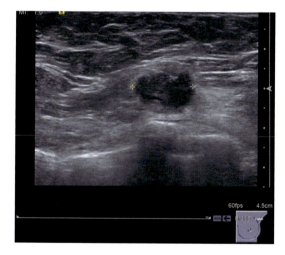

Fig. 10 Complete replacement of metastatic lymph node by a hypoechoic ill-defined mass

5 Clinical Utility of Axillary US

Ultrasound and axillary core needle biopsy have a positive impact on the management of patients with breast cancer, as preoperative identification of axillary metastases allows the surgeon to proceed directly to full axillary lymph node dissection and avoid an unnecessary sentinel lymph node biopsy. A meta-analysis performed by Houssami estimated the clinical utility of axillary US and biopsy as triaging 19.8% of patients directly to ALND (Houssami et al. 2011). However, the performance characteristics of axillary US vary widely in the literature. The underlying prevalence of axillary metastases within the study population will influence results, as will inclusion of only patients undergoing ultrasound-guided biopsy as opposed to all patients undergoing US imaging. In addition, criteria for classifying axillary lymph nodes as positive or negative have not been clearly defined. Three large meta-analyses looking at diagnostic accuracy report a pooled estimate for sensitivity of axillary US and biopsy of approximately 50% (Diepstraten et al. 2014; Houssami and Turner 2014; Van Wely et al. 2015). There is better utility in women who have higher underlying nodal risk, e.g., larger tumors.

When considering why we are not able to detect more axillary nodes which are involved with metastatic disease, the answer is likely threefold. Most metastases are too small to be seen on conventional axillary grayscale US,

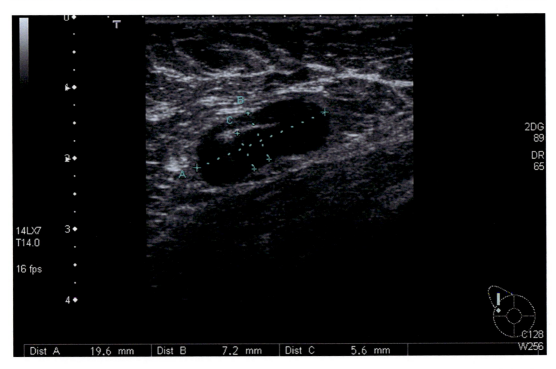

Fig. 11 Axillary lymph node with diffusely thickened cortex of 6 mm, which could represent either metastatic involvement or a reactive node

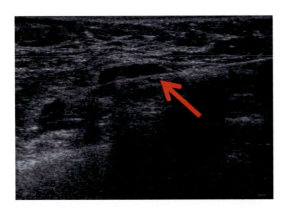

Fig. 12 US of axillary lymph node undergoing percutaneous core biopsy, with the needle seen to pass through the cortex (arrow)

given that micrometastases at less than 2 mm will cause no apparent nodal morphological change. One in four women with a negative/normal axillary US will still be proven to have axillary metastases at subsequent SLNB (Diepstraten et al. 2014). Secondly, we are only able to identify the sentinel node using US in 64–78% of cases (Britton et al. 2009a, b), and finally even using core needle biopsy as opposed to FNA we are only able to sample part of the node.

More "intelligent" targeting of the SLN using a gamma probe, fluorescence imaging, and ultrasound-guided contrast agents such as microbubbles has been investigated. The use of contrast-enhanced US (CEUS) to localize the SLN has shown it to be both safe and feasible. In comparison to traditional isotope SLNB, the sensitivity of CEUS to detect the SLN correctly was shown in studies to be 89%. In clinically node-negative patients, the sensitivity of CEUS-guided biopsy was 61–66.7% (Sever et al. 2012; Suvi et al. 2015).

However, the clinical utility of preoperative axillary US was called into question with the advent of the American College of Surgeons Oncology Group Z0011 trial, a large prospective randomized control trial in which SLNB-positive patients with small tumors were randomized to ALND versus no further surgery. They reported that ALND was not associated with any survival benefit and that both groups had an extremely low regional recurrence rate (0.9% for SNB alone and 0.5% for ALND), confirming that ALND provided minimal benefit while exposing a substantial number of patients to long-term morbidity, specifically lymphedema (Giuliano et al. 2011).

A number of concerns were raised regarding the trial, including a high proportion of patients with low burden of axillary disease, failure to meet accrual targets, and lack of detail on radiation therapy. The POSNOC trial in the UK (Goyal and Dodwell 2015) is currently underway and designed to overcome some of the limitations of Z0011 with respect to patient selection and statistical power.

However, the results of the Z0011 trial led to a significant change in surgical practice (Gainer et al. 2012), with the majority of surgeons in the USA now omitting completion ALND in patients who fulfill Z0011 criteria (stage T1 or T2 tumor, one or two positive SLNs only, undergoing breast conservation treatment and planned for whole-breast irradiation). The changing algorithm of axillary surgical treatment means that ultrasound-guided biopsy will have less utility if surgeons omit ALND for minimal nodal metastatic disease. Positive findings on preoperative axillary US and biopsy identifying nodal involvement would commit patients to ALND who may have not required this if they fulfilled Z0011 criteria.

The focus has therefore shifted from trying to improve identification of any nodal metastatic disease to discriminating between limited and advanced nodal disease, given that this has the greatest impact on patient management of the axilla post-Z0011. While axillary US alone is inadequate for excluding axillary metastases given its false-negative rate of 25% (Diepstraten et al. 2014), preoperative negative axillary US can exclude 96% of stage N2 and N3 axillary metastases (Neal et al. 2010; Schipper et al. 2013a, b). Characteristics associated with false negatives in this study included invasive lobular carcinoma, larger tumor size, and multifocality of the primary tumor. The prospective randomized controlled multicenter SOUND (Sentinel node versus Observation after axillary UltrasouND) trial is currently underway to compare SLN surgery to observation when axillary US is negative in patients with small breast cancers (Gentilini and Veronesi 2012).

Conversely, when at least two abnormal lymph nodes are identified on axillary US, pN2 or higher disease is highly likely (PPV 82%) and is even more likely when the tumor is larger than 10 mm (Abe et al. 2013). A correlation between increasing number of abnormal nodes identified on axillary US and mean number of abnormal nodes on final histology has been demonstrated (Van Wely et al. 2015). Therefore, when multiple nodes are seen on US, it is unlikely that these patients will fulfill Z0011 criteria and have only two lymph nodes positive on final histology, and therefore these patients will still benefit from preoperative biopsy and triaging to ALND.

However, a more usual scenario in both symptomatic and screen-detected breast cancer patients is the identification on axillary US of just one abnormal node. This poses a greater diagnostic dilemma, as biopsy proving metastatic involvement will commit the patient to ALND when they may have had no more than two nodes in total involved. Furthermore, in the Z0011 trial, the patients did not require axillary imaging, and final nodal number was determined on SLNB. The question therefore arises if women who are detected as lymph node positive on axillary US are more likely to have more extensive nodal disease burden than those detected by SLNB. Studies by Caudle et al. and Verheuvel et al. compared node-positive patients identified by axillary US and needle biopsy to women with negative axillary imaging found to have a positive node with SLNB (Caudle et al. 2014; Verheuvel et al. 2016). While women identified as being node positive by US and needle biopsy were at higher risk for heavy nodal disease burden, 37–52% had only 1–2 total positive LNs and were therefore potentially Z0011 "eligible." Furthermore, while survival was expectedly worse in the needle biopsy cohort reported by Verheuvel et al. that presented with more advanced-stage disease, there was no difference in regional recurrence, with only one isolated regional relapse in each group. Other studies (Cools-Lartigue et al. 2013; Schipper et al. 2013a, b) have demonstrated similar findings. Various authors have attempted to clarify the degree of "overtreatment" of patients who undergo routine axillary US and biopsy, with estimations of 38% (Farrell et al. 2015), 47% (Pilewskie et al. 2016a, b), and 53% (Wallis et al. 2017). On this basis, it is debated as to whether women presenting with small T1 or T2 breast cancer should undergo preoperative axillary biopsy if only one abnormal node is identified on axillary US and instead proceed to SLNB, with some centers such as Memorial Sloan Kettering Cancer Center abandoning all preoperative axillary imaging to avoid direct triage to ALND (Pilewskie et al. 2016a, b).

6 Neoadjuvant Chemotherapy and Imaging of Axillary Lymph Nodes

Neoadjuvant chemotherapy (NAC) has been shown to be as effective as adjuvant treatment, and to decrease disease burden to allow less extensive surgery. Furthermore, it also affects axillary nodes achieving pathological complete response (pCR) in up to 40–60% of previously node-positive patients with new anti-Her2 therapies. The extent of persistent axillary disease following NAC is a prognostic marker for locoregional recurrence and survival (Kuerer et al. 1999). Historically, ALND was always performed after NAC, but as neoadjuvant chemotherapy is increasingly offered in early-stage and clinically node-negative breast cancer usually to improve breast conservation outcomes, the timing of SLNB in the setting of NAC has been a subject of much debate.

There are advantages and disadvantages to performing SLNB either prior to or post-NAC. The strongest argument for SLNB before NAC is that knowing the pathological status of the axilla before NAC may influence subsequent radiotherapy. However, several studies have suggested that accurate staging after NAC is a more meaningful predictor of locoregional recurrence than accurate staging before NAC. The main indication for performing SLNB after NAC is to take advantage of the pCR resulting in more con-

servative axillary surgery. However, the concern has been whether performing SLNB post-NAC results in an unacceptably high false-negative rate (FNR). Various studies have documented the FNR to be higher than the generally accepted 10% cutoff (Fu et al. 2014). Three prospective studies ACOSOG Z0171, SENTINA, and SN FNAC (Boughey et al. 2013; Kuehn et al. 2013; Boileau et al. 2015) aimed to address this issue, and the conclusions were that by using dual-tracer mapping and immunohistochemistry and removing ≥ 3 SLNs at surgery, the FNR could be lowered to less than 10%. Importantly for radiologists, it has also been shown that post-NAC assessment of the axilla with US can lower the FNR. A secondary analysis of Z1071 trial assessed axillary US as a selection criterion to stratify women for risk of residual axillary involvement following NAC, with the goal of identifying those who could be safely spared a full ALND in the setting of negative SLNB. An abnormal axillary US after neoadjuvant chemotherapy was also associated with more positive nodes (75.4%) compared with patients with a normal axillary US (63.9%). A key point is that if combined, normal axillary US following NAC and SLNB had a FNR of 9.8%, under the 10% threshold for clinical care (Boughey et al. 2015).

Also of importance to radiologists is that preoperative clip placement in the positive axillary node at the time of US-guided biopsy, allowing documentation of its excision at the SLNB procedure, also results in reduced FNR. The MD Anderson researchers developed targeted axillary dissection (TAD), which includes placing a clip at the time of the axillary node biopsy, and after NAC and before surgery a I^{125} seed was placed in the clip node to guide the surgical excision of this node. Initial reports show that the seeds do not interfere with the radioisotope for the axillary surgery, and in 80% the node that had the clip was the SLN (Caudle et al. 2015). Other groups have tried other techniques for marking and removing the axillary nodes, including wire placement and black carbon tattooing (Choy et al. 2015). With more patients undergoing NAC for breast cancer and improvements in pCR, there is increasing importance of research to improve prediction of pCR and to determine which patients can feasibly be spared ALND and its associated morbidity.

7 Multimodality Imaging of Axillary Lymph Nodes

While US is the most widely used technique for the assessment of axillary lymph nodes given its high specificity and ease of use, given the shift towards less aggressive management of the axilla, imaging techniques that may have sufficient negative predictive value to omit surgical staging of the axilla by SLNB have been investigated. Breast MRI, as well as CT and whole-body PET/CT, is often obtained in newly diagnosed breast cancer patients for clinical staging and can be used to provide regional nodal staging information.

Breast MRI often includes the axillary region in the field of view (FOV), with the additional benefit that both axillae can be compared easily (Fig. 13). However, examination of the axillary region is technically challenging since respiratory motion can cause artifacts from the adjacent thoracic wall, and pulsation artifact from the heart may obscure the axillary region due to the phase-encoding direction often being from left to right (Hieken et al. 2013). The use of additional coils to the standard breast MRI coil or performing a separate dedicated axillary MRI can overcome this (Baltzer et al. 2011; Schipper et al. 2013a, b). Although this requires an additional MRI examination, it does have the advantage of facilitating the use of a dedicated lymph node contrast agent, for example gadofosveset or ultrasmall superparamagnetic iron oxide (USPIO).

On MRI, the nodal cortex demonstrates decreased signal intensity with T1W and intermediate to increased signal with T2W (Fig. 14). Usually at least one nonfat-sat sequence is performed where the hilar fat is shown to demonstrate increased signal. As with US, features that are seen with metastatic involvement of lymph nodes include cortical irregularity, loss of fatty hilum, and round shape (Luciani et al. 2004) (Fig. 15). Similar to US, a short-axis threshold of 4 mm yielded the best predictive value for metastatic nodal involvement with a sensitivity and specificity of 78.6% and 62.3%, respectively (Luciani et al. 2004). Two MRI-specific imaging features that have been reported to have potential diagnostic utility are perifocal edema, presence of areas with marked T2 prolongation in the fat surrounding a lymph node (Baltzer et al. 2011), and comet-tail sign, an imaging finding first described in breast lesions and hypothesized to represent infiltration or angiogenesis (Arslan et al. 2016).

Regarding the addition of diffusion-weighted imaging, while some authors have demonstrated high reproducibility and reliability of measurements of ADCs and shown metastatic nodes to have mean ADC lower than that of benign nodes (Fornasa et al. 2012), DWI has not yet convincingly been shown to improve diagnostic performance (Scaranelo et al. 2012; Schipper et al. 2015).

Lymph nodes enhance rapidly on dynamic enhanced contrast sequences, and a type 3 curve is usually seen and is not useful for predicting metastatic involvement (Fig. 16). However, nodes

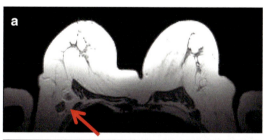

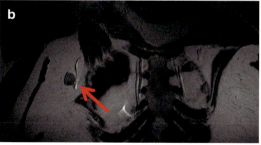

Fig. 13 (**a**) Axial T2W breast MRI demonstrating morphologically abnormal enlarged right axillary node (arrow). This is also clearly demonstrated on the coronal view (**b**)

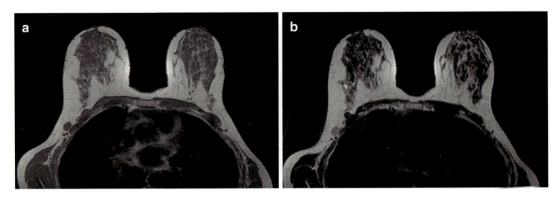

Fig. 14 Axial T1w (**a**) and T2W (**b**) breast MRI demonstrating decreased signal intensity of abnormal right-sided axillary node on T1W imaging and intermediate signal on T2W imaging

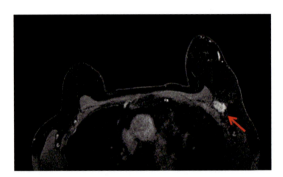

Fig. 15 T1W fat-sat post-IV gadolinium breast MRI demonstrating an enhancing enlarged and irregular left-sided axillary lymph node (arrow) with metastatic involvement

with less intense enhancement have been shown to have a high negative predictive value for metastatic involvement (Murray et al. 2002). The presence of rim enhancement, defined as signal intensity that is higher at the periphery of a node than at its center on DCE MR images at delayed imaging, has also been reported to have a high positive predictive value for the detection of metastases (Baltzer et al. 2011).

Diagnostic performance of unenhanced axillary MR imaging for nodal staging in patients with breast cancer has shown a negative predictive value (NPV) of 86–91% (Scaranelo et al. 2012; Schipper et al. 2015). As the NPV of enhanced MRI is not close enough to that of SLNB to substitute, lymph node-specific contrast agents have been investigated to improve the diagnostic performance of MRI.

After intravenous injection of superparamagnetic iron oxide USPIO, normal nodes accumulate iron-containing nanoparticles, which reduce the nodal signal due to susceptibility effects, while metastatic nodes that do not accumulate the nanoparticles maintain a high signal intensity in T2- or T2*-weighted images. USPIO-enhanced MRI has shown superior sensitivity compared to normal MRI (Will et al. 2006) and high diagnostic accuracy for identifying axillary lymph node metastases in patients with early-stage breast cancer. However, this conclusion is based on limited articles, and additional studies are required to further validate these findings.

18F-fluoro-2-deoxy-D-glucose (FDG) positron-emission tomography/computed tomography (PET/CT) has proven useful in the evaluation of distant metastatic disease. Despite lower sensitivity, specificity of PET/CT in the detection of lymph node metastases is high, ranging from 95% to 100%. Lymph node morphology as well as increased FDG avidity can be assessed on PET/CT. Previous authors have reported high specificity for metastasis for all visually FDG-avid lymph nodes, and it can be used to identify internal mammary chain and supraclavicular metastases, which may be incompletely included or difficult to evaluate by MRI (Aukema et al. 2010) (Fig. 17).

A pitfall of PET/CT is its relatively high false-negative rate due to its inability to detect small metastatic deposits (Challa et al. 2013). While comparisons of diagnostic performance of MRI

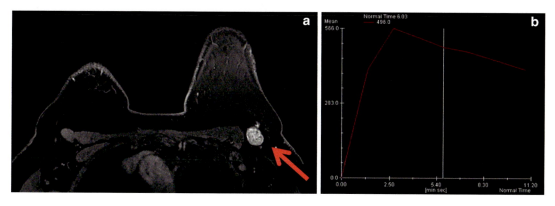

Fig. 16 (**a**, **b**) T1W fat-sat post-IV gadolinium breast MRI demonstrating an enhancing left-sided axillary lymph node (arrow) with a type 3 curve. The abnormal enlarged morphology of the lymph node indicates suspicion for metastatic involvement, rather than enhancement curve

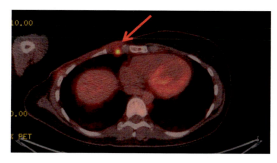

Fig. 17 FDG PET/CT demonstrating tracer uptake within the right internal mammary region (arrow) in a metastatic node. No morphologic abnormality was appreciated on conventional CT

versus PET/CT have suggested that MRI has a higher sensitivity than PET/CT for axillary lymph node metastatic diagnosis (Liang et al. 2017), it is possible that a combination of USPIO-enhanced MRI and FDG PET may provide high enough sensitivity, specificity, PPV, and NPV to be clinically useful in identifying patients who should undergo direct ALND.

ing. While there are significant limitations to US assessment of the axilla, it is important to remember that axillary US and biopsy have the ideal characteristics of an accurate triage test in axillary staging given its consistently high specificity and PPV, as well as its ease of use. Advances in ultrasound technology and newer generation microbubble agents may potentially allow improved accuracy in the preoperative axillary staging setting and may identify patients who are likely to have no or limited axillary disease and therefore be spared ALND and potentially any surgical intervention. Implementation of parameters from imaging techniques and tumor biology into nomograms predicting the probability of lymph node metastasis is another approach to improve preoperative assessment (Qiu et al. 2016). This, along with the accurate identification of axillary status after NAC, remains the great challenge for axillary imaging and patient care, and where future research should be directed.

8 Summary

The movement to reduce surgical treatment of the axilla in breast cancer patients is continuing. It is now established that ALND is overtreatment in a significant subset of patients with early breast cancer. As surgical staging of the axilla continues to evolve, so too must the role of axillary imag-

References

Abe H, Schmidt RA, Kulkarni K et al (2009) Axillary lymph nodes suspicious for breast cancer metastasis: sampling with US-guided 14-gauge core-needle biopsy—clinical experience in 100 patients. Radiology 250(1):41–49

Abe H, Schacht D, Sennett C (2013) Utility of preoperative ultrasound for predicting pN2 or higher stage axillary lymph node involvement in patients with newly diagnosed breast cancer. AJR Am J Roentgenol 200:696–702

Ahmed RL, Prizment A, Lazovich D et al (2008) Lymphedema and quality of life in breast cancer survivors: the Iowa Women's Health Study. J Clin Oncol 26(35):5689–5696

American Society of Breast Surgeons (2011) Position statement on management of the axilla in patients with invasive breast cancer. https://www.breastsurgeons. org/new_layout/about/statements/PDF_Statements/ Axillary_Management.pdf. Accessed 16 Jun 2017

Amin MB, Edge SB, Greene FL (2017) AJCC (American Joint Committee on Cancer) cancer staging manual, 8th edn. Springer, New York

Arslan G, Altintoprak K, Yirgin IK et al (2016) Diagnostic accuracy of metastatic axillary lymph nodes in breast MRI. Springerplus 5:735

Aukema S, Straver M, Peeters M et al (2010) Detection of extra-axillary lymph node involvement with FDG PET/CT in patients with stage II-III breast cancer. Eur J Cancer 46:3205–3210

Baltzer P, Dietzel M, Burmeister H et al (2011) Application of MR mammography beyond local staging: is there a potential to accurately assess axillary lymph nodes? Evaluation of an extended protocol in an initial prospective study. Am J Roentgenol 196(5):W641–W647

Banerjee M, George J, Song EY et al (2004) Tree based model for breast cancer prognostication. J Clin Oncol 22:2567–2575

Bedi DG, Krishnamurthy R, Krishnamurthy S et al (2008) Cortical morphologic features of axillary lymph nodes as a predictor of metastasis in breast cancer: in vitro sonographic study. AJR Am J Roentgenol 191(3):646–652

Benson JR, Della Rovere GQ, Axilla Management Consensus Group (2007) Management of the axilla in patients with breast cancer. Lancet Oncol 8:331–348

Boileau JF, Poirier B, Basik M et al (2015) Sentinel node biopsy after neo-adjuvant chemotherapy in biopsy-proven node-positive breast cancer: the SN FNAC Study. J Clin Oncol 33:258–264

Boughey JC, Suman VJ, Mittendorf EA et al (2013) Sentinel lymph node surgery after neoadjuvant chemotherapy in patients with node-positive breast cancer: the ACOSOG Z1071 (Alliance) clinical trial. JAMA 310:1455–1461

Boughey J, Suman V, Mittendorf E et al (2015) Factors affecting sentinel lymph node identification rate after neoadjuvant chemotherapy for breast cancer patients enrolled in ACOSOG Z0171 (Alliance). Ann Surg 261(3):547–552

Britton PD, Gould A, Godward S et al (2009a) Use of ultrasound guided axillary node core biopsy in staging of early breast cancer. Eur Radiol 19:561–569

Britton PD, Provenzano E, Barter S (2009b) Ultrasound guided percutaneous axillary lymph node core biopsy: how often is the sentinel lymph node being biopsied? Breast 18:13–16

Britton PD, Moyle P, Benson J et al (2010) Ultrasound of the axilla: where to look for the sentinel lymph node. Clin Radiol 65:373–376

Caudle A, Kuerer H, Le-Petross H et al (2014) Predicting the extent of nodal disease in early-stage breast cancer. Ann Surg Oncol 21:3440–3447

Caudle A, Yang WT, Mittendorf EA et al (2015) Selective surgical localization of axillary nodes containing metastases in patients with breast cancer. A prospective feasibility trial. JAMA Surg 150(2):137

Challa VR, Srivastava A, Dhar A et al (2013) Role of fluorine-18-labeled 2-fluoro-2-deoxy-d-glucose positron emission tomography-computed tomography in the evaluation of axillary lymph node involvement in operable breast cancer in comparison with sentinel lymph node biopsy. Indian J Nucl Med 28(3):138–143

Chen L, Gu Y, Leaw S et al (2010) Internal mammary lymph node recurrence: rare but characteristic metastasis site in breast cancer. BMC Cancer 10:479

Ching CD, Edge SB, Krishnamurthy S et al (2010) Initial AJCC staging. In: Kuerer HM (ed) Kuerer's breast surgical oncology. McGraw-Hill, New York, pp 141–144

Choi YJ, Ko EY, Han BK, Shin JH, Kang SS, Hahn SY (2009) High-resolution ultrasonographic features of axillary lymph node metastasis in patients with breast cancer. Breast 18(2):119–122

Choy N, Lipson J, Porter C et al (2015) Initial results with preoperative tattooing of biopsied axillary lymph nodes and correlation to sentinel lymph nodes in breast cancer patients. Ann Surg Oncol 22(2):377–382

Cools-Lartigue J, Sinclair A, Trabulsi N et al (2013) Preoperative axillary ultrasound and fine-needle aspiration biopsy in the diagnosis of axillary metastases in patients with breast cancer: predictors of accuracy and future implications. Ann Surg Oncol 20:819–827

Deurloo EE, Tanis PJ, Gilhuijs KGA et al (2003) Reduction in the number of sentinel lymph node procedures by preoperative ultrasonography of the axilla in breast cancer. Eur J Cancer 39:1068–1073

Dialani V, James D, Slanetz P (2015) A practical approach to imaging the axilla. Insights Imaging 6:217–229

Diepstraten S, Sever A, Constantinus F et al (2014) Value of preoperative ultrasound-guided axillary lymph node biopsy for preventing completion axillary lymph node dissection in breast cancer: a systematic review and meta-analysis. Ann Surg Oncol 21:51–59

Farrell TP, Adams NC, Stenson M et al (2015) The Z0011 trial: is this the end of axillary ultrasound in the preoperative assessment of breast cancer patients? Eur Radiol 25(9):2682–2687

Feu J, Tresserra F, Fábregas R et al (1997) Metastatic breast carcinoma in axillary lymph nodes: in vitro US detection. Radiology 205(3):831–835

Fleissig A, Fallowfield LJ, Langridge CI et al (2005) Postoperative arm morbidity and quality of life: results of the ALMANAC randomised trial comparing sentinel node biopsy with standard axillary treatment in the management of patients with early breast cancer. Breast Cancer Res Treat 95:279–293

Fornasa F, Nesoti MV, Bovo C et al (2012) Diffusion-weighted magnetic resonance imaging in the characterization of axillary lymph nodes in patients with breast cancer. J Magn Reson Imaging 36:858–864

Fu JF, Chen HL, Yang J et al (2014) Feasibility and accuracy of sentinel lymph node biopsy in clinically node-positive breast cancer after neoadjuvant chemotherapy: a meta-analysis. PLoS One 9:e105316

Gainer S, Hunt K, Beitsch P (2012) Changing behavior in clinical practice in response to the ACOSOG Z0011 trial: a survey of the American Society of Breast Surgeons. Ann Surg Oncol 19:3152–3158

Gentilini O, Veronesi U (2012) Abandoning sentinel lymph node biopsy in early breast cancer? A new trial in progress at the European Institute of Oncology of Milan (SOUND: Sentinel node vs Observation after axillary UltraSouND). Breast 21:678–681

Giuliano AE, Hunt KK, Ballman KV et al (2011) Axillary dissection vs no axillary dissection in women with invasive breast cancer and sentinel node metastasis: a randomized clinical trial. JAMA 305(6):569–575

Goyal A, Dodwell D (2015) POSNOC: a randomised trial looking at axillary treatment in women with one or two sentinel nodes with macrometastases. Clin Oncol 27(12):692–695

Hieken TJ, Boughey JC, Jones KN et al (2013) Imaging response and residual metastatic axillary lymph node disease after neoadjuvant chemotherapy for primary breast cancer. Ann Surg Oncol 20:3199–3204

Houssami N, Turner RM (2014) Staging the axilla in women with breast cancer: the utility of preoperative ultrasound n-guided biopsy. Cancer Biol Med 11:69–77

Houssami N, Ciatto S, Turner RM et al (2011) Preoperative ultrasound guided needle biopsy of axillary nodes in invasive breast cancer: meta-analysis of its accuracy and utility in staging the axilla. Ann Surg 254:243–251

Hyun SJ, Kim EK, Moon HJ et al (2016) Preoperative axillary lymph node evaluation in breast cancer patients by magnetic resonance imaging (MRI): can breast MRI exclude advanced nodal disease. Eur Radiol 236:3865–34873

Kleer CG, Sabel MS (2010) Prognostic and predictive factors in breast cancer. In: Kuerer HM (ed) Kuerer's breast surgical oncology. McGraw-Hill, New York, p 244

Krishnamurthy S et al (2002) Role of ultrasound-guided fine-needle aspiration of indeterminate and suspicious axillary lymph nodes in the initial staging of breast carcinoma. Cancer 95(5):982–988

Kuehn T, Bauerfeind I, Fehm T et al (2013) Sentinel-lymph-node biopsy in patients with breast cancer before and after neoadjuvant chemotherapy (SENTINA): a prospective, multicenter cohort study. Lancet Oncol 14(7):609–618

Kuerer H, Sahin A, Hunt K et al (1999) Incidence and impact of documented eradication of breast cancer axillary lymph node metastases before surgery in patients treated with neoadjuvant chemotherapy. Ann Surg 230:72–78

Liang X, Yu J, Wen B et al (2017) MRI and FDG-PET/CT based assessment of axillary lymph node metastasis in early breast cancer: a meta-analysis. Clin Radiol 72:295–301

Liu CQ, Guo Y, Shi JY et al (2009) Late morbidity associated with a tumour-negative sentinel lymph node biopsy in primary breast cancer patients: a systematic review. Eur J Cancer 45(9):1560–1568

Lucci A, McCall LM, Beitsch PD et al (2007) Surgical complications associated with sentinel lymph node dissection (SLND) plus axillary lymph node dissection compared with SLND alone in the American College of Surgeons Oncology Group trial Z0011. J Clin Oncol 25:3657–3663

Luciani A, Dao TH, Lapeyre M et al (2004) Simultaneous bilateral breast and high-resolution axillary MRI of patients with breast cancer: preliminary results. AJR Am J Roentgenol 182(4):1059–1067

Lyman GH, Giulano AE, Somerfieled MR et al (2005) American Society of Clinical Oncology guideline recommendations for sentinel lymph node biopsy in early-stage breast cancer. J Clin Oncol 23(30):7703–7720

Mainiero MB et al (2010) Axillary ultrasound and fine-needle aspiration in the preoperative evaluation of the breast cancer patient: an algorithm based on tumour size and lymph node appearance. AJR Am J Roentgenol 195(5):1261–1267

Moore KL (1985) The upper limb. In: Clinically oriented anatomy, vol 660, 2nd edn. Williams & Wilkins, Baltimore, Md

Murray AD, Staff RT, Redpath TW et al (2002) Dynamic contrast enhanced MRI of the axilla in women with breast cancer: comparison with pathology of excised nodes. Br J Radiol 75(891):220–228

Nathanson SD, Burke M, Slater R et al (2007) Preoperative identification of the sentinel lymph node in breast cancer. Ann Surg Oncol 14:3102–3110

National Institute for Clinical excellence (2009) Early and locally advanced breast cancer: diagnosis and treatment Clinical guideline. www.nice.org.uk/guidance/cg80

Neal C, Daly P, Nees A (2010) Can preoperative axillary US help exclude N2 and N3 metastatic breast cancer? Radiology 257:2

Pilewskie M, Mautner SK, Stempel M et al (2016a) Does a positive axillary lymph node needle biopsy result predict the need for an axillary lymph node dissection in clinically node-negative breast cancer patients in the ACOSOG Z0011 era? Ann Surg Oncol 23(4):1123–1128

Pilewskie M, Jochelson M, Gooch J (2016b) Is preoperative axillary imaging beneficial in identifying clinically node-negative patients requiring axillary lymph node dissection? J Am Coll Surg 222(2):138–145

Qiu SQ, Zeng HC, Zhang F et al (2016) A nomogram to predict the probability of axillary lymph node metastasis in early breast cancer patients with positive axillary ultrasound. Sci Rep 6:21196

Rautiainen S, Masarwah A, Sudah M et al (2013) Axillary lymph node biopsy in newly diagnosed invasive breast cancer: comparative accuracy of fine-needle aspiration biopsy versus core-needle biopsy. Radiology 269:1

Saffar B, Bennett M, Metcalf C et al (2015) Retrospective preoperative assessment of the axillary lymph nodes in patients with breast cancer and literature review. Clin Radiol 70:954–959

Scaranelo A, Eiada R, Jacks L et al (2012) Accuracy of unenhanced MR imaging in the detection of axillary lymph node metastasis: study of reproducibility and reliability. Radiology 262:2

Schipper R, van Roozendaal L, de Vries B et al (2013a) Axillary ultrasound for preoperative nodal staging in breast cancer patients: is it of added value? Breast 22:1108–1113

Schipper RJ, Smidt ML, van Roozendaal LM et al (2013b) Noninvasive nodal staging in patients with breast cancer using gadofosveset-enhanced magnetic resonance imaging: a feasibility study. Invest Radiol 48(3):134–139

Schipper R, Paiman ML, Beets-Tan R et al (2015) Diagnostic performance of dedicated axillary T2- and diffusion-weighted MR imaging for nodal staging in breast cancer. Radiology 275:2

Sever A, Mills P, Jones S et al (2012) Sentinel node identification using microbubbles and contrast-enhanced ultrasonography. Clin Radiol 67(7):687–694

Siesling S, van Dijck JA, Visser O et al (2003) Trends in incidence of and mortality from cancer in The Netherlands in the period 1989–1998. Eur J Cancer 39(17):2521–2530

Suvi R, Mazena S, Sarianna J et al (2015) Contrast-enhanced ultrasound-guided axillary lymph node core biopsy: diagnostic accuracy in preoperative staging of invasive breast cancer. Eur J Radiol 84:2130–2136

Taylor K, O'Keeffe S, Britton PD et al (2011) Ultra-sound elastography as an adjuvant to conventional ultrasound in the preoperative assessment of axillary lymph nodes in suspected breast cancer: a pilot study. Clin Radiol 66:1064–1071

Van Wely BJ, de Wilt JH, Francissen C et al (2015) Meta-analysis of ultrasound-guided biopsy of suspicious axillary lymph nodes in the selection of patients with extensive axillary tumour burden in breast cancer. Br J Surg 102(3):159–168

Verheuvel N, Ooms H, Tjan-Heijnen V (2016) Predictors for extensive nodal involvement in breast cancer patients with axillary lymph node metastases. Breast 27:175–181

Veronesi U, Paganelli G, Viale G et al (2003) A randomised comparison of sentinel node biopsy with routine axillary dissection in breast cancer. N Engl J Med 349:546–553

Wallis M, Kilburn-Toppin F, Taylor-Phillips S (2017) Does preoperative axillary staging lead to overtreatment of women with screen detected breast cancer. Clin Radiol 73(5):467–472

Will O, Purkayastha S, Chan C et al (2006) Diagnostic precision of nanoparticle-enhanced MRI for lymph-node metastases: a meta-analysis. Lancet Oncol 7(1):52–60

Wojcinski S, Dupont J, Schmidt W et al (2012) Real-time ultrasound elastography in 180 axillary lymph nodes: elasticity distribution in healthy lymph nodes and prediction of breast cancer metastases. BMC Med Imaging 12:35

Imaging of Ductal Carcinoma In Situ (DCIS)

Paola Clauser, Marianna Fanizza,
and Pascal A. T. Baltzer

Contents

1 **Background** 288

2 **Diagnosis of DCIS** 288
  2.1 Mammography and Digital Breast Tomosynthesis 289
  2.2 Ultrasound 291
  2.3 Contrast-Enhanced Breast Magnetic Resonance Imaging and Contrast-Enhanced Mammography 293

3 **Comparative Sensitivity of Mammography and MRI** 296

4 **Risk Stratification in DCIS** 296

5 **Preoperative and Intraoperative Management of DCIS** 297

6 **Conclusion** 299

References 299

Abstract

The term ductal carcinoma in situ (DCIS) indicates a heterogeneous spectrum of disease with different prognosis and behavior. In most of the cases, DCIS is diagnosed in asymptomatic women during screening, though in some cases women might present with nipple discharge or a palpable mass. Typically, DCIS presents on mammography as microcalcifications with or without an associated mass or architectural distortion. Digital breast tomosynthesis has limited additional value for the evaluation of microcalcifications, but it can help in the identification and characterization

---

P. Clauser · P. A. T. Baltzer (✉)
Division of Molecular and Gender Imaging,
Department of Biomedical Imaging and Image-
Guided Therapy, Medical University of Vienna,
Vienna, Austria
e-mail: pascal.baltzer@meduniwien.ac.at

M. Fanizza
Division of Molecular and Gender Imaging,
Department of Biomedical Imaging and Image-
Guided Therapy, Medical University of Vienna,
Vienna, Austria

Radiology Department, Fondazione IRCCS
Policlinico San Matteo, Pavia, Italy

© Springer Nature Switzerland AG 2022
M. Fuchsjäger et al. (eds.), *Breast Imaging*, Medical Radiology Diagnostic Imaging,
https://doi.org/10.1007/978-3-030-94918-1_14

of the concomitant soft-tissue modifications. DCIS is rarely primarily detected on ultrasound, though in some cases it might present as mass or with ductal abnormalities. Contrast-enhanced magnetic resonance imaging (MRI) is playing an increasingly relevant role in the diagnosis and management of DCIS. MRI has a higher sensitivity than mammography for DCIS, as it is able to identify also noncalcified lesions, and can more accurately assess the extent of disease. Whether this same role could be true for contrast-enhanced mammography as well is not yet established.

1 Background

Ductal carcinoma in situ (DCIS) is defined as a neoplastic deregulation of epithelial cell proliferation within the breast ducts, typically affecting the whole terminal ductolobular unit. It does not permeate the basal membrane and is thus noninvasive (or in situ) (Ellis 2010). While many authors still consider DCIS as a precursor lesion in the development of invasive carcinoma, others have suggested that DCIS may have a direct possibility to progress and metastasize. This theory is supported by the evidence of DCIS-related breast cancer mortality and of a lacking statistical connection between successful local treatment— to avoid local recurrence—and mortality in case of primary DCIS (Ellis 2010; Barrio and Van Zee 2017; Narod and Sopik 2018; Thompson et al. 2018).

As all neoplastic lesions, DCIS represents a heterogeneous spectrum of disease. While some DCIS can progress and even cause death, others will never progress into a clinically manifest disease. In autopsy studies on women who died of other reasons than breast cancer, the prevalence of undiagnosed DCIS has been reported as being around 8.9% (0–14.7%) while the rate of previously undiagnosed invasive cancer was 1.3% (0–1.8%) (Duffy et al. 2003; Erbas et al. 2006). Studies on initially misdiagnosed DCIS suggest that 14–53% may progress to invasive breast cancer within 10–15 years (Erbas et al. 2006). In

addition, 3% of all DCIS present with lymph node metastasis at diagnosis, and 1.5–22.5% of all DCIS will recur with an invasive component, though recurrence was also found to be correlated with resection margins (Narod and Sopik 2018). The risk of a DCIS progressing in an aggressive disease seems to be related to its grade, with high-grade tumors being associated with a worse prognosis (Buerger et al. 1999; Simpson et al. 2005). According to some authors, the more aggressive forms of DCIS are also characterized by multiple localization in the same lobe as well as aberrant branching and lobularization, defined as neoductgenesis (Tot 2005; Zhou et al. 2014). The identification of these patterns at imaging and pathology should help distinguish cancer aggressiveness and tailor therapy accordingly.

2 Diagnosis of DCIS

Imaging has played a central role in the understanding and management of DCIS. The diagnosis of DCIS increased significantly with the introduction of breast cancer screening programs, and about 20% of all cancers diagnosed when screening with mammography are DCIS (Duffy et al. 2005; Virnig et al. 2010; Siegel et al. 2018). In the majority of the cases, DCIS is asymptomatic but in approximately 20% of DCIS cases, patients may present with nipple discharge or a palpable lesion (Schouten van der Velden et al. 2006). As a majority of DCIS presents with microcalcifications, mammography plays a central role in the diagnosis of this entity (Virnig et al. 2010). With the improvement of ultrasound (US) technology, it became evident that some lesions present with associated soft-tissue alterations that can be detected by using US (Gwak et al. 2011; Jin et al. 2015). The introduction of contrast-enhanced magnetic resonance imaging (MRI) led to new insights into DCIS, in particular revealing that at least 10% and up to 40% of DCIS do not present with or as mammographic microcalcifications (Stomper et al. 1989; Kuhl et al. 2007), and that the identification of hypervascularization rather than microcalcifications could help guiding the management of these lesions (Esserman et al. 2006; Kuhl et al. 2007).

2.1 Mammography and Digital Breast Tomosynthesis

The detection of microcalcifications and, consequently, the diagnosis of DCIS increased with the spread of screening programs for breast cancer and also with the transition from screen-film to digital mammography. Improvements in image quality led to an increase in cancer detection through better visualization of smaller calcification clusters (Pisano et al. 2005; Bluekens et al. 2012; Luiten et al. 2017). Currently, approximately 42–72% of DCIS are initially diagnosed as asymptomatic microcalcifications visible on mammography. DCIS is detected in approximately 1.5 per 1000 women screened and accounts for 20–25% of cancers detected at screening (Duffy et al. 2003; Luiten et al. 2017; Siegel et al. 2018). However, about one-third of all lesions detected by mammography are microcalcifications: thus, microcalcifications are a rather common finding, but not necessarily associated with breast cancer (Wilkinson et al. 2017).

To stratify the risk of malignancy in these lesions, the Breast Imaging-Reporting And Data System (BI-RADS) committee of the American College of Radiology (ACR) has suggested semantic descriptors that define morphology and distribution of mammographic microcalcifications and assist in risk stratification (D'Orsi et al. 2013).

The most characteristic features of DCIS on mammography are fine microcalcifications with linear, linear-branching, or pleomorphic morphology and a linear or segmental distribution (Fig. 1). Approximately 80–100% of microcalcifications presenting with these characteristics are associated with malignancy (Liberman et al. 1998; Kim et al. 2015). The fine linear microcalcifications in DCIS are usually thin, irregular, and discontinuous (D'Orsi 2010). DCIS can also appear as amorphous or coarse heterogeneous microcalcifications. Amorphous calcifications (Fig. 2) are hazy and less conspicuous in com-

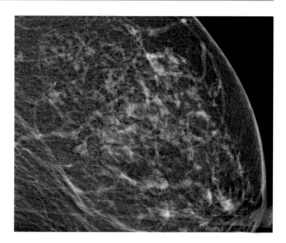

Fig. 1 Postmenopausal asymptomatic woman presenting with pleomorphic microcalcifications. Stereotactic vacuum-assisted breast biopsy revealed DCIS, G2, Her2/neu positive

parison to pleomorphic and coarse heterogeneous (D'Orsi 2010; D'Orsi et al. 2013) and might represent DCIS in up to 20% of the cases (Berg et al. 2001; Kim et al. 2015). Coarse heterogeneous microcalcifications are larger than amorphous and pleomorphic microcalcifications (Fig. 3) and are associated with malignancy in 12–20% of the cases (Bent et al. 2010; Kim et al. 2015, 2018). DCIS usually does not present with a diffuse distribution, but it can be characterized by a regional or clustered/grouped distribution. In these cases, the positive predictive value ranges between 8% and 15% (Bent et al. 2010; Kim et al. 2015, 2018).

While BI-RADS features indeed help stratifying the risk of underlying breast cancer, a meta-analysis has highlighted one major issue: there is practically no combination of BI-RADS features that does not exceed BI-RADS 3 benchmarks (Rominger et al. 2012). This implies that formally the vast majority of microcalcifications would require invasive workup, leading to a large amount of unnecessary biopsies for benign microcalcifications. Besides adverse effects of the minimal invasive biopsy procedure, the stereotactic biopsy procedure is technically demanding and expensive. Therefore, various alternatives have been proposed to manage suspicious microcalcifications classified as BI-RADS 3 and 4a. The option

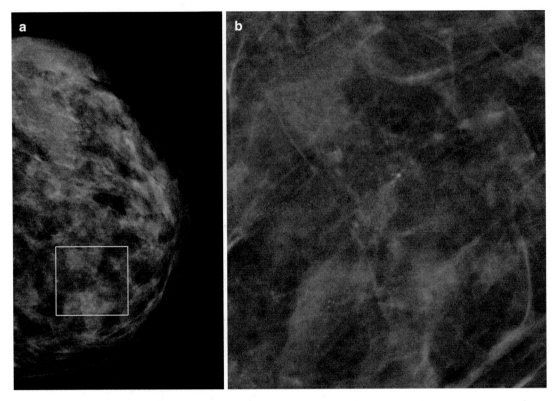

Fig. 2 Perimenopausal asymptomatic woman presenting with amorphous microcalcifications. Stereotactic vacuum-assisted breast biopsy revealed DCIS, G2, Her2/neu positive

of offering short-term follow-up is probably least favorable, as DCIS lesions may remain stable over years and unchanged imaging appearance does not exclude breast cancer (Coleman 2019). Additional tests, such as breast magnetic resonance imaging (MRI), can identify associated suspicious enhancement with a very high accuracy (see Sect. 2.3). The large-scale feasibility and cost-effectiveness of additional breast MRI examinations in this setting, though, remain unproven.

The role of digital breast tomosynthesis (DBT) for the diagnosis of DCIS is also limited. The majority of the studies showed that DBT increased the detection rate of invasive cancers, but not that of DCIS (Gilbert et al. 2015; Caumo et al. 2018; Skaane et al. 2019). This can be clearly explained by the technical characteristics of DBT: the reconstruction of quasi-3D images on the two mammographic views improves soft-tissue evaluation but does not add relevant information on the distribution or characteristics of microcalcifications. On the contrary, it might hinder the detection of small clusters of microcalcifications, though most studies agree that the performance of DBT and mammography to diagnose microcalcifications is comparable (Kopans et al. 2011; Clauser et al. 2015; Tagliafico and Houssami 2015). DBT can be helpful in detecting additional signs suggestive of malignancy, as the intraductal location of microcalcifications or the association with masses or architectural distortions, which might indicate the presence of associated invasive disease. DBT can also improve the detection of noncalcified DCIS and the evaluation of lesion extent (Fig. 4) (Berger et al. 2016; Su et al. 2017).

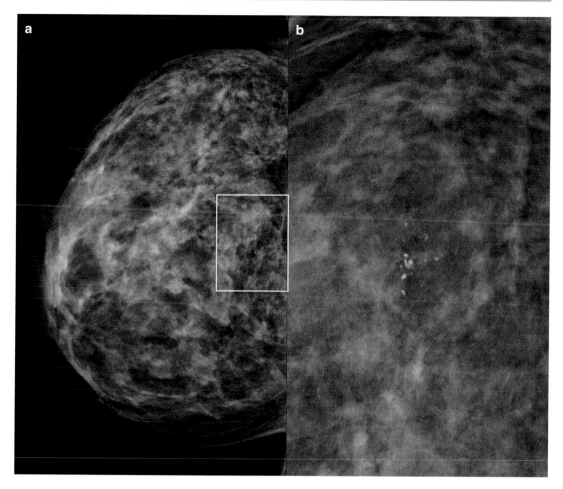

Fig. 3 Premenopausal asymptomatic woman presenting with coarse heterogeneous microcalcifications. Stereotactic vacuum-assisted breast biopsy revealed DCIS, G1, luminal A type

Synthetic mammography images, reconstructed from the DBT dataset, have been introduced as a method to avoid the increase in radiation dose due to the double acquisition of mammography and DBT. While the first studies indicated comparable results when using synthetic or digital mammography (Skaane et al. 2014; Bernardi et al. 2016; Clauser et al. 2016), further analyses suggested that the use of synthetic mammography does not provide the diagnostic performance achievable with combined mammography and DBT in screening (Caumo et al. 2017; Hofvind et al. 2019). In addition, microcalcifications might not be optimally visualized on synthetic mammography, and image characteristics vary between vendors (Nelson et al. 2016; Baldelli et al. 2018). Until more evidence is available, digital mammography remains the preferred examination technique to evaluate microcalcifications (Bae and Moon 2018).

2.2 Ultrasound

As DCIS usually presents with microcalcifications, the initial diagnosis of DCIS rarely occurs when using ultrasound.

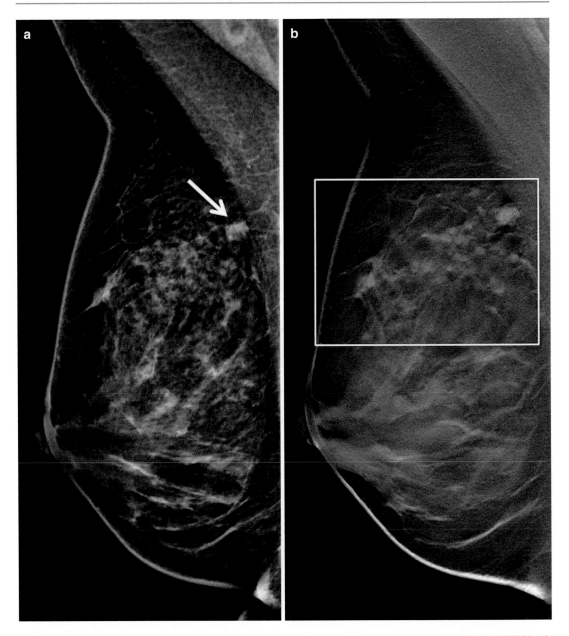

Fig. 4 Perimenopausal asymptomatic woman with a mammography detected mass (**a**). (**b**) The additional DBT identified the extensive associated architectural distortion, corresponding to DCIS, G2

If DCIS is visible on US, more than 50% of the findings appear as a hypoechoic mass lesion with indistinct margins, alone or with associated US-visible microcalcifications (Fig. 5). Other less common features, detected in 10–20% of the cases, can be microcalcifications alone or ductal abnormalities, in particular the identification of intraductal hypervascularized lesions, with or without microcalcifications (Londero et al. 2007; Scoggins et al. 2015). The presence of an US-visible lesion, as opposed to DCIS visible on mammography only, seems to be associated with a worse prognosis (Yoon et al. 2019).

Ultrasound can serve as image guidance for biopsy, when the lesion can be detected.

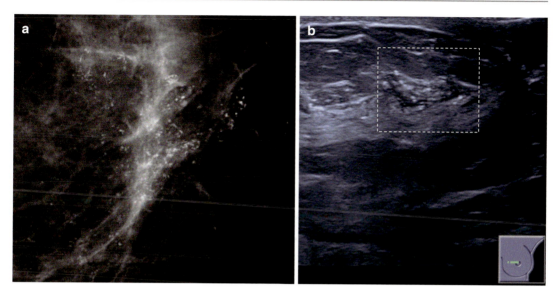

Fig. 5 Postmenopausal asymptomatic woman presenting with extensive pleomorphic microcalcifications on mammography (**a**). US (**b**) demonstrates an intraductal hypoechoic lesion (dashed margins) with evident hyperechoic calcifications. US-guided core needle biopsy revealed a calcified DCIS, G3

2.3 Contrast-Enhanced Breast Magnetic Resonance Imaging and Contrast-Enhanced Mammography

Breast MRI cannot directly visualize mammographic microcalcifications, but it is able to detect contrast enhancement associated with tumor growth and likely depict biologically active breast cancer (Kuhl 2009). Breast cancer growth leads to an increasing demand of nutrients that cannot be met by diffusion alone. The resulting lack of nutrients, including oxygen, leads to a hypoxia-induced and cytokine-mediated neovascularization, referred to as the angiogenetic switch. Consequently, biologically active neoplastic lesions enhance starting from about 2 to 3 mm in size (Jansen et al. 2009). Despite a regularly encountered opinion, this process not only is present in invasive cancer, but also affects all kinds of neoplastic growth including DCIS, lesions of uncertain malignant potential, and benign proliferations as well as inflammations. Consequently, a biologically active DCIS should present with contrast enhancement, whereas the absence of enhancement should allow to largely exclude an active neoplasm in case of mammographic microcalcifications.

MRI has been investigated by several studies as an additional examination technique to differentiate benign from malignant microcalcifications and avoid unnecessary biopsies. A meta-analysis investigating the use of contrast-enhanced breast MRI to diagnose malignancy in lesions presenting as mammographic microcalcifications reported a general negative predictive value of 90%, which increased to 99% when considering only the performance of breast MRI to exclude invasive cancers (Bennani-Baiti and Baltzer 2016; Baltzer et al. 2018). Despite the high negative predictive value, the best diagnostic criteria for the detection of malignancy in case of microcalcifications are still unclear. While the differentiation between presence and absence of enhancement may be the best predictor to exclude malignancy, its application would potentially yield a high rate of false-positive findings. Encouraging results regarding the application of the Kaiser score in lesions presenting as mammographic microcalcifications have recently been published (Wengert et al. 2019).

Diagnosis of malignancy, however, is not the only use of breast MRI in case of a diagnosed or suspected DCIS. MRI can be able to better depict the extent of disease, particularly in women with dense breast parenchyma. In addition, it can better evaluate the involvement of the nipple as well as the distance from the skin, and thus help in pre-surgical planning (Balleyguier et al. 2019; Preibsch et al. 2019). The imaging characteristics of DCIS can be subtle, and a certain level of expertise for image interpretation and accurate preoperative evaluation is needed (Dietzel et al. 2017; Lam et al. 2019).

In the majority of the cases, DCIS presents as a non-mass enhancement (60–80%). The detection of a mass lesion is less frequent for pure DCIS lesions and can be seen in 14–40% of the cases. In less than 10% of the cases, DCIS presents at breast MRI as a focus (Greenwood et al. 2013; Dietzel et al. 2017).

When presenting as non-mass enhancement, DCIS is typically characterized by a linear or segmental distribution. The internal enhancement is usually heterogeneous or clumped: in particular in advanced cases, the more specific clustered ring pattern can be seen (Fig. 6).

The imaging characteristics of DCIS presenting as mass are variable but fulfill the criteria of malignancy (as given in Dietzel and Baltzer 2018): typically, the lesion presents with non-circumscribed margins and oval or round shape

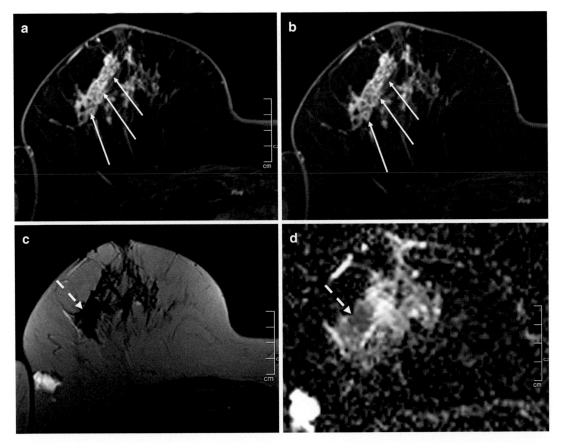

Fig. 6 Premenopausal asymptomatic woman with screen-detected parenchymal asymmetry and without definite lesion at US. Contrast-enhanced breast MRI (**a**: early enhanced, **b**: late enhanced, **c**: T2w-TSE, **d**: ADC map derived from diffusion-weighted-imaging) shows an early and distinct enhancement (**a**) with washout (loss of signal) in the late phase (**b**). The internal morphology of this non-mass enhancement is "clustered ring," a finding specific for DCIS. Note that both lesions correlated on T2w (**c**) and the ADC map (**d**) are hypointense, hinting at a biologically more aggressive lesion. Histology revealed DCIS G3, Her2/neu positive

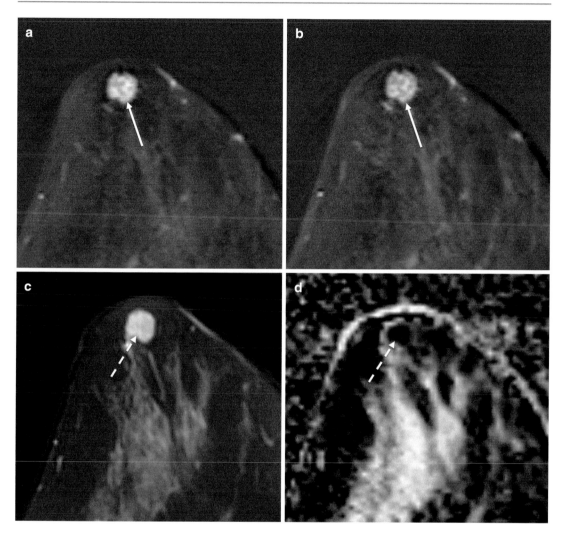

Fig. 7 Perimenopausal woman presenting with a new palpable lesion in the retroareolar region of the right breast. Contrast-enhanced breast MRI (**a**: early enhanced, **b**: late enhanced, **c**: T2w-STIR, **d**: ADC map derived from diffusion-weighted-imaging) shows a mass lesion (arrows) with non-circumscribed margins, washout in the late phase, and heterogeneous internal enhancement. STIR image shows high signal intensity (**c**), while the ADC map shows a low signal intensity (dashed arrows). US-guided core needle biopsy revealed a noncalcified DCIS, G1, luminal A type

(Fig. 7). Irregular masses with spiculated margins have also been described in the literature (Greenwood et al. 2013; Dietzel et al. 2017).

Not many studies evaluated the role of contrast-enhanced digital mammography (CEDM) for DCIS. As microcalcifications are clearly visible on CEDM, the additional value of CEDM compared to MRI could be the concomitant evaluation of both microcalcifications and associated contrast.

To date, only one small study analyzed the usefulness of CEDM for DCIS. The authors showed that not all pure DCIS showed a detectable enhancement on CEDM, while enhancement could be identified in lesions with microinvasion (Vignoli et al. 2019). The future adoption of CEDM in clinical practice, however, will largely depend on its ability to detect subtle lesions such as DCIS in order to match the superior sensitivity of MRI (Baltzer et al. 2017).

3 Comparative Sensitivity of Mammography and MRI

A number of studies have compared the sensitivity of mammography with that of MRI. Both methods can claim an advantage over the other: while MRI cannot visualize microcalcifications, mammography does not provide functional information. Advocates of MRI regularly point out that the functional information on tissue vascularization would rather detect biologically aggressive high-risk DCIS while mammography inherently tends to diagnose less aggressive, probably even biologically insignificant disease (Kuhl et al. 2007; Kuhl 2009). While it seems to be true that MRI has a higher sensitivity for detection of DCIS than mammography (Fig. 8), results are somewhat controversial as some studies report a higher sensitivity for DCIS using mammography as compared to MRI. A definite bias towards mammography-detected DCIS may be assumed as only mammography is used in national screening programs for imaging-based secondary prevention. This assumption is confirmed by the higher absolute and relative rates of DCIS in mammography-screened populations. While a negative contrast-enhanced MRI scan can indeed largely rule out (invasive) breast cancer, the hypothesis that only low-grade and low-risk DCIS are missed by breast MRI is not backed up by the current empirical evidence (Facius et al. 2007; Kuhl et al. 2007; Vag et al. 2008).

4 Risk Stratification in DCIS

When DCIS is diagnosed, two main factors have to be taken into consideration: the risk for this lesion to be high grade and thus associated with a worse prognosis, and the risk for this lesion to be associated with invasive cancer, requiring a more aggressive therapy including axillary lymph node sampling.

Mammography is of limited use in differentiating low- from high-grade lesions. Some studies suggested that DCIS presenting as linear-branching and casting-type calcifications as well as with an associated mass and larger lesion size are more often high-grade tumors (Dinkel et al. 2000; Barreau et al. 2005; Zhou et al. 2017). However, all these scarce reports showed a large overlap between lesion characteristics and grade, suggesting a limited role of mammography in this respect.

MRI seems to be the best tool for both detection of high-grade DCIS and identification of previously missed invasive cancers associated with DCIS lesions. Low-grade, estrogen receptor-

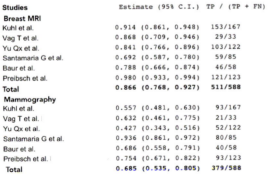
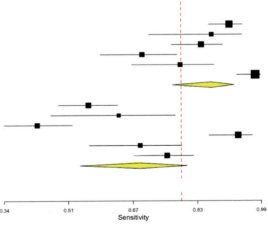
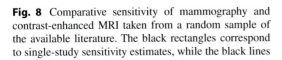

Fig. 8 Comparative sensitivity of mammography and contrast-enhanced MRI taken from a random sample of the available literature. The black rectangles correspond to single-study sensitivity estimates, while the black lines denote the 95% confidence intervals of these findings. The yellow diamonds represent pooled (random effects model) subgroup estimates with their 95% confidence intervals

positive tumors more often present as focal enhancement, while high-grade, estrogen receptor-negative tumors are usually larger in size and present with a clumped, segmental enhancement (Esserman et al. 2006). In addition, low-grade lesions more often lack enhancement on MRI (Facius et al. 2007; Kuhl et al. 2007; Vag et al. 2008), though this is not a robust predictor (see Fig. 7). Some authors investigated the use of diffusion-weighted imaging (DWI) and peak enhancement to distinguish low- from high-grade tumors. High-grade DCIS is characterized by lower apparent diffusion coefficient (DWI) value and higher peak initial enhancement (Iima et al. 2011; Rahbar et al. 2012). If FDG PET might also play a role in identifying DCIS with a worse prognosis by identifying an increased uptake of radioactive labeled glucose as suggested by preliminary evidence is yet unclear (Graña-López et al. 2019).

Mammography and ultrasound can play a role in diagnosing the presence of an invasive component after a histological diagnosis of DCIS. The presence of a mass, architectural distortion, or focal asymmetry should always raise the suspicion of an associated invasive component (Sim et al. 2015). In addition, the presence of a palpable mass and a large diameter and the presence of BI-RADS 5 characteristics at imaging can indicate the presence of an invasive component. In these cases, the use of a larger needle or the acquisition of more samples at biopsy might be indicated to ensure a correct diagnosis (Schulz et al. 2013; Hogue et al. 2014).

Elastography has also been proposed as a method to identify DCIS at higher risk of being associated with an invasive carcinoma. The size of the US finding and an increased stiffness have been associated with an increased risk of an associated invasive carcinoma, but the published results are rather heterogeneous (Evans et al. 2016; Bae et al. 2017; Shin et al. 2019). Currently, while US may suggest the presence of an invasive component, it is not possible to reliably distinguish DCIS from invasive breast cancer based on mammography and ultrasound (Londero et al. 2007; Scoggins et al. 2015; Shin et al. 2019).

In addition to a superior lesion extent mapping during preoperative evaluation, MRI can also suggest the presence of an invasive component associated with DCIS. The presence of a spiculated mass as opposed to non-mass enhancement only, the size of the lesion, and a presence of a heterogeneous enhancement in a non-mass lesion are all factors associated with a higher percentage of an associated invasive component (Hahn et al. 2013; Lee et al. 2016; Lamb et al. 2019). In addition, DWI may play a role in this setting: despite an inter-study variability in ADC values, the presence of an invasive breast cancer component is associated with significantly lower ADC values (Bickel et al. 2015).

5 Preoperative and Intraoperative Management of DCIS

Chemotherapy and hormonal therapy currently have no role in the preoperative management of DCIS (NICE 2018; Morrow et al. 2016; Ditsch et al. 2019), and after diagnosis and evaluation of the extension of disease (Kandel et al. 2020), surgery is performed.

In case with larger area of microcalcifications or enhancement, extending for more than one quadrant, mastectomy is generally indicated (Sakorafas and Farley 2003). Mastectomy should also be preferred in patients with multiple tumors and persistent positive margins after re-excision and in all the cases in which irradiation after surgery is contraindicated (Sakorafas and Farley 2003). For the cases in which breast-conserving surgery (BCS) with or without radiation therapy is feasible, a precise localization of the malignant area is mandatory prior to surgery.

Three methods are mostly used for the preoperative localization of DCIS (Chan et al. 2015):

- Wire-guided localization
- Radioactive seed localization (RSL)
- Radioguided occult lesion localization (ROLL)

Depending on the localization and the extension of the tumor, one or more wires can be placed, to ensure a complete resection of the tumor with sufficient free margins to reduce the risk of recurrence (Mannu et al. 2020).

Both wire localization and localization methods with radioactive tracers showed a high accuracy (Chan et al. 2015), and the choice of how to perform the preoperative localization is currently mostly guided by surgeons and radiologists' expertise and preferences (Niinikoski et al. 2019; Agahozo et al. 2020).

The intraoperative evaluation of the resection margins is advised in order to reduce the number of reoperations (Harness et al. 2014). The intraoperative histological evaluation of the surgical margins seems to be the most effective technique to evaluate margin status (Laws et al. 2016). In DCIS presenting with microcalcifications, the evaluation of the surgical specimen with mammography can help determining the complete excision of the malignant lesion. In the last years, the classical mammography of the surgical specimen has been progressively substituted with remote intraoperative specimen mammography, performed in the surgical block instead of the radiology unit, thus saving time and facilitating the procedure and communication between radiologists and surgeons (Mariscotti et al. 2020) (Fig. 9). In addition, digital breast tomosynthesis systems have been implemented for intraoperative specimen imaging, which improves the evaluation of soft tissues and the overall accuracy of the specimen evaluation (Garlaschi et al. 2019).

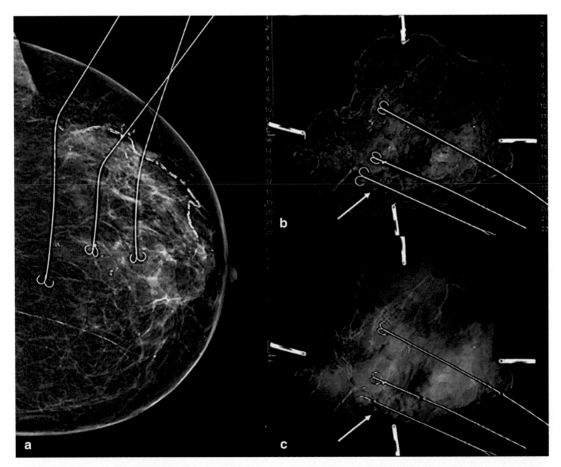

Fig. 9 Postmenopausal asymptomatic woman with a high-grade ductal carcinoma in situ. A preoperative stereotactic guided wire localization was performed. Three hook wires were used to precisely circumscribe the area with microcalcifications (**a**, craniocaudal control mammography). Mammography (**b**) and DBT (**c**) of the surgical specimen were performed, which showed close margins in the anterior margin of the specimen (arrow in **b** and **c**). This finding was confirmed at the histological evaluation

6 Conclusion

In conclusion, imaging plays a major role in the diagnosis of DCIS, a non-obligate precursor lesion to invasive DCIS. Currently, digital mammography remains the most important imaging method in diagnosing DCIS due to its implementation in national screening programs and its ability to detect microcalcifications as an imaging hallmark of DCIS. However, its lack of specificity causes problems: diagnosis of microcalcifications requiring unnecessary invasive and expensive biopsies that ultimately turn out as benign and diagnosis of biologically irrelevant disease that will never progress into invasive breast cancer. Further imaging tests have been investigated to resolve this issue with varying success: while the use of additional breast MRI can largely exclude breast cancer in general and specifically invasive breast cancer with very high NPVs and may thus obviate the need for biopsies of mammographic microcalcifications, the ability of different modalities to distinguish biologically aggressive from less aggressive DCIS is—though encouraging results have been published in particular for diagnosing invasive breast cancer associated with DCIS—less well explored.

References

Agahozo MC et al (2020) Radioactive seed versus wire-guided localization for ductal carcinoma in situ of the breast: comparable resection margins. Ann Surg Oncol. https://doi.org/10.1245/s10434-020-08744-8

Bae MS, Moon WK (2018) Is synthetic mammography comparable to digital mammography for detection of microcalcifications in screening? Radiology 289(3):639–640. https://doi.org/10.1148/radiol.2018181961

Bae JS et al (2017) Prediction of invasive breast cancer using shear-wave elastography in patients with biopsy-confirmed ductal carcinoma in situ. Eur Radiol 27(1):7–15. https://doi.org/10.1007/s00330-016-4359-6

Baldelli P et al (2018) A comparative study of physical image quality in digital and synthetic mammography from commercially available mammography systems. Phys Med Biol 63(16):165020. https://doi.org/10.1088/1361-6560/aad106

Balleyguier C et al (2019) Preoperative breast magnetic resonance imaging in women with local ductal carcinoma in situ to optimize surgical outcomes: results from the randomized phase III trial IRCIS. J Clin Oncol 37(11):885–892. https://doi.org/10.1200/JCO.18.00595

Baltzer PAT et al (2017) New diagnostic tools for breast cancer. Memo 10(3):175–180. https://doi.org/10.1007/s12254-017-0341-5

Baltzer PAT et al (2018) Is breast MRI a helpful additional diagnostic test in suspicious mammographic microcalcifications? Magn Reson Imaging 46:70–74. https://doi.org/10.1016/j.mri.2017.10.012

Barreau B et al (2005) Mammography of ductal carcinoma in situ of the breast: review of 909 cases with radiographic-pathologic correlations. Eur J Radiol 54(1):55–61. https://doi.org/10.1016/j.ejrad.2004.11.019

Barrio AV, Van Zee KJ (2017) Controversies in the treatment of ductal carcinoma in situ. Annu Rev Med 68:197–211. https://doi.org/10.1146/annurev-med-050715-104920

Bennani-Baiti B, Baltzer PA (2016) MR imaging for diagnosis of malignancy in mammographic microcalcifications: a systematic review and meta-analysis. Radiology 2016:161106. https://doi.org/10.1148/radiol.2016161106

Bent CK et al (2010) The positive predictive value of BI-RADS microcalcification descriptors and final assessment categories. AJR Am J Roentgenol 194(5):1378–1383. https://doi.org/10.2214/AJR.09.3423

Berg WA et al (2001) Biopsy of amorphous breast calcifications: pathologic outcome and yield at stereotactic biopsy. Radiology 221(2):495–503. https://doi.org/10.1148/radiol.2212010164

Berger N et al (2016) Assessment of the extent of microcalcifications to predict the size of a ductal carcinoma in situ: comparison between tomosynthesis and conventional mammography. Clin Imaging 40(6):1269–1273. https://doi.org/10.1016/j.clinimag.2016.09.003

Bernardi D et al (2016) Breast cancer screening with tomosynthesis (3D mammography) with acquired or synthetic 2D mammography compared with 2D mammography alone (STORM-2): a population-based prospective study. Lancet Oncol 17(8):1105–1113. https://doi.org/10.1016/S1470-2045(16)30101-2

Bickel H et al (2015) Quantitative apparent diffusion coefficient as a noninvasive imaging biomarker for the differentiation of invasive breast cancer and ductal carcinoma in situ. Invest Radiol 50(2):95–100. https://doi.org/10.1097/RLI.0000000000000104

Bluekens AMJ et al (2012) Comparison of digital screening mammography and screen-film mammography in the early detection of clinically relevant cancers: a multicenter study. Radiology 265(3):707–714. https://doi.org/10.1148/radiol.12111461

Buerger H et al (1999) Different genetic pathways in the evolution of invasive breast cancer are associated with distinct morphological subtypes. J Pathol 189(4):521–526. https://doi.org/10.1002/(SICI)1096-9896(199912)189:4<521::AID-PATH472>3.0.CO;2-B

Caumo F et al (2017) Digital breast tomosynthesis with synthesized two-dimensional images versus full-field digital mammography for population screening: outcomes from the Verona screening program.

Radiology 2017:170745. https://doi.org/10.1148/radiol.2017170745

Caumo F et al (2018) Comparison of breast cancers detected in the Verona screening program following transition to digital breast tomosynthesis screening with cancers detected at digital mammography screening. Breast Cancer Res Treat 170(2):391–397. https://doi.org/10.1007/s10549-018-4756-4

Chan BKY et al (2015) Localization techniques for guided surgical excision of non-palpable breast lesions. Cochrane Database Syst Rev (12):CD009206. https://doi.org/10.1002/14651858.CD009206.pub2

Clauser P et al (2015) Comparison of digital breast tomosynthesis vs full field digital mammography for the detection and characterisation of calcifications in the breast in ECR 2015 Book of abstracts - B - Scientific sessions and late-breaking clinical trials. Insights Imaging 6(1):159–445. https://doi.org/10.1007/s13244-015-0387-z

Clauser P et al (2016) Diagnostic performance of digital breast tomosynthesis with a wide scan angle compared to full-field digital mammography for the detection and characterization of microcalcifications. Eur J Radiol 85(12):2161–2168. https://doi.org/10.1016/j.ejrad.2016.10.004

Coleman WB (2019) Breast ductal carcinoma in situ: precursor to invasive breast cancer. Am J Pathol 189(5):942–945. https://doi.org/10.1016/j.ajpath.2019.03.002

D'Orsi CJ (2010) Imaging for the diagnosis and management of ductal carcinoma in situ. J Natl Cancer Inst Monogr 2010(41):214–217. https://doi.org/10.1093/jncimonographs/lgq037

D'Orsi CJ et al (2013) ACR BI-RADS® atlas, breast imaging reporting and data system, 5th edn. American College of Radiology, Reston, VA

Dietzel M, Baltzer PAT (2018) How to use the Kaiser score as a clinical decision rule for diagnosis in multiparametric breast MRI: a pictorial essay. Insights Imaging 9(3):325–335. https://doi.org/10.1007/s13244-018-0611-8

Dietzel M et al (2017) Differentiation of ductal carcinoma in situ versus fibrocystic changes by magnetic resonance imaging: are there pathognomonic imaging features? Acta Radiol 58(10):1206–1214. https://doi.org/10.1177/0284185117690420

Dinkel HP, Gassel AM, Tschammler A (2000) Is the appearance of microcalcifications on mammography useful in predicting histological grade of malignancy in ductal cancer in situ? Br J Radiol 73(873):938–944. https://doi.org/10.1259/bjr.73.873.11064645

Ditsch N et al (2019) AGO recommendations for the diagnosis and treatment of patients with early breast cancer: update 2019. Breast Care 14(4):224–245. https://doi.org/10.1159/000501000

Duffy SW et al (2003) The relative contributions of screen-detected in situ and invasive breast carcinomas in reducing mortality from the disease. Eur J Cancer 39(12):1755–1760. https://doi.org/10.1016/s0959-8049(03)00259-4

Duffy SW et al (2005) Overdiagnosis and overtreatment of breast cancer: estimates of overdiagnosis from two trials of mammographic screening for breast cancer. Breast Cancer Res 7(6):258–265. https://doi.org/10.1186/bcr1354

Ellis IO (2010) Intraductal proliferative lesions of the breast: morphology, associated risk and molecular biology. Mod Pathol 23(Suppl 2):S1–S7. https://doi.org/10.1038/modpathol.2010.56

Erbas B et al (2006) The natural history of ductal carcinoma in situ of the breast: a review. Breast Cancer Res Treat 97(2):135–144. https://doi.org/10.1007/s10549-005-9101-z

Esserman LJ et al (2006) Magnetic resonance imaging captures the biology of ductal carcinoma in situ. J Clin Oncol 24(28):4603–4610. https://doi.org/10.1200/JCO.2005.04.5518

Evans A et al (2016) Stiffness at shear-wave elastography and patient presentation predicts upgrade at surgery following an ultrasound-guided core biopsy diagnosis of ductal carcinoma in situ. Clin Radiol 71(11):1156–1159. https://doi.org/10.1016/j.crad.2016.07.004

Facius M et al (2007) Characteristics of ductal carcinoma in situ in magnetic resonance imaging. Clin Imaging 31(6):394–400. https://doi.org/10.1016/j.clinimag.2007.04.030

Garlaschi A et al (2019) Intraoperative digital breast tomosynthesis using a dedicated device is more accurate than standard intraoperative mammography for identifying positive margins. Clin Radiol 74(12):974.e1–974.e6. https://doi.org/10.1016/j.crad.2019.08.004

Gilbert FJ et al (2015) The TOMMY trial: a comparison of TOMosynthesis with digital MammographY in the UK NHS Breast Screening Programme—a multicentre retrospective reading study comparing the diagnostic performance of digital breast tomosynthesis and digital mammography with digital mammography alone. Health Technol Assess 19(4):i–xxv, 1–136. https://doi.org/10.3310/hta19040

Graña-López L et al (2019) Can dedicated breast PET help to reduce overdiagnosis and overtreatment by differentiating between indolent and potentially aggressive ductal carcinoma in situ? Eur Radiol. https://doi.org/10.1007/s00330-019-06356-9

Greenwood HI et al (2013) Ductal carcinoma in situ of the breasts: review of MR imaging features. Radiographics 33(6):1569–1588. https://doi.org/10.1148/rg.336125055

Gwak YJ et al (2011) Ultrasonographic detection and characterization of asymptomatic ductal carcinoma in situ with histopathologic correlation. Acta Radiol 52(4):364–371. https://doi.org/10.1258/ar.2011.100391

Hahn SY et al (2013) MR features to suggest microinvasive ductal carcinoma of the breast: can it be differentiated from pure DCIS? Acta Radiol 54(7):742–748. https://doi.org/10.1177/0284185113484640

Harness JK et al (2014) Margins: a status report from the Annual meeting of the American Society of Breast Surgeons. Ann Surg Oncol 21(10):3192–3197. https://doi.org/10.1245/s10434-014-3957-2

Hofvind S et al (2019) Two-view digital breast tomosynthesis versus digital mammography in a population-based breast cancer screening programme (To-Be): a randomised, controlled trial. Lancet Oncol 20(6):795–805. https://doi.org/10.1016/S1470-2045(19)30161-5

Hogue J-C et al (2014) Characteristics associated with upgrading to invasiveness after surgery of a DCIS diagnosed using percutaneous biopsy. Anticancer Res 34(3):1183–1191

Iima M et al (2011) Apparent diffusion coefficient as an MR imaging biomarker of low-risk ductal carcinoma in situ: a pilot study. Radiology 260(2):364–372. https://doi.org/10.1148/radiol.11101892

Jansen SA et al (2009) Ductal carcinoma in situ: X-ray fluorescence microscopy and dynamic contrast-enhanced MR imaging reveals gadolinium uptake within neoplastic mammary ducts in a murine model. Radiology 253(2):399–406. https://doi.org/10.1148/radiol.2533082026

Jin Z-Q et al (2015) Diagnostic evaluation of ductal carcinoma in situ of the breast: ultrasonographic, mammographic and histopathologic correlations. Ultrasound Med Biol 41(1):47–55. https://doi.org/10.1016/j.ultrasmedbio.2014.09.023

Kandel M et al (2020) Cost-effectiveness of preoperative magnetic resonance imaging to optimize surgery in ductal carcinoma in situ of the breast. Eur J Radiol 129:109058. https://doi.org/10.1016/j.ejrad.2020.109058

Kim S-Y et al (2015) Evaluation of malignancy risk stratification of microcalcifications detected on mammography: a study based on the 5th edition of BI-RADS. Ann Surg Oncol 22(9):2895–2901. https://doi.org/10.1245/s10434-014-4362-6

Kim J et al (2018) "Category 4A" microcalcifications: how should this subcategory be applied to microcalcifications seen on mammography? Acta Radiol 59(2):147–153. https://doi.org/10.1177/0284185117709036

Kopans D et al (2011) Calcifications in the breast and digital breast tomosynthesis. Breast J 17(6):638–644. https://doi.org/10.1111/j.1524-4741.2011.01152.x

Kuhl CK (2009) Why do purely intraductal cancers enhance on breast MR images? Radiology 253(2):281–283. https://doi.org/10.1148/radiol.2532091401

Kuhl CK et al (2007) MRI for diagnosis of pure ductal carcinoma in situ: a prospective observational study. Lancet 370(9586):485–492. https://doi.org/10.1016/S0140-6736(07)61232-X

Lam DL et al (2019) The impact of preoperative breast MRI on surgical management of women with newly diagnosed ductal carcinoma in situ. Acad Radiol. https://doi.org/10.1016/j.acra.2019.05.013

Lamb LR et al (2019) Ductal carcinoma in situ (DCIS) at breast MRI: predictors of upgrade to invasive carcinoma. Acad Radiol. https://doi.org/10.1016/j.acra.2019.09.025

Laws A et al (2016) Intraoperative margin assessment in wire-localized breast-conserving surgery for invasive cancer: a population-level comparison of techniques. Ann Surg Oncol 23(10):3290–3296. https://doi.org/10.1245/s10434-016-5401-2

Lee C-W et al (2016) Preoperative clinicopathologic factors and breast magnetic resonance imaging features can predict ductal carcinoma in situ with invasive components. Eur J Radiol 85(4):780–789. https://doi.org/10.1016/j.ejrad.2015.12.027

Liberman L et al (1998) The breast imaging reporting and data system: positive predictive value of mammographic features and final assessment categories. AJR Am J Roentgenol 171(1):35–40. https://doi.org/10.2214/ajr.171.1.9648759

Londero V et al (2007) Role of ultrasound and sonographically guided core biopsy in the diagnostic evaluation of ductal carcinoma in situ (DCIS) of the breast. Radiol Med 112(6):863–876. https://doi.org/10.1007/s11547-007-0183-z

Luiten JD et al (2017) Trends in incidence and tumour grade in screen-detected ductal carcinoma in situ and invasive breast cancer. Breast Cancer Res Treat 166(1):307–314. https://doi.org/10.1007/s10549-017-4412-4

Mannu GS et al (2020) Invasive breast cancer and breast cancer mortality after ductal carcinoma in situ in women attending for breast screening in England, 1988–2014: population based observational cohort study. BMJ 369:m1570. https://doi.org/10.1136/bmj.m1570

Mariscotti G et al (2020) Intraoperative breast specimen assessment in breast conserving surgery: comparison between standard mammography imaging and a remote radiological system. Br J Radiol 93(1109):20190785. https://doi.org/10.1259/bjr.20190785

Morrow M et al (2016) Society of Surgical Oncology-American Society for Radiation Oncology-American Society of Clinical Oncology consensus guideline on margins for breast-conserving surgery with whole-breast irradiation in ductal carcinoma in situ. Pract Radiat Oncol 6(5):287–295. https://doi.org/10.1016/j.prro.2016.06.011

Narod SA, Sopik V (2018) Is invasion a necessary step for metastases in breast cancer? Breast Cancer Res Treat 169(1):9–23. https://doi.org/10.1007/s10549-017-4644-3

Nelson JS et al (2016) How does c-view image quality compare with conventional 2D FFDM? Med Phys 43(5):2538. https://doi.org/10.1118/1.4947293

NICE (2018) Recommendations. Early and locally advanced breast cancer: diagnosis and management. Guidance. NICE. https://www.nice.org.uk/guidance/ng101/chapter/Recommendations. Accessed 15 Aug 2020

Niinikoski L et al (2019) Resection margins and local recurrences of impalpable breast cancer: comparison between radioguided occult lesion localization (ROLL) and radioactive seed localization (RSL). Breast 47:93–101. https://doi.org/10.1016/j.breast.2019.07.004

Pisano ED et al (2005) Diagnostic performance of digital versus film mammography for breast-cancer screening. N Engl J Med 353(17):1773–1783. https://doi.org/10.1056/NEJMoa052911

Preibsch H et al (2019) Accuracy of breast magnetic resonance imaging compared to mammography in the preoperative detection and measurement of pure ductal carcinoma in situ: a retrospective analysis. Acad Radiol 26(6):760–765. https://doi.org/10.1016/j.acra.2018.07.013

Rahbar H et al (2012) In vivo assessment of ductal carcinoma in situ grade: a model incorporating dynamic contrast-enhanced and diffusion-weighted breast MR imaging parameters. Radiology 263(2):374–382. https://doi.org/10.1148/radiol.12111368

Rominger M, Wisgickl C, Timmesfeld N (2012) Breast microcalcifications as type descriptors to stratify risk of malignancy: a systematic review and meta-analysis of 10665 cases with special focus on round/punctate microcalcifications. Rofo 184(12):1144–1152. https://doi.org/10.1055/s-0032-1313102

Sakorafas GH, Farley DR (2003) Optimal management of ductal carcinoma in situ of the breast. Surg Oncol 12(4):221–240. https://doi.org/10.1016/S0960-7404(03)00031-8

Schouten van der Velden AP et al (2006) Clinical presentation and surgical quality in treatment of ductal carcinoma in situ of the breast. Acta Oncol 45(5):544–549. https://doi.org/10.1080/02841860600617068

Schulz S et al (2013) Prediction of underestimated invasiveness in patients with ductal carcinoma in situ of the breast on percutaneous biopsy as rationale for recommending concurrent sentinel lymph node biopsy. Breast 22(4):537–542. https://doi.org/10.1016/j.breast.2012.11.002

Scoggins ME et al (2015) Correlation between sonographic findings and clinicopathologic and biologic features of pure ductal carcinoma in situ in 691 patients. AJR Am J Roentgenol 204(4):878–888. https://doi.org/10.2214/AJR.13.12221

Shin YJ et al (2019) Predictors of invasive breast cancer in patients with ductal carcinoma in situ in ultrasound-guided core needle biopsy. J Ultrasound Med 38(2):481–488. https://doi.org/10.1002/jum.14722

Siegel RL, Miller KD, Jemal A (2018) Cancer statistics, 2018. CA Cancer J Clin 68(1):7–30. https://doi.org/10.3322/caac.21442

Sim YT et al (2015) Upgrade of ductal carcinoma in situ on core biopsies to invasive disease at final surgery: a retrospective review across the Scottish Breast Screening Programme. Clin Radiol 70(5):502–506. https://doi.org/10.1016/j.crad.2014.12.019

Simpson PT et al (2005) Molecular evolution of breast cancer. J Pathol 205(2):248–254. https://doi.org/10.1002/path.1691

Skaane P et al (2014) Two-view digital breast tomosynthesis screening with synthetically reconstructed projection images: comparison with digital breast tomosynthesis with full-field digital mammographic images. Radiology 271(3):655–663. https://doi.org/10.1148/radiol.13131391

Skaane P et al (2019) Digital mammography versus digital mammography plus tomosynthesis in breast cancer screening: the Oslo Tomosynthesis Screening Trial. Radiology 291(1):23–30. https://doi.org/10.1148/radiol.2019182394

Stomper PC et al (1989) Clinically occult ductal carcinoma in situ detected with mammography: analysis of 100 cases with radiologic-pathologic correlation. Radiology 172(1):235–241. https://doi.org/10.1148/radiology.172.1.2544922

Su X et al (2017) Non-calcified ductal carcinoma in situ of the breast: comparison of diagnostic accuracy of digital breast tomosynthesis, digital mammography, and ultrasonography. Breast Cancer 24(4):562–570. https://doi.org/10.1007/s12282-016-0739-7

Tagliafico A, Houssami N (2015) Digital breast tomosynthesis might not be the optimal modality for detecting microcalcification. Radiology 275(2):618–619. https://doi.org/10.1148/radiol.2015142752

Thompson AM et al (2018) Management and 5-year outcomes in 9938 women with screen-detected ductal carcinoma in situ: the UK Sloane Project. Eur J Cancer 101:210–219. https://doi.org/10.1016/j.ejca.2018.06.027

Tot T (2005) DCIS, cytokeratins, and the theory of the sick lobe. Virchows Arch 447(1):1–8. https://doi.org/10.1007/s00428-005-1274-7

Vag T et al (2008) Diagnosis of ductal carcinoma in situ using contrast-enhanced magnetic resonance mammography compared with conventional mammography. Clin Imaging 32(6):438–442. https://doi.org/10.1016/j.clinimag.2008.05.005

Vignoli C et al (2019) Role of preoperative breast dual-energy contrast-enhanced digital mammography in ductal carcinoma in situ. Breast J 25(5):1034–1036. https://doi.org/10.1111/tbj.13408

Virnig BA et al (2010) Ductal carcinoma in situ of the breast: a systematic review of incidence, treatment, and outcomes. J Natl Cancer Inst 102(3):170–178. https://doi.org/10.1093/jnci/djp482

Wengert GJ et al (2019) Impact of the Kaiser score on clinical decision-making in BI-RADS 4 mammographic calcifications examined with breast MRI. Eur Radiol 30(3):1451–1459

Wilkinson L, Thomas V, Sharma N (2017) Microcalcification on mammography: approaches to interpretation and biopsy. Br J Radiol 90(1069):20160594. https://doi.org/10.1259/bjr.20160594

Yoon JH et al (2019) Outcomes of ductal carcinoma in situ according to detection modality: a multicenter study comparing recurrence between mammography and breast US. Ultrasound Med Biol 45(10):2623–2633. https://doi.org/10.1016/j.ultrasmedbio.2019.06.420

Zhou W et al (2014) Breast cancer with neoductgenesis: histopathological criteria and its correlation with mammographic and tumour features. Int J Breast Cancer 2014:581706. https://doi.org/10.1155/2014/581706

Zhou W et al (2017) Ductal breast carcinoma in situ: mammographic features and its relation to prognosis and tumour biology in a population based cohort. Int J Breast Cancer 2017:4351319. https://doi.org/10.1155/2017/4351319

Cystic and Complex Cystic and Solid Lesions

Panagiotis Kapetas and Thomas Helbich

Contents

1	**Introduction: About the Nature of Cystic Lesions of the Breast**	303
2	**Imaging Classification of Cystic Lesions of the Breast**	304
	2.1 Simple Cysts	305
	2.2 Complicated Cysts	309
	2.3 Complex Cystic and Solid Lesions	313
	2.4 Clustered Microcysts	317
3	**Differential Diagnosis of Cystic Breast Lesions**	321
	3.1 Benign Lesions	321
	3.2 Malignant Lesions	330
4	**Conclusion**	331
	References	333

Abstract

The BI-RADS lexicon classifies cystic breast lesions as simple cysts, complicated cysts, and complex cystic and solid lesions. In addition, the role of clustered microcysts will be described. Different types of cystic lesions reflect different underlying pathologies, probabilities of malignancy, as well as management recommendations. This chapter summarizes the pathophysiology behind the development, imaging findings, management recommendations, and differential diagnosis of the different types of cystic breast lesions.

1 Introduction: About the Nature of Cystic Lesions of the Breast

Cystic lesions represent the most common breast pathology. A prevalence between 50% and 90% is estimated (Rinaldi et al. 2010). Several studies have tried to explore a potential correlation of breast cysts with malignancy. However, literature

P. Kapetas (✉) · T. Helbich
Department of Biomedical Imaging and Image-Guided Therapy, Medical University of Vienna, Vienna, Austria
e-mail: panagiotis.kapetas@meduniwien.ac.at; thomas.helbich@meduniwien.ac.at

© Springer Nature Switzerland AG 2022
M. Fuchsjäger et al. (eds.), *Breast Imaging*, Medical Radiology Diagnostic Imaging,
https://doi.org/10.1007/978-3-030-94918-1_15

is ambiguous, with some authors finding cysts to be a true risk factor, whereas others regard them as a non-obligate precursor lesion of apocrine carcinoma or even as benign lesions with no correlation with malignancy (Celis et al. 2006; Dixon et al. 1999; Mannello et al. 2006; Yates and Ahmed 1988). Moreover, an increased risk of subsequent malignancy with increasing number of cyst aspirations in a woman's life has been suggested (ten or more cyst aspirations correlated to a sixfold relative risk in one study) (Bodian et al. 1992). Overall, cysts appear to be correlated with a small increase of relative risk for subsequent breast cancer (RR: 1.5–2) (Berg et al. 2003; Mannello et al. 2006).

The frequency of breast cysts reaches its peak in the third and fourth decades of life and sharply diminishes after menopause, except for women under hormone replacement therapy (HRT) (Rinaldi et al. 2010). Regarding their development mechanism, different cyst types are pathologically identified: apocrine (or secretory) cysts and transudative cysts, both arising in the terminal ductal lobular unit (TDLU), while intermediate types are also encountered (Dixon et al. 1985; Mannello et al. 2006; Rinaldi et al. 2010). It has to be noted that simultaneous or sequential, multiple cysts in the same woman are usually of the same type (Rinaldi et al. 2010). Imaging cannot differentiate between these two different pathological cyst types (Rinaldi et al. 2010).

Apocrine (or secretory) cysts are lined with metabolically active, apocrine epithelial cells, similar to the ones found in sweat glands. The prevailing theory regarding their origin is that the epithelial lining of the TDLU undergoes an apocrine metaplastic change (Chinyama 2014; Haagensen 1991). Lobules tend then to expand due to secretions, "unfold," and finally fuse, creating larger cystic spaces (Chinyama 2014; Warner et al. 1998; Wellings and Alpers 1987) (Fig. 1). The epithelial cells show tight cell-cell junctions and proliferate and are thus prone to the development of hyperplasia, atypia, or even preneoplastic alterations (Mannello et al. 2006; Rinaldi et al. 2010). The fluid in apocrine cysts shows a low Na^+/K^+ ratio (<3) and contains several secretory products (Dixon et al. 1985).

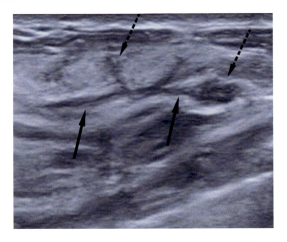

Fig. 1 Ultrasound image, depicting dilated and fused acini along a duct (arrows) to form different sized cystic spaces (dashed arrows)

Apocrine epithelial cells lack estrogen-α and progesterone receptors, while they express androgen receptors (Chinyama 2014). Finally, this type of cysts has been suggested to have a tendency towards multiplicity and recurrence (Berg et al. 2003; Dixon et al. 1985).

Transudative cysts on the other hand are lined with flattened epithelium that does not show any metabolic hypertrophy. The biochemical composition of their fluid content is similar to that of plasma (Na^+/K^+ ratio >3) (Dixon et al. 1985), and the epithelial cells are strongly positive for estrogen-α and progesterone receptors and demonstrate open cell-cell junctions (Celis et al. 2006). Transudative cysts are more often solitary and have a lower tendency to recur (Mannello et al. 2006; Rinaldi et al. 2010). Finally, transudative cysts are postulated to occur due to fibrosis of a duct, leading to a retention of fluid, which derives from plasma (Mannello et al. 2006; Rinaldi et al. 2010).

2 Imaging Classification of Cystic Lesions of the Breast

Cysts can be seen on mammography (MG), ultrasound (US), and magnetic resonance imaging (MRI). However, US is the modality of choice for the characterization of cystic lesions, whereas MG and MRI have a more limited role.

The BI-RADS lexicon (Mendelson et al. 2013) classifies cystic breast lesions as simple cysts, complicated cysts, and complex cystic and solid lesions, while clustered microcysts form a further special case.

Cystic lesions have a different appearance according to their type, and thus their imaging findings are of importance for their correct characterization.

2.1 Simple Cysts

2.1.1 Imaging Findings

2.1.1.1 Ultrasound

Simple breast cysts have a typical morphology in ultrasound (US). They present as an oval or round, anechoic lesion with an imperceptible wall, circumscribed margin, and posterior enhancement (Fig. 2). They tend to flatten with compression (Berg et al. 2010) and usually show a lateral edge refraction (Venta et al. 1994).

Sometimes simple cysts do not present with their typical features. Posterior enhancement may be absent (Berg et al. 2010), and due to reverberation artifacts false echoes may appear in a simple cyst. They may even demonstrate lobulations or thin (<0.5 mm) septa. In these cases, one should consider the presence of two or more abutting simple cysts. Wall thickness of 0.5 mm corresponds to the combined thickness of two myoepithelial and epithelial cell layers (Rinaldi et al. 2010).

With currently available, high-frequency linear array transducers, most simple cysts with a size of at least 5–8 mm, lying at a depth of less than 4 cm, can be accurately characterized. It has been shown that the characterization of cysts is more accurate between different examiners for lesions with a diameter of at least 8 mm (Berg et al. 2006b). For deeper lying lesions, it is possible to reduce the transducer frequency, in order to ensure an adequate penetration of the beam (Athanasiou et al. 2014) and consequent recognition of a lesion as a simple cyst.

Decreasing the dynamic range may also prove beneficial for a correct diagnosis of a simple cyst (Fig. 3). A narrow dynamic range essentially means that less shades of gray are used, leading to a decrease in false intracystic echoes (e.g., due to reverberation artifacts) (Berg et al. 2003; Vargas et al. 2004). However, a too narrow dynamic range may lead to hypoechoic solid lesions presenting as anechoic ones and thus be falsely interpreted as simple cysts (Berg et al. 2010; Kim et al. 2011).

Several complementary US techniques, besides B-mode, can be used to facilitate the correct diagnosis of a simple cyst in problematic cases. These include harmonic imaging, spatial compounding, elastography, Doppler, as well as administration of a contrast medium (Balleyguier et al. 2013b; Berg et al. 2003; Gulati et al. 2015; Rinaldi et al. 2010).

Harmonic imaging uses the resonance of tissue, due to the transmission of the US beam. This leads to the generation of harmonic waves, whose frequency is a higher integer multiple of the transmission frequency. For image generation, the transmitted frequency spectrum is filtered out. Currently, the second harmonic (that is twice the transmitted frequency) is used for imaging (Choudhry et al. 2000; Rosen and Soo 2001). Harmonic imaging leads to an improved spatial resolution and contrast as well as a reduction in artifacts (e.g., reverberation artifact) and false internal echoes, allowing for a higher operator

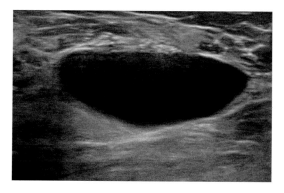

Fig. 2 Typical appearance of a simple cyst at B-mode US, presenting as an oval, circumscribed, anechoic lesion with posterior enhancement. This is a BI-RADS 2 finding

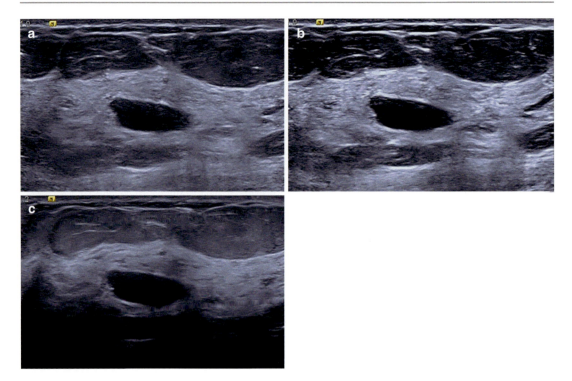

Fig. 3 Forty-nine-year-old woman, screening US. B-mode (**a**) shows a simple cyst with artifactual internal echoes. By reducing the dynamic range from 75 to 50 dB (**b**) or use of harmonic imaging (**c**), its anechoic nature can be better appreciated (BI-RADS 2)

confidence in diagnosing a lesion as cystic (Berg et al. 2003; Rinaldi et al. 2010; Rosen and Soo 2001) (Fig. 3). However, harmonics are attenuated at bigger depths, and their role for the evaluation of deep-lying cysts may be limited.

Spatial compounding averages several images taken from different perspectives (Kern et al. 2004). This leads to a higher signal-to-noise ratio and a decrease of speckle artifacts and background noise. The internal structure and the tumor margins can be characterized better, and calcifications are recognized more accurately (Athanasiou et al. 2014; Cha et al. 2005). However, posterior features become less conspicuous with compound imaging (Fig. 4).

Elastography is a relatively recent development, which enables an evaluation of tissue stiffness. Two different forms of elastography are currently in use: strain elastography, which is based on tissue compression, and elastography based on the propagation of shear waves (shear wave elastography—SWE—and acoustic radiation force impulse—ARFI). Cystic lesions tend to present with characteristic patterns in strain elastography, either as a triple-layered lesion (blue-green-red) due to an aliasing artifact in systems that deploy a color-coded elastogram (Cho et al. 2011) (Fig. 5) or with a typical "bull's-eye" appearance (hyperechoic center and hypoechoic periphery) due to subtle fluid motion in devices that use a black-and-white elastogram (Balleyguier et al. 2013a; Barr 2018) (Fig. 6). On the other hand, in SWE and ARFI technology, cysts present a central void, since shear waves do not propagate in nonviscous fluids (Balleyguier et al. 2013b) (Fig. 7). More details on further US techniques can be found in Chapter "Breast Ultrasound-Advanced Techniques."

Doppler imaging may also be particularly helpful in the diagnosis of simple cysts. Doppler is used for the characterization of flow. Since by definition simple cysts lack any solid internal compo-

Cystic and Complex Cystic and Solid Lesions

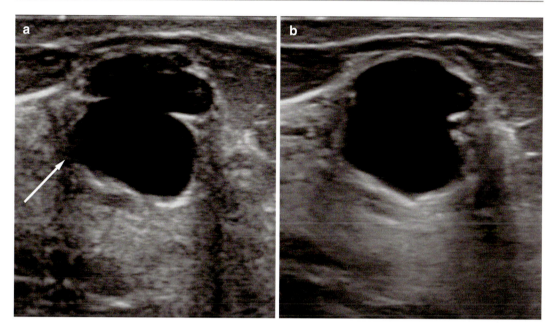

Fig. 4 Thirty-eight-year-old woman referred for a palpable lump in the left breast. B-mode US (**a**) shows a cystic lesion with internal echoes and a partially indistinct margin (arrow). With the use of compound imaging (**b**), the artifactual internal echoes are reduced and the margin is better delineated, proving this to be a simple cyst (BI-RADS 2). However, the posterior enhancement becomes less apparent with compound imaging

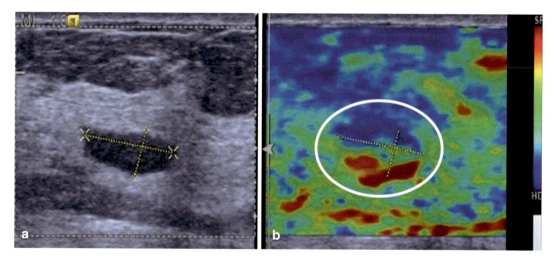

Fig. 5 Twenty-seven-year-old woman presenting with pain in the left breast. In B-mode, US (**a**) shows a hypoechoic lesion, which may be mistaken for a solid mass. However, the color-coded elastogram (**b** strain elastography) demonstrates a triple-layered (blue-green-red) appearance (white circle), which is typical of a cystic lesion. Fine needle aspiration yielded green fluid. No residual mass remained post-interventionally. In 6-month follow-up, the cyst was not visible

nent, no internal vascularization should be evident in Doppler examination (Busilacchi et al. 2012). However, in cases of an inflamed cyst, a peripheral hyperemia is possible (Athanasiou et al. 2014).

In some cases, Doppler can be false negative, despite the presence of vessels inside a lesion. The detection of internal vasculature can be significantly improved by the application of a con-

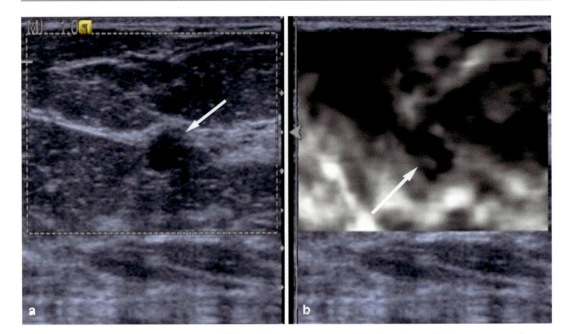

Fig. 6 Thirty-two-year-old woman, recalled from screening for a lesion in the right breast. In B-mode US (**a**) it is partially anechoic; however, it also shows artifactual echoes and a partially indistinct margin (arrow). Strain elastography with a device applying a black-and-white elastogram (**b**) demonstrates a typical "bull's-eye" appearance corresponding to a cystic lesion (arrow). Fine needle aspiration yielded only some drops of black fluid. No residual mass remained post-interventionally. In 6-month follow-up, the cyst was visible neither at US nor at MG

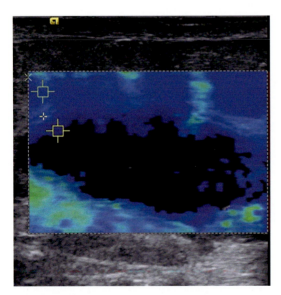

Fig. 7 Shear wave elastogram of a simple cyst in the left breast of a 38-year-old woman. The central void is due to the lack of shear wave propagation in nonviscous fluid and is a typical finding of simple cysts, classified as BI-RADS 2

trast medium. Again, a simple cyst should not demonstrate any internal enhancement at contrast-enhanced US, whereas an increased peripheral enhancement may be encountered in cases of an inflamed cyst (Barnard et al. 2008; Gulati et al. 2015).

2.1.1.2 Mammography

At MG, simple cysts present as round or oval, hypo- to isodense, circumscribed or obscured masses. Obviously, MG cannot reliably distinguish cystic from solid lesions. They are often multiple and bilateral, while a fluctuation over consecutive controls is possible, with some regressing and others developing (Berg et al. 2006a) (Figs. 8 and 9).

2.1.1.3 Magnetic Resonance Imaging

At magnetic resonance imaging (MRI), simple cysts also have typical features. Their signal intensity is similar to that of water (hyperintense

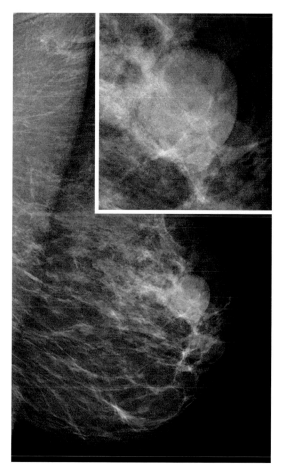

Fig. 8 A 44-year-old woman presenting with a palpable lump in the left breast. MG (MLO projection) demonstrates a round, isodense, partially circumscribed, and partially obscured mass (close-up inside the white frame). Cystic and solid lesions cannot be differentiated in MG, resulting in a BI-RADS 0 score. Further workup consisted of US, which demonstrated a simple cyst (not shown)

on T2w and STIR and hypointense on T1w sequences), and they do not show any enhancement after application of a contrast medium (Berg et al. 2010) (Figs. 9 and 10).

2.1.2 Management

If the imaging findings are that of a typical simple cyst, no further action is necessary. The lesion can be classified as a BI-RADS 2 (benign findings), and the patient can be returned to normal screening (Cohen et al. 2019; Mendelson et al. 2013).

An US-guided fine needle aspiration (FNA) can be considered for symptomatic relief, if the cyst is large and palpable or painful. In this case it is not necessary to change the overall BI-RADS 2 classification (Mendelson et al. 2013). The management of the acquired fluid depends on its color. If it is cloudy or clear yellow or greenish-black, then it can be safely discarded (Ciatto et al. 1987; Hindle et al. 2000; Smith et al. 1997). This kind of fluid may be sent for cytological examination at the patient's request or if the patient has a personal history of breast cancer or atypias (Rinaldi et al. 2010). However, if bloody fluid is aspirated and this is not attributable to the puncture itself, then it should be sent to cytology and a subsequent US-guided biopsy should be considered (Athanasiou et al. 2014; Smith et al. 1997). If a biopsy is not performed immediately after the FNA, the location of the cyst needs to be marked with a clip for future reference.

2.2 Complicated Cysts

2.2.1 Imaging Findings

2.2.1.1 Ultrasound

The term complicated describes the US appearance of a cyst, which fulfills all the criteria of a simple cyst (circumscribed margin, imperceptible wall, posterior enhancement) besides the internal echogenicity. Complicated cysts are not anechoic and may present with either homogeneous low-level echoes (due to the presence of proteins, blood, or pus) (Fig. 11) or a fluid-debris level (Fig. 12) or even bright echogenic foci, corresponding to cholesterol crystals or milk of calcium (Athanasiou et al. 2014; Berg et al. 2010; Mendelson et al. 2013; Rinaldi et al. 2010).

Turning the patient to the oblique position during the examination may be especially helpful to demonstrate the movement of debris that does not adhere to the cystic wall, thus ruling out the presence of a solid intracystic component. Furthermore, the observation of debris movement inside a cyst can be facilitated by examining it with color or power Doppler. The energy transmitted during the application of Doppler is higher

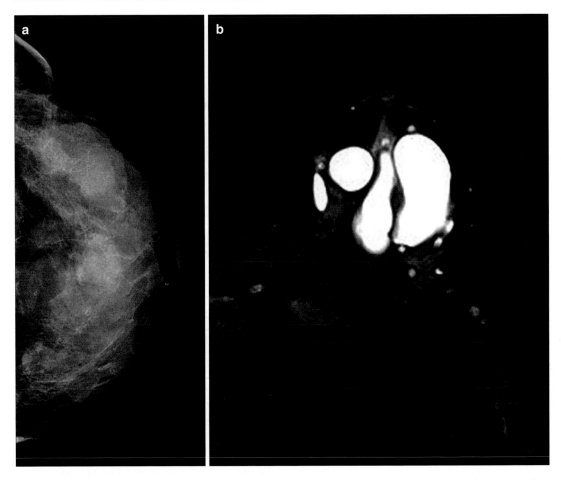

Fig. 9 Screening MG (**a** CC projection) of a 52-year-old woman demonstrates extremely dense (BI-RADS composition D) parenchyma of the left breast with several iso- to hypodense lesions, which are partially obscured because of overlapping breast parenchyma (BI-RADS 0). Axial MRI scan (**b** STIR, TR: 5360, TE: 188) shows multiple hyperintense simple cysts of different sizes. The final assessment taking into account the MRI findings is BI-RADS 2

than that of B-mode US, which makes fluid particles move away from the transducer due to an acoustic streaming phenomenon (Clarke et al. 2005; Nightingale et al. 1995). The observation of this movement can prove the cystic nature of a lesion (Fig. 13). To rule out an intracystic solid component, administration of a contrast medium can be useful in selected cases (Fig. 14).

2.2.1.2 Mammography

The MG appearance of complicated cysts is similar to that of simple ones. They typically present as round or oval, hypo- to isodense, circumscribed or obscured masses. They may also be solitary or multiple, uni- or bilateral, and fluctuating over consecutive controls (Berg et al. 2006a). Occasionally, they may demonstrate milk of calcium or even rim calcifications. As with simple cysts, they cannot be differentiated from a solid lesion on MG (Fig. 15).

2.2.1.3 Magnetic Resonance Imaging

At MRI, the signal intensity of a complicated cyst depends on the nature of its content. Blood or protein-rich fluid will be hyperintense on T1w and hypointense on STIR and T2w sequences (Fig. 16). Fatty content will be hyperintense in T1w, isointense in T2w, and hypointense in fat-

Cystic and Complex Cystic and Solid Lesions

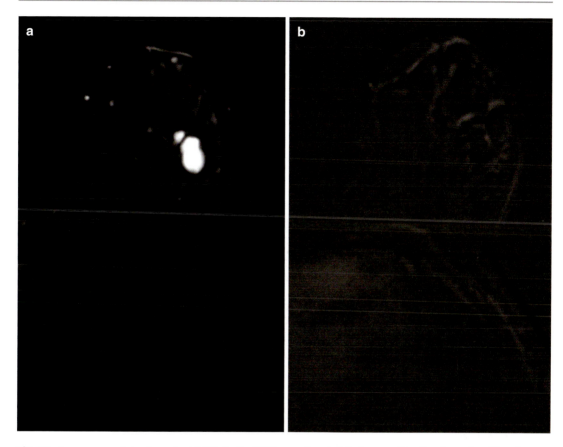

Fig. 10 Appearance of simple cysts at MRI. In the STIR image (**a** TR: 5360, TE: 188), the cyst content is homogeneously hyperintense. After IV contrast administration (**b** early arterial phase, subtraction image), neither the cyst contents nor the walls demonstrate any enhancement. These findings are consistent with a BI-RADS 2 score

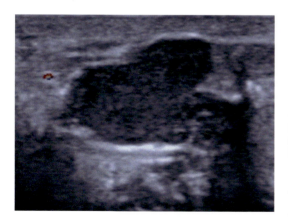

Fig. 11 Twenty-three-year-old woman referred for pain in the right breast. B-mode US demonstrates a complicated cyst, presenting with homogeneous low-level echoes. Complicated cysts like this are classified as BI-RADS 3

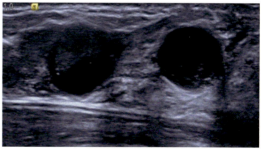

Fig. 12 Forty-six-year-old woman referred for pain in the left breast. B-mode US performed on both breasts showed two complicated cysts with evident fluid-debris levels as an incidental finding in the right breast. These were asymptomatic and were classified as BI-RADS 2

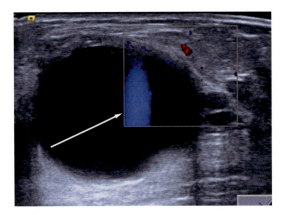

Fig. 13 Doppler US of a complicated cyst in the left breast of a 47-year-old woman, referred for a painful lump. Doppler imparts more energy than B-mode US and thus brings fluid to motion, something that can be demonstrated as large color artifacts (arrow)

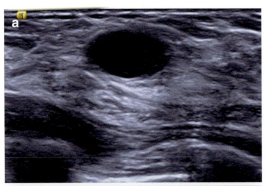

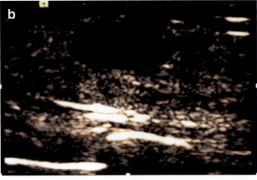

Fig. 14 B-mode US (**a**) demonstrating a cystic lesion with internal echoes in the left breast of a 46-year-old woman. To rule out a complex cystic and solid lesion, contrast-enhanced US (**b**) with a sonographic contrast medium (SonoVue®, Bracco, Milan, Italy) was performed. Here, no enhancement of the lesion is observed, thus proving the content to be debris and the lesion to be a complicated cyst

suppressed sequences. The presence of pus will lead to an internal diffusion restriction, typical for abscesses. The observation of a fluid-debris level is possible. After application of a contrast medium, some complicated cysts may demonstrate a rim enhancement of their wall. However, this will be thin (<2 mm) and smooth and demonstrate persistent kinetics (Figs. 15 and 17). If the enhancing rim is thick or irregular or shows a washout, then the lesion should be regarded as suspicious.

2.2.2 Management

Asymptomatic complicated cysts, which present with homogeneous low-level echoes or fluid-debris levels and are an incidental finding, may be classified as BI-RADS 3, and a short-term follow-up (in 6, 12, and 24 months) can be safely initiated (Berg et al. 2010). The probability of a malignancy of such lesions is very low, well under the 2% cutoff required for the BI-RADS 3 category (0.2–1%) (Berg et al. 2010; Graf et al. 2007; Gruber et al. 2013). If the lesion size increases by more than 20% in the 6-month follow-up, a biopsy is required (Gordon et al. 2003).

In contrast, a lesion should be classified as BI-RADS 4 in the following cases: (1) if it is possibly solid and new or enlarging, (2) if a complex cystic and solid lesion cannot be confidently excluded, or (3) if there are any other suspicious features in US, MG, and MRI. In these cases, a FNA (possibly followed by an US-guided biopsy, if the lesion proves to be solid) is warranted.

Special caution should be taken if a new or developing, solitary lesion resembling a complicated cyst is found in a postmenopausal woman who is not on HRT. Since it is quite unusual for postmenopausal women to develop breast cysts, such a lesion should be viewed with suspicion and a short-term follow-up or even a histologic workup may be appropriate (Aujero et al. 2019; Markopoulos et al. 2002).

FNA may be performed even in non-suspicious lesions for symptomatic relief in case of a palpable or tender cyst. There is no need for a BI-RADS upgrade in such a case (Mendelson et al. 2013). The management of the acquired fluid is similar to that of a simple cyst FNA. If pus is aspirated, it should be sent to bacteriology.

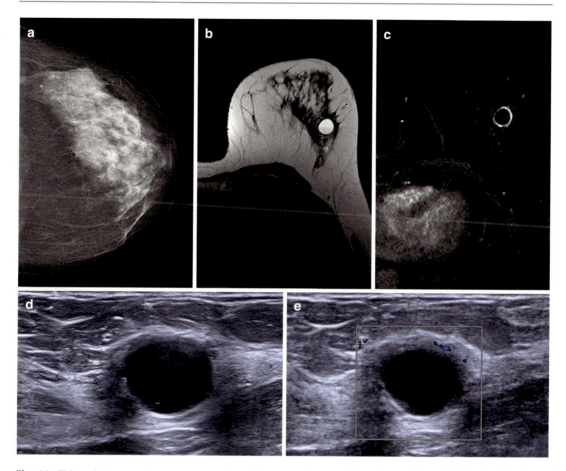

Fig. 15 Thirty-eight-year-old woman presenting with a new, painful, palpable lesion in the lateral left breast. In MG (**a** CC projection), an isodense mass can be seen; however, the margin cannot be sufficiently evaluated due to overlapping with breast parenchyma. B-mode US (**d**) shows a cystic lesion with a prominent wall, internal echoes, and peripheral edema, whereas Doppler (**e**) demonstrates peripheral vascularity. In MRI, the T2w image (**b** TR: 5360, TE: 188) shows a round, circumscribed hyperintense mass with a fluid-debris level. After IV application of contrast medium (**c** early arterial phase, subtraction image), a thin and smooth enhancement rim is evident. The imaging findings correspond with an inflamed cyst

2.3 Complex Cystic and Solid Lesions

Complex cystic and solid lesions present with both cystic and solid components. According to Berg et al. (2003, 2010), four different types of these lesions can be identified, based on their imaging findings: type I comprises cysts with a thick (≥0.5 mm) wall, type II cysts with thick (≥0.5 mm) septations, type III predominantly cystic lesions (>50%) with solid parts (otherwise called intracystic masses), and type IV predominantly solid (>50%) lesions with central or peripheral cystic parts.

2.3.1 Imaging Findings

2.3.1.1 Ultrasound

The US appearance of complex cystic and solid breast lesions depends on their subtype. They demonstrate either as cystic masses with a thick wall (Fig. 18) or thick septations (Fig. 19) or as an intracystic mass (Fig. 20) or even as solid lesions with cystic components (Fig. 21). Due to the cystic part, they may show posterior enhancement. Especially in cases of malignant lesions, they are at least partially non-circumscribed and may have microlobulated, indistinct, angular, or less often spiculated margins (Yao et al. 2017).

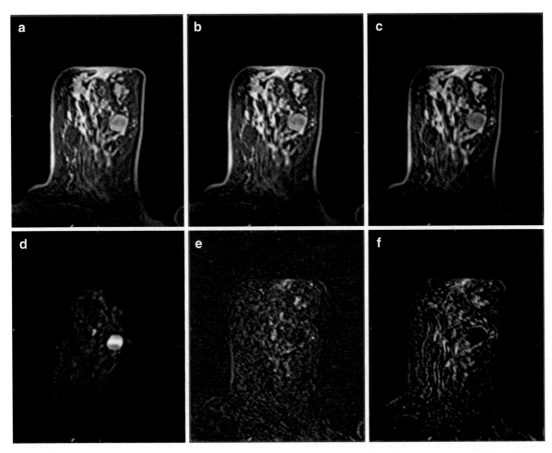

Fig. 16 Forty-eight-year-old woman, recall from screening for a lesion in the left breast. US (not shown) showed a possibly complex cystic and solid lesion; therefore, the woman was referred to MRI. In the pre-contrast T1w image (**a** TR: 4.68, TE: 1.65, DIXON technique, water-only image), it is heterogeneously hypointense with a fluid-debris level. After IV contrast administration (**b** + **e**: early arterial phase, **c** + **f** venous phase, subtraction images), it does not show any enhancement. The fluid-debris level is better appreciated in the STIR sequence (**d** TR: 5360, TE: 188). The MRI findings are typical of a complicated cyst

Their shape and orientation may be variable. Sometimes solid parts may bleed, and hemorrhagic material may mask the actual intracystic mass. In these cases, repositioning the patient will usually aid in the recognition of a solid, intracystic component (Athanasiou et al. 2014; Berg et al. 2010; Xiang et al. 2020).

Doppler imaging may be very useful for the characterization of complex cystic and solid lesions, since it will often demonstrate vascularity in solid components (Fig. 22). In case of intraductal or intracystic papillomas, their vascular stalk may also be demonstrated (Jagmohan et al. 2013) (Fig. 23). However, lack of intralesional vascularization in Doppler does not preclude a solid lesion (Doshi et al. 2007). Elastography will also sometimes point out a stiff solid part of the lesion, which is more usual in case of malignancies (Athanasiou et al. 2014). Finally, contrast-enhanced US may be helpful in the correct identification of a complex cystic and solid breast lesion. In such a case, the solid lesion parts will usually demonstrate an avid contrast enhancement (Liu et al. 2009) (Figs. 24 and 25).

2.3.1.2 Mammography

The MG appearance of complex cystic and solid lesions may be variable, and the demonstration of a circumscribed mass is possible. However, some suspicious features (e.g., a partially indistinct

Cystic and Complex Cystic and Solid Lesions 315

Fig. 17 Different appearances of simple and complicated cysts at MRI. The medially located (complicated cyst) is less hypointense than the other two simple cysts in the pre-contrast T1w (**a** TR: 4.68, TE: 1.65, DIXON technique, fat-only image) and shows a persistent, thin, smooth rim enhancement after IV contrast administration (**b** early arterial phase, **c** venous phase). In the T2w image (**d** TR: 5360, TE: 188), all cysts are markedly hyperintense

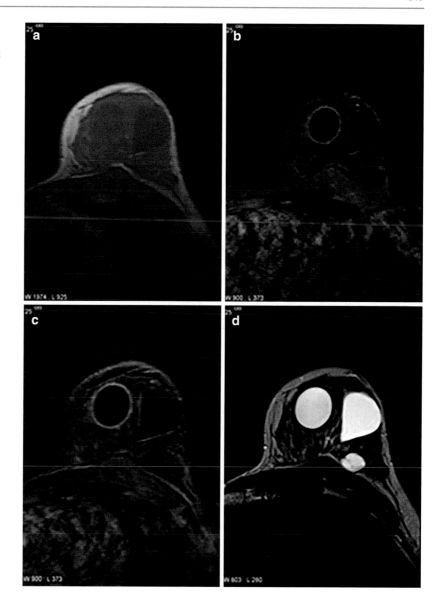

margin or an evident hyperdensity) may be present and point to a malignancy (Berg et al. 2010) (Fig. 26). Complex cystic and solid lesions will often present with associated microcalcifications, either amorphous, punctate, or even coarse heterogeneous (Berg et al. 2010; Doshi et al. 2007; Jagmohan et al. 2013) (Fig. 27).

2.3.1.3 Magnetic Resonance Imaging

At MRI, complex cystic and solid lesions will also show a variable appearance according to their subtype. An irregular shape and a non-circumscribed margin are often seen in malignancies. The cystic part may be hypo-, iso-, or hyperintense in T1w sequences, depending on its composition (bloody or proteinaceous fluid will be iso- to hyperintense), and generally hyperintense in STIR and T2w sequences (Popli et al. 2016) (Fig. 28). The presence of peritumoral edema is also highly suggestive of a malignancy, although it may be seen around inflammatory lesions (Kaiser et al. 2015; Wang et al. 2014). After contrast administration, a rim enhancement is typical of complex cystic and solid lesions.

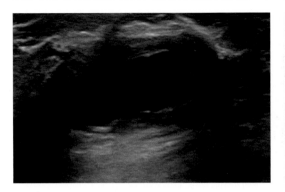

Fig. 18 Fifty-six-year-old woman presenting with a palpable lump in the left breast, 6 months after breast-conserving surgery. B-mode US demonstrates a thick-walled complex cystic and solid lesion, corresponding to a postoperative, organizing hemato-seroma. Without knowledge of the history of the patient and comparison with previous examinations, ruling out a necrotic tumor may be difficult in such a case. The lesion did not change in follow-up examinations over 4 years

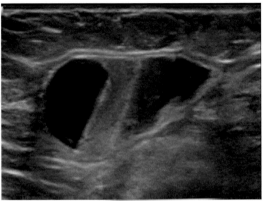

Fig. 19 Sixty-seven-year-old woman with a history of breast-conserving surgery of the left breast 4 years ago. B-mode US shows a complex cystic and solid lesion with a thick wall and thick septations. US-guided biopsy resulted in a postoperative oil cyst

Whereas benign lesions will usually show a smooth, thin, slowly, and persistently enhancing rim, malignancies typically demonstrate a nodular, irregular, thick rim, with rapid enhancement and a plateau or washout (Berg et al. 2010; Popli et al. 2016; Wang et al. 2014) (Fig. 26). More details on the MRI imaging findings of complex cystic and solid lesions can be found in Chapter "Breast MRI: Multiparametric and Advanced Techniques."

2.3.2 Management

Due to the high rate of underlying malignancy, complex cystic and solid lesions of the breast should be classified as BI-RADS 4 and need to be histopathologically examined. A 14G large core needle biopsy is adequate for sampling predominantly solid lesions with small cystic parts (Fig. 29). However, for lesions with a thick wall or thick septations as well as for small intracystic masses, biopsy should ideally be performed with an 7–11G vacuum-assisted needle (VAB) (Athanasiou et al. 2014; Heywang-Köbrunner et al. 2009) (Fig. 30). In any case, the biopsy area should be marked with a clip, to ensure adequate recognition of the lesion in future (Athanasiou et al. 2014; Doshi et al. 2007).

After biopsy of a complex cystic and solid lesion of the breast, a thorough radiologic-pathologic correlation has to be performed (Athanasiou et al. 2014; Doshi et al. 2007; Heywang-Köbrunner et al. 2009). It is important that the pathologic findings can explain the imaging appearance, and a detailed description of the lesion should be provided to the pathologist (Doshi et al. 2007). If the results are benign and are deemed concordant, a 6-month follow-up is suggested (Athanasiou et al. 2014; Doshi et al. 2007).

In case pathology demonstrates a benign papilloma, the case should be discussed in the multi-disciplinary board. If the biopsy was performed using a large core needle, the risk of upgrade to atypia or even malignancy due to undersampling is up to 24% (Cyr et al. 2011). Therefore, a surgical excision is usually warranted (Athanasiou et al. 2014; Berg et al. 2010). However, if a VAB was performed, the risk of an upgrade is less than 2% due to the larger tissue sample size (Lee et al. 2014). Therefore, it is considered as a safe alternative to open surgical biopsy (Brookes and Bourke 2008; Lee et al. 2014; Rageth et al. 2016), and follow-up may be an adequate option (Rageth et al. 2016).

If an atypical lesion is diagnosed at pathology, then an open surgical biopsy should be performed,

Cystic and Complex Cystic and Solid Lesions

Fig. 20 Fifty-year-old woman, referred from screening. B-mode US (**a**) shows a type III complex cystic and solid lesion, with a solid, intracystic mass adhering at the cyst wall. In MRI of the same patient, the pre-contrast T1w image (**b**) TR: 4.68, TE: 1.65, DIXON technique, fat-only image) shows the cyst to be hypointense and the T2w image (**c**) TR: 5360, TE: 188) heterogeneously hyperintense. After IV administration of contrast medium (**d**) late arterial phase, DIXON technique, fat-only image; (**e**) late arterial phase, subtraction image), the "intracystic mass" does not show any enhancement, proving it to be tumefactive, wall-adherent debris. The lesion regressed in the next follow-up round

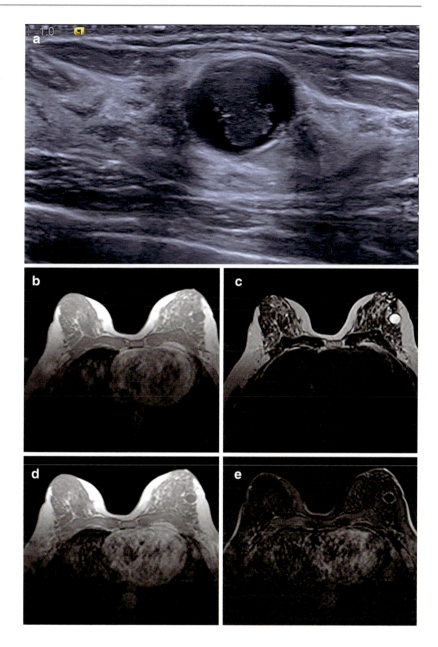

since the upgrade rate ranges between 17% and 38% at final pathology (Athanasiou et al. 2014; Mooney et al. 2016). In any case of discordance between imaging findings and pathology, a re-biopsy is recommended. If the initial biopsy was performed with a core needle, VAB could be considered. Alternatively, an open surgical biopsy is the appropriate management in these cases.

2.4 Clustered Microcysts

Clustered microcysts arise due to a cystic dilatation of a part or all acini of a TDLU and are most commonly seen perimenopausally (Berg 2005; Berg et al. 2010). They are the typical imaging finding of apocrine metaplasia, while they also often represent fibrocystic changes (Berg 2005;

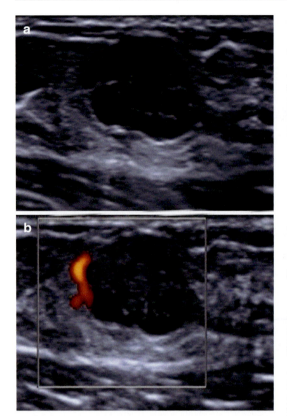

Fig. 21 Thirty-seven-year-old woman referred for a palpable abnormality in the left breast. B-mode US (**a**) demonstrates a type IV complex cystic and solid lesion with peripheral cystic spaces. Power Doppler (**b**) identifies a vessel in the rim of the lesion. US-guided biopsy showed an area of fibrocystic changes

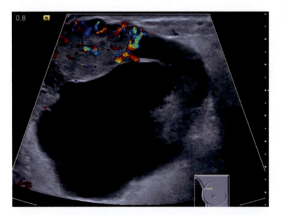

Fig. 22 Grade 3 invasive carcinoma of no special type in a 34-year-old woman with a palpable, rapid enlarging lump in the right breast, presenting as a complex cystic and solid lesion. Doppler demonstrates avid vascularization in the solid lesion parts

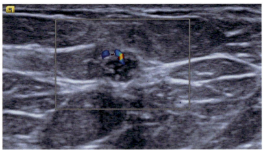

Fig. 23 Doppler US of a biopsy-proven intraductal papilloma in the right breast of a 46-year-old woman. Doppler may enable the identification of the vascular stalk of papillary lesions

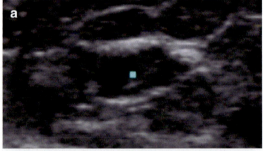

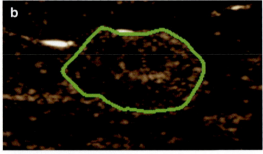

Fig. 24 US images of an incidental finding in the right breast of a 42-year-old woman, referred for a palpable lesion in the left breast. B-mode US (**a**) demonstrates a small complex cystic and solid lesion. In contrast-enhanced US with a sonographic contrast medium (SonoVue®, Bracco, Milan, Italy) (**b**), the solid lesion components are enhanced, as opposed to the cystic parts (green line demarcates the lesion boundaries). US-guided biopsy proved this lesion to be an area of apocrine metaplasia with small papillary lesions

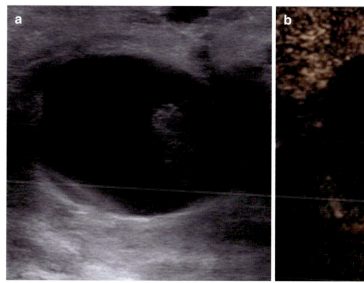
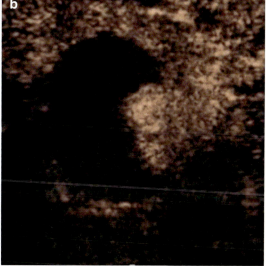

Fig. 25 Sixty-eight-year-old woman, referred for bloody secretion from the left nipple. B-mode US of the left breast (**a**) shows an intracystic mass, which enhances avidly after IV contrast administration (**b** contrast-enhanced US with a sonographic contrast medium (SonoVue®, Bracco, Milan, Italy)). The lesion proved to be a papillary carcinoma in situ after vacuum-assisted ultrasound-guided biopsy

Berg et al. 2003; Warner et al. 1998). Less usually, they may correspond to fibroadenomas, whereas malignant lesions rarely (if at all) present as true clusters of microcysts (Berg 2005; Berg et al. 2003, 2010; Chang et al. 2007; Daly et al. 2008; Tanaka et al. 2016).

2.4.1 Imaging Findings

2.4.1.1 Ultrasound

At US, clustered microcysts present as oval, circumscribed, or microlobulated (but not indistinct) masses, consisting of several adjacent anechoic foci (usually 1–7 mm each) (Berg 2005; Goldbach et al. 2020; Warner et al. 1998). The latter are separated by thin (<0.5 mm), possibly fuzzy septations, which represent the combination of two myoepithelial and epithelial cell layers (Rinaldi et al. 2010). Posterior enhancement may be present or absent. The individual cysts may contain milk of calcium (evident as bright echogenic foci) or be complicated (Fig. 31). In this case, their differentiation from solid components may be difficult.

With Doppler, no internal vascularization should be evident in the septations. Compound imaging may allow a better delineation of the individual septa, whereas harmonics may help depict the single cysts as truly anechoic areas (Fig. 32).

2.4.1.2 Mammography

At MG, clustered microcysts usually appear as oval, microlobulated, circumscribed, or obscured, hypo- to isoechoic masses, possibly with milk of calcium (Berg 2005; Warner et al. 1998). However, presentation as a focal asymmetry, with or without amorphous or coarse heterogeneous calcifications, is also possible (Tanaka et al. 2016).

2.4.1.3 Magnetic Resonance Imaging

The typical appearance of clustered microcysts at MRI is that of an oval lobulated mass, which is hypointense in T1w sequences. In STIR and T2w sequences, the cystic components will be hyper- whereas the septa hypointense. After application of a contrast medium, only the septa may demonstrate enhancement.

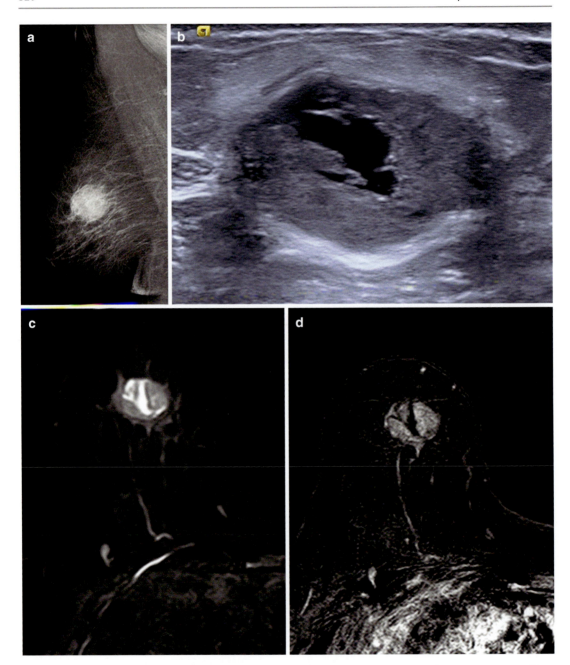

Fig. 26 Fifty-four-year-old woman presenting with a palpable lump in the right breast. MG (**a** MLO projection) shows a round, hyperdense mass which has a partially indistinct margin. In B-mode US (**b**), a type IV complex cystic and solid lesion with indistinct margins and peripheral edema is demonstrated. In MRI (**c** STIR, TR: 5360, TE: 188; **d** early arterial phase, post-contrast subtraction image), the solid parts show an avid enhancement, whereas the cystic ones do not. US-guided biopsy showed a grade 3 invasive carcinoma of no special type

Cystic and Complex Cystic and Solid Lesions

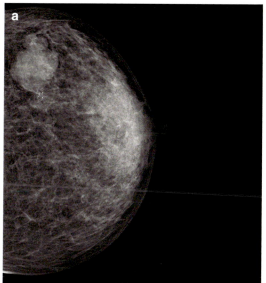

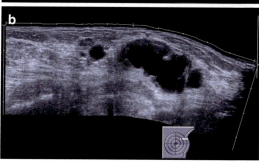

Fig. 27 Forty-eight-year-old woman presenting with a palpable lump in the left breast. MG (**a** CC projection) shows an irregular, polylobulated, hyperdense mass with a partially indistinct margin and associated pleomorphic microcalcifications. In B-mode US (**b**), a panoramic image demonstrates two abutting complex cystic and solid masses, one with a thick wall and thick septations and the other predominantly solid with cystic parts. US-guided biopsy showed a grade 2 invasive carcinoma of no special type

2.4.2 Management

The management of incidentally found clustered microcysts depends on the menopausal status of the woman. In premenopausal women, clusters with a typical, circumscribed appearance may be considered as BI-RADS 2 findings. Small lesions, which may be difficult to characterize or lesions containing individual complicated cysts, should be classified as BI-RADS 3 and a short-term follow-up should be suggested. However, if a cluster of microcysts presents with any suspicious findings (either in US or MG or MRI), a rapid growth, or a presumable solid component, an US-guided biopsy should be performed (BI-RADS 4) (Berg 2020; Berg et al. 2010; Goldbach et al. 2020; Greenwood et al. 2017; Tanaka et al. 2016).

In postmenopausal women, especially if they are not on HRT, newly formed clustered microcysts should be regarded with caution. If a lesion is new and has a typical circumscribed appearance, then it should be classified as BI-RADS 3 and a short-term follow-up should be performed. Again, any suspicious imaging or clinical findings, a rapid growth, or solid lesion components should prompt a classification of BI-RADS 4 and an US-guided biopsy (Berg et al. 2010).

3 Differential Diagnosis of Cystic Breast Lesions

The most usual benign and malignant differential diagnoses of cystic breast lesions are presented in the following section and summarized in Table 1:

3.1 Benign Lesions

Abscesses may present as either complicated cysts or complex cystic and solid lesions, with a thick wall and/or thick septations (Chang et al. 2007). They are more frequent in breastfeeding and smoking women (Schafer et al. 1988) and will typically present with clinical symptoms like erythema and tenderness. Accompanying reactive axillary lymph nodes are often encountered. A perilesional hyperechogenicity due to edema and/or hyperemia (on Doppler) can be usually observed (Fig. 33). A rim enhancement is typical at MRI. This may be irregular, while the putrid content normally shows a restricted diffusion (Fig. 28).

Adenomyoepitheliomas are benign breast lesions characterized by a biphasic proliferation of epithelial and myoepithelial cells and may recur after surgical excision (Lee et al. 2010). Due to the compression or obstruction of an adjacent duct space, these lesions sometimes present

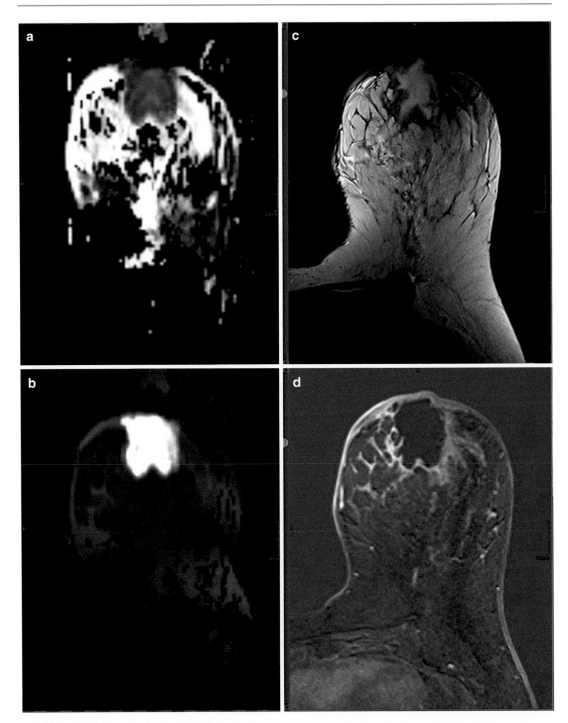

Fig. 28 Thirty-eight-year-old woman with a history of recurrent abscesses in the left breast. MRI demonstrates a complex cystic and solid lesion with a thick wall (type I). The ADC map (**a**) shows low values inside the abscess, correlating to restricted diffusion due to pus (**b** DWI, hyperintense in the b800 image, TR: 6700, TE: 60). In the T2w image (**c** TR: 5360, TE: 188), the abscess wall is hypo- and the content hyperintense. After IV contrast administration (**d** late arterial phase, subtraction image), the abscess wall shows a thick, irregular rim enhancement. US-guided aspiration yielded 25 mL of pus

Cystic and Complex Cystic and Solid Lesions

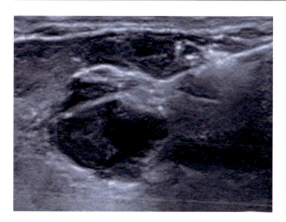

Fig. 29 Fifty-six-year-old woman, referred from screening for a lesion in the right breast. In US, this proved to be a predominantly solid (type IV) complex cystic and solid lesion, classified as BI-RADS 4. US-guided biopsy with a 14 G core needle was performed. The lesion proved to be a benign papilloma

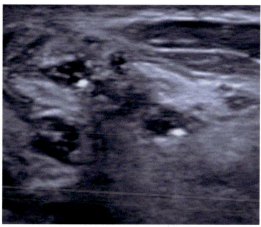

Fig. 31 Clustered microcysts, with individual cysts containing milk of calcium, which appears as bright echogenic foci

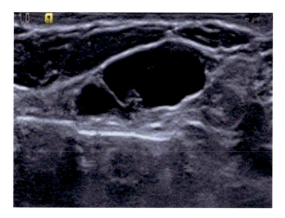

Fig. 30 Fifty-three-year-old woman, presenting with a palpable lump in the left breast. US demonstrated a type III complex cystic and solid lesion with a small intracystic mass, classified as BI-RADS 4. US-guided biopsy was performed with a 9 G vacuum-assisted needle, rendering a benign papilloma. If a usual 14 G core needle biopsy had been used in this case, the cystic part would have most likely collapsed after the first passage, rendering this small papilloma very hard to identify. Notice that the needle opening is placed right under the solid mass, thus facilitating its proper sampling

as complex cystic and solid lesions (Hikino et al. 2007; Lee et al. 2010). At MG, they may show microcalcifications and an associated architectural distortion, whereas in MRI, a type III enhancement curve is possible.

Apocrine metaplasia originates at the lobular part of the TDLU and is associated with a dilatation of fluid-filled acini. Epithelial changes are also present—however, at the absence of atypias, this lesion is not considered premalignant and carries a breast cancer risk, similar to that of other fibrocystic changes (Warner et al. 1998). Clustered microcysts are the imaging hallmark of apocrine metaplasia (Fig. 32), whereas thick-walled complex cystic and solid lesions may also be encountered (Doshi et al. 2007). The usual MG appearance is that of a circumscribed, micro- or microlobulated, hypodense mass, while the presence of milk of calcium is possible. *Papillary apocrine metaplasia* represents a specific subtype of apocrine metaplasia, where the apocrine cells form papillary projections into the ducts (Ha et al. 2018). This condition is considered as an early, premalignant lesion (Kosemehmetoglu and Guler 2010). At US, it may sometimes have the appearance of a cluster of microcysts; however, it more usually presents with solid components or an intracystic mass, in the sense of a complex cystic and solid lesion.

Small (<8 mm) or deep-lying simple cysts may present with *artifactual internal echoes* (Berg et al. 2006b), making the differentiation from a complicated cyst difficult. Harmonic or

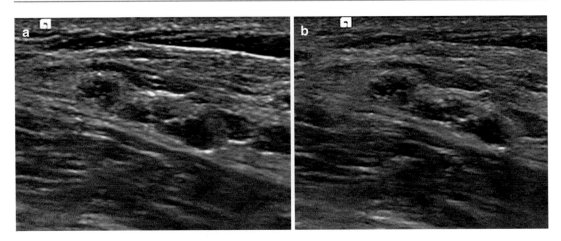

Fig. 32 Clustered microcysts. B-mode US without (**a**) and with (**b**) harmonic imaging. Harmonics aid in the characterization of the individual cystic components

compound imaging may help reduce these artifactual echoes, aiding in establishing the correct diagnosis. Moreover, adjacent simple cysts may sometimes be difficult to differentiate from clustered microcysts, although this differentiation is of little clinical importance (Fig. 34).

The *debris* inside a complicated cyst may sometimes adhere to its wall, thus resembling an intracystic mass. Moving the patient to the lateral decubitus position will sometimes make the debris to move (Athanasiou et al. 2014). If this does not happen, a contrast medium (either in US or in MRI) may be applied. In that case, solid components will demonstrate enhancement whereas debris not (Fig. 20).

Fibroadenomas are the most usual US differential diagnosis of complicated cysts with homogeneous, low-level echogenicity. They typically present as oval, circumscribed hypo- or isoechoic lesions, possibly with posterior enhancement. The detection of internal vascularity or coarse calcifications can help differentiate them from a truly cystic lesion. Less often, they may present as predominantly solid masses with smaller cystic parts and thus resemble a type IV complex cystic and solid lesion (Fig. 35).

Fibrocystic changes have a wide imaging spectrum, including simple and complicated cysts or clustered microcysts, or even complex cystic and solid lesions of all four types (Fig. 31) (Berg et al. 2003).

Galactoceles typically present as complicated cysts (Fig. 36). They arise due to the retention of milklike, fat-containing fluid, resulting from the obstruction of a duct, and are commonly found during pregnancy or breastfeeding (Salvador et al. 1990). At US, they usually contain echogenic fat plugs, whereas a fat-fluid level is common, with fat in the nondependent portion of the cyst. Sometimes, they may appear as a homogeneous iso- to hypoechoic lesion, which makes differentiation from a solid mass difficult. In MG, the demonstration of a fat-fluid level on a true lateral projection, with radiolucent fat in the cranial portion of the lesion, is pathognomonic. At MRI, the presence of fat leads to hyperintense parts in T1w sequences, which are hypointense with fat suppression.

Postoperative or posttraumatic *hematomas* usually present as complicated or even complex cystic and solid lesions (Fig. 18). Their appearance changes over time due to different degrees of blood liquefaction, and they contain different amounts of both serum and clot, while fibrin strands may also be seen (Athanasiou et al. 2014). In the hyperacute phase, they are anechoic, while they demonstrate increasingly echogenic content as the clot develops in the acute phase. In the subacute phase, they usually become heterogeneous

Cystic and Complex Cystic and Solid Lesions

Table 1 The most usual benign and malignant differential diagnoses according to each breast cyst type (simple cysts, complicated cysts, type I–IV complex cystic and solid lesions, and clustered microcysts)

	Simple cysts	Complicated cysts	Complex cystic and solid lesions			Clustered microcysts
			Types I/II	Type III	Type IV	
Benign	Fibrocystic changes	Simple cyst with artifactual echoes	Abscess	Complicated cyst with wall-adherent debris	Fibrocystic changes	Apocrine metaplasia
	Oil cyst	Proteinaceous cyst	Ruptured/inflamed cyst	Oil cyst	Fibroadenoma	Papillary apocrine metaplasia
	Seroma	Abscess	Hematoma	Adenomyoepithelioma	Oil cyst	Fibrocystic changes
		Galactocele	Seroma	Hematoma	Abscess	Abutting simple cysts
		Fibroadenoma	Fibrocystic changes	Seroma	Hematoma	
		Hemorrhagic cyst	Juvenile papillomatosis	Papillary apocrine metaplasia	Phyllodes tumor (benign, borderline)	
		Hematoma	Oil cyst	Fibrocystic changes	Papillary tumors (benign, atypical)	
		Seroma	Apocrine metaplasia	Papillary tumors (benign, atypical)		
		Oil cyst				
		Ruptured/inflamed cyst				
		Fibrocystic changes				
Malignant	Markedly hypoechoic malignancy	Markedly hypoechoic malignancy	High-grade, necrotic malignancy	Papillary tumors (malignant)	Phyllodes tumor (malignant)	
	Infiltrated lymph node	Infiltrated lymph node	Medullary carcinoma	High-grade, necrotic malignancy	Papillary tumors (malignant)	
			Metastasis from other malignancies	Malignant myoepithelial tumor	High-grade, necrotic malignancy	
				Medullary carcinoma	DCIS	
				Metaplastic carcinoma	Mucinous carcinoma	
					Sarcoma	

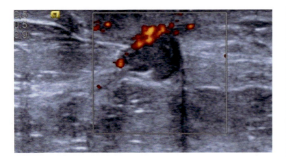

Fig. 33 Forty-two-year-old woman presenting with a palpable, painful lump in the left breast with associated skin thickening and redness. Doppler US demonstrates a subcutaneous abscess, presenting as a complicated cyst with peripheral hyperemia. Fine needle aspiration yielded pus

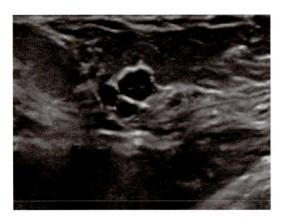

Fig. 34 Abutting simple cysts, presenting as clustered microcysts

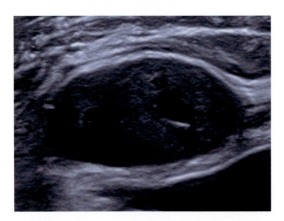

Fig. 35 Twenty-three-year-old woman with bilateral breast implants and a new palpable lump in the right breast. B-mode US shows a type IV complex cystic and solid lesion with central cystic spaces. The lesion proved to be a fibroadenoma after US-guided biopsy

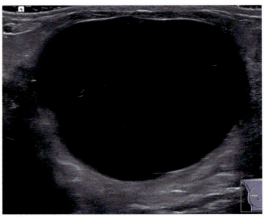

Fig. 36 Twenty-seven-year-old lactating woman presenting with a palpable lump in the right breast. B-mode US shows a complicated cyst with small echogenic foci due to lipid content. The imaging findings are typical of a galactocele

hyperechoic lesions, possibly with mural nodules, while their appearance in the chronic phase is variable (Berg et al. 2006a). The signal intensity of hematomas on MRI follows that of aging blood products. Without the appropriate history of a recent trauma or intervention, differentiation from a malignancy may prove difficult.

Juvenile papillomatosis usually presents as clusters of multiple cysts with thick walls and thick septations, an appearance which has given rise to the term "Swiss cheese disease" (Chung et al. 2009). Since papillomatosis presents a high-risk lesion, surgical removal is indicated (Athanasiou et al. 2014; Chung et al. 2009) (Fig. 37).

Oil cysts (or fat necrosis) occur after trauma or surgery and contain liquefied fat, due to a local destruction of adipocytes. Their most usual US appearance is that of a heterogeneous complex cystic and solid lesion (Fig. 19), although they may occasionally appear as complicated cysts (with either homogeneous low-level echoes or a fluid-debris level) and—sometimes—a rim calcification. They may even be anechoic, resembling a simple cyst. The variable US morphology correlates with the degree of liquefaction of their fatty content (Harvey et al. 1997) and usually makes the correct diagnosis challenging. The accompanying postoperative scar and the lack of

Cystic and Complex Cystic and Solid Lesions

Fig. 37 A case of biopsy-proven juvenile papillomatosis in a 23-year-old woman with a palpable abnormality in the right breast. B-mode US (**a**) demonstrates an area with multiple small cysts, with internal echoes and thick septations between them. In MRI, the pre-contrast T1w (**b** TR: 4.68, TE: 1.65, DIXON technique, water-only image) and the T2w (**c** TR: 5360, TE: 188) images show the small cysts with different signal intensities, due to the bloody content of some. After IV contrast administration (**d** venous phase, DIXON technique, water-only image and **e** venous phase, subtraction image), the same area shows a diffuse non-mass enhancement and some of the cystic walls enhance. However, no signs of intracystic enhancement are evident. This appearance has given rise to the term "Swiss cheese disease"

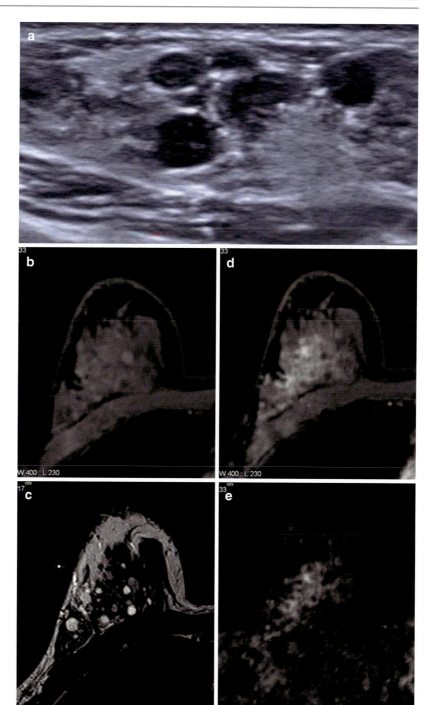

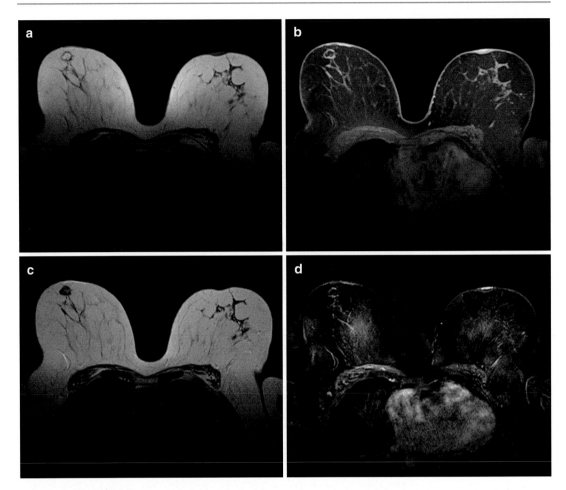

Fig. 38 MRI appearance of an oil cyst in the right breast of a 46-year-old woman with a history of a car accident 2 years ago. The pre-contrast T1w image (**a** TR: 4.68, TE: 1.65, DIXON technique, fat-only image) shows a hyperintense lesion (due to the presence of fat) with a smooth hypointense rim. With fat suppression (**b** TR: 4.68, TE: 1.65, DIXON technique, water-only image), the fatty content appears hypointense, whereas in the T2w image (**c** TR: 5360, TE: 188), it is heterogeneously hyperintense, however less than in the T1w image. After IV contrast administration (**d** late arterial phase, subtraction image), there is a smooth, thin rim enhancement with no enhancement of the fatty content

internal vascularization may be helpful in order to establish the diagnosis of an oil cyst. At MG, they typically appear as a lucent mass with a thin wall, which over time calcifies. MRI can also be helpful in detecting the fatty content of an oil cyst, in cases of a diagnostic dilemma (Fig. 38).

Papillary breast lesions usually appear as intracystic or intraductal solid masses (Figs. 39 and 40). These comprise a wide pathological spectrum, from benign papillomas to papillomas with atypias or DCIS or even papillary carcinomas (Collins and Schnitt 2008). Papillary lesions may be solitary or multiple and usually present with bloody or clear nipple discharge (Jagmohan et al. 2013). Both benign and atypical papillomas represent lesions of unknown malignant potential. Therefore, the current standard practice is their complete surgical excision (Athanasiou et al. 2014; Jagmohan et al. 2013). Intracystic papillary carcinomas are quite unusual, representing 0.6–1% of all breast cancers (Athanasiou et al. 2014). The imaging differentiation between benign, atypical, and malignant papillary lesions is usually very difficult. Older age, large size, ill-

Cystic and Complex Cystic and Solid Lesions

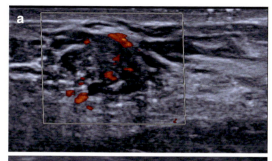

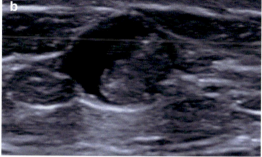

Fig. 39 US images of a benign (**a**) and an atypical (**b**) papilloma, both presenting as complex cystic and solid lesions in two different patients. An accurate differentiation between benign, atypical, and malignant papillary lesions is often not possible by imaging

defined margins, nonparallel orientation, increased vascularity with Doppler, areas of increased stiffness in elastography, and associated calcifications are more usual in malignant lesions (Jagmohan et al. 2013; Kim et al. 2008; Lam et al. 2006).

Occasionally, a papilloma may bleed inside a cystic formation. In such a case, blood may obscure the solid part and the lesion may present as a complicated cyst. Doppler will sometimes demonstrate internal vascularity inside the solid papillary lesion; however, setting the correct diagnosis may prove difficult. MG cannot aid in the differentiation of intracystic masses, which appear as circumscribed tumors. However, at MRI, the solid parts demonstrate an avid enhancement and can be easily differentiated from the hemorrhagic component (Jiang et al. 2018).

Phyllodes tumors typically present as predominantly solid masses with peripheral macrocysts or slit-like cystic clefts (Liberman et al. 1996; McCarthy et al. 2014) (Fig. 41). They can be

Fig. 40 Fifty-two-year-old woman presenting with bloody discharge from the right nipple. MRI demonstrates an intracystic mass (type III complex cystic and solid lesion). The T2w image (**a** TR: 5360, TE: 188) shows the cystic part of the lesion as hyperintense and the solid one as isointense. After IV contrast administration (**b** late arterial phase, subtraction image), only the solid part enhances. US-guided biopsy showed a benign papilloma

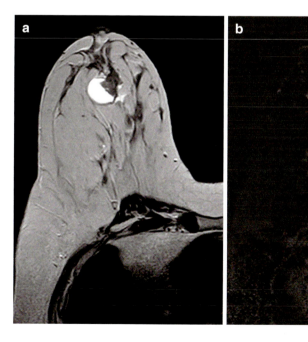

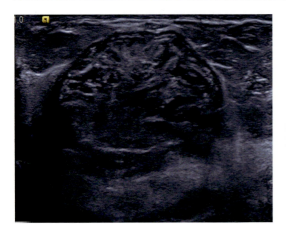 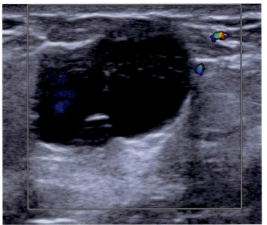

Fig. 41 Fifty-six-year-old woman presenting with a palpable lump in the left breast. B-mode US shows a type IV complex cystic and solid lesion with several slit-like cystic clefts. US-guided biopsy showed a benign phyllodes tumor

Fig. 42 Forty-seven-year-old woman presenting with a palpable, painful lump in the left breast. US shows a complex cystic and solid lesion with thick septations, possibly an intracystic mass, and an indistinct margin. Notice the movement of fluid demonstrated as an artifact (blue color) due to the energy imparted by color Doppler. US-guided biopsy demonstrated a ruptured and inflamed cyst

benign, borderline, or malignant and are characterized by a rapid growth. In imaging, the first two categories can usually not be differentiated from fibroadenomas, while malignant tumors usually have an indistinct or microlobulated margin and high vascularity in Doppler. Surgical management is until today the mainstay (Mishra et al. 2013).

Ruptured or inflamed cysts may sometimes present as complicated cysts with internal echoes. However, the cystic wall is usually—at least partially—thickened and the lesion margin indistinct, thus resembling a complex cystic and solid lesion (Figs. 15 and 42). Doppler usually demonstrates peripheral hyperemia. At MRI, the presence of a smooth, thin rim enhancement is typical, differentiating them from a malignant necrotic tumor (Wang et al. 2014).

Postoperative *seromas* usually present as simple cystic lesions at the lumpectomy or mastectomy site, possibly with floating fibrin strands (Berg et al. 2006a). However, a thick, irregular wall or thick internal septations may also be evident, thus having the appearance of a complex cystic and solid lesion (Fig. 18) (Athanasiou et al. 2014). Clinical information will aid in establishing the correct diagnosis in cases of a diagnostic dilemma.

3.2 Malignant Lesions

Malignancies are normally easily differentiated from *simple or complicated cysts*. High-grade invasive ductal carcinomas are often markedly hypoechoic and may resemble a cystic lesion. However, the tumor margins are usually indistinct. Doppler will also often demonstrate vessels inside the tumor. At MG, a hyperdense mass with (usually partially) non-circumscribed or even spiculated margins will be seen. Suspicious microcalcifications may also be evident within or around the tumor. At MRI, rim enhancement and washout kinetics in a partially non-circumscribed or spiculated mass will point to the malignant diagnosis. More details on the MG and MRI findings of breast malignancies can be found in the corresponding chapters.

On the other hand, *complex cystic and solid lesions* have a considerable probability of corresponding to a malignant tumor, variable according to their type (up to 30% for types I and II, 22% for type III, and 18–62% for type IV) (Berg et al. 2003; Chang et al. 2007). They usually represent high-grade, necrotic invasive ductal or (rarely) lobular carcinomas (Figs. 22, 26, 43, 44,

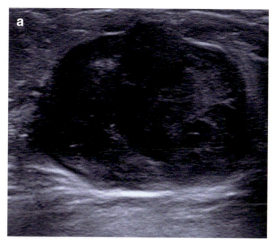

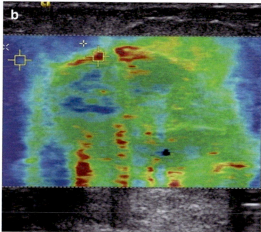

Fig. 43 Seventy-four-year-old woman presenting with a palpable lump in the left breast. B-mode US (**a**) shows a type IV complex cystic and solid lesion with central cystic areas corresponding to necrosis. Elastography (**b**) demonstrates high stiffness in the solid parts and softer necrotic parts of the tumor. US-guided biopsy showed a grade 2 invasive carcinoma of no special type

and 45), DCIS, as well as other, less usual types of breast cancer [medullary, mucinous, metaplastic, or papillary (Fig. 46) carcinomas, malignant myoepithelial or phyllodes tumors, etc.], sarcomas, infiltrated lymph nodes, and breast metastases from other tumors (Athanasiou et al. 2014; Berg et al. 2003; Chang et al. 2007; Rinaldi et al. 2010).

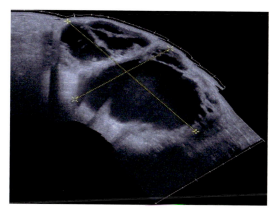

Fig. 44 Thirty-eight-year-old woman presenting with a rapidly growing palpable tumor in the left breast. B-mode US shows a large complex cystic and solid lesion with indistinct margins, a thick wall, and thick septations. US-guided biopsy demonstrated a triple-negative grade 3 necrotic invasive carcinoma of no special type. In cases of very large tumors (larger than the footprint of the transducer), a panoramic image can aid in depicting the whole mass

4 Conclusion

Cysts are the most usual breast pathology, usually presenting as a mass in MG. However, MG cannot differentiate between cystic and solid lesions. US has been traditionally used for the identification of breast cysts with a high diagnostic accuracy. MRI is not usually necessary for the characterization of cystic breast lesions. In cases of doubt regarding the presence of solid parts, an US-guided FNA and/or biopsy should be performed.

Simple breast cysts are benign findings and should be classified as BI-RADS 2, whereas for complicated cysts and clustered microcysts BI-RADS 3 is an appropriate recommendation. Finally, complex cystic and solid lesions should be classified as BI-RADS 4, since they are potentially malignant. In this case, an image-guided biopsy is warranted. For small intracystic masses or lesions with a thick wall or thick septations, VAB should be considered. The biopsy site should always be marked with a clip for future reference.

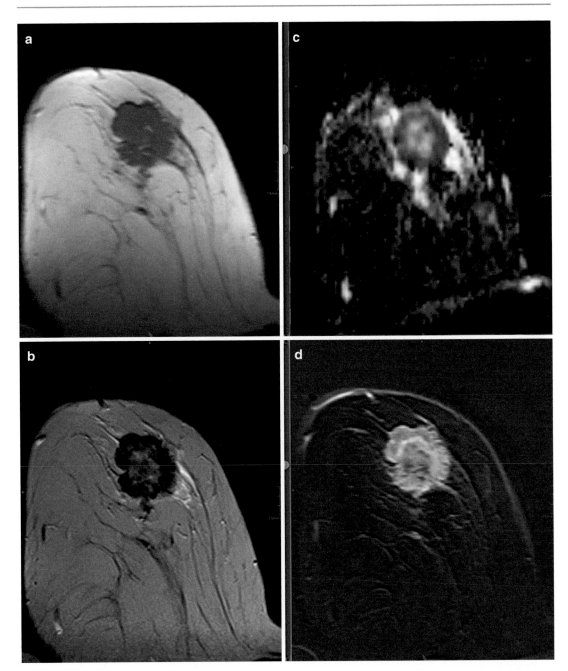

Fig. 45 Forty-seven-year-old woman presenting with a palpable lump in the medial right breast. At MRI, the pre-contrast T1w image (**a** TR: 4.68, TE: 1.65, DIXON technique, fat-only image) shows a lobulated, heterogeneous lesion. The necrotic center and the surrounding edema are better appreciated in the T2w image (**b** TR: 5360, TE: 188). In the ADC map (**c**), the solid peripheral parts of the tumor demonstrate low values, due to restricted diffusion, whereas the necrotic center is more hyperintense. After IV contrast administration (**d** early arterial phase, subtraction image), areas of necrosis do not enhance, in contrast to the tumor periphery. US-guided biopsy showed a necrotic, grade 3 invasive carcinoma of no special type

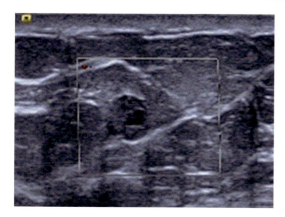

Fig. 46 US image of a type IV complex cystic and solid lesion corresponding to a small invasive papillary carcinoma in the left breast of a 56-year-old woman, referred from screening. Doppler fails to demonstrate any vascularity inside or around the tumor

Acknowledgements We would like to thank Mrs. Ines Foetschl for the processing of the images of this chapter. Funding was provided in part by the European Union's Horizon 2020 Research and Innovation Programme under grant agreement Nr. 688188.

References

Athanasiou A, Aubert E, Vincent Salomon A, Tardivon A (2014) Complex cystic breast masses in ultrasound examination. Diagn Interv Imaging 95:169–179

Aujero MP, Tirada N, Khorjekar G (2019) Asymptomatic complicated cysts in postmenopausal women: is tissue sampling unnecessarily high? Acad Radiol 26:900–906

Balleyguier C, Canale S, Ben Hassen W, Vielh P, Bayou EH, Mathieu MC, Uzan C, Bourgier C, Dromain C (2013a) Breast elasticity: principles, technique, results: an update and overview of commercially available software. Eur J Radiol 82:427–434

Balleyguier C, Ciolovan L, Ammari S, Canale S, Sethom S, Al Rouhbane R, Vielh P, Dromain C (2013b) Breast elastography: the technical process and its applications. Diagn Interv Imaging 94:503–513

Barnard S, Cooke T, Angerson W, Leen E (2008) A contrast-enhanced ultrasound study of benign and malignant breast tissue. S Afr Med J 98:386–391

Barr RG (2018) The role of sonoelastography in breast lesions. Semin Ultrasound CT MR 39:98–105

Berg WA (2005) Sonographically depicted breast clustered microcysts: is follow-up appropriate? AJR Am J Roentgenol 185:952–959

Berg WA (2020) Reducing unnecessary biopsy and follow-up of benign cystic breast lesions. Radiology 295:52–53

Berg WA, Campassi CI, Ioffe OB (2003) Cystic lesions of the breast: sonographic-pathologic correlation. Radiology 227:183–191

Berg WA, Birdwell RL, Gombos E, Wang S-C, Parkinson BT, Raza S, Green GE, Kennedy A, Kettler M (2006a) Diagnostic imaging: breast, 1st edn. Amirsys Inc., Salt Lake City, UT

Berg WA, Blume JD, Cormack JB, Mendelson EB (2006b) Operator dependence of physician-performed whole-breast US: lesion detection and characterization. Radiology 241:355–365

Berg WA, Sechtin AG, Marques H, Zhang Z (2010) Cystic breast masses and the ACRIN 6666 experience. Radiol Clin North Am 48:931–987

Bodian CA, lattes R, Perzin KH (1992) The epidemiology of gross cystic disease of the breast confirmed by biopsy or by aspiration of cyst fluid. Cancer Detect Prev 16:7–15

Brookes MJ, Bourke AG (2008) Radiological appearances of papillary breast lesions. Clin Radiol 63:1265–1273

Busilacchi P, Draghi F, Preda L, Ferranti C (2012) Has color Doppler a role in the evaluation of mammary lesions? J Ultrasound 15:93–98

Celis JE, Gromov P, Moreira JMA, Cabezón T, Friis E, Vejborg IMM, Proess G, Rank F, Gromova I (2006) Apocrine cysts of the breast: biomarkers, origin, enlargement, and relation with cancer phenotype. Mol Cell Proteomics 5:462–483

Cha JH, Moon WK, Cho N, Chung SY, Park SH, Park JM, Han BK, Choe YH, Cho G, Im J-G (2005) Differentiation of benign from malignant solid breast masses: conventional US versus spatial compound imaging. Radiology 237:841–846

Chang Y-W, Kwon KH, Goo DE, Choi DL, Lee HK, Yang SB (2007) Sonographic differentiation of benign and malignant cystic lesions of the breast. J Ultrasound Med 26:47–53

Chinyama CN (2014) Benign breast diseases. Radiology - pathology - risk assessment, 2nd edn. Springer, Berlin

Cho N, Moon WK, Chang JM, Kim SJ, Lyou CY, Choi HY (2011) Aliasing artifact depicted on ultrasound (US)-elastography for breast cystic lesions mimicking solid masses. Acta Radiol 52:3–7

Choudhry S, Gorman B, Charboneau JW, Tradup DJ, Beck RJ, Kofler JM, Groth DS (2000) Comparison of tissue harmonic imaging with conventional US in abdominal disease. Radiographics 20:1127–1135

Chung EM, Cube R, Hall GJ, Gonzalez C, Stocker JT, Glassman LM (2009) From the archives of the AFIP: breast masses in children and adolescents: radiologic-pathologic correlation. Radiographics 29:907–931

Ciatto S, Cariaggi P, Bulgaresi P (1987) The value of routine cytologic examination of breast cyst fluids. Acta Cytol 31:301–304

Clarke L, Edwards A, Pollard K (2005) Acoustic streaming in ovarian cysts. J Ultrasound Med 24:617–621

Cohen EO, Tso HH, Leung JWT (2019) Multiple bilateral circumscribed breast masses detected at imaging:

review of evidence for management recommendations. AJR Am J Roentgenol 214:276–281

Collins LC, Schnitt SJ (2008) Papillary lesions of the breast: selected diagnostic and management issues. Histopathology 52:20–29

Cyr AE, Novack D, Trinkaus K, Margenthaler JA, Gillanders WE, Eberlein TJ, Ritter J, Aft RL (2011) Are we overtreating papillomas diagnosed on core needle biopsy? Ann Surg Oncol 18:946–951

Daly CP, Bailey JE, Klein KA, Helvie MA (2008) Complicated breast cysts on sonography: is aspiration necessary to exclude malignancy? Acad Radiol 15:610–617

Dixon JM, Scott WN, Miller WR (1985) Natural history of cystic disease. the importance of cyst type. Br J Surg 72:190–192

Dixon JM, McDonald C, Elton RA, Miller WR (1999) Risk of breast cancer in women with palpable breast cysts: a prospective study. Lancet 353:1742–1745

Doshi DJ, March DE, Crisi GM, Coughlin BF (2007) Complex cystic breast masses: diagnostic approach and imaging-pathologic correlation. Radiographics 27(Suppl 1):S53–S64

Goldbach AR, Tuite CM, Ross E (2020) Clustered microcysts at breast US: outcomes and updates for appropriate management recommendations. Radiology 295:44–51

Gordon PB, Gagnon FA, Lanzkowsky L (2003) Solid breast masses diagnosed as fibroadenoma at fine-needle aspiration biopsy: acceptable rates of growth at long-term follow-up. Radiology 229:233–238

Graf O, Helbich TH, Hopf G, Graf C, Sickles EA (2007) Probably benign breast masses at US: is follow-up an acceptable alternative to biopsy? Radiology 244:87–93

Greenwood HI, Lee AY, Lobach IV, Carpentier BM, Freimanis RI, Strachowski LM (2017) Clustered microcysts on breast ultrasound: what is an appropriate management recommendation? AJR Am J Roentgenol 209:W395–W399

Gruber R, Jaromi S, Rudas M, Pfarl G, Riedl CC, Flory D, Graf O, Sickles EA, Helbich TH (2013) Histologic work-up of non-palpable breast lesions classified as probably benign at initial mammography and/or ultrasound (BI-RADS category 3). Eur J Radiol 82:398–403

Gulati M, King KG, Gill IS, Pham V, Grant E, Duddalwar VA (2015) Contrast-enhanced ultrasound (CEUS) of cystic and solid renal lesions: a review. Abdom Imaging 40:1982–1996

Ha T, Yim H, Park SY, Kang DK, Kim TH (2018) Papillary apocrine metaplasia of the breast mimicking papillary neoplasm: a case report. J Korean Soc Radiol 78:103–106

Haagensen DEJ (1991) Is cystic disease related to breast cancer? Am J Surg Pathol 15:687–694

Harvey JA, Moran RE, Maurer EJ, DeAngelis GA (1997) Sonographic features of mammary oil cysts. J Ultrasound Med 16:719–724

Heywang-Köbrunner SH, Heinig A, Hellerhoff K, Holzhausen HJ, Nährig J (2009) Use of ultrasound-guided percutaneous vacuum-assisted breast biopsy for selected difficult indications. Breast J 15:348–356

Hikino H, Kodama K, Yasui K, Ozaki N, Nagaoka S, Miura H (2007) Intracystic adenomyoepithelioma of the breast—case report and review. Breast Cancer 14:429–433

Hindle WH, Arias RD, Florentine B, Whang J (2000) Lack of utility in clinical practice of cytologic examination of nonbloody cyst fluid from palpable breast cysts. Am J Obstet Gynecol 182:1300–1305

Jagmohan P, Pool FJ, Putti TC, Wong J (2013) Papillary lesions of the breast: imaging findings and diagnostic challenges. Diagn Interv Radiol 19:471–478

Jiang T, Tang W, Gu Y, Xu M, Yang W, Peng W (2018) Magnetic resonance imaging features of breast encapsulated papillary carcinoma. J Comput Assist Tomogr 42:536–541

Kaiser CG, Herold M, Baltzer PA, Dietzel M, Krammer J, Gajda M, Camara O, Schoenberg SO, Kaiser WA, Wasser K (2015) Is "prepectoral edema" a morphologic sign for malignant breast tumors? Acad Radiol 22:684–689

Kern R, Szabo K, Hennerici M, Meairs S (2004) Characterization of carotid artery plaques using real-time compound B-mode ultrasound. Stroke 35:870–875

Kim TH, Kang DK, Kim SY, Lee EJ, Jung YS, Yim H (2008) Sonographic differentiation of benign and malignant papillary lesions of the breast. J Ultrasound Med 27:75–82

Kim MJ, Kim JY, Yoon JH, Youk JH, Moon HJ, Son EJ, Kwak JY, Kim E-K (2011) How to find an isoechoic lesion with breast US. Radiographics 31:663–676

Kosemehmetoglu K, Guler G (2010) Papillary apocrine metaplasia and columnar cell lesion with atypia: is there a shared common pathway? Ann Diagn Pathol 14:425–431

Lam WW, Chu WC, Tang AP, Tse G, Ma TK (2006) Role of radiologic features in the management of papillary lesions of the breast. AJR Am J Roentgenol 186:1322–1327

Lee JH, Kim SH, Kang BJ, Lee AW, Song BJ (2010) Ultrasonographic features of benign adenomyoepithelioma of the breast. Korean J Radiol 11:522–527

Lee SH, Kim EK, Kim MJ, Moon HJ, Yoon JH (2014) Vacuum-assisted breast biopsy under ultrasonographic guidance: analysis of a 10-year experience. Ultrasonography 33:259–266

Liberman L, Bonaccio E, Hamele-Bena D, Abramson AF, Cohen MA, Dershaw DD (1996) Benign and malignant phyllodes tumors: mammographic and sonographic findings. Radiology 198:121–124

Liu H, Jiang Y-X, Liu J-B, Zhu Q-L, Sun Q, Chang X-Y (2009) Contrast-enhanced breast ultrasonography. J Ultrasound Med 28:911–920

Mannello F, Tonti GAM, Papa S (2006) Human gross cyst breast disease and cystic fluid: bio-molecular, morphological, and clinical studies. Breast Cancer Res Treat 97:115–129

Markopoulos C, Kouskos E, Gogas H, Kakisis J, Kyriakou V, Gogas J, Kostakis A (2002) Diagnosis and treatment of intracystic breast carcinomas. Am Surg 68:783–786

McCarthy E, Kavanagh J, O'Donoghue Y, McCormack E, D'Arcy C, O'Keeffe SA (2014) Phyllodes tumours of the breast: radiological presentation, management and follow-up. Br J Radiol 87:20140239

Mendelson EB, Böhm-Vélez M, Berg WA, Whitman GJ, Feldman MI, Madjar H, Rizzatto G, Baker JA, Zuley M, Stavros AT, Comstock C, Van Duyn Wear V (2013) ACR BI-RADS® ultrasound. In: D'Orsi CJ, Sickles EA, Mendelson EB, Morris EA (eds) ACR BI-RADS® atlas, breast imaging reporting and data system, 5th edn. American College of Radiology, Reston, VA, pp 216–355

Mishra SP, Tiwary SK, Mishra M, Khanna AK (2013) Phyllodes tumor of breast: a review article. ISRN Surg 2013:361469

Mooney KL, Bassett LW, Apple SK (2016) Upgrade rates of high-risk breast lesions diagnosed on core needle biopsy: a single-institution experience and literature review. Mod Pathol 29:1471–1484

Nightingale KR, Kornguth PJ, Walker WF, McDermott BA, Trahey GE (1995) A novel ultrasonic technique for differentiating cysts from solid lesions: preliminary results in the breast. Ultrasound Med Biol 21:745–751

Popli MB, Gupta P, Arse D, Kumar P, Kaur P (2016) Advanced MRI techniques in the evaluation of complex cystic breast lesions. Breast Cancer Basic Clin Res 10:71–76

Rageth CJ, O'Flynn EAM, Comstock C, Kurtz C, Kubik R, Madjar H, Lepori D, Kampmann G, Mundinger A, Baege A, Decker T, Hosch S, Tausch C, Delaloye J-F, Morris E, Varga Z (2016) First International Consensus Conference on lesions of uncertain malignant potential in the breast (B3 lesions). Breast Cancer Res Treat 159:203–213

Rinaldi P, Ierardi C, Costantini M, Magno S, Giuliani M, Belli P, Bonomo L (2010) Cystic breast lesions: sonographic findings and clinical management. J Ultrasound Med 29:1617–1626

Rosen EL, Soo MS (2001) Tissue harmonic imaging sonography of breast lesions: improved margin analysis, conspicuity, and image quality compared to conventional ultrasound. Clin Imaging 25:379–384

Salvador R, Salvador M, Jimenez JA, Martinez M, Casas L (1990) Galactocele of the breast: radiologic and ultrasonographic findings. Br J Radiol 63:140–142

Schafer P, Furrer C, Mermillod B (1988) An association of cigarette smoking with recurrent subareolar breast abscess. Int J Epidemiol 17:810–813

Smith DN, Kaelin CM, Korbin CD, Ko W, Meyer JE, Carter GR (1997) Impalpable breast cysts: utility of cytologic examination of fluid obtained with radiologically guided aspiration. Radiology 204: 149–151

Tanaka A, Imai A, Goto M, Konishi E, Shinkura N (2016) Which patients require or can skip biopsy for breast clustered microcysts? Predictive findings of breast cancer and mucocele-like tumor. Breast Cancer 23:590–596

Vargas HI, Vargas MP, Gonzalez KD, Eldrageely K, Khalkhali I (2004) Outcomes of sonography-based management of breast cysts. Am J Surg 188: 443–447

Venta LA, Dudiak CM, Salomon CG, Flisak ME (1994) Sonographic evaluation of the breast. Radiographics 14:29–50

Wang L, Wang D, Fei X, Ruan M, Chai W, Xu L, Li X (2014) A rim-enhanced mass with central cystic changes on MR imaging: how to distinguish breast cancer from inflammatory breast diseases? PLoS One 9:e90355

Warner JK, Kumar D, Berg WA (1998) Apocrine metaplasia: mammographic and sonographic appearances. AJR Am J Roentgenol 170:1375–1379

Wellings SR, Alpers CE (1987) Apocrine cystic metaplasia: subgross pathology and prevalence in cancer-associated versus random autopsy breasts. Hum Pathol 18:381–386

Xiang H, Tang G, Li Y, Liu Y, Liu L, Lin X (2020) Value of hand-held ultrasound in the differential diagnosis and accurate breast imaging reporting and data system subclassification of complex cystic and solid breast lesions. Ultrasound Med Biol 46:1111–1118

Yao J-P, Hao Y-Z, Chang Q, Geng C-Y, Chen Y, Zhao W-P, Song Y, Zhou X (2017) Value of ultrasonographic features for assessing malignant potential of complex cystic breast lesions. J Ultrasound Med 36: 699–704

Yates AJ, Ahmed A (1988) Apocrine carcinoma and apocrine metaplasia. Histopathology 13:228–231

High-Risk Lesions of the Breast: Diagnosis and Management

Maria Adele Marino, Katja Pinker, and Thomas Helbich

Contents

1   **Introduction** 338

2   **Histopathologic Characteristics, Prognosis, Diagnosis, and Management of High-Risk Lesions of the Breast** 339
    2.1   Atypical Ductal Hyperplasia 339
    2.2   Flat Epithelial Atypia 342
    2.3   Lobular Neoplasia 343
    2.4   Papillary Lesions 346
    2.5   Phyllodes Tumor 348
    2.6   Radial Scar and Complex Sclerosing Lesion 350

3   **Chemoprevention in High-Risk Lesions** 352

4   **Conclusion** 352

References 352

M. A. Marino (✉)
Department of Biomedical Sciences and Morphologic and Functional Imaging, University of Messina, Messina, Italy

K. Pinker
Breast Imaging Service, Department of Radiology, Memorial Sloan Kettering Cancer Center, New York, NY, USA
e-mail: pinkerdk@mskcc.org

T. Helbich
Division of Molecular and Gender Imaging, Department of Biomedical Imaging and Image-Guided Therapy, Medical University of Vienna, Vienna, Austria
e-mail: thomas.helbich@meduniwien.ac.at

Abstract

High-risk lesions of the breast comprise a broad variety of diseases, which remain poorly understood. These lesions include atypical ductal hyperplasia, flat epithelial atypia, lobular neoplasia, papillary lesions, phyllodes tumor, radial scar, complex sclerosing lesions, and other rare entities. Diagnosis is frequently made by needle biopsy under ultrasound, stereotactic, or

© Springer Nature Switzerland AG 2022
M. Fuchsjäger et al. (eds.), *Breast Imaging*, Medical Radiology Diagnostic Imaging,
https://doi.org/10.1007/978-3-030-94918-1_16

magnetic resonance imaging guidance as these lesions lack specific diagnostic imaging features. They are also referred to as B3 lesions, which histopathologically are lesions of unknown biological potential; that is, they are non-obligate precursors of malignancy and risk indicators with an increased possibility of developing breast cancer in any location of the same or the contralateral breast. The management of these lesions is challenging; a wide spectrum of therapeutic options are available to women to limit potential overtreatment in patients at low risk. The aim of this chapter is to provide a comprehensive overview of the different high-risk lesions. We review their characteristics with respect to histopathology and imaging phenotypes and discuss the role of the individual imaging modalities in this context. We detail the prognosis for the different high-risk lesions and current guidelines for management. We further discuss other therapeutic options for the women diagnosed with these lesions, such as chemoprevention. Finally, we discuss the strategies the multidisciplinary team may adopt to find an individually adapted and optimized treatment for each patient diagnosed with a high-risk lesion.

Abbreviations

ADH	Atypical ductal hyperplasia
ALH	Atypical lobular hyperplasia
CNB	Core needle biopsy
CSL	Complex sclerosing lesion
DBT	Digital breast tomosynthesis
FEA	Flat epithelial atypia
LCIS	Lobular carcinoma in situ
LN	Classical lobular neoplasia
MRI	Magnetic resonance imaging
PL	Papillary lesions
PT	Phyllodes tumor
RS	Radial scar
VAB	Vacuum-assisted biopsy
VAE	Vacuum-assisted excision

1 Introduction

High-risk lesions are a heterogeneous group of breast diseases that carry a low risk of malignancy, ranging between 0.2% and 5% (Vizcaíno et al. 2001; D'Orsi et al. 2013).

Systematic mammography screening has contributed to a two- to fourfold increase in the incidence of these lesions over the last few decades (Fisher et al. 1996; Philpotts et al. 2000; Li et al. 2006; Portschy et al. 2013; Hoffmann et al. 2016). Based on suspicious findings, image-guided biopsies are performed by either core needle biopsy (CNB) or vacuum-assisted biopsy (VAB) under ultrasound, stereotactic, or magnetic resonance imaging (MRI) guidance. Up to 14% of these biopsies yield the definitive diagnosis of lesions of uncertain potential, i.e., histopathological B3 lesions. B3 lesions are also found on surgically excised specimens sporadically (Bahl et al. 2017; Allison et al. 2015; Eby et al. 2009; Graf et al. 2004, 2007; Gruber et al. 2013; Riedl et al. 2007).

Following the diagnosis of a high-risk lesion, due to their variable biologic profiles and their potential to be histologically upgraded to ductal carcinoma in situ (DCIS) or invasive cancer, surgical excision is frequently adopted to treat these lesions (Kohr et al. 2010; Liberman et al. 1999; Foster et al. 2004; Lourenco et al. 2014). However, a lack of consensus exists regarding the proper management of these lesions, and the final treatment decision remains a challenging task for the multidisciplinary team. The steady development in percutaneous breast biopsy procedures, from VAB in the late 1990s to percutaneous excisional devices such as the intact breast lesion excision system since, has questioned the role of surgery as the uniquely available treatment for these lesions (Kohr et al. 2010; Liberman et al. 1999; Foster et al. 2004; Lourenco et al. 2014). Vacuum-assisted excision (VAE), i.e., excision of a breast lesion with VAB, is currently considered the method of choice for secondary assessment of most B3 lesions. The aim of VAE is to remove the lesion in its entirety, but in lesions larger than 20 mm, it is difficult to ensure complete sampling. Thus, in many high-risk lesions, these less

High-Risk Lesions of the Breast: Diagnosis and Management

invasive procedures might be sufficient for therapeutic excision (Alonso-Bartolomé et al. 2004; Saladin et al. 2016; Rageth et al. 2016).

The aim of this chapter is to provide the reader with a complete overview on the diagnosis and management of lesions classified as borderline (B3) with an uncertain potential of malignancy. We treat each entity separately according to its histologic diagnosis, giving insight into the histopathologic aspects, immunoprofile features, when possible, and prognosis. We outline the salient diagnostic features of these lesions on mammography, ultrasound, and MRI. Further, we review the recently published literature and introduce guidelines proposed by the First International Consensus Conference on B3 lesions and the NHS Breast Screening multidisciplinary working group (Rageth et al. 2016; Pinder et al. 2018). Finally, we stress the importance of strategies that multidisciplinary team could adopt to allow optimized treatment to avoid overtreatment in women with low-risk B3 lesions.

2 Histopathologic Characteristics, Prognosis, Diagnosis, and Management of High-Risk Lesions of the Breast

High-risk lesions are represented by a broad variety of histologic diagnoses including atypical ductal hyperplasia (ADH), flat epithelial atypia (FEA), lobular neoplasia (LN), papillary lesions (PLs), phyllodes tumor (PT), radial scar (RS), complex sclerosing lesions (CLS), and some other rare entities (Rageth et al. 2016; Lakhani et al. 2012). According to European guidelines, the term B3 should be used when the entities are diagnosed at needle biopsy. The categories B1–B5 provide a systematic communication between pathologists, clinicians, and radiologists (Perry et al. 2008).

B3 lesions are defined as *benign lesions of unknown biological potential* because they may occur within or in the periphery of DCIS or invasive breast cancer. B3 lesions are also considered

a *non-obligate precursor of malignancy* because they might develop into higher grade lesions. Finally, some B3 lesions function as *risk indicators* with an increased possibility of a breast cancer diagnosis in any location within the same breast or within the contralateral breast (Heywang-Köbrunner et al. 2010).

2.1 Atypical Ductal Hyperplasia

Atypical ductal hyperplasia (ADH) is an intraductal proliferative lesion. In this respect, it bears similarities to usual ductal hyperplasia (UDH) and DCIS. ADH is found in up to 4% of breast biopsies for palpable masses and in 31% for microcalcifications (Purushothaman et al. 2016). ADH is seen in women spanning a wide age range of seven to eight decades postadolescence (Lakhani et al. 2012). Despite being exceedingly rare (<1%) in males undergoing reduction mammoplasty for gynecomastia, ADH is also seen (Myers and Bhimji 2017).

Histopathology ADH typically originates in the terminal-duct lobular unit, similar to UDH and DCIS, and is confined to the mammary ductal-lobular system (Lakhani et al. 2012). Usually, homogeneous involvement of less than two membrane-bound spaces and a size ≤2 mm serve as the histopathologic diagnostic criteria for ADH (Clauser et al. 2016). The pathologic distinction between ADH and either low-grade DCIS or FEA can be challenging. Over the last decade, the ductal intraepithelial neoplasia (DIN) system classification has slowly gained ground and has shown to be useful for decreasing the confusion in distinguishing between these different lesion types; for instance, DIN limits the term "carcinoma" to invasive tumors (Tavassoli and Devilee 2003; Galimberti et al. 2013). DIN1A corresponds to FEA, which has an extremely low risk of local recurrence and progression to invasive cancer; DIN1B corresponds to ADH, which shares some but not all the features of low- or intermediate-grade DCIS; and DIN1C corresponds to grade 1 DCIS. DIN2

Table 1 Histopathological classification of ductal intraepithelial neoplasia (DIN) and lobular intraepithelial neoplasia (LIN)

Traditional histopathological classification	Ductal intraepithelial neoplasia (DIN) classification
Flat epithelial atypia	DIN1A
Atypical ductal hyperplasia (ADH)	DIN1B
Low-grade DCIS (G1) cribriform or micropapillary	DIN1C
Intermediate-grade DCIS (G2) cribriform or micropapillary with necrosis or atypia or other types	DIN2
High grade (G3) with or without necrosis	DIN3
Traditional histopathological classification	Lobular intraepithelial neoplasia (LIN) classification
Atypical lobular hyperplasia	LIN1
Classic-type LCIS	LIN2
High-grade or pleomorphic LCIS	LIN3

corresponds to grade 2 DCIS. DIN3 corresponds to grade 3 DCIS (Galimberti et al. 2013) (Table 1). At the same time, morphologic and molecular studies have supported a model of breast cancer development in which ADH is a non-obligate precursor of low-grade DCIS and invasive carcinoma (Nutter et al. 2017; Buckley et al. 2015; Collins et al. 2007, 2016; Hartmann et al. 2015, 2014).

Immunoprofile A variety of biomarkers have been studied, but none have been validated for clinical use for ADH. ADH typically shows cells that are positive for estrogen receptor but negative for high-molecular-weight keratins (such as keratin 5/6) (Lakhani et al. 2012). ADH shows an identical immunoprofile and low number of chromosomal abnormalities to low-grade DCIS, which confirms a progression between the two entities, i.e., from ADH to DCIS. ADH may be contained in fibroadenomas, papillomas, radial scars, or benign changes (Heywang-Köbrunner et al. 2010).

Prognosis ADH is associated with a moderately increased risk for invasive breast cancer, with a relative risk between 3.0 and 5.0 for both breasts (Kohr et al. 2010; Clauser et al. 2016). It is thus more likely to be a precursor lesion than UDH, which has a relative risk of 1.5. In up to 69% of cases, moderate- or high-grade invasive ductal breast cancers are associated with ADH. The risk is twice as high in the ipsilateral as in the contralateral breast (Hartmann et al. 2014).

Imaging Findings ADH has been reported in 2–11% of abnormal mammographic findings; ADH most commonly presents as microcalcifications on the mammogram (Clauser et al. 2016; Jackman et al. 2002). Often, the microcalcifications are amorphous; sporadically, they are coarse heterogeneous or fine pleomorphic (Fig. 1a–c). Their distribution may be grouped, linear, or regional. ADH may also present as a mass with or without associated microcalcifications (Heywang-Köbrunner et al. 2010). On ultrasound, the evidence concerning ADH is limited. According to Mesurolle et al. (2014), ADH may present as a hypoechoic mass with an irregular shape, microlobulated margins, no posterior acoustic feature, abrupt interface, and parallel orientation. Usually, however, there is no clear ultrasound correlate (Clauser et al. 2016) (Fig. 1d). With the increasing use of breast MRI, ADH is now a relatively common finding at MRI-guided biopsy, found in up to 21% (Riedl et al. 2007; Lourenco et al. 2014). On MRI, a mass or non-mass enhancement might be associated with ADH, with ADH having a slight predilection for non-mass enhancement (Lourenco et al. 2014; Heller et al. 2013, 2014).

Management Currently, open surgery remains the recommended option to rule out concomitant malignant lesions when there is a histologic diagnosis of ADH (Rageth et al. 2016). This is mainly due to the still high underestimation rate for ADH, ranging from 9% to 65% for all needle biopsies, either CNB or VAB (Jackman et al.

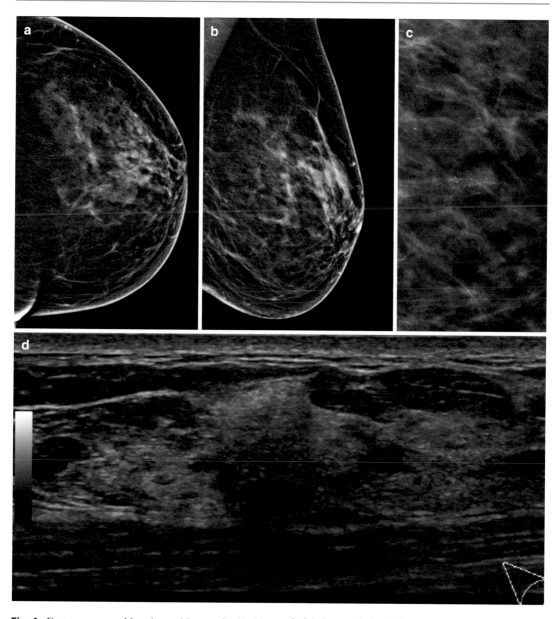

Fig. 1 Forty-one-year-old patient without a family history of breast cancer. (**a–c**) Screening mammography of the left breast: (**a**) craniocaudal projection, (**b**) mediolateral-oblique projection, and (**c**) magnification view. (**a, b**) There are scattered areas of fibroglandular density (ACR BI-RADS density class *b*) demonstrating fine linear and fine pleomorphic microcalcification (red circle) better depicted in (**c**) the magnification view (BI-RADS 4b). (**d**) B-mode ultrasound shows no correlate to the microcalcifications seen in the mammogram. Therefore, a vacuum-assisted biopsy under stereotactic guidance was performed. Final histopathology: areas of usual ductal hyperplasia (DIN1A) and atypical ductal hyperplasia (DIN1B)

2002; Houssami et al. 2007; AGO 2016). Although the rate is lower for VAB, studies demonstrated underestimation rates of up to 17% even when no residual microcalcifications are present (Kohr et al. 2010; Forgeard et al. 2008; McGhan et al. 2012; Villa et al. 2011). Several studies have investigated the possible histopathologic and imaging characteristics that can safely warrant a follow-up and spare open surgery (Hong et al. 2011; Allison et al. 2011; Elsheikh and Silverman 2005; Ancona et al. 2011; Caplain et al. 2014; Linda et al. 2010). In order to suggest follow-up instead of open surgery, several histopathologic characteristics should be considered such as the number of ADH foci related to the number of specimens involved, size of ADH, and micropapillary type. On imaging, especially mammography, factors that should be considered are the lesion type (microcalcifications versus mass), lesion diameter, complete removal of microcalcification clusters or complete removal of the target lesion, type of needle used to perform the biopsy, and age of the patient at the time of diagnosis (Clauser et al. 2016; Ancona et al. 2011; Caplain et al. 2014). The First International Consensus Conference on B3 lesions and the NHS working group stated that in cases of a completely removed unifocal ADH, a careful follow-up is justified. In all other cases, diagnostic surgical excision is mandatory (Table 2) (Rageth et al. 2016).

Table 2 Consensus recommendations for the management of B3 lesions (Modified from Rageth CJ et al. Breast Cancer Res Treat (2016) 159:203–213)

High-risk lesion	Management
Lobular neoplasia (LN)	Open excision or VAB If after VAB, the lesion has been radiologically removed, follow up
Atypical ductal hyperplasia (ADH)	Open excision or VAB. VAB is suggested in unifocal ADH in small lesions If the lesion has been removed completely and only focal ADH with calcifications exists, surveillance could be justified
Flat epithelial atypia (FEA)	Open excision or VAB. If after VAB, the lesion has been radiologically removed, follow up
Papillary lesion (PL)	VAB or open excision Open excision recommended for large, symptomatic, and peripheric papillomas
Phyllodes tumor (PT)	Open excision If diagnosis made by VAB and the lesion has been radiologically removed, follow up
Radial scars (RS)	VAB or open excision If after VAB, the lesion has been radiologically removed, follow up

2.2 Flat Epithelial Atypia

Flat epithelial atypia (FEA) is also known as "columnar cell change with atypia" or "cell hyperplasia with atypia." It is found in 1–2% of benign breast biopsies and is thus fairly rare (Mooney et al. 2016; Said et al. 2015). When diagnosed, it is frequently associated with other high-risk lesions such as ADH, atypical lobular hyperplasia (ALH), and lobular neoplasia (LN). It can co-occur in "in situ" or in invasive breast cancers, typically tubular carcinoma (Schnitt and Vincent-Salomon 2003; Rudin et al. 2017).

Histopathology FEA is a neoplastic alteration characterized by a replacement of native epithelial cells that lack polarity in the terminal-duct lobular unit. The atypical cells may be cuboidal or columnar; bridges and micropapillary formations are usually absent, hence the name "flat." Involved terminal-duct lobular units have acini that are variably distended and that may contain secretory or floccular material with microcalcifications (Lakhani et al. 2012). According to the degree of architectural atypia, i.e., no atypia, atypia, or DCIS, several entities can be identified: columnar cell change, composed of a single layer of columnar cells; columnar cell hyperplasia, made of multiple layers with stratification and apical tufting; and FEA (Schnitt and Vincent-Salomon 2003; Pandey et al. 2007).

Immunoprofile The cells of FEA are strongly and diffusely positive for estrogen receptor and are negative for low-molecular-weight cytokeratins (Rageth et al. 2016; Lakhani et al. 2012; Tavassoli and Devilee 2003).

Prognosis FEA is of great scientific interest as the morphologic spectrum of intraductal proliferations shows a continuum from FEA to ADH and low-grade DCIS. The relative risk of breast cancer is 1–2 times for women with FEA compared with women without FEA, which is substantially lower than that of ADH and ALH. In up to 40% of cases, FEA is eventually upgraded, and usually ADH and DCIS are the most frequent pathologies following surgical excision (Darvishian et al. 2009; Ingegnoli et al. 2010; Senetta et al. 2009; Piubello et al. 2009). The underestimation rate of FEA at both CNB and VAB ranges from 0% to 21% (Rageth et al. 2016).

Imaging Findings FEA is usually detected as fine amorphous or branching microcalcifications with associated marked duct dilatation (Heywang-Köbrunner et al. 2010; Pandey et al. 2007; Senetta et al. 2009; Fraser et al. 1998) (Fig. 2). On ultrasound, the evidence concerning FEA is limited. Occasionally, FEA can appear as a nonspecific mass with or without microcalcifications. Yu et al. investigated possible predictors of underestimation of malignancy after core needle biopsy of FEA or ADH. In their cohort of 128 FEA, they found that masses with calcifications discovered on ultrasound were associated with an underestimation rate of up to 46.2% (Yu et al. 2015). No specific predictive morphologic or kinetic MRI characteristics or imaging features have been found that could reliably exclude malignancy (Crystal et al. 2011; Malhaire et al. 2010; Heller and Moy 2012).

Management Currently, several guidelines recommend that surgical excision for FEA is only needed under specific conditions (Rageth et al. 2016; AGO 2016; National Comprehensive Cancer Center 2017). The Arbeitsgemeinschaft Gynäkologische Onkologie (AGO) recommends surgery if there is radio-pathological discrepancy, if the lesion is visible on imaging and the imaging classification is BI-RADS 4, if the lesion involves more than two terminal-duct lobular units, and if an imaging abnormality remains after VAB (AGO 2016). The First International Consensus Conference on B3 lesions recommended therapeutic excision with VAB (Table 2) (Rageth et al. 2016). For the NHS group, surgical excision should be considered in the presence of architectural atypia at VAE (Pinder et al. 2018).

2.3 Lobular Neoplasia

Lobular neoplasia (LN) is both a risk indicator and a non-obligate precursor for breast cancer. LN is found in 0.5–4% of breast biopsies and occurs in premenopausal women predominantly (Lakhani et al. 2012; Choi et al. 2012). The lesion is multicentric in 85% of cases and bilateral in up to 67% of cases (Liberman et al. 1999).

Histopathology The term LN is used to characterize all atypical epithelial lesions arising from the terminal-duct lobular unit that are characterized by a proliferation of generally small, non-cohesive cells, with or without pagetoid involvement of the terminal ducts (Lakhani et al. 2012). The term was introduced after two studies found that subdividing these findings into LCIS or ALH did not have prognostic significance. The

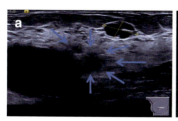
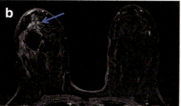
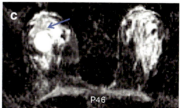

Fig. 2 Forty-three-year-old patient without a family history of breast cancer. Ultrasound of the right breast (**a**). In the retroareolar region, ultrasound shows several simple cysts associated with a hypoechoic area, non-circumscribed with nonparallel orientation and no posterior features. Dynamic multiparametric magnetic resonance imaging (MRI) of the breast: (**b**) dynamic contrast-enhanced subtracted MRI and (**c**) apparent diffusion coefficient (ADC) map. There is a clumped non-mass enhancement with fast wash-in in the early phase and decreased ADC values (<1.2 × 10^{-3} mm^2/s). Final histology: atypical ductal hyperplasia and ductal carcinoma in situ

World Health Organization (WHO) differentiates LCIS and ALH based on the extent of individual lobular unit involvement: LCIS involves more than half of the acini of a terminal-duct lobular unit, while ALH is typically less extended. Several variants of LCIS have been reported: (a) classic LCIS (type A or B); (b) florid LCIS, characterized by marked cell expansion of the terminal-duct lobular unit with accompanying necrosis and calcifications; and (c) pleomorphic LCIS, characterized by marked nuclear pleomorphism. Classic LCIS is the most frequent variant and is considered to have an indolent behavior (Lakhani et al. 2012). Florid LCIS is associated with invasive cancer, commonly lobular cancer, in 40–67% of the cases (Bagaria et al. 2011). Pleomorphic LCIS is considered the most aggressive and has a similar biologic behavior to that of DCIS and therefore should not be considered as a B3 lesion (Rageth et al. 2016; Guo et al. 2017). The WHO more recently proposed the term lobular intraepithelial lesion (LIN), which can be classified as LIN1, -2, and -3, with LIN1 being equivalent to ALH, LIN2 to LCIS, and LIN3 to pleomorphic or extensive LN variants with or without necrosis. Current international recommendations endorse the use of classical LN as B3 and pleomorphic LCIS as B5a (Rageth et al. 2016; Lakhani et al. 2012; Thill et al. 2016). LN may also be associated with a variety of lesions, including sclerosing adenosis, radial scars, papillary lesions, and fibroadenomas, and in some cases may be associated with collagenous spherulosis.

Immunoprofile Classic LN has an immunoprofile similar to that of invasive lobular carcinoma and low-grade DCIS. The majority of classic LNs (up to 90%) are positive for estrogen and progesterone receptors without overexpression of HER2 or p53 protein. Conversely, pleomorphic LCIS is usually negative for ER and positive for HER2 and p53 and Ki67 proliferative index (Lakhani et al. 2012). LN typically lacks E-cadherin expression; hence, the absence of E-cadherin may be useful to differentiate LCIS from DCIS or to classify indeterminate lesions.

As LN can express E-cadherin in rare cases, when a case cannot be definitively classified as LCIS or DCIS, a designation of "carcinoma in situ with mixed ductal and lobular features" should be rendered (Lakhani et al. 2012; Breier et al. 2014; Dabbs et al. 2013).

Prognosis Molecular analysis has demonstrated that LN is a clonal neoplastic proliferation and a precursor for invasive cancer. The relative risk of developing breast cancer for women with LN and women without LN is different for LCIS and ALH, 4–12 times and 4–5 times, respectively. According to several studies, the possibility of LCIS coexisting with DCIS is approximately 21–22%, and the likelihood of LCIS developing into infiltrating ductal or lobular carcinoma is 15% (Clauser et al. 2016; Choi et al. 2012; Guo et al. 2017; Stein et al. 2005). After the diagnosis of LN, the relative risk of developing cancer is 1–2% per year, 15–17% after 15 years, and 35% after 35 years, with relatively equal rates in the ipsi- and contralateral breast (8.7% and 6.7%, respectively) (Rageth et al. 2016; Heller et al. 2014; Choi et al. 2012; Rendi et al. 2012). The risk doubles with a family history of breast cancer (London et al. 1992). Although all types of invasive carcinoma have been observed after a diagnosis of LN, invasive lobular carcinoma or special-type carcinomas are seen with higher frequency than in the general breast cancer population (Page et al. 1985).

Imaging Findings LN has been historically reported as an incidental lesion found on specimens acquired for other reasons (Rageth et al. 2016). It does not show any specific features according to the BI-RADS lexicon (Ferré et al. 2017). LN is frequently mammographically occult and an incidental finding at routine screening mammograms, usually because of microcalcifications which can be seen in up to 84% of the cases (Rendi et al. 2012; Choi et al. 2011) (Fig. 3a, b). Microcalcifications associated with LN are usually amorphous with a grouped distribution (D'Orsi et al. 2013; Clauser et al. 2016;

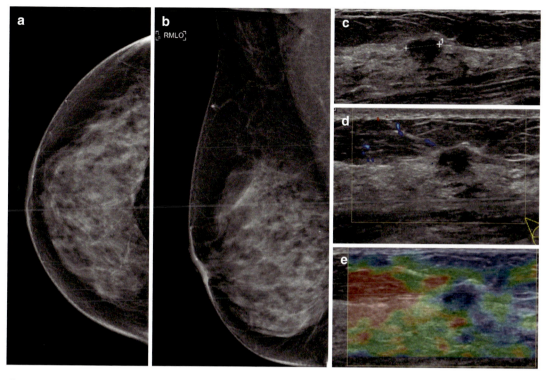

Fig. 3 Forty-nine-year-old woman at her second screening mammography round. (**a**) Craniocaudal and (**b**) mediolateral-oblique projections of the right breast show it to be heterogeneously dense (ACR-BI-RADS density class *c*). No lesions or suspicious microcalcifications are identified (BI-RADS 1). Ultrasound (**c**) B-mode, (**d**) color Doppler, and (**e**) elastography. (**c**) At 12'o clock of the right breast, B-mode ultrasound shows a 6 mm irregular-shaped lesion with non-circumscribed margins, vertical (nonparallel) orientation, and no posterior feature associated. (**d**) Color Doppler demonstrates absent vascularity. (**e**) Elasticity assessment with shear wave elastography shows stiffness of the small mass. The lesion is suspicious (BI-RADS 4c). Final histopathology: classic lobular carcinoma in situ (LCIS)

Cutuli et al. 2015). Less frequently, LN can be seen as mass, architectural distortion, or asymmetry. On ultrasound, LN may appear as an avascular, irregular, hypoechoic mass with posterior shadowing (Choi et al. 2011; Cutuli et al. 2015; Scoggins et al. 2013) (Fig. 3c–e). On contrast-enhanced breast MRI, the evidence is limited for LN, but non-mass enhancement seems to be the most frequent finding (Lourenco et al. 2014; Heller et al. 2014; Sung et al. 2011).

Management The management of patients with LN diagnosed at core needle biopsy remains controversial. Reported rates of an upgrade to cancer on excision vary widely due to variations in study design, ranging from 0% to 50% (Rageth et al. 2016; Lakhani et al. 2012). Current international recommendations suggest open surgical excision in the following cases:

1. If there is another lesion which by itself would warrant excision
2. If there is radio-pathological discordance
3. If there is presence of another B3 lesion
4. If there is a mass lesion on imaging

In addition, excision should be performed for classic LCIS with comedo-necrosis, bulky mass-forming LCIS lesions, and pleomorphic LCIS (Rageth et al. 2016; Lakhani et al. 2012).

Open surgical excision is not necessary if there is a complete concordance between histopathology and imaging, if the imaging finding is classified as BI-RADS 3, or if LN is a focal finding and not associated with calcifications (Rageth et al. 2016; Lakhani et al. 2012; Thill et al. 2016).

The First International Consensus Conference on B3 lesions recommended that a lesion containing a classical LN lesion, which is visible on imaging, should undergo therapeutic VAE (Rageth et al. 2016) (Table 2). For the NHS multidisciplinary group, diagnostic surgery is proposed in case of radiological-pathological discordance or in cases of an upgrade to DCIS or invasive cancer. Otherwise, surveillance is justified.

2.4 Papillary Lesions

Papillary lesions (PLs) constitute less than 10% of benign and less than 1% of malignant breast disease. They are mostly seen in women between 30 and 50 years and rarely in adolescents (Lakhani et al. 2012).

Histopathology PLs are breast lesions growing in the milk ducts. They are characterized by fingerlike fibrovascular cores covered by an epithelial and myoepithelial cell layer (Lakhani et al. 2012). The best-known entities of this heterogeneous group of lesions are papilloma; atypical papilloma; papillomatosis; papillary hyperplasia without atypia; papillary carcinoma, encysted; papillary carcinoma, invasive; micropapillary hyperplasia with atypia (ADH); micropapillary DCIS; and micropapillary invasive carcinoma (Rageth et al. 2016; Lakhani et al. 2012; Thill et al. 2016). The histological distinction between these entities is not always straightforward. Usually, they are divided into two main groups: central (solitary) papillomas that originate in the ducts of the subareolar region, sparing the terminal-duct lobular unit, and peripheral (multiple) papillomas arising from the terminal-duct lobular unit and extending into the ducts (Nakhlis 2018).

Prognosis For women with PLs, the risk of developing invasive breast cancer is twofold for central lesions and threefold for peripheral lesions. The risk can increase up to 7.5-fold in cases of papillomas with atypia (Lakhani et al. 2012). The risk of subsequent carcinoma and local recurrence is mostly associated with the coexistence of ADH or DCIS within the breast parenchyma surrounding the PL (Fisher et al. 2005). For PLs without atypia, the upgrade rate to malignancy after surgical excision ranges from 0% to 12% when initially diagnosed at core needle biopsy (Nakhlis 2018; Nakhlis et al. 2015), while no upgrade has been reported for when initially diagnosed at VAB (Wyss et al. 2014; Youk et al. 2012; Mosier et al. 2013). For PLs with atypia, the upgrade rate ranges from 21% to 72% when initially diagnosed at core needle biopsy and 0% to 28% when initially diagnosed at VAB (Yamaguchi et al. 2015; Rizzo et al. 2012).

Imaging Findings PLs can clinically present as palpable masses near the nipple or as serous, colored, or hemorrhagic nipple discharge in 20–50% of cases (Hussain et al. 2006). Papillomas can cause bloody nipple discharge as a result of the rotation of its stalk or as a result of irritation of the papilloma duct (Lakhani et al. 2012). Frequently, PLs can be asymptomatic and detected randomly at routine breast cancer screening. Mammography has a low diagnostic sensitivity and specificity for PLs, with reported positive findings in less than 50% of patients (Hirose et al. 2007). Mammographic findings are nonspecific when visible: areas of increased density, a dilated duct, or a solitary mass with benign or malignant features. Therefore, the main role of mammography is to depict the presence of malignant calcifications that may accompany a papillary malignant lesion (Wei 2016). Galactography, which directly shows the discharging duct cannulated and opacified through contrast medium injection, has long been the gold standard for assessing nipple discharge (Van Zee et al. 1998; Tabár et al. 1983). However, its use has decreased due to the often aspecific findings, technical difficulties to cannulate the duct especially in patients with intermittent discharge or nipple retraction, low level of tolerance for patients, and issues related to radiation (Hou et al. 2001;

Dawes et al. 1998). Breast ultrasound is of great value in the diagnosis of PLs, combining conventional ultrasound, Doppler ultrasound, and elastography (Ciurea et al. 2015). US may demonstrate a solid round mass or masses with well-defined borders, an intracystic mass, or a hypoechoic, well-defined mass in a dilated duct (Fig. 4a). The fibrovascular stalk of a PL can further be assessed at Color Doppler and power Doppler (Fig. 4b). Elastography can show increased stiffness of the area within the duct and can help in differential diagnosis, increasing the degree of suspicion for malignancy (Ballesio et al. 2007). MRI is useful when a papillary lesion is suspected based on other imaging techniques because of its ability to demonstrate ductal relation of the lesions and also its superior accuracy in diagnosing the extension of malignant lesions. MRI can be performed using a standard protocol including both unenhanced and contrast-enhanced sequences (Clauser et al. 2016).

Moreover, with 3D MRI ductography, dilated ducts are imaged as tubular structures with high signal intensity, and abnormalities are seen as a signal defect (Hirose et al. 2007). On contrast-enhanced sequences, PLs often present as strongly enhancing, small, and well-defined mass lesions (Fig. 4c). In a retrospective study of 53 patients with unilateral nipple discharge, Manganaro et al. (2015) demonstrated that contrast-enhanced MRI is a valid tool to detect ductal pathologies in patients presenting with bloody or serous-bloody discharge with a higher sensitivity and specificity compared to galactography.

Management The management of PLs relies on many different factors, such as the time of diagnosis, lesion type, and presence of atypia, i.e., the presence or absence of atypia and coexistence of other high-risk lesions such as ADH or even con-

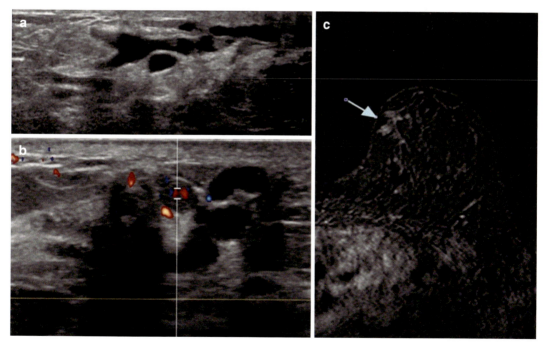

Fig. 4 Fifty-five-year-old patient with a bloody nipple discharge of the left breast. (**a**) B-mode ultrasound shows dilated ducts filled with fluid and small (<6 mm) solid nodules at 7 o'clock of the left breast. (**b**) Power Doppler demonstrates a vascular stalk within one of these solid nodules. Ultrasound findings are suggestive of intraductal lesions with low suspicion of malignancy (BI-RADS 4a). (**c**) Dynamic contrast-enhanced subtracted MRI, axial plane. The oval-shaped masses are visible in the post-contrast images as enhancing masses (BI-RADS 4). Final histopathology: intraductal papillomas and papillomatosis

comitant invasive or ductal in situ cancer. When PL with atypia is diagnosed by core needle biopsy, excision is generally recommended to rule out a concurrent malignant neoplasm (Wen and Cheng 2013; Khan et al. 2017). For PL without atypia, recommendations for excision versus observation are variable (Wen and Cheng 2013; Khan et al. 2017). Glenn et al. (2015) investigated the role of the size of the papilloma as an indicator for the need of surgery. They found that there is no size threshold below which a papilloma of the breast can be safely watched or ignored without risking a missed diagnosis of atypia or cancer. The First International Conference on B3 lesions recommended that in the case of a papillary lesion visible on imaging, a therapeutic excision with VAB should be performed. Thereafter, surveillance is justified (Table 2). The suggested pathway for management of patients with papillary lesions proposed by the NHS multidisciplinary group offers surgical excision after the first diagnosis.

2.5 Phyllodes Tumor

Phyllodes tumors (PTs) account for less than 1% of all primary tumors of the breast (Lakhani et al. 2012; Buchanan 1995). Commonly, they occur in women aged 40–51 years, although in Asian countries the average age of occurrence is about 25–30 years (Chua et al. 1988). Malignant PTs develop on average 2–5 years later than benign PTs and are usually more frequent among Hispanics, especially those born in Central and South America. In men, isolated cases of PT have been found (Lakhani et al. 2012).

Histopathology PTs are considered part of fibro-epithelial neoplasms, together with fibroadenomas and hamartomas. PTs are thought to derive from the intralobular or peri-ductal stroma. Although the evidence for the direct evolution of PT from fibroadenomas is limited (Noguchi et al. 1995), both PT and fibroadenomas possess molecular similarities in addition to bearing a

striking morphological resemblance in some cases (Tan et al. 2016). PTs are classified into benign, borderline, malignant, and peri-ductal stromal tumors based on the combination of histological features, i.e., the degree of stromal cellularity and atypia, stromal overgrowth, mitotic count, and nature of their tumor borders/margins (Lakhani et al. 2012). Benign and borderline PTs are considered as high-risk lesions, categorized as B3, and account for 63–78% and 11–30% of diagnosed PTs, respectively (Rageth et al. 2016). Benign PTs usually present higher stromal cellularity than fibroadenomas, and necrosis may be seen in large tumors (Tan et al. 2005). Benign lipomatous, cartilaginous, and osseous metaplasias have been reported in benign PTs. Benign PTs have well-circumscribed margins with protrusive expansions, which may be left behind after surgical removal and serve as a source of local recurrence (Buchanan 1995; Duman et al. 2016). Malignant PTs show marked nuclear pleomorphism of stromal cells, stromal overgrowth, increased diffuse stromal cellularity, and infiltrative borders. Borderline PTs show a combination of histological characteristics found in malignant and benign PTs (Tan et al. 2012, 2016; Duman et al. 2016).

PTs have the potential for local recurrence but usually do not metastasize (Tan et al. 2012). Any PT that has recognizable epithelial elements may harbor DCIS, LN, or their invasive counterparts, although this is an uncommon finding (Lakhani et al. 2012).

Prognosis Most PTs behave in a benign fashion; the rate of potential metastases is about 2% or less. Local recurrences can occur in all PTs at an overall rate of 21%, ranging from 10% to 17%, 14% to 25%, and 23% to 30% for benign, borderline, and malignant PTs, respectively (Tan et al. 2012). Excision margins have been reported to be the most reliable predictor for local recurrence, while stromal overgrowth, classification grade, and necrosis are less consistent predictors (Tan et al. 2016; Barrio et al. 2007).

Imaging Findings Usually, patients are symptomatic, showing a unilateral, firm, painless breast mass not attached to the skin. Large PTs may stretch the skin, and distention of superficial veins may be seen (Lakhani et al. 2012). Due to screening programs, very large lesions (>10 cm) are rare nowadays and the average size of PTs at diagnosis ranges from 2 to 5 cm (Tan et al. 2016). Mammographic and ultrasound imaging findings reveal overlapping features with benign fibroadenomas. On mammography, PTs usually have an oval shape, high density, irregular margins, and larger size compared to fibroadenomas (Plaza et al. 2015). Due to their rapid growth, calcifications are rare. However, cases of coarse intratumoral calcifications have been reported (Jorge Blanco et al. 1999). The fat compound of PTs can be seen as a lucent halo of the margins, and digital breast tomosynthesis is of added value in these cases to better discriminate the solid homogeneous dense appearance of the PT (Freer et al. 2014). On ultrasound, PTs can show both well-defined and ill-defined (i.e., microlobulated) margins (Plaza et al. 2015). Usually, PTs are heterogeneous masses with foci of degeneration and necrosis, posterior acoustic enhancement, and internal vessels (Yilmaz et al. 2002) (Fig. 5). On MRI, PTs do not show differences in signal intensity/time or in kinetic assessment compared with fibroadenomas. Occasionally, suspicious enhancement can be seen in up to 18% of PTs (Duman et al. 2016; Boetes et al. 1997; Kuhl et al. 1999).

Management Available data suggest that the most common management for all PT subtypes is open surgical excision (Rageth et al. 2016; Youk et al. 2015; Ouyang et al. 2016; Choi and Koo 2012; Youn et al. 2013) (Table 2). In PTs diagnosed by CNB, mean underestimation rates are documented at around 20%, whereas in PTs diagnosed by VAB, an underestimation happens in up to 8.7% of cases (Youk et al. 2015). Based on these evidences, the First International Conference on B3 lesions recommended that a PT lesion visible on imaging should undergo open surgical excision with clear margins. Similar recommendations are proposed by the NHS group. Only in cases of benign PT, following VAB, surveillance is justified.

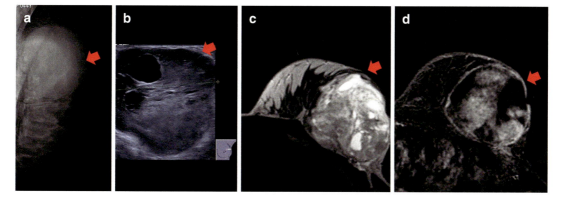

Fig. 5 A 28-year-old patient with a palpable lump in the left breast that has subjectively grown in size over the past 2 months. Digital mammography (**a**) mediolateral-oblique projections of the left side. The breast is extremely dense (ACR-BI-RADS density class *d*). In the upper-outer quadrant of the left breast, an oval mass with obscured margins can be discerned. No suspicious microcalcifications within the mass or in the breast are seen, and ultrasound was performed for further assessment. (**b**) B-mode ultrasound shows at 10/11 o'clock of the left side a round oval shaped, microlobulated complex mass and without any posterior features associated. (**c**, **d**) Magnetic resonance imaging (MRI) of the left breast: (**c**) T2-weighted and (**d**) dynamic contrast-enhanced (DCE) MRI. The lesion shows a round-shaped mass, with circumscribed margins and rim enhancement. Final histopathology: malignant phyllodes tumor, high grade

2.6 Radial Scar and Complex Sclerosing Lesion

Radial scar (RS) is a breast lesion that may mimic an invasive carcinoma because of its stellate configuration. RS is a small (<1 cm) focus, while "complex sclerosing lesion" (CSL) refers to a lesion larger than 1 cm that is accompanied by more complex features (Rageth et al. 2016; Lakhani et al. 2012; Chou et al. 2018). The frequency of RSs and CSLs ranges from 14% to 28%. RS may be multiple and bilateral. RS is uncommon in women younger than 30 years and is seen most frequently in women 30–60 years old (Cohen and Newell 2017).

Histopathology RS and CSL are characterized by a central fibroelastic core with radiating spokes of ducts and lobules. At the lesion periphery, there are a multitude of benign changes, such as cysts, UDH, and sclerosing adenosis. The variable proportion of these additional entities contributes to the imaging features of RS (Lakhani et al. 2012; Cohen and Newell 2017).

Prognosis There is no firm evidence that these lesions may be premalignant (Rageth et al. 2016; Lakhani et al. 2012; Cohen and Newell 2017). RS and CSL are proliferative lesions that frequently can be associated with other high-risk lesions and proliferative lesions, such as atypia that may itself contribute to the high frequency of associated cancers and to the upgrade rate to malignancy at excision (Chai and Brown 2009). Therefore, the prognosis of RS and CSL depends on the presence of associated atypia (Linda et al. 2010; Cohen and Newell 2017; Douglas-Jones et al. 2007). In RS and CSL without atypia, there is up to 3.0% relative risk of developing breast cancer (Rageth et al. 2016; Linda et al. 2010; Douglas-Jones et al. 2007). In RS and CSL with atypia, the relative risk ranges from 2.8% to 6.7% particularly in patients over 50 years of age (Berg et al. 2008; Sanders et al. 2006; Jacobs et al. 1999). Underestimation rates for pure RS and CSL vary from 1% to 28% following core needle biopsy and 8% following VAB (Rageth et al. 2016; Lakhani et al. 2012).

Imaging Findings On mammography, RS and CSL mostly appear as a stellate lesion mimicking invasive carcinoma. Different mammographic features have been suggested by Tabar et al. for the diagnosis of RS and CSL (Teaching Atlas of Mammography 2018). Usually, RS presents as radiolucent linear structures paralleling radiopaque spicules, hence the nomenclature "black stars" for RS in contradistinction to the "white stars" of breast cancers. Further, the distortion varies in different projections; no skin thickening/retraction or palpable lump is present over the lesion (Cohen and Newell 2017; Teaching Atlas of Mammography 2018) (Fig. 6a, b). Calcifications are common in RS, but their morphologic features are often nonspecific; therefore, they may be the only imaging finding prompting a biopsy in some cases (Rageth et al. 2016; AGO 2016). Digital breast tomosynthesis has shown great potential for differentiating breast lesions from normal overlapping tissue, leading to an improved detection in breast cancer (Freer et al. 2014). Partyka et al. (2014) investigated its role for assessing architectural distortion compared with digital mammography. They reviewed 26 cases of architectural distortion detected on breast tomosynthesis only and found that it provided better visualization and identification of architectural distortion than digital mammography with an increased cancer detection rate (Fig. 6c, d). The sonographic appearance of RS is variable, ranging from no clear correlate to a hypoechoic, irregular mass with indistinct margins or as a focal area of shadowing with no associated mass (Cohen and Newell 2017; Shetty 2002). In some cases, RS may show inherent stiffness at elastography; however, at present there is no ultrasound imaging finding that appears to be reliable for differentiating RS from malignant lesions. RS has a broadly variable MRI appearance ranging from being invisible to presenting as an enhancing, irregular, malignant-appearing mass. The negative predictive value for non-enhancing RS across studies is high, ranging from 97% to 100% (Linda et al. 2010; Pediconi et al. 2005). With respect to the management of enhancing lesions diagnosed as RS at MRI-guided biopsy, recent studies have

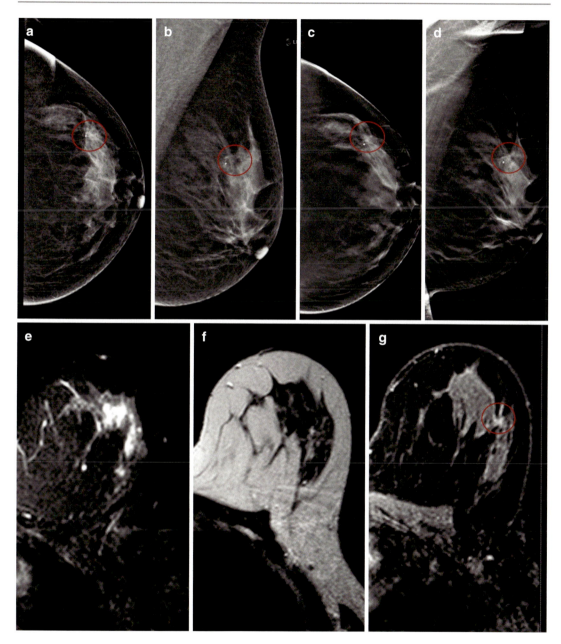

Fig. 6 A 55-year-old patient with left-breast pain. Digital mammography: (**a**) craniocaudal and (**b**) mediolateral-oblique projections of the left side and digital breast tomosynthesis; (**c**) craniocaudal and (**d**) mediolateral-oblique projections of the same breast. The breasts are characterized by scattered areas of fibroglandular tissue (ACR-BI-RADS density class *b*). In the upper-outer quadrant of the left breast (**a–d**), an architectural distortion can be seen without an associated mass or suspicious microcalcification. An oval mass with obscured margins is visible. No suspicious microcalcifications within the mass or in the breast are seen. B-mode ultrasound did not demonstrate any lesion (not shown). (**e–g**) Magnetic resonance imaging (MRI). (**e**) Short tau inversion recovery (STIR) axial image, (**f**) T2-weighted image, and (**g**) DCE-MRI (delayed phase). Only on the delayed DCE-MRI a subtle uptake of contrast enhancement can be seen in the upper-outer quadrant of the left breast as a 5 mm focal area of non-mass enhancement with slow and persistent kinetics (BI-RADS 4a). Final histopathology: sclerosing ductal hyperplasia compatible with radial scar

shown a high upgrade rate to malignancy, ranging from 20% to 23% (Lourenco et al. 2014; Heller and Moy 2012). Therefore, the current consensus in cases of enhancing RS, visible at MRI only, is excision (Fig. 6e–g).

Management The management of RS diagnosed at CNB is controversial. Different studies demonstrated that breast cancer is often present in the periphery of the RS and CSL and this eccentric location may be conceivably the reason of sampling errors (Alvarado-Cabrero and Tavassoli 2000; López-Medina et al. 2006). Currently, the WHO 2012 guidelines recommend surveillance if the imaging findings have been completely excised at VAB and no atypia is found in the histological examination. A similar approach is recommended by the NHS group. However, in case of RS and CSL with atypia on histology following either core needle biopsy or VAB, open surgical excision is mandatory (Rageth et al. 2016; Pinder et al. 2018; Lakhani et al. 2012; AGO 2016) (Table 2).

3 Chemoprevention in High-Risk Lesions

Breast cancer chemoprevention with tamoxifen has been recommended by the National Comprehensive Cancer Network since relevant data was published in 2005 demonstrating up to 80% risk reduction of invasive breast cancer in patients with ADH, LCIS, ALH, or FEA with a 5-year breast cancer risk assessment of 1.7% and a life expectancy of 10 years (Fisher et al. 2005). Thereafter, other chemopreventive agents, i.e., raloxifene, exemestane, and anastrozole, have been validated as alternative drugs with similar efficacy to tamoxifen in postmenopausal women at high risk for breast cancer (Goss et al. 2011; Cuzick et al. 2014). However, only a small minority of high-risk women accept the use of chemopreventive agents, most likely due to concerns about thromboembolism as a side effect of the treatment and lack of knowledge and awareness (Clauser et al. 2016).

4 Conclusion

Based on the current evidence, the most recent international guidelines (Rageth et al. 2016; Pinder et al. 2018) on high-risk breast lesion (B3), i.e., lesions of uncertain malignant potential, recommend VAE for the majority, opting for a more conservative approach and sparing open surgery if this can be avoided (Table 2). Thereafter, annual screening mammography is justified, whereas screening MRI in these patients is still controversially seen, as it has not yet been demonstrated to improve clinical outcomes.

The more conservative approach has been adopted because of the continued concerns regarding potential harms associated with unnecessary surgeries in case of suspicious imaging findings. Prior to these guidelines, surgical excision has been typically recommended for these lesions because of the low but present potential for upgrade to malignancy. However, this often leads to overtreatment, with unnecessary surgery for high-risk lesions that are not associated with malignancy.

All guidelines stress the importance of the management of high-risk lesions in a multidisciplinary team approach. The multidisciplinary team has to develop a personalized strategy related to the individual risk of developing cancer in each patient to limit surgery to only those patients who need it. Overtreatment in women with B3 lesions at low risk should be avoided.FundingFunding was provided in part by the 2020 Research and Innovation Framework Programme PHC-11-2015 Nr. 667211-2 and under grant agreement Nr. 688188.

References

AGO (2016) Guidelines of the AGO breast committee: lesions of uncertain malignant potential (B3) (ADH, LIN, FEA, Papilloma, Radial Scar). http://www.ago-onlinede/fileadmin/downloads/leitlinien/mamma/Maerz2016/en/2016E%2006_Lesions%20of%20Uncertain%20Malignant%20Potential%20%28B3%29pdf

Allison KH, Eby PR, Kohr J et al (2011) Atypical ductal hyperplasia on vacuum-assisted breast biopsy: suspicion for ductal carcinoma in situ can stratify patients at high risk for upgrade. Hum Pathol 42:41–50. https://doi.org/10.1016/j.humpath.2010.06.011

Allison KH, Abraham LA, Weaver DL et al (2015) Trends in breast tissue sampling and pathology diagnoses among women undergoing mammography in the U.S.: a report from the Breast Cancer Surveillance Consortium. Cancer 121:1369–1378. https://doi.org/10.1002/cncr.29199

Alonso-Bartolomé P, Vega-Bolívar A, Torres-Tabanera M et al (2004) Sonographically guided 11-G directional vacuum-assisted breast biopsy as an alternative to surgical excision: utility and cost study in probably benign lesions. Acta Radiol 45:390–396

Alvarado-Cabrero I, Tavassoli FA (2000) Neoplastic and malignant lesions involving or arising in a radial scar: a clinicopathologic analysis of 17 cases. Breast J 6:96–102

Ancona A, Capodieci M, Galiano A et al (2011) Vacuum-assisted biopsy diagnosis of atypical ductal hyperplasia and patient management. Radiol Med 116:276–291. https://doi.org/10.1007/s11547-011-0626-9

Bagaria SP, Shamonki J, Kinnaird M et al (2011) The florid subtype of lobular carcinoma in situ: marker or precursor for invasive lobular carcinoma? Ann Surg Oncol 18:1845–1851. https://doi.org/10.1245/s10434-011-1563-0

Bahl M, Barzilay R, Yedidia AB et al (2017) High-risk breast lesions: a machine learning model to predict pathologic upgrade and reduce unnecessary surgical excision. Radiology 2017:170549. https://doi.org/10.1148/radiol.2017170549

Ballesio L, Maggi C, Savelli S et al (2007) Adjunctive diagnostic value of ultrasonography evaluation in patients with suspected ductal breast disease. Radiol Med 112:354–365. https://doi.org/10.1007/s11547-007-0146-4

Barrio AV, Clark BD, Goldberg JI et al (2007) Clinicopathologic features and long-term outcomes of 293 phyllodes tumors of the breast. Ann Surg Oncol 14:2961–2970. https://doi.org/10.1245/s10434-007-9439-z

Berg WA, Blume JD, Cormack JB et al (2008) Combined screening with ultrasound and mammography vs mammography alone in women at elevated risk of breast cancer. JAMA 299:2151–2163. https://doi.org/10.1001/jama.299.18.2151

Boetes C, Strijk SP, Holland R et al (1997) False-negative MR imaging of malignant breast tumors. Eur Radiol 7:1231–1234. https://doi.org/10.1007/s003300050281

Breier G, Grosser M, Rezaei M (2014) Endothelial cadherins in cancer. Cell Tissue Res 355:523–527. https://doi.org/10.1007/s00441-014-1851-7

Buchanan EB (1995) Cystosarcoma phyllodes and its surgical management. Am Surg 61:350–355

Buckley E, Sullivan T, Farshid G et al (2015) Risk profile of breast cancer following atypical hyperplasia detected through organized screening. Breast 24:208–212. https://doi.org/10.1016/j.breast.2015.01.006

Caplain A, Drouet Y, Peyron M et al (2014) Management of patients diagnosed with atypical ductal hyperplasia by vacuum-assisted core biopsy: a prospective assessment of the guidelines used at our institution. Am J Surg 208:260–267. https://doi.org/10.1016/j.amjsurg.2013.10.029

Chai H, Brown RE (2009) Field effect in cancer-an update. Ann Clin Lab Sci 39:331–337

Choi J, Koo JS (2012) Comparative study of histological features between core needle biopsy and surgical excision in phyllodes tumor. Pathol Int 62:120–126. https://doi.org/10.1111/j.1440-1827.2011.02761.x

Choi BB, Kim SH, Park CS et al (2011) Radiologic findings of lobular carcinoma in situ: mammography and ultrasonography. J Clin Ultrasound 39:59–63. https://doi.org/10.1002/jcu.20772

Choi BB, Kim SH, Shu KS (2012) Lobular lesions of the breast: imaging findings of lobular neoplasia and invasive lobular carcinoma. J Reprod Med 57:26–34

Chou WYY, Veis DJ, Aft R (2018) Radial scar on image-guided breast biopsy: is surgical excision necessary? Breast Cancer Res Treat. https://doi.org/10.1007/s10549-018-4741-y

Chua CL, Thomas A, Ng BK (1988) Cystosarcoma phyllodes—Asian variations. Aust N Z J Surg 58:301–305

Ciurea A, Calin A, Ciortea C, Dudea SM (2015) Ultrasound in the diagnosis of papillary breast lesions. Med Ultrason 17:392–397

Clauser P, Marino MA, Baltzer PAT et al (2016) Management of atypical lobular hyperplasia, atypical ductal hyperplasia, and lobular carcinoma in situ. Expert Rev Anticancer Ther 16:335–346. https://doi.org/10.1586/14737140.2016.1143362

Cohen MA, Newell MS (2017) Radial scars of the breast encountered at core biopsy: review of histologic, imaging, and management considerations. AJR Am J Roentgenol 209:1168–1177. https://doi.org/10.2214/AJR.17.18156

Collins LC, Baer HJ, Tamimi RM et al (2007) Magnitude and laterality of breast cancer risk according to histologic type of atypical hyperplasia: results from the Nurses' Health Study. Cancer 109:180–187. https://doi.org/10.1002/cncr.22408

Collins LC, Aroner SA, Connolly JL et al (2016) Breast cancer risk by extent and type of atypical hyperplasia: an update from the Nurses' Health Studies. Cancer 122:515–520. https://doi.org/10.1002/cncr.29775

Crystal P, Sadaf A, Bukhanov K et al (2011) High-risk lesions diagnosed at MRI-guided vacuum-assisted breast biopsy: can underestimation be predicted? Eur Radiol 21:582–589. https://doi.org/10.1007/s00330-010-1949-6

Cutuli B, De Lafontan B, Kirova Y et al (2015) Lobular carcinoma in situ (LCIS) of the breast: is long-term outcome similar to ductal carcinoma in situ (DCIS)? Analysis of 200 cases. Radiat Oncol 10:110. https://doi.org/10.1186/s13014-015-0379-7

Cuzick J, Sestak I, Forbes JF et al (2014) Anastrozole for prevention of breast cancer in high-risk postmenopausal women (IBIS-II): an international, double-blind, randomised placebo-controlled trial.

Lancet 383:1041–1048. https://doi.org/10.1016/S0140-6736(13)62292-8

D'Orsi CJ, Sickles EA, Mendelson EB, Morris EA et al (2013) ACR BI-RADS® Atlas, Breast Imaging Reporting and Data System. American College of Radiology, Reston, VA

Dabbs DJ, Schnitt SJ, Geyer FC et al (2013) Lobular neoplasia of the breast revisited with emphasis on the role of E-cadherin immunohistochemistry. Am J Surg Pathol 37:e1–e11. https://doi.org/10.1097/PAS.0b013e3182918a2b

Darvishian F, Singh B, Simsir A et al (2009) Atypia on breast core needle biopsies: reproducibility and significance. Ann Clin Lab Sci 39:270–276

Dawes LG, Bowen C, Venta LA, Morrow M (1998) Ductography for nipple discharge: no replacement for ductal excision. Surgery 124:685–691. https://doi.org/10.1067/msy.1998.91362

Douglas-Jones AG, Denson JL, Cox AC et al (2007) Radial scar lesions of the breast diagnosed by needle core biopsy: analysis of cases containing occult malignancy. J Clin Pathol 60:295–298. https://doi.org/10.1136/jcp.2006.037069

Duman L, Gezer NS, Balcı P et al (2016) Differentiation between phyllodes tumors and fibroadenomas based on mammographic sonographic and MRI features. Breast Care (Basel) 11:123–127. https://doi.org/10.1159/000444377

Eby PR, Ochsner JE, DeMartini WB et al (2009) Frequency and upgrade rates of atypical ductal hyperplasia diagnosed at stereotactic vacuum-assisted breast biopsy: 9-versus 11-gauge. AJR Am J Roentgenol 192:229–234. https://doi.org/10.2214/AJR.08.1342

Elsheikh TM, Silverman JF (2005) Follow-up surgical excision is indicated when breast core needle biopsies show atypical lobular hyperplasia or lobular carcinoma in situ: a correlative study of 33 patients with review of the literature. Am J Surg Pathol 29:534–543

Ferré R, Omeroglu A, Mesurolle B (2017) Sonographic appearance of lesions diagnosed as lobular neoplasia at sonographically guided biopsies. AJR Am J Roentgenol 208:669–675. https://doi.org/10.2214/AJR.15.15056

Fisher ER, Costantino J, Fisher B et al (1996) Pathologic findings from the National Surgical Adjuvant Breast Project (NSABP) Protocol B-17. Five-year observations concerning lobular carcinoma in situ. Cancer 78:1403–1416. https://doi.org/10.1002/(SICI)1097-0142(19961001)78:7<1403::AID-CNCR6>3.0.CO;2-L

Fisher B, Costantino JP, Wickerham DL et al (2005) Tamoxifen for the prevention of breast cancer: current status of the National Surgical Adjuvant Breast and Bowel Project P-1 study. J Natl Cancer Inst 97:1652–1662. https://doi.org/10.1093/jnci/dji372

Forgeard C, Benchaib M, Guerin N et al (2008) Is surgical biopsy mandatory in case of atypical ductal hyperplasia on 11-gauge core needle biopsy? A retrospective study of 300 patients. Am J Surg 196:339–345. https://doi.org/10.1016/j.amjsurg.2007.07.038

Foster MC, Helvie MA, Gregory NE et al (2004) Lobular carcinoma in situ or atypical lobular hyperplasia at core-needle biopsy: is excisional biopsy necessary? Radiology 231:813–819. https://doi.org/10.1148/radiol.2313030874

Fraser JL, Raza S, Chorny K et al (1998) Columnar alteration with prominent apical snouts and secretions: a spectrum of changes frequently present in breast biopsies performed for microcalcifications. Am J Surg Pathol 22:1521–1527

Freer PE, Wang JL, Rafferty EA (2014) Digital breast tomosynthesis in the analysis of fat-containing lesions. Radiographics 34:343–358. https://doi.org/10.1148/rg.342135082

Galimberti V, Monti S, Mastropasqua MG (2013) DCIS and LCIS are confusing and outdated terms. They should be abandoned in favor of ductal intraepithelial neoplasia (DIN) and lobular intraepithelial neoplasia (LIN). Breast 22:431–435. https://doi.org/10.1016/j.breast.2013.04.010

Glenn ME, Throckmorton AD, Thomison JB, Bienkowski RS (2015) Papillomas of the breast 15 mm or smaller: 4-year experience in a community-based dedicated breast imaging clinic. Ann Surg Oncol 22:1133–1139. https://doi.org/10.1245/s10434-014-4128-1

Goss PE, Ingle JN, Alés-Martínez JE et al (2011) Exemestane for breast-cancer prevention in postmenopausal women. N Engl J Med 364:2381–2391. https://doi.org/10.1056/NEJMoa1103507

Graf O, Helbich TH, Fuchsjaeger MH et al (2004) Follow-up of palpable circumscribed noncalcified solid breast masses at mammography and US: can biopsy be averted? Radiology 233:850–856. https://doi.org/10.1148/radiol.2333031845

Graf O, Helbich TH, Hopf G et al (2007) Probably benign breast masses at US: is follow-up an acceptable alternative to biopsy? Radiology 244:87–93. https://doi.org/10.1148/radiol.2441060258

Gruber R, Jaromi S, Rudas M et al (2013) Histologic work-up of non-palpable breast lesions classified as probably benign at initial mammography and/or ultrasound (BI-RADS category 3). Eur J Radiol 82:398–403. https://doi.org/10.1016/j.ejrad.2012.02.004

Guo T, Wang Y, Shapiro N, Fineberg S (2017) Pleomorphic lobular carcinoma in situ diagnosed by breast core biopsy: clinicopathologic features and correlation with subsequent excision. Clin Breast Cancer. https://doi.org/10.1016/j.clbc.2017.10.004

Hartmann LC, Radisky DC, Frost MH et al (2014) Understanding the premalignant potential of atypical hyperplasia through its natural history: a longitudinal cohort study. Cancer Prev Res (Phila) 7:211–217. https://doi.org/10.1158/1940-6207.CAPR-13-0222

Hartmann LC, Degnim AC, Santen RJ et al (2015) Atypical hyperplasia of the breast—risk assessment and management options. N Engl J Med 372:78–89. https://doi.org/10.1056/NEJMsr1407164

Heller SL, Moy L (2012) Imaging features and management of high-risk lesions on contrast-enhanced dynamic breast MRI. AJR Am J Roentgenol 198:249–255. https://doi.org/10.2214/AJR.11.7610

Heller SL, Hernandez O, Moy L (2013) Radiologic-pathologic correlation at breast MR imaging: what is the appropriate management for high-risk lesions? Magn Reson Imaging Clin N Am 21:583–599. https://doi.org/10.1016/j.mric.2013.03.001

Heller SL, Elias K, Gupta A et al (2014) Outcome of high-risk lesions at MRI-guided 9-gauge vacuum-assisted breast biopsy. AJR Am J Roentgenol 202:237–245. https://doi.org/10.2214/AJR.13.10600

Heywang-Köbrunner SH, Nährig J, Hacker A et al (2010) B3 lesions: radiological assessment and multidisciplinary aspects. Breast Care (Basel) 5:209–217. https://doi.org/10.1159/000319326

Hirose M, Nobusawa H, Gokan T (2007) MR ductography: comparison with conventional ductography as a diagnostic method in patients with nipple discharge. Radiographics 27(Suppl 1):S183–S196. https://doi.org/10.1148/rg.27si075501

Hoffmann O, Stamatis GA, Bittner A-K et al (2016) B3-lesions of the breast and cancer risk - an analysis of mammography screening patients. Mol Clin Oncol 4:705–708. https://doi.org/10.3892/mco.2016.790

Hong Z-J, Chu C-H, Fan H-L et al (2011) Factors predictive of breast cancer in open biopsy in cases with atypical ductal hyperplasia diagnosed by ultrasound-guided core needle biopsy. Eur J Surg Oncol 37:758–764. https://doi.org/10.1016/j.ejso.2011.06.014

Hou MF, Huang TJ, Liu GC (2001) The diagnostic value of galactography in patients with nipple discharge. Clin Imaging 25:75–81

Houssami N, Ciatto S, Ellis I, Ambrogetti D (2007) Underestimation of malignancy of breast core-needle biopsy: concepts and precise overall and category-specific estimates. Cancer 109:487–495. https://doi.org/10.1002/cncr.22435

Hussain AN, Policarpio C, Vincent MT (2006) Evaluating nipple discharge. Obstet Gynecol Surv 61:278–283. https://doi.org/10.1097/01.ogx.0000210242.44171.f6

Ingegnoli A, d'Aloia C, Frattaruolo A et al (2010) Flat epithelial atypia and atypical ductal hyperplasia: carcinoma underestimation rate. Breast J 16:55–59. https://doi.org/10.1111/j.1524-4741.2009.00850.x

Jackman RJ, Birdwell RL, Ikeda DM (2002) Atypical ductal hyperplasia: can some lesions be defined as probably benign after stereotactic 11-gauge vacuum-assisted biopsy, eliminating the recommendation for surgical excision? Radiology 224:548–554. https://doi.org/10.1148/radiol.2242011528

Jacobs TW, Byrne C, Colditz G et al (1999) Radial scars in benign breast-biopsy specimens and the risk of breast cancer. N Engl J Med 340:430–436. https://doi.org/10.1056/NEJM199902113400604

Jorge Blanco A, Vargas Serrano B, Rodríguez Romero R, Martínez Cendejas E (1999) Phyllodes tumors of the breast. Eur Radiol 9:356–360. https://doi.org/10.1007/s003300050680

Khan S, Diaz A, Archer KJ et al (2017) Papillary lesions of the breast: to excise or observe? Breast J. https://doi.org/10.1111/tbj.12907

Kohr JR, Eby PR, Allison KH et al (2010) Risk of upgrade of atypical ductal hyperplasia after stereotactic breast biopsy: effects of number of foci and complete removal of calcifications. Radiology 255:723–730. https://doi.org/10.1148/radiol.09091406

Kuhl CK, Mielcareck P, Klaschik S et al (1999) Dynamic breast MR imaging: are signal intensity time course data useful for differential diagnosis of enhancing lesions? Radiology 211:101–110. https://doi.org/10.1148/radiology.211.1.r99ap38101

Lakhani SREI, Schnitt SJ, Tan PH, van de Vijver MJ (2012) WHO classification of tumours of the breast, 4th edn. International Agency for Research on Cancer, Lyon

Li CI, Malone KE, Saltzman BS, Daling JR (2006) Risk of invasive breast carcinoma among women diagnosed with ductal carcinoma in situ and lobular carcinoma in situ, 1988–2001. Cancer 106:2104–2112. https://doi.org/10.1002/cncr.21864

Liberman L, Sama M, Susnik B et al (1999) Lobular carcinoma in situ at percutaneous breast biopsy: surgical biopsy findings. AJR Am J Roentgenol 173:291–299. https://doi.org/10.2214/ajr.173.2.10430122

Linda A, Zuiani C, Furlan A et al (2010) Radial scars without atypia diagnosed at imaging-guided needle biopsy: how often is associated malignancy found at subsequent surgical excision, and do mammography and sonography predict which lesions are malignant? AJR Am J Roentgenol 194:1146–1151. https://doi.org/10.2214/AJR.09.2326

London SJ, Connolly JL, Schnitt SJ, Colditz GA (1992) A prospective study of benign breast disease and the risk of breast cancer. JAMA 267:941–944

López-Medina A, Cintora E, Múgica B et al (2006) Radial scars diagnosed at stereotactic core-needle biopsy: surgical biopsy findings. Eur Radiol 16:1803–1810. https://doi.org/10.1007/s00330-006-0196-3

Lourenco AP, Khalil H, Sanford M, Donegan L (2014) High-risk lesions at MRI-guided breast biopsy: frequency and rate of underestimation. AJR Am J Roentgenol 203:682–686. https://doi.org/10.2214/AJR.13.11905

Malhaire C, El Khoury C, Thibault F et al (2010) Vacuum-assisted biopsies under MR guidance: results of 72 procedures. Eur Radiol 20:1554–1562. https://doi.org/10.1007/s00330-009-1707-9

Manganaro L, D'Ambrosio I, Gigli S et al (2015) Breast MRI in patients with unilateral bloody and serous-bloody nipple discharge: a comparison with galactography. Biomed Res Int 2015:806368. https://doi.org/10.1155/2015/806368

McGhan LJ, Pockaj BA, Wasif N et al (2012) Atypical ductal hyperplasia on core biopsy: an automatic trigger for excisional biopsy? Ann Surg Oncol 19:3264–3269. https://doi.org/10.1245/s10434-012-2575-0

Mesurolle B, Perez JCH, Azzumea F et al (2014) Atypical ductal hyperplasia diagnosed at sonographically guided core needle biopsy: frequency, final surgical outcome, and factors associated with underestimation. AJR Am J Roentgenol 202:1389–1394. https://doi.org/10.2214/AJR.13.10864

Mooney KL, Bassett LW, Apple SK (2016) Upgrade rates of high-risk breast lesions diagnosed on core needle biopsy: a single-institution experience and literature review. Mod Pathol 29:1471–1484. https://doi.org/10.1038/modpathol.2016.127

Mosier AD, Keylock J, Smith DV (2013) Benign papillomas diagnosed on large-gauge vacuum-assisted core needle biopsy which span <1.5 cm do not need surgical excision. Breast J 19:611–617. https://doi.org/10.1111/tbj.12180

Myers DJ, Bhimji SS (2017) Breast, atypical hyperplasia. In: StatPearls. StatPearls Publishing, Treasure Island, FL

Nakhlis F (2018) How do we approach benign proliferative lesions? Curr Oncol Rep 20:34. https://doi.org/10.1007/s11912-018-0682-1

Nakhlis F, Ahmadiyeh N, Lester S et al (2015) Papilloma on core biopsy: excision vs. observation. Ann Surg Oncol 22:1479–1482. https://doi.org/10.1245/s10434-014-4091-x

National Comprehensive Cancer Center (2017) National Comprehensive Cancer Network Clinical Guidelines, Breast cancer risk reduction, v1. https://www.nccn.org/professionals/physician_gls/PDF/breast_risk.pdf

Noguchi S, Yokouchi H, Aihara T et al (1995) Progression of fibroadenoma to phyllodes tumor demonstrated by clonal analysis. Cancer 76:1779–1785

Nutter EL, Weiss JE, Marotti JD et al (2017) Personal history of proliferative breast disease with atypia and risk of multifocal breast cancer. Cancer. https://doi.org/10.1002/cncr.31202

Ouyang Q, Li S, Tan C et al (2016) Benign phyllodes tumor of the breast diagnosed after ultrasound-guided vacuum-assisted biopsy: surgical excision or wait-and-watch? Ann Surg Oncol 23:1129–1134. https://doi.org/10.1245/s10434-015-4990-5

Page DL, Dupont WD, Rogers LW, Rados MS (1985) Atypical hyperplastic lesions of the female breast. A long-term follow-up study. Cancer 55:2698–2708

Pandey S, Kornstein MJ, Shank W, de Paredes ES (2007) Columnar cell lesions of the breast: mammographic findings with histopathologic correlation. Radiographics 27(Suppl 1):S79–S89. https://doi.org/10.1148/rg.27si075515

Partyka L, Lourenco AP, Mainiero MB (2014) Detection of mammographically occult architectural distortion on digital breast tomosynthesis screening: initial clinical experience. AJR Am J Roentgenol 203:216–222. https://doi.org/10.2214/AJR.13.11047

Pediconi F, Occhiato R, Venditti F et al (2005) Radial scars of the breast: contrast-enhanced magnetic resonance mammography appearance. Breast J 11:23–28. https://doi.org/10.1111/j.1075-122X.2005.21530.x

Perry N, Broeders M, de Wolf C et al (2008) European guidelines for quality assurance in breast cancer screening and diagnosis. Fourth edition—summary document. Ann Oncol 19:614–622. https://doi.org/10.1093/annonc/mdm481

Philpotts LE, Shaheen NA, Jain KS et al (2000) Uncommon high-risk lesions of the breast diagnosed at stereotactic core-needle biopsy: clinical importance. Radiology 216:831–837. https://doi.org/10.1148/radiology.216.3.r00se31831

Pinder SE, Shaaban A, Deb R et al (2018) NHS Breast Screening multidisciplinary working group guidelines for the diagnosis and management of breast lesions of uncertain malignant potential on core biopsy (B3 lesions). Clin Radiol 73:682–692. https://doi.org/10.1016/j.crad.2018.04.004

Piubello Q, Parisi A, Eccher A et al (2009) Flat epithelial atypia on core needle biopsy: which is the right management? Am J Surg Pathol 33:1078–1084. https://doi.org/10.1097/PAS.0b013e31819d0a4d

Plaza MJ, Swintelski C, Yaziji H et al (2015) Phyllodes tumor: review of key imaging characteristics. Breast Dis 35:79–86. https://doi.org/10.3233/BD-150399

Portschy PR, Marmor S, Nzara R et al (2013) Trends in incidence and management of lobular carcinoma in situ: a population-based analysis. Ann Surg Oncol 20:3240–3246. https://doi.org/10.1245/s10434-013-3121-4

Purushothaman HN, Lekanidi K, Shousha S, Wilson R (2016) Lesions of uncertain malignant potential in the breast (B3): what do we know? Clin Radiol 71:134–140. https://doi.org/10.1016/j.crad.2015.10.008

Rageth CJ, O'Flynn EA, Comstock C et al (2016) First International Consensus Conference on lesions of uncertain malignant potential in the breast (B3 lesions). Breast Cancer Res Treat 159:203–213. https://doi.org/10.1007/s10549-016-3935-4

Rendi MH, Dintzis SM, Lehman CD et al (2012) Lobular in-situ neoplasia on breast core needle biopsy: imaging indication and pathologic extent can identify which patients require excisional biopsy. Ann Surg Oncol 19:914–921. https://doi.org/10.1245/s10434-011-2034-3

Riedl CC, Ponhold L, Flöry D et al (2007) Magnetic resonance imaging of the breast improves detection of invasive cancer, preinvasive cancer, and premalignant lesions during surveillance of women at high risk for breast cancer. Clin Cancer Res 13:6144–6152. https://doi.org/10.1158/1078-0432.CCR-07-1270

Rizzo M, Linebarger J, Lowe MC et al (2012) Management of papillary breast lesions diagnosed on core-needle biopsy: clinical pathologic and radiologic analysis of 276 cases with surgical follow-up. J Am Coll Surg 214:280–287. https://doi.org/10.1016/j.jamcollsurg.2011.12.005

Rudin AV, Hoskin TL, Fahy A et al (2017) Flat epithelial atypia on core biopsy and upgrade to cancer: a systematic review and meta-analysis. Ann Surg Oncol 24:3549–3558. https://doi.org/10.1245/s10434-017-6059-0

Said SM, Visscher DW, Nassar A et al (2015) Flat epithelial atypia and risk of breast cancer: a Mayo cohort study. Cancer 121:1548–1555. https://doi.org/10.1002/cncr.29243

Saladin C, Haueisen H, Kampmann G et al (2016) Lesions with unclear malignant potential (B3) after minimally invasive breast biopsy: evaluation of vacuum biopsies performed in Switzerland and recommended further management. Acta Radiol 57:815–821. https://doi.org/10.1177/0284185115610931

Sanders ME, Page DL, Simpson JF et al (2006) Interdependence of radial scar and proliferative disease with respect to invasive breast carcinoma risk in patients with benign breast biopsies. Cancer 106:1453–1461. https://doi.org/10.1002/cncr.21730

Schnitt SJ, Vincent-Salomon A (2003) Columnar cell lesions of the breast. Adv Anat Pathol 10:113–124

Scoggins M, Krishnamurthy S, Santiago L, Yang W (2013) Lobular carcinoma in situ of the breast: clinical, radiological, and pathological correlation. Acad Radiol 20:463–470. https://doi.org/10.1016/j.acra.2012.08.020

Senetta R, Campanino PP, Mariscotti G et al (2009) Columnar cell lesions associated with breast calcifications on vacuum-assisted core biopsies: clinical, radiographic, and histological correlations. Mod Pathol 22:762–769. https://doi.org/10.1038/modpathol.2009.21

Shetty MK (2002) Radial scars of the breast: sonographic findings. Ultrasound Q 18:203–207

Stein LF, Zisman G, Rapelyea JA et al (2005) Lobular carcinoma in situ of the breast presenting as a mass. AJR Am J Roentgenol 184:1799–1801. https://doi.org/10.2214/ajr.184.6.01841799

Sung JS, Malak SF, Bajaj P et al (2011) Screening breast MR imaging in women with a history of lobular carcinoma in situ. Radiology 261:414–420. https://doi.org/10.1148/radiol.11110091

Tabár L, Dean PB, Péntek Z (1983) Galactography: the diagnostic procedure of choice for nipple discharge. Radiology 149:31–38. https://doi.org/10.1148/radiology.149.1.6611939

Tan P-H, Jayabaskar T, Chuah K-L et al (2005) Phyllodes tumors of the breast: the role of pathologic parameters. Am J Clin Pathol 123:529–540. https://doi.org/10.1309/U6DV-BFM8-1MLJ-C1FN

Tan PH, Thike AA, Tan WJ et al (2012) Predicting clinical behaviour of breast phyllodes tumours: a nomogram based on histological criteria and surgical margins. J Clin Pathol 65:69–76. https://doi.org/10.1136/jclinpath-2011-200368

Tan BY, Acs G, Apple SK et al (2016) Phyllodes tumours of the breast: a consensus review. Histopathology 68:5–21. https://doi.org/10.1111/his.12876

Tavassoli FA, Devilee P (eds) (2003) Pathology and genetics of tumours of the breast and female genital organs. IARC, Lyon

Teaching Atlas of Mammography (2018). https://www.thieme.com/books-main/radiology/product/80-teaching-atlas-of-mammography. Accessed 22 Mar 2018

Thill M, Liedtke C, AGO Breast Committee (2016) AGO recommendations for the diagnosis and treatment of patients with advanced and metastatic breast cancer: update 2016. Breast Care (Basel) 11:216–222. https://doi.org/10.1159/000447030

Van Zee KJ, Ortega Pérez G, Minnard E, Cohen MA (1998) Preoperative galactography increases the diagnostic yield of major duct excision for nipple discharge. Cancer 82:1874–1880

Villa A, Tagliafico A, Chiesa F et al (2011) Atypical ductal hyperplasia diagnosed at 11-gauge vacuum-assisted breast biopsy performed on suspicious clustered microcalcifications: could patients without residual microcalcifications be managed conservatively? AJR Am J Roentgenol 197:1012–1018. https://doi.org/10.2214/AJR.11.6588

Vizcaíno I, Gadea L, Andreo L et al (2001) Short-term follow-up results in 795 nonpalpable probably benign lesions detected at screening mammography. Radiology 219:475–483. https://doi.org/10.1148/radiology.219.2.r01ma11475

Wei S (2016) Papillary lesions of the breast: an update. Arch Pathol Lab Med 140:628–643. https://doi.org/10.5858/arpa.2015-0092-RA

Wen X, Cheng W (2013) Nonmalignant breast papillary lesions at core-needle biopsy: a meta-analysis of underestimation and influencing factors. Ann Surg Oncol 20:94–101. https://doi.org/10.1245/s10434-012-2590-1

Wyss P, Varga Z, Rössle M, Rageth CJ (2014) Papillary lesions of the breast: outcomes of 156 patients managed without excisional biopsy. Breast J 20:394–401. https://doi.org/10.1111/tbj.12283

Yamaguchi R, Tanaka M, Tse GM et al (2015) Management of breast papillary lesions diagnosed in ultrasound-guided vacuum-assisted and core needle biopsies. Histopathology 66:565–576. https://doi.org/10.1111/his.12477

Yilmaz E, Sal S, Lebe B (2002) Differentiation of phyllodes tumors versus fibroadenomas. Acta Radiol 43:34–39

Youk JH, Kim MJ, Son EJ et al (2012) US-guided vacuum-assisted percutaneous excision for management of benign papilloma without atypia diagnosed at US-guided 14-gauge core needle biopsy. Ann Surg Oncol 19:922–928. https://doi.org/10.1245/s10434-011-2033-4

Youk JH, Kim H, Kim E-K et al (2015) Phyllodes tumor diagnosed after ultrasound-guided vacuum-assisted excision: should it be followed by surgical excision? Ultrasound Med Biol 41:741–747. https://doi.org/10.1016/j.ultrasmedbio.2014.11.004

Youn I, Choi SH, Moon HJ et al (2013) Phyllodes tumors of the breast: ultrasonographic findings and diagnostic performance of ultrasound-guided core needle biopsy. Ultrasound Med Biol 39:987–992. https://doi.org/10.1016/j.ultrasmedbio.2013.01.004

Yu C-C, Ueng S-H, Cheung Y-C et al (2015) Predictors of underestimation of malignancy after image-guided core needle biopsy diagnosis of flat epithelial atypia or atypical ductal hyperplasia. Breast J 21:224–232. https://doi.org/10.1111/tbj.12389

Minimal Invasive Therapy

Gabriel Adelsmayr, Gisela Sponner,
and Michael Fuchsjäger

Contents

1   **Introduction** 360

2   **Cryotherapy** 360
    2.1 Cryotherapy in Fibroadenomas 363
    2.2 Cryotherapy in Breast Cancer 363

3   **Radiofrequency Ablation** 364

4   **Microwave Ablation** 366

5   **High-Intensity Focused Ultrasound Ablation** 366

6   **Potential Complications of Minimally Invasive Therapies for Breast Tumors** 367
    6.1 Cryotherapy 367
    6.2 Radiofrequency Ablation 368
    6.3 Microwave Ablation 368
    6.4 High-Intensity Focused Ultrasound Ablation 368

7   **Potential Advantages** 369

8   **Limitations** 369

9   **Summary and Outlook** 369

References 369

Abstract

Minimally invasive therapies of breast tumors are emerging techniques in selected patients and specific indications potentially changing the treatment and management of benign and malignant breast lesions.

At *cryotherapy*, a probe for alternating cycles of freezing and thawing is inserted into the lesion to damage tumor tissue under local

G. Adelsmayr (✉) · M. Fuchsjäger
Division of General Radiology, Department of
Radiology, Medical University of Graz, Graz, Austria
e-mail: gabriel.adelsmayr@medunigraz.at; michael.
fuchsjaeger@medunigraz.at

G. Sponner
Department of Medicine, LKH Weststeiermark,
Voitsberg, Austria

© Springer Nature Switzerland AG 2022
M. Fuchsjäger et al. (eds.), *Breast Imaging*, Medical Radiology Diagnostic Imaging,
https://doi.org/10.1007/978-3-030-94918-1_17

anesthesia and guidance of real-time ultrasound, CT, or MRI. Promising results of this method were reported for treatment of fibroadenomas and breast cancer.

Radiofrequency ablation destroys tumor tissue by frictional heat using alternating current, most commonly under ultrasound-guidance. Since this treatment is generally more painful, deep sedation or general anesthesia is required.

Microwave ablation uses electromagnetic waves of at least 900 MHz and is commonly guided by CT or ultrasound. Deep sedation or general anesthesia is required.

High-intensity focused ultrasound ablation is a noninvasive method for treatment of breast tumors and utilizes higher energy ultrasound waves of lower frequency than that in diagnostic ultrasound. Tissue is heated at a cigar-shaped focus zone under ultrasound or MRI guidance. With up to 3 h, this procedure is rather time consuming.

Requirements for successful minimally invasive therapies of breast tumors include tumor size below 2 cm; visibility of the tumor at MRI, CT, or ultrasound; and a minimum distance between tumor and skin/muscle of 1 cm. Partly due to lack of evidence, limitations of minimally invasive breast tumor ablation are large and/or multicentric tumors, tumors close to skin and/or muscle, and invasive lobular carcinomas and DCIS.

Success rates of minimally invasive therapies were found to be 96% with relatively low minor and major complication rates, such as pain, skin burns, edema and necrosis, and pneumothorax.

1 Introduction

Minimally invasive therapies of breast tumors are emerging techniques in selected patients and specific indications potentially changing the treatment and management of benign and malignant breast lesions.

Therapeutic interventions that aim at minimally invasive tumor ablation utilize direct application of chemical or thermal therapies for eradication or substantial structural damage of tumors. Techniques that will be discussed in this chapter include cryoablation, radiofrequency ablation, microwave ablation, and high-frequency ultrasound ablation.

Since the implementation of breast cancer screening, more breast tumors are detected at an early stage and with small size (Berry et al. 2005). Small breast tumors can potentially be eliminated with excellent cosmetic results by surgery; however, this treatment requires general anesthesia. Minimally invasive therapies on the other hand can be performed without general anesthesia, and in most cases, local anesthesia is sufficient for pain control. Therefore, this therapeutic option can be carried out on an outpatient basis that generally is preferred by patients to an inpatient setting. Moreover, the minimally invasive therapeutic approach is time and resource saving, reducing costs for health-care providers.

Generally accepted requirements for successful minimally invasive therapies of breast tumors include tumor size below 2 cm; visibility of the tumor at MRI, CT, or ultrasound; and a minimum distance between tumor and skin/muscle of 1 cm to avoid freezing and burning injuries. Limitations of minimally invasive breast tumor ablation are large and/or multicentric tumors, tumors close to skin and/or muscle, and invasive lobular carcinomas and DCIS, the latter two due to lack of evidence (Roubidoux et al. 2014).

Pooled technical success rate of percutaneous ablation with radiofrequency, microwaves, cryoablation, laser, and high-intensity focused ultrasound was found to be 96% with a pooled major complication rate of 6% and minor complication pooled rate of 8% (Mauri et al. 2017).

2 Cryotherapy

Already in antiquity, Hippocrates recommended cold for hemostasis as well as to reduce the swelling of painful joints. In the eleventh century, cold was used as a local anesthetic, and in the nineteenth century, malignant diseases were successfully treated with cold with a reduction in morbidity.

The development of adiabatic expansion systems, which allow a change of state without heat exchange, led to the liquification of oxygen, air, and nitrogen. Carbon dioxide, hydrogen, and helium were also liquified at the beginning of the twentieth century. By liquid nitrogen, temperatures of −160 °C were reached and applied in the course of the century on different organ systems. Finally, the Joule-Thomson cryoprobe, which achieves cooling by expansion of liquid nitrogen or argon gas, was developed (Korpan 2007).

According to its freezing profile (size and shape of originating ice ball to guarantee for a complete ablation with safety margins of at least 5 mm), the needle probe to be used has to be specifically chosen to perfectly fit for the respective lesion.

One or more cryoprobes are placed under imaging guidance and local anesthesia through a small skin incision in the center of the tumor (Tarkowski and Rzaca 2014; Huston and Simmons 2005).

Imaging guiding can be achieved by ultrasound (Fig. 1), computed tomography (CT), or magnetic resonance imaging (MRI).

By means of liquid nitrogen or argon gas, tissue is cooled around the cryoprobe to −160 to −187 °C, and a sonographically visible ice ball is formed.

First-generation cryoprobes cool along the entire stem, and the second-generation are vacuum isolated and become cold only at the distal tip, making skin protection easier to achieve (Kaufman et al. 2004). Different numbers of freeze-thaw cycles can be used; however, the most commonly used method is two freeze-thawing cycles of 10-min freezing with a 10-min thawing intermission, in which fast freezing and relatively slow thawing seem to be most effective. Using ultrasound, the procedure can be observed in real time (Gage et al. 1985; Huston and Simmons 2005).

Methods to prevent cold-induced skin necrosis during ice ball formation are warmed saline bags placed on the skin at the site of the ice ball or rubbing of the skin (Korpan 2007).

With regard to tissue destruction, there is an immediate and a delayed mechanism.

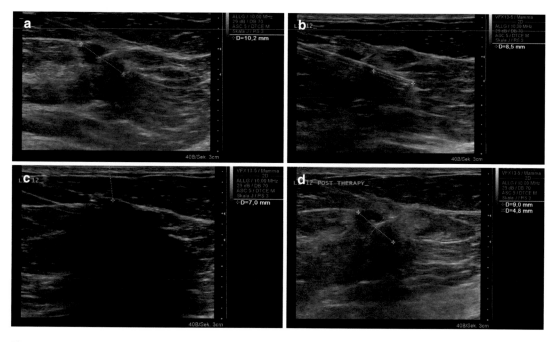

Fig. 1 Pre-cryoablation ultrasound image of a 10 mm invasive ductal carcinoma (**a**), ultrasound-guided positioning of the cryoprobe into the target lesion (**b**), formation of an ice ball around the tip of the cryoprobe (**c**), and post-interventional ultrasound image of the target lesion after thawing of the ice ball (**d**)

The immediate mechanism is triggered by damaging effects of cooling and thawing of the cells, which are delayed by the progressive failure of the microcirculation and ultimately the vascular stasis. Tissue ischemia after the dew point, however, obscures the effect of direct cell damage.

With a drop in temperature, the cell metabolism is disturbed. By freezing the tissue, the contained water crystallizes. Ice crystals first form extracellularly because the cell is better protected by the lipid membrane. The extracellular freezing of water leads to an osmotic shift, and water is drawn out of the cell into the extracellular space. This happens mainly at temperatures around −20 °C. Due to the dehydration, the cell shrinks, electrolyte concentrations increase, and membrane and cell contents are damaged (Gage and Baust 1998).

The so-called solution effect is not always fatal for the cell, in contrast to intracellular ice, which forms mainly by rapid cooling to temperatures below −40 °C and tears cell organelles and membranes. During the thaw cycle, the crystals fuse into larger formations. This so-called recrystallization occurs especially at temperatures between −20 and −25 °C and ruptures cell membranes. By melting, the extracellular space becomes hypotonic, water is drawn into the cell, its volume increases, and it bursts.

By thawing the tissue, a microcirculatory stasis develops at −20 °C. By cooling the tissue in the freezing phase, vasoconstriction and reduced blood flow result. As soon as the temperature rises again above 0 °C, the circulation starts again and vasodilation sets in. The vascular permeability increases; edema, platelet aggregation, and microthrombi arise; and the circulation stagnates after about 30–45 min. Due to lack of blood flow, the tissue becomes necrotic (Gage and Baust 1998).

As the tissue near the probe freezes faster and in the periphery of the probe more slowly, intracellular ice forms near the probe and extracellular ice forms on the edge of the ice ball. Decisive for cell destruction, however, is above all the change in temperature over time. For a single freeze-thaw cycle, cells will be destroyed at −40 to −50 °C. With temperatures below −40 °C, the duration of the freezing should be correspondingly longer, if compared to, e.g., −160 °C. Thawing should always be as slow as possible to achieve greater ice formation and maximum cell destruction. Depending on the system used, active thawing can be achieved by supplying helium to the cryoprobe.

The destructive changes and the size of the ice formations increase with further freeze-thaw cycles. Usually, two freeze-thaw cycles are used. In the periphery of the ice ball, the osmotic and hypothermic stress is often insufficient to allow uniform cell destruction. However, studies have shown that some of these cells undergo apoptosis after a few days (Gage and Baust 1998).

Multiple cryoprobes give rise to thermal synergies that fuse lethal isotherms (connecting lines between sites of the same temperature) and continue to expand. For example, the percentage of lethal ice increases in a diameter from 35% to more than 70% for three or more cryoprobes. The nonlethal rim described in the in vitro studies has been consistently below 1 cm (Littrup et al. 2009a). With the combination of several cryoprobes, larger size tumors can be successfully treated (Gage and Baust 1998).

An interesting aspect of cryotherapy is cryoimmunology: the ability to create an immune response to tumor-specific antigens. However, the experiences of cryotherapy in animal models with different tumors are diverse. It turns out that cryotherapy can have both positive effects on tumor-specific defense and immunosuppressive effects. The predominant mechanism depends on the type of tumor, the body's immune competence before treatment, the method of freezing, the ablated tumor volume, and the site where the immune response is sought. Crucial for immunomodulatory effects of cryotherapy is the relation of induced apoptosis and necrosis: apoptosis induces immunotolerance, and necrosis stimulates a humoral immune response (Sabel et al. 2005, 2006, 2010; Sabel 2009; Koido et al. 2014; McArthur et al. 2016). Promising results of a small trial investigating the feasibility of preoperative cryoablation and the administration of a checkpoint inhibitor in breast cancer suggest further studies of this therapy strategy in patients with operable breast cancer (McArthur et al. 2016). The combination of cryotherapy and immunotherapy also showed auspicious results in patients with metastatic breast cancer with failed radical surgery (Niu et al. 2013) and HER2-positive breast cancer (Liang et al. 2017).

T-cell receptor sequencing may serve as a biomarker for immune response to cryoimmunotherapy (Page et al. 2016).

2.1 Cryotherapy in Fibroadenomas

Cryotherapy has the potential to successfully reduce the volume of fibroadenomas in an outpatient setting with low complication rates. After cryoablation of fibroadenomas, the necrotic tumor is slowly absorbed with a residual tumor volume depending on the initial tumor size. The procedure is performed with high patient's satisfaction and good to excellent cosmetic results. Artifacts in mammography after cryotherapy of fibroadenomas are rare (Kaufman et al. 2004, 2005; Caleffi et al. 2004; Hahn et al. 2013; Littrup et al. 2005; Nurko et al. 2005).

2.2 Cryotherapy in Breast Cancer

Cryotherapy was performed in several studies both in a curative setting, in women with localized disease, and in a palliative setting, in women with generalized disease.

The effects of freezing may make subsequent surgical removal of breast tumors easier than with normal surgery, minimizing bleeding (Tafra et al. 2003).

In a study excluding invasive lobular and colloidal carcinomas and tumors with more than 25% DCIS component, a complete ablation was achieved in carcinomas up to 1.5 cm (Sabel et al. 2004).

Another study observed that in none of the 29 completed treatments with cryotherapy of invasive breast cancer up to 1.5 cm diameter, living invasive tumor cells were detected at histopathologic assessment. In 5 of 30 patients (16.7%), however, DCIS was found outside the ablation area (Pfleiderer et al. 2005).

A trial including 87 unifocal, invasive, ductal breast cancers up to 2 cm diameter, with less than 25% intraductal component and MRI contrast media enhancement, found a complete cryoablation in 75.9% and in the remaining cases invasive residual tumor and/or DCIS components. If the multifocality discovered in histology is not considered a cryoablation failure, successful tumor ablation was achieved in 92% of the 87 tumors (Simmons et al. 2016).

Even in multifocal and bulky breast cancer, cryoablation may yield desired effects through large treatment zones. Combined guidance with ultrasound and CT seems appropriate in this patient group (Littrup et al. 2009b).

In patients who refuse or are not fit for surgical treatment of malignant breast tumors, cryotherapy offers a potential alternative to reduce tumor load, with decreasing efficiency of tumor size control over time (Simmons et al. 2016; Cazzato et al. 2015; Pusceddu et al. 2011, 2014; Li et al. 2014).

In metastatic breast cancer, cryotherapy, especially in combination with immunotherapy, may even extend overall survival (Niu et al. 2013).

A limitation in assessing the role of cryotherapy in recent literature is the relatively small number of patients included in most studies, missing long-term follow-up data and the study setting where the procedure was mostly performed under purely research "treat and resect" protocols. Moreover, success rates vary among studies, declining with increasing tumor size (Bergin et al. 2008; Manenti et al. 2011; Gajda et al. 2014; Poplack et al. 2015; Pusztaszeri et al. 2007; Morin et al. 2004).

For assessment of residual tumor load after cryotherapy, MRI is considered the method of choice (Figs. 2 and 3) (Simmons et al. 2016; Manenti et al. 2013).

In mammography and ultrasound, increased density and echogenicity are observed following cryoablation, corresponding to the size and location of the ice ball (Roubidoux et al. 2004).

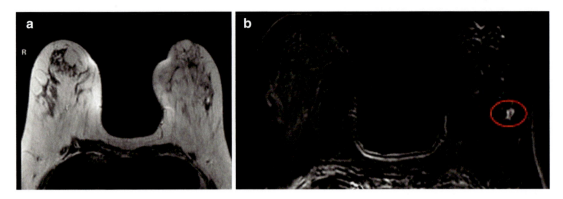

Fig. 2 Pre-cryoablation axial T2-weighted MR image (**a**) and axial contrast-enhanced T1-weighted MR image (**b**) of an enhancing spiculated lesion in the left breast (red circle). (Reprinted by permission from Springer Nature Customer Service Centre GmbH: Springer Nature, European Radiology, Percutaneous local ablation of unifocal subclinical breast cancer: clinical experience and preliminary results of cryotherapy, Guglielmo Manenti et al., ©2011)

Fig. 3 One-month post-cryoablation of the same lesion as in Fig. 2. Axial T1-weighted MR image (**a**), axial T2-weighted MR image (**a′**), and axial contrast-enhanced MR image (**b**). Disappearance of the previously enhancing lesion with a new area of necrosis can be appreciated (red circle). (Reprinted by permission from Springer Nature Customer Service Centre GmbH: Springer Nature, European Radiology, Percutaneous local ablation of unifocal subclinical breast cancer: clinical experience and preliminary results of cryotherapy, Guglielmo Manenti et al., ©2011)

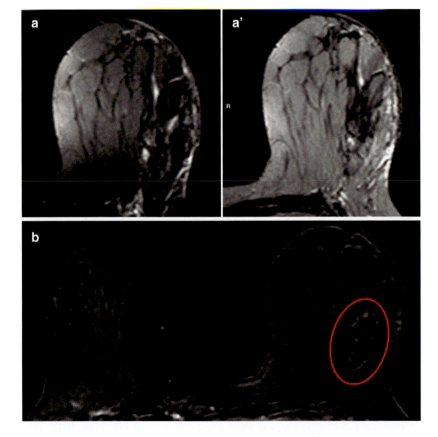

3 Radiofrequency Ablation

Radiofrequency ablation is a minimally invasive technique for destroying solid tumors by frictional heat generated by intracellular ions set in motion via alternating current (AC). The current flows from the electrode placed in the tumor in the direction of a grounding plate, which is attached to the skin. High-frequency electrical power (400–500 kHz) is used at up to 200 W.

The ablation zone can be increased either by increasing the conductivity of the tissue by introducing saline or by enlarging the electrode by flipping several secondary electrodes out of the tip of the primary electrode to form a star or screen shape. The size of the ablation zone can thus be increased to 3–5 cm (Dowlatshahi et al. 2001).

Most commonly, ultrasound is used to guide and visualize the procedure because the frequency of radiofrequency ablation used interferes with MRI. MRI-compatible probes are available, but extremely expensive.

The treatment is painful; therefore, deep sedation or general anesthesia is required (Fornage and Hunt 2015).

After ablation, ultrasound depicts a hyperechogenic coagulated zone (Vlastos and Verkooijen 2007). However, visualization during treatment is difficult as it causes rapid and diffuse hyperechogenicity in the vicinity of the tumor from the beginning, rendering the tumor unrecognizable.

There are three ways to perform this treatment.

The most common technique is impedance based. A gradual increase in power is performed in 5 or 10 W increments every 1 or 2 min until there is a so-called power roll-off, an impedance increase of at least 20 Ω, which is indicative of total tissue coagulation. If this "impedance jump" is not achieved, treatment is usually stopped after 15 min (Jeffrey et al. 1999; Izzo et al. 2001).

Another possibility is treatment at a constant temperature for a certain time. Temperatures of 75 °C (Head and Elliott 2009) to 100 °C (Mackey et al. 2012), but usually 90–95 °C, are held over 10–20 min (temperature/time based).

The third option is assessment based on imaging where the treatment is continued until the entire tumor appears to be coagulated under ultrasound guidance (imaging based) (Lamuraglia et al. 2005; Medina-Franco et al. 2008).

At histopathology, coagulation necrosis and protein denaturation are seen; therefore, accurate histological analysis including receptor status should be performed prior to radiofrequency ablation. The cell-destroying changes are often only found after 48 h; hence, immediate resection after radiofrequency ablation requires immunohistochemical analysis (for example by NADH staining) in addition to standard HE staining to assess the viability of the tumor cells (Huston and Simmons 2005). CK8 immunohistochemistry showed promising results as a potential alternative to NADH diaphoresis (Schassburger et al. 2014).

Successful radiofrequency ablation with screen- or star-shaped electrodes (Manenti et al. 2013; Fornage and Hunt 2015; Head and Elliott 2009; Burak Jr. et al. 2003; Noguchi et al. 2006; Earashi et al. 2007; Imoto et al. 2009; Hung et al. 2011) or a single electrode (Schassburger et al. 2014; Susini et al. 2007; Khatri et al. 2007; Oura et al. 2007; Nagashima et al. 2009; Wiksell et al. 2010; Yamamoto et al. 2011; Waaijer et al. 2014; Ohtani et al. 2011) was demonstrated in several studies in breast tumors up to 2 cm diameter.

Data on success rates of radiofrequency ablation in breast tumors greater than 2 cm are scarce, and in larger trials it has been reported to be between 30% and 55% (Medina-Franco et al. 2008; Kinoshita et al. 2011).

Postsurgical radiofrequency ablation of the resection cavity is a novel approach with promising results and may offer an alternative to radiation in certain patients (Mackey et al. 2012; Wilson et al. 2012; Klimberg et al. 2014).

For assessment following radiofrequency ablation, MRI examinations are recommended (Manenti et al. 2009, 2013; Vilar et al. 2012). After radiofrequency ablation, altered signal intensity with peripheral enhancement in MRI can be observed, which decreases in size over time. Correspondingly, in mammography a halo surrounding an area equal to that found in MRI may be discerned, representing fat necrosis (Nagashima et al. 2009; Hayashi et al. 2003).

In long-term follow-up, a residual nodular resistance may remain after radiofrequency ablation (Manenti et al. 2009; Noguchi et al. 2012).

4   Microwave Ablation

Microwaves lie between infrared radiation and radio waves at a frequency between 900 and 2450 MHz. The microwaves vibrate the polar water molecules up to two billion times a second, creating friction and heat, causing cell death through coagulation necrosis.

Percutaneous microwave ablation can be ultrasound or CT targeted and is usually performed under local anesthesia with sedation or under general anesthesia. The microwave antenna is placed directly in the center of the tumor, and the electromagnetic microwaves are applied at up to 60 W and at 915 MHz (Vilar et al. 2012). Grounding is not necessary.

The high energy density zone is larger at 2 cm around the antenna than at the radio frequency, which actively heats a larger zone and makes the cell destruction more uniform. In addition, microwave ablation does not cause the tissue to cook and char, which would act as an insulator and limit imaging. Without this restriction, the tissue can be heated to higher degrees.

Experimental studies have shown that tumor cells die when heated at 43 °C for 60 min. For each degree of temperature increase, the duration can be reduced by a factor of 2. The thermal energy necessary for a 120-min treatment at 43 °C can be reduced to approximately 3.75 min at 48 °C and is referred to as a thermal equivalent dose (CEM 43 °C = cumulative equivalent minutes relative to 43 °C) (Simon et al. 2005; Vargas et al. 2004).

Studies on microwave ablation in breast tumors are rare. Included were mostly patients in the palliative setting with breast tumors up to 8 cm diameter, where control of the tumor load or preoperative downsizing was the main objective. In one larger trial, the extent of tumor necrosis depended on the CEM applied, ranging from below 50% to 84% (Vargas et al. 2004; Zhou et al. 2012, 2014). Ultrasound and MRI images of a fibroadenoma before and after microwave ablation are shown in Fig. 4.

5   High-Intensity Focused Ultrasound Ablation

High-intensity focused ultrasound ablation, strictly speaking, is not a minimal but a noninvasive ablation method.

Higher energy ultrasound waves of lower frequency (0.8–3.5 MHz) are used than in diagnostic ultrasound. The waves pass through the skin and the tissue without damage; only at the focal point, heat is generated and the target tissue is destroyed. The focus zone is typically cigar shaped with up to 3 × 15 mm diameter. In order to treat larger volumes, several of these so-called sonification zones have to be lined up side by side. Within a few seconds, the tissue is heated to 60–95 °C and undergoes localized protein denaturation and coagulation necrosis. In addition to the thermal energy, mechanical stress (Vargas et al. 2004) develops, which also leads to cell destruction. The heat leads to cell death at over 56 °C for over 1 s. Wave motion and heat create microbubbles that cause intracellular mechanical disruption (Brenin 2011). Antiangiogenic effects of high-intensity focused ultrasound ablation may also play a role in the treatment of breast cancer (Guan and Xu 2016).

The ablation procedure is performed under MRI or ultrasound guidance, with ultrasound having the advantage of showing the treatment in real time. Temperature can also be measured by means of MRI (Fig. 5) (Brenin 2011; Peek et al. 2015).

The procedure is time consuming with a duration of up to 3 h, which makes optimal patient positioning necessary (Furusawa et al. 2006; Wu et al. 2005). Therefore, deep sedation or general anesthesia is generally required (Wu et al. 2003, 2005, 2007).

Repeated high-intensity focused ultrasound ablation was performed in patients with breast cancer up to 2.5 cm diameter and contraindication to surgery or who refused surgery, with post-ablation tumor-free biopsies in 79% and promising long-term results (Gianfelice et al. 2003).

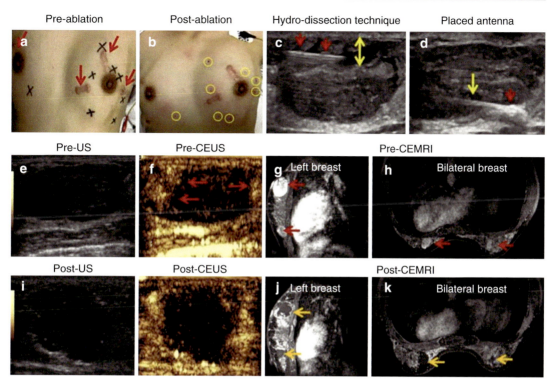

Fig. 4 Technical success of MWA in one representative case (20-year-old woman with eight fibroadenomas in bilateral breast). (**a**) Appearance of the skin before MWA. Red arrow is pointing to the scar from the surgery for fibroadenoma 9 months ago. The black marker indicates the location of the breast lesions. (**b**) The yellow ring indicates the needle site after MWA. (**c**) The needle (red arrows) was inserted into the space between the lesion margin and the skin to infuse saline, which increased the distance (yellow arrow) between the lesion and the skin. (**d**) US scan shows that the antenna tip placed in the deepest site of lesion increased echogenicity (red arrow) near the irradiating segment of the antenna (yellow arrow) at the beginning of the MWA session. (**e**) US scan shows the hypoechoic lesion before MWA. (**f**) CEUS shows the hyper-enhancement (red arrow) at the margin of the lesion. (**g, h**) CEMRI shows early enhancing lesions bilaterally (arrows) before MWA. (**i**) B-mode (left) and CEUS (right) after MWA show decreased enhancement of the lesion. (**j, k**) Contrast-enhanced MRI shows hypointense treatment zones and peripheral nodular enhancement in the arterial phase. *MWA* microwave ablation, *CEMRI* contrast-enhanced magnetic resonance imaging, *CEUS* contrast-enhanced ultrasound, *US* ultrasound. (Reprinted by permission from Springer Nature Customer Service Centre GmbH: Springer Nature, European Radiology, Ultrasound-guided percutaneous microwave ablation for 755 benign breast lesions: a prospective multicenter study, Qi Yang et al., ©2020)

Another study found a complete tumor ablation in 54% of patients with breast cancer up to T2 stage (Furusawa et al. 2006). Success rates of ablation however decrease with larger tumors (Wu et al. 2007; Gianfelice et al. 2003).

Preoperative high-intensity focused ultrasound ablation may constitute an additional field of use (Guan and Xu 2016).

6 Potential Complications of Minimally Invasive Therapies for Breast Tumors

6.1 Cryotherapy

Complication rates are very low, and side effects include pain, hematoma, thermal skin reaction,

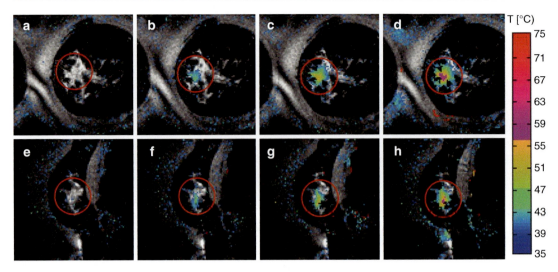

Fig. 5 Magnitude images (grayscale) overlaid with MR thermometry data (color coded) during sonification (50 W and a duration of 24.5 s) with a maximum temperature of 56.4 °C. Figures show coronal (**a–d**) and sagittal (**e–h**) images through the focal point. (Reprinted by permission from Springer Nature Customer Service Centre GmbH: Springer Nature, European Radiology, First clinical experience with a dedicated MRI-guided high-intensity focused ultrasound system for breast cancer ablation, Laura G. Merckel et al., ©2016)

infection, skin ulceration/necrosis and pigmentation disorders, bleeding, and potentially fatal "cryoshock," which is a systemic cytokine-mediated reaction with hypotension, dyspnea, and disseminated intravascular coagulation. Tenderness and swelling normally resolve within a few weeks (Kaufman et al. 2004; Caleffi et al. 2004; Cazzato et al. 2016; Mahnken et al. 2018).

Major complications (grade 2 or 3 skin burns, skin necrosis, and pneumothorax) were found in 2% and minor complications (local discomfort and grade 1 skin burns) in 8% (Mauri et al. 2017).

6.2 Radiofrequency Ablation

Complication rates are low with ecchymosis (Burak Jr. et al. 2003), combustion of pectoral muscle, nipple-areola complex (Imoto et al. 2009; Wiksell et al. 2010; Yoshinaga et al. 2013) or at the skin attachment site of the ground plate (Yamamoto et al. 2011; Yoshinaga et al. 2013), granulomatous mastitis (Yamamoto et al. 2011), and pneumothorax (Waaijer et al. 2014).

Bipolar needle electrodes can potentially minimize burns as a complication of radiofrequency ablation (Waaijer et al. 2014).

Overall, major complications (grade 2 or 3 skin burns, skin necrosis, and pneumothorax) were found in 6% and minor complications (local discomfort and grade 1 skin burns) in 7% (Mauri et al. 2017).

6.3 Microwave Ablation

Side effects include pain, edema, thermal skin reaction/burns, and postsurgical necrosis (Vargas et al. 2004; Gardner et al. 2002). It seems that microwave ablation does not destroy the lymphatics as suspected and thus does not interfere with sentinel node marking (Vargas et al. 2003).

Major complications (grade 2 or 3 skin burns, skin necrosis, and pneumothorax) were found in 4% and minor complications (local discomfort and grade 1 skin burns) in 14% (Mauri et al. 2017).

6.4 High-Intensity Focused Ultrasound Ablation

Complications of high-intensity focused ultrasound ablation are mild fever, edema, skin burns, and pain, potentially requiring sedation (Guan and Xu 2016; Gianfelice et al. 2003; Zippel and

Papa 2005). Complication rates were among the highest compared to the previously discussed ablation techniques with a major complication (grade 2 or 3 skin burns, skin necrosis, and pneumothorax) rate of 10% and a minor complication (local discomfort and grade 1 skin burns) rate of 15% (Mauri et al. 2017).

7 Potential Advantages

Minimally invasive therapy of breast tumors offers an alternative therapy strategy to surgical interventions in breast tumors predominantly due to its reduced morbidity and mortality. Especially patients with multiple comorbidities are eligible, since no general anesthesia is required in most minimally invasive therapy options.

The procedure can be performed in supine position with patients awake; consequently, patient's comfort is considered superior to surgical interventions.

Good cosmetic outcomes and an outpatient basis with the potential to reduce costs are additional advantages of implementing minimally invasive therapy strategies.

8 Limitations

Minimally invasive breast tumor therapies are limited by the tumor size and extent of tumor burden. Most of the research has been done on cryotherapy of breast cancer with promising results in selected patients. Large and multicentric tumors are not suitable for cryotherapy. Moreover, cryotherapy should not be performed on tumors close to the skin or muscle because of the danger of necrosis. Invasive lobular cancer and DCIS with associated microcalcifications also preclude cryotherapy.

To date, there are no large randomized multicenter trials investigating the effects of minimally invasive therapy options on patient's outcome and further treatment. Data of a prospective trial in progress investigating the effect of cryoablation on early breast cancer

are expected soon (IceCure Medical Ltd. 2014).

More data and close cooperation with clinical partners (i.e., surgery, gynecology, oncology, radiation therapy) are needed before minimally invasive therapy of breast tumors may be implemented on a larger scale as a standard treatment option.

9 Summary and Outlook

Minimally invasive therapies of breast tumors have shown to be effective as a primary treatment option and an alternative to invasive therapies in selected patients with benign and malignant breast tumors. The rate of adverse events and complication severity are considered to be low with the benefit of a possible outpatient setting and high feasibility of the various techniques.

Minimally invasive therapy of breast cancer might lead to several paradigm shifts for both physicians and patients:

A surgical incision may not be necessary in selected patients with breast tumors, and a lesion might remain palpable even after successful therapy. Moreover, minimally invasive therapy for breast tumors offers a potential alternative therapy strategy that can be performed in the awake and supine-positioned patient. And last, when assessing therapeutic success, post-interventional imaging and not histopathology might determine a "R0 resection."

To achieve optimum patient selection and to make the right choice of technique, further studies with long-term follow-up and larger patient cohorts are necessary.

References

Bergin JT, Sisney GA, Lee FT Jr, Burnside ES, Salkowski LR (2008) Unresected breast cancer: evolution of imaging findings following cryoablation. Radiol Case Rep 3(1):150

Berry DA, Cronin KA, Plevritis SK, Fryback DG, Clarke L, Zelen M, Mandelblatt JS, Yakovlev AY, Habbema JD, Feuer EJ et al (2005) Effect of screening and adjuvant therapy on mortality from breast cancer. N Engl J Med 353(17):1784–1792

Brenin DR (2011) Focused ultrasound ablation for the treatment of breast cancer. Ann Surg Oncol 18(11):3088–3094

Burak WE Jr, Agnese DM, Povoski SP, Yanssens TL, Bloom KJ, Wakely PE, Spigos DG (2003) Radiofrequency ablation of invasive breast carcinoma followed by delayed surgical excision. Cancer 98(7):1369–1376

Caleffi M, Filho DD, Borghetti K, Graudenz M, Littrup PJ, Freeman-Gibb LA, Zannis VJ, Schultz MJ, Kaufman CS, Francescatti D et al (2004) Cryoablation of benign breast tumors: evolution of technique and technology. Breast 13(5):397–407

Cazzato RL, de Lara CT, Buy X, Ferron S, Hurtevent G, Fournier M, Debled M, Palussiere J (2015) Single-centre experience with percutaneous cryoablation of breast cancer in 23 consecutive non-surgical patients. Cardiovasc Intervent Radiol 38(5):1237–1243

Cazzato RL, Garnon J, Ramamurthy N, Koch G, Tsoumakidou G, Caudrelier J, Arrigoni F, Zugaro L, Barile A, Masciocchi C et al (2016) Percutaneous image-guided cryoablation: current applications and results in the oncologic field. Med Oncol 33(12):140

Dowlatshahi K, Francescatti DS, Bloom KJ, Jewell WR, Schwartzberg BS, Singletary SE, Robinson D (2001) Image-guided surgery of small breast cancers. Am J Surg 182(4):419–425

Earashi M, Noguchi M, Motoyoshi A, Fujii H (2007) Radiofrequency ablation therapy for small breast cancer followed by immediate surgical resection or delayed mammotome excision. Breast Cancer 14(1):39–47

Fornage BD, Hunt KK (2015) Image-guided percutaneous ablation of small breast cancer: which technique is leading the pack? Technol Cancer Res Treat 14(2):209–211

Furusawa H, Namba K, Thomsen S, Akiyama F, Bendet A, Tanaka C, Yasuda Y, Nakahara H (2006) Magnetic resonance-guided focused ultrasound surgery of breast cancer: reliability and effectiveness. J Am Coll Surg 203(1):54–63

Gage AA, Baust J (1998) Mechanisms of tissue injury in cryosurgery. Cryobiology 37(3):171–186

Gage AA, Guest K, Montes M, Caruana JA, Whalen DA Jr (1985) Effect of varying freezing and thawing rates in experimental cryosurgery. Cryobiology 22(2):175–182

Gajda MR, Mireskandari M, Baltzer PA, Pfleiderer SO, Camara O, Runnebaum IB, Kaiser WA, Petersen I (2014) Breast pathology after cryotherapy. Histological regression of breast cancer after cryotherapy. Pol J Pathol 65(1):20–28

Gardner RA, Vargas HI, Block JB, Vogel CL, Fenn AJ, Kuehl GV, Doval M (2002) Focused microwave phased array thermotherapy for primary breast cancer. Ann Surg Oncol 9(4):326–332

Gianfelice D, Khiat A, Boulanger Y, Amara M, Belblidia A (2003) Feasibility of magnetic resonance imaging-guided focused ultrasound surgery as an adjunct to tamoxifen therapy in high-risk surgical patients with breast carcinoma. J Vasc Interv Radiol 14(10):1275–1282

Guan L, Xu G (2016) Damage effect of high-intensity focused ultrasound on breast cancer tissues and their vascularities. World J Surg Oncol 14(1):153

Hahn M, Pavlista D, Danes J, Klein R, Golatta M, Harcos A, Wallwiener D, Gruber I (2013) Ultrasound guided cryoablation of fibroadenomas. Ultraschall Med 34(1):64–68

Hayashi AH, Silver SF, van der Westhuizen NG, Donald JC, Parker C, Fraser S, Ross AC, Olivotto IA (2003) Treatment of invasive breast carcinoma with ultrasound-guided radiofrequency ablation. Am J Surg 185(5):429–435

Head JF, Elliott RL (2009) Stereotactic radiofrequency ablation: a minimally invasive technique for nonpalpable breast cancer in postmenopausal patients. Cancer Epidemiol 33(3–4):300–305

Hung WK, Mak KL, Ying M, Chan M (2011) Radiofrequency ablation of breast cancer: a comparative study of two needle designs. Breast Cancer 18(2):124–128

Huston TL, Simmons RM (2005) Ablative therapies for the treatment of malignant diseases of the breast. Am J Surg 189(6):694–701

IceCure Medical Ltd. (2014) Cryoablation of low risk small breast cancer- Ice3 trial. ClinicalTrials.gov Identifier: NCT02200705

Imoto S, Wada N, Sakemura N, Hasebe T, Murata Y (2009) Feasibility study on radiofrequency ablation followed by partial mastectomy for stage I breast cancer patients. Breast 18(2):130–134

Izzo F, Thomas R, Delrio P, Rinaldo M, Vallone P, DeChiara A, Botti G, D'Aiuto G, Cortino P, Curley SA (2001) Radiofrequency ablation in patients with primary breast carcinoma: a pilot study in 26 patients. Cancer 92(8):2036–2044

Jeffrey SS, Birdwell RL, Ikeda DM, Daniel BL, Nowels KW, Dirbas FM, Griffey SM (1999) Radiofrequency ablation of breast cancer: first report of an emerging technology. Arch Surg 134(10):1064–1068

Kaufman CS, Littrup PJ, Freman-Gibb LA, Francescatti D, Stocks LH, Smith JS, Henry CA, Bailey L, Harness JK, Simmons R (2004) Office-based cryoablation of breast fibroadenomas: 12-month follow-up. J Am Coll Surg 198(6):914–923

Kaufman CS, Littrup PJ, Freeman-Gibb LA, Smith JS, Francescatti D, Simmons R, Stocks LH, Bailey L, Harness JK, Bachman BA et al (2005) Office-based cryoablation of breast fibroadenomas with long-term follow-up. Breast J 11(5):344–350

Khatri VP, McGahan JP, Ramsamooj R, Griffey S, Brock J, Cronan M, Wilkendorf S (2007) A phase II trial of image-guided radiofrequency ablation of small invasive breast carcinomas: use of saline-cooled tip electrode. Ann Surg Oncol 14(5):1644–1652

Kinoshita T, Iwamoto E, Tsuda H, Seki K (2011) Radiofrequency ablation as local therapy for early breast carcinomas. Breast Cancer 18(1):10–17

Klimberg VS, Ochoa D, Henry-Tillman R, Hardee M, Boneti C, Adkins LL, McCarthy M, Tummel E, Lee J, Malak S et al (2014) Long-term results of phase II ablation after breast lumpectomy added to extend intraoperative margins (ABLATE l) trial. J Am Coll Surg 218(4):741–749

Koido S, Kinoshita S, Mogami T, Kan S, Takakura K, Okamoto M, Homma S, Ohkusa T, Tajiri H, Harada J (2014) Immunological assessment of cryotherapy in breast cancer patients. Anticancer Res 34(9):4869–4876

Korpan NN (2007) A history of cryosurgery: its development and future. J Am Coll Surg 204(2):314–324

Lamuraglia M, Lassau N, Garbay JR, Mathieu MC, Rouzier R, Jaziri S, Roche A, Leclere J (2005) Doppler US with perfusion software and contrast medium injection in the early evaluation of radiofrequency in breast cancer recurrences: a prospective phase II study. Eur J Radiol 56(3):376–381

Li J, Niu L, Mu F, Chen J, Zuo J, Xu K (2014) Comprehensive cryotherapy for recurrent breast cancer with distant metastases after failure of radical surgery. Breast J 20(3):327–328

Liang S, Niu L, Xu K, Wang X, Liang Y, Zhang M, Chen J, Lin M (2017) Tumor cryoablation in combination with natural killer cells therapy and Herceptin in patients with HER2-overexpressing recurrent breast cancer. Mol Immunol 92:45–53

Littrup PJ, Freeman-Gibb L, Andea A, White M, Amerikia KC, Bouwman D, Harb T, Sakr W (2005) Cryotherapy for breast fibroadenomas. Radiology 234(1):63–72

Littrup PJ, Jallad B, Vorugu V, Littrup G, Currier B, George M, Herring D (2009a) Lethal isotherms of cryoablation in a phantom study: effects of heat load, probe size, and number. J Vasc Interv Radiol 20(10):1343–1351

Littrup PJ, Jallad B, Chandiwala-Mody P, D'Agostini M, Adam BA, Bouwman D (2009b) Cryotherapy for breast cancer: a feasibility study without excision. J Vasc Interv Radiol 20(10):1329–1341

Mackey A, Feldman S, Vaz A, Durrant L, Seaton C, Klimberg VS (2012) Radiofrequency ablation after breast lumpectomy added to extend intraoperative margins in the treatment of breast cancer (ABLATE): a single-institution experience. Ann Surg Oncol 19(8):2618–2619

Mahnken AH, Konig AM, Figiel JH (2018) Current technique and application of percutaneous cryotherapy. Rofo 190(9):836–846

Manenti G, Bolacchi F, Perretta T, Cossu E, Pistolese CA, Buonomo OC, Bonanno E, Orlandi A, Simonetti G (2009) Small breast cancers: in vivo percutaneous US-guided radiofrequency ablation with dedicated cool-tip radiofrequency system. Radiology 251(2):339–346

Manenti G, Perretta T, Gaspari E, Pistolese CA, Scarano L, Cossu E, Bonanno E, Buonomo OC, Petrella G, Simonetti G et al (2011) Percutaneous local ablation of unifocal subclinical breast cancer: clinical experience and preliminary results of cryotherapy. Eur Radiol 21(11):2344–2353

Manenti G, Scarano AL, Pistolese CA, Perretta T, Bonanno E, Orlandi A, Simonetti G (2013) Subclinical breast cancer: minimally invasive approaches. Our experience with percutaneous radiofrequency ablation vs. cryotherapy. Breast Care 8(5):356–360

Mauri G, Sconfienza LM, Pescatori LC, Fedeli MP, Ali M, Di Leo G, Sardanelli F (2017) Technical success, technique efficacy and complications of minimally-invasive imaging-guided percutaneous ablation procedures of breast cancer: a systematic review and meta-analysis. Eur Radiol 27(8):3199–3210

McArthur HL, Diab A, Page DB, Yuan J, Solomon SB, Sacchini V, Comstock C, Durack JC, Mayhody M, Sung J et al (2016) A pilot study of preoperative single-dose ipilimumab and/or cryoablation in women with early-stage breast cancer with comprehensive immune profiling. Clin Cancer Res 22(23):5729–5737

Medina-Franco H, Soto-Germes S, Ulloa-Gomez JL, Romero-Trejo C, Uribe N, Ramirez-Alvarado CA, Robles-Vidal C (2008) Radiofrequency ablation of invasive breast carcinomas: a phase II trial. Ann Surg Oncol 15(6):1689–1695

Morin J, Traore A, Dionne G, Dumont M, Fouquette B, Dufour M, Cloutier S, Moisan C (2004) Magnetic resonance-guided percutaneous cryosurgery of breast carcinoma: technique and early clinical results. Can J Surg 47(5):347–351

Nagashima T, Sakakibara M, Sangai T, Kazama T, Fujimoto H, Miyazaki M (2009) Surrounding rim formation and reduction in size after radiofrequency ablation for primary breast cancer. Jpn J Radiol 27(5):197–204

Niu L, Mu F, Zhang C, Li Y, Liu W, Jiang F, Li L, Liu C, Zeng J, Yao F et al (2013) Cryotherapy protocols for metastatic breast cancer after failure of radical surgery. Cryobiology 67(1):17–22

Noguchi M, Earashi M, Fujii H, Yokoyama K, Harada K, Tsuneyama K (2006) Radiofrequency ablation of small breast cancer followed by surgical resection. J Surg Oncol 93(2):120–128

Noguchi M, Motoyoshi A, Earashi M, Fujii H (2012) Long-term outcome of breast cancer patients treated with radiofrequency ablation. Eur J Surg Oncol 38(11):1036–1042

Nurko J, Mabry CD, Whitworth P, Jarowenko D, Oetting L, Potruch T, Han L, Edwards MJ (2005) Interim results from the FibroAdenoma Cryoablation Treatment Registry. Am J Surg 190(4):647–651; discussion 651–642

Ohtani S, Kochi M, Ito M, Higaki K, Takada S, Matsuura H, Kagawa N, Hata S, Wada N, Inai K et al (2011) Radiofrequency ablation of early breast cancer followed by delayed surgical resection—a promising alternative to breast-conserving surgery. Breast 20(5):431–436

Oura S, Tamaki T, Hirai I, Yoshimasu T, Ohta F, Nakamura R, Okamura Y (2007) Radiofrequency ablation therapy in patients with breast cancers two centimeters or less in size. Breast Cancer 14(1):48–54

Page DB, Yuan J, Redmond D, Wen YH, Durack JC, Emerson R, Solomon S, Dong Z, Wong P, Comstock C et al (2016) Deep sequencing of T-cell receptor DNA as a biomarker of clonally expanded TILs in breast cancer after immunotherapy. Cancer Immunol Res 4(10):835–844

Peek MC, Ahmed M, Napoli A, ten Haken B, McWilliams S, Usiskin SI, Pinder SE, van Hemelrijck M, Douek M (2015) Systematic review of high-intensity focused ultrasound ablation in the treatment of breast cancer. Br J Surg 102(8):873–882; discussion 882

Pfleiderer SO, Marx C, Camara O, Gajda M, Kaiser WA (2005) Ultrasound-guided, percutaneous cryotherapy of small (< or = 15 mm) breast cancers. Invest Radiol 40(7):472–477

Poplack SP, Levine GM, Henry L, Wells WA, Heinemann FS, Hanna CM, Deneen DR, Tosteson TD, Barth RJ Jr (2015) A pilot study of ultrasound-guided cryoablation of invasive ductal carcinomas up to 15 mm with MRI follow-up and subsequent surgical resection. AJR Am J Roentgenol 204(5):1100–1108

Pusceddu C, Capobianco G, Meloni F, Valle E, Dessole S, Cherchi PL, Meloni GB (2011) CT-guided cryoablation of both breast cancer and lymph node axillary metastasis. Eur J Gynaecol Oncol 32(2):224–225

Pusceddu C, Sotgia B, Amucano G, Fele RM, Pilleri S, Meloni GB, Melis L (2014) Breast cryoablation in patients with bone metastatic breast cancer. J Vasc Interv Radiol 25(8):1225–1232

Pusztaszeri M, Vlastos G, Kinkel K, Pelte MF (2007) Histopathological study of breast cancer and normal breast tissue after magnetic resonance-guided cryotherapy ablation. Cryobiology 55(1):44–51

Roubidoux MA, Sabel MS, Bailey JE, Kleer CG, Klein KA, Helvie MA (2004) Small (<2.0-cm) breast cancers: mammographic and US findings at US-guided cryoablation--initial experience. Radiology 233(3):857–867

Roubidoux MA, Yang W, Stafford RJ (2014) Image-guided ablation in breast cancer treatment. Tech Vasc Interv Radiol 17(1):49–54

Sabel MS (2009) Cryo-immunology: a review of the literature and proposed mechanisms for stimulatory versus suppressive immune responses. Cryobiology 58(1):1–11

Sabel MS, Kaufman CS, Whitworth P, Chang H, Stocks LH, Simmons R, Schultz M (2004) Cryoablation of early-stage breast cancer: work-in-progress report of a multi-institutional trial. Ann Surg Oncol 11(5):542–549

Sabel MS, Nehs MA, Su G, Lowler KP, Ferrara JL, Chang AE (2005) Immunologic response to cryoablation of breast cancer. Breast Cancer Res Treat 90(1):97–104

Sabel MS, Arora A, Su G, Chang AE (2006) Adoptive immunotherapy of breast cancer with lymph node cells primed by cryoablation of the primary tumor. Cryobiology 53(3):360–366

Sabel MS, Su G, Griffith KA, Chang AE (2010) Rate of freeze alters the immunologic response after cryoablation of breast cancer. Ann Surg Oncol 17(4):1187–1193

Schassburger KU, Lofgren L, Lagerstedt U, Leifland K, Thorneman K, Sandstedt B, Auer G, Wiksell H (2014) Minimally-invasive treatment of early stage breast cancer: a feasibility study using radiofrequency ablation under local anesthesia. Breast 23(2):152–158

Simmons RM, Ballman KV, Cox C, Carp N, Sabol J, Hwang RF, Attai D, Sabel M, Nathanson D, Kenler A et al (2016) A phase II trial exploring the success of cryoablation therapy in the treatment of invasive breast carcinoma: results from ACOSOG (Alliance) Z1072. Ann Surg Oncol 23(8):2438–2445

Simon CJ, Dupuy DE, Mayo-Smith WW (2005) Microwave ablation: principles and applications. Radiographics 25(Suppl 1):S69–S83

Susini T, Nori J, Olivieri S, Livi L, Bianchi S, Mangialavori G, Branconi F, Scarselli G (2007) Radiofrequency ablation for minimally invasive treatment of breast carcinoma. A pilot study in elderly inoperable patients. Gynecol Oncol 104(2):304–310

Tafra L, Smith SJ, Woodward JE, Fernandez KL, Sawyer KT, Grenko RT (2003) Pilot trial of cryoprobe-assisted breast-conserving surgery for small ultrasound-visible cancers. Ann Surg Oncol 10(9):1018–1024

Tarkowski R, Rzaca M (2014) Cryosurgery in the treatment of women with breast cancer-a review. Gland Surg 3(2):88–93

Vargas HI, Dooley WC, Gardner RA, Gonzalez KD, Heywang-Kobrunner SH, Fenn AJ (2003) Success of sentinel lymph node mapping after breast cancer ablation with focused microwave phased array thermotherapy. Am J Surg 186(4):330–332

Vargas HI, Dooley WC, Gardner RA, Gonzalez KD, Venegas R, Heywang-Kobrunner SH, Fenn AJ (2004) Focused microwave phased array thermotherapy for ablation of early-stage breast cancer: results of thermal dose escalation. Ann Surg Oncol 11(2):139–146

Vilar VS, Goldman SM, Ricci MD, Pincerato K, Oliveira H, Abud TG, Ajzen S, Baracat EC, Szejnfeld J (2012) Analysis by MRI of residual tumor after radiofrequency ablation for early stage breast cancer. AJR Am J Roentgenol 198(3):W285–W291

Vlastos G, Verkooijen HM (2007) Minimally invasive approaches for diagnosis and treatment of early-stage breast cancer. Oncologist 12(1):1–10

Waaijer L, Kreb DL, Fernandez Gallardo MA, Van Rossum PS, Postma EL, Koelemij R, Van Diest PJ, Klaessens JH, Witkamp AJ, Van Hillegersberg R (2014) Radiofrequency ablation of small breast tumours: evaluation of a novel bipolar cool-tip application. Eur J Surg Oncol 40(10):1222–1229

Wiksell H, Lofgren L, Schassburger KU, Grundstrom H, Janicijevic M, Lagerstedt U, Leifland K, Nybom R, Rotstein S, Saracco A et al (2010) Feasibility study on the treatment of small breast carcinoma using percutaneous US-guided preferential radiofrequency ablation (PRFA). Breast 19(3):219–225

Wilson M, Korourian S, Boneti C, Adkins L, Badgwell B, Lee J, Suzanne Klimberg V (2012) Long-term results of excision followed by radiofrequency ablation as the sole means of local therapy for breast cancer. Ann Surg Oncol 19(10):3192–3198

Wu F, Wang ZB, Cao YD, Chen WZ, Bai J, Zou JZ, Zhu H (2003) A randomised clinical trial of high-intensity focused ultrasound ablation for the treatment of patients with localised breast cancer. Br J Cancer 89(12):2227–2233

Wu F, Wang ZB, Zhu H, Chen WZ, Zou JZ, Bai J, Li KQ, Jin CB, Xie FL, Su HB (2005) Extracorporeal high intensity focused ultrasound treatment for patients with breast cancer. Breast Cancer Res Treat 92(1):51–60

Wu F, Wang ZB, Cao YD, Zhu XQ, Zhu H, Chen WZ, Zou JZ (2007) "Wide local ablation" of localized breast cancer using high intensity focused ultrasound. J Surg Oncol 96(2):130–136

Yamamoto N, Fujimoto H, Nakamura R, Arai M, Yoshii A, Kaji S, Itami M (2011) Pilot study of radiofrequency ablation therapy without surgical excision for T1 breast cancer: evaluation with MRI and vacuum-assisted core needle biopsy and safety management. Breast Cancer 18(1):3–9

Yoshinaga Y, Enomoto Y, Fujimitsu R, Shimakura M, Nabeshima K, Iwasaki A (2013) Image and pathological changes after radiofrequency ablation of invasive breast cancer: a pilot study of nonsurgical therapy of early breast cancer. World J Surg 37(2):356–363

Zhou W, Zha X, Liu X, Ding Q, Chen L, Ni Y, Zhang Y, Xu Y, Chen L, Zhao Y et al (2012) US-guided percutaneous microwave coagulation of small breast cancers: a clinical study. Radiology 263(2):364–373

Zhou W, Jiang Y, Chen L, Ling L, Liang M, Pan H, Wang S, Ding Q, Liu X, Wang S (2014) Image and pathological changes after microwave ablation of breast cancer: a pilot study. Eur J Radiol 83(10):1771–1777

Zippel DB, Papa MZ (2005) The use of MR imaging guided focused ultrasound in breast cancer patients; a preliminary phase one study and review. Breast Cancer 12(1):32–38

Post-therapy Evaluation (Including Breast Implants)

Silvia Pérez Rodrigo and Julia Camps-Herrero

Contents

1 **Introduction** 376

2 **Post-therapy Changes Without Reconstruction** 377
  2.1 The Basis for Iatrogenic Changes in the Breast 377
  2.2 Timeline for Iatrogenic Changes in Breast 381
  2.3 Mastectomy 382
  2.4 Breast-Conserving Treatment 383

3 **Heterologous and Implant-Based Breast Reconstruction (IBR)** 390
  3.1 Breast Implants 391
  3.2 Complementary Meshes 406

4 **Autologous Breast Reconstruction (ABR)** 407
  4.1 Autologous Flaps 407
  4.2 Lipofilling, Lipomodeling, or Free-Fat Injection 413

References 414

Abstract

Breast cancer treatment has evolved over time being the breast conservative surgery with adyuvant radiation therapy the gold standard treatment. However the mastectomy rates have also increased and new reconstructive techniques have been developed achieving not only a safe oncological result but also a greast cosmetic results result. The radiologist should be aware of the radiological findings that can be observed after the different types of surgery and reconstruction and how to combine the different imaging techniques to fo that purpose.

S. P. Rodrigo (✉)
Head of Breast Radiology Department,
MD Anderson Cancer Center, Madrid, Spain

J. Camps-Herrero
Chief of Breast Health, Ribera Salud Hospitals,
Valencia, Spain
e-mail: jcamps@riberasalud.es

© Springer Nature Switzerland AG 2022
M. Fuchsjäger et al. (eds.), *Breast Imaging*, Medical Radiology Diagnostic Imaging,
https://doi.org/10.1007/978-3-030-94918-1_18

Table 1 Diagnostic accuracy of clinical examination and radiologic diagnostic methods in the evaluation of the treated patient

Clinical examination	Mammography	Ultrasound	MRI
• Worse prognosis when the lesion is palpable	• Limited sensitivity and specificity		• Highest sensitivity and specificity
	• Difficult compression	• Posterior shadowing	• Morphology and function
	• Difficult differentiating scar from recurrence; difficult differentiating edema post-RT from lymphatic vessel involvement	• Difficult differentiating scar from recurrence	• Benign lesions may enhance after IVC administration

1 Introduction

Breast cancer treatment has evolved over time, and currently the gold standard is breast-conservative surgery with adjuvant radiation therapy (RT). This approach has decreased the morbidity with the same survival rates and has improved the aesthetic outcomes. Another therapeutic option is mastectomy, considered until recently a second-choice technique. However, diagnostic improvements with increased detection of additional lesions, as well as better surgical reconstruction techniques, have recently increased mastectomy rates. In any case, one of the most important issues is to obtain free margins, in spite of which recurrence is still possible, even after a mastectomy. In addition, many patients undergo aesthetic procedures with endogenous and exogenous material, not only for reconstructive reasons but also for aesthetic reasons. Therefore, the radiologist should be aware of the radiological findings that can be seen after the different types of surgery and reconstruction and should also know the most reliable imaging techniques for that purpose (Perez et al. 2017; Siegel et al. 2016) (Table 1).

Mammography is the technique of choice to detect early breast cancer. Nevertheless, it has limited sensitivity, from 55% to 68%. In addition, after a surgical intervention the performance of the test is more limited, due to the fact that it is difficult to obtain an adequate compression and to achieve visualization of the whole breast and the axillary region. In spite of this fact, there may be some radiological findings that can be misinterpreted, as for example the presence of distortion that requires a differential diagnosis between recurrence and scar changes, or the presence of edema that requires a differential diagnosis between post-radiotherapy changes and lymphatic involvement.

Clinical examination has proved to be complementary to mammography in detecting recurrence, but tumors detected only at screening mammography are less likely to develop metastases during follow-up because they usually present at an early stage. In cases of mastectomy, in which mammography cannot be performed, the clinical examination has high sensitivity.

Ultrasound has also a limited sensitivity for small or noninvasive lesions. The presence of posterior acoustic shadowing requires a differential diagnosis between fibrous scar and recurrence.

Breast MRI has high sensitivity and high specificity compared to mammography and clinical examination (from 90% to 100% and 83% to 93%, respectively). At 12–18 months posttreatment, it is the most reliable technique to differentiate scar from recurrence. The absence of enhancement after intravenous contrast (IVC) suggests fibrous scar. However, the presence of enhancement is not always indicative of malignancy since there are many benign processes that can cause uptake, such as fat necrosis.

2 Post-therapy Changes Without Reconstruction

2.1 The Basis for Iatrogenic Changes in the Breast

Iatrogenic changes that take place in the breast can be explained in terms of

1. Changes due to fluid collections
   (a) Seroma
   (b) Hematoma
   (c) Abscess
2. Changes due to fat necrosis
   (a) Edema and skin-thickening phase
   (b) Scar formation and inflammatory phase (architectural distortions)
   (c) Lipid cyst formation phase
   (d) Chronic granulomatous phase or foreign bodies (calcifications)

Most clinical contexts that will be shown in this chapter share the same iatrogenic changes due to the fact that the underlying mechanisms are the same (i.e., fluid collections, fat necrosis, foreign bodies, and anatomical changes). The following text will deal mainly with the causes, the timeline, and the influence of these changes on the radiological study of the breast (Fig. 1).

The imaging appearance of the breast following surgery or radiation therapy reflects the specific surgical methods employed, the amount of radiation delivered, the temporal facts, the proportion of glandular-to-fatty tissue, and the overall breast size (Mendelson 1989).

Routine follow-up of patients treated for breast cancer does not include breast MRI. However, because of the limitations of mammography and ultrasound in these patients, MRI may be a valuable addition in the case of these patients. It certainly is a very helpful tool in the workup of a possible recurrence when the conventional techniques are equivocal.

2.1.1 Changes Due to Fluid Collections

1. Seromas are fluid collections as a result that in closing the surgical wound, only the skin is sutured. The breast parenchyma, fatty tissue, and subcutaneous elements are not re-approximated surgically. Although surgical drains are placed, sometimes the surgical cav-

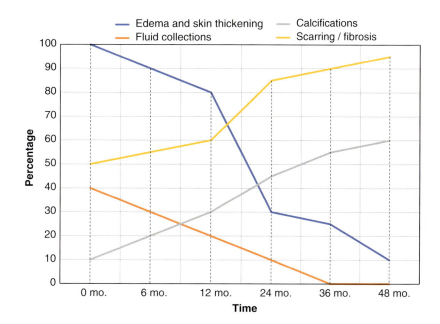

Fig. 1 Graph depicts the frequency of characteristic mammographic findings in 6- and 12-month intervals after breast conservation therapy. (Khrisnamurythy et al. Mammographic findings after breast conservation therapy. Radiographics 1999:19:S53–S62)

ity fills up with fluid (serum), forming a seroma. Seromas are usually simple cystic masses with a well-defined border but can also contain septa. They disappear frequently after 9–12 months, although they can also remain in the breast for longer. Seromas are hyperintense on T2 sequences and do not enhance (Figs. 2 and 3).
2. Hematomas: Acute hemorrhagic collections may contain debris, but after the first week or 2, most are simple fluid collections (Fig. 4). Signal intensity in T2-weighted images and unenhanced T1-weighted sequences varies depending on the timing; most frequently, chronic hematomas are hypointense on T2 and hyperintense on T1 unenhanced images. Hematomas show a subtle rim enhancement which is thin. The timeline of hematomas is identical to that of seromas.

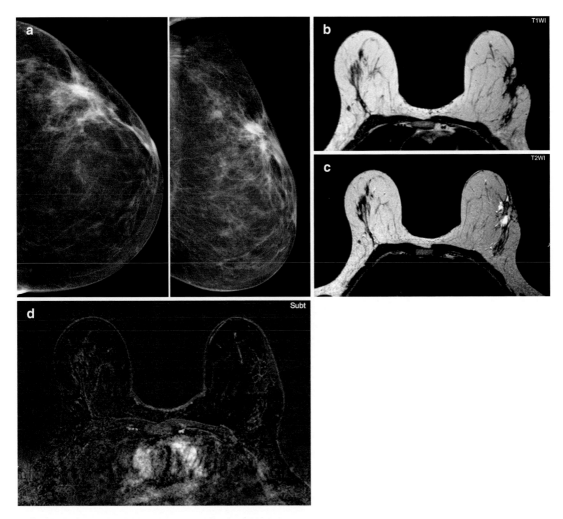

Fig. 2 Fifty-two-year-old woman with an IDC in UOQ of left breast treated with surgery and chemotherapy. An MRI was performed 9 months after the surgery and chemotherapy and before the radiotherapy. (**a**) Left-breast mammography. Skin thickening is seen in that quadrant. (**b, c**) T1 and T2 sequences show an evolved hematoma with hyperintense areas in both sequences (blue circle) combined with hyperintense in T1 sequence and hypointense in T2 sequence areas (red circle). (**d**) Subtracted images do not show any enhancement

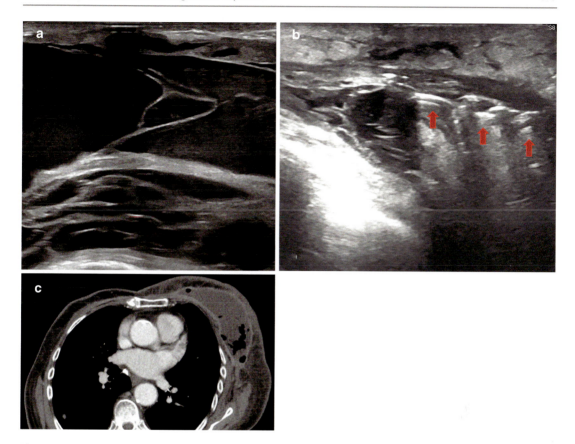

Fig. 3 Seroma 2 months after a mastectomy in a 74-year-old patient. (**a**) It showed an atypical appearance with multiple thick and irregular septa. Due to the large size (all the mastectomy bed) and the associated clinical symptoms, the patient underwent several drainages. Sometime later, the seroma did not disappear and additionally the patient had skin thickening, edema, and redness. (**b**) The ultrasound showed a more complex lesion with multiple hyperechogenic areas (red arrows) suggesting gas. (**c**) The CT also showed the collection, confirming the presence of gas inside, which obliged to rule out an abscess or infection

3. Abscesses are formed as a result of an infected cavity, usually rare, as less than 5–10% of the fluid collections become infected (Fig. 3). Abscesses usually show a thick rim enhancement, with a cystic central component. This rim enhances in a similar way to breast neoplasms.

2.1.2 Changes Due to Fat Necrosis

The pathogenesis of fat necrosis is very helpful to explain the radiological features (edema, skin thickening, architectural distortion, and calcifications) (Ganau et al. 2009). The interaction between the adipocytes and the microvessels is the key to all the findings and undergoes different phases that may overlap:

1. Phase 1: Edema formation:

   During this phase, vessel damage generates an inflammatory reaction that initially causes vasoconstriction of arterioles (to prevent bleeding) with posterior vasodilatation. This increases the intravessel pressure and plasma leaks into the tissue, causing edema and fluid collections (hematomas and seromas), which can be seen in different forms depending on the imaging technique. In breast MRI, it is usually high signal intensity on T2WI and hypointense in T1WI. This edema does not enhance after contrast injection.

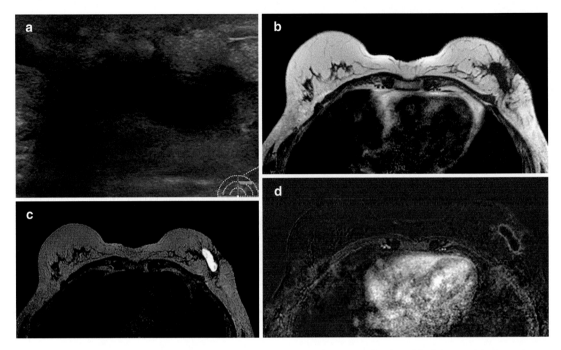

Fig. 4 Woman with conservative surgery some days ago with positive margins and hemorrhagic collection in UOQ of left breast. (**a**) Ultrasound shows a fluid collection. (**b**) T1-WI shows a hypointense collection. (**c**) T2-WI shows a hyperintense collection. (**d**) Subtracted images show a peripheral and thin rim enhancement. There was no macroscopic evidence of residual tumor

2. Phase 2: Scar formation and inflammatory changes:

    Damage to the vessels activates a cascade that ends with the production of fibrin, a protein that forms a meshwork with platelets with the aim of controlling bleeding. This meshwork also serves as a scaffold for fibroblasts and angioblasts. Fibroblasts create the extracellular matrix of granulation, and angioblasts are necessary for angiogenesis. The association with leukocytes and macrophages will form the granulation tissue that will mature into a scar. Findings on MRI will vary depending on the stage of the scar formation, and the main point is that angiogenesis is the cause for peripheral contrast enhancement in this phase, to be taken into account in order to differentiate it from cancer recurrence. Scarring in breast MRI, mammography, or ultrasound will be seen as an architectural distortion (Fig. 5).

3. Phase 3: Lipid cyst formation:

    Rupture of fat cells causes lipid contents to be released into the interstitium, which in turn causes chemical irritation and inflammation. A fibrous capsule may form around the oily fatty acids forming a lipid cyst. In case of precipitation of calcium salts along the capsule, a lipid cyst with "eggshell calcifications" may form. These are seen in MRI as well-defined nodules that are hyperintense on T1WI and hypo- or hyperintense on T2WI. Enhancement of the capsule might be seen depending on the phase of the granulation tissue.

4. Phase 4: Foreign body and chronic granulomatous change:

    Another pathway for released fatty acids is to form a chronic granulomatous reaction in case of interaction with the immune system. Over time, a fibrous reaction or calcification may appear. MRI findings may be similar to those of both phases described above (Fig. 6).

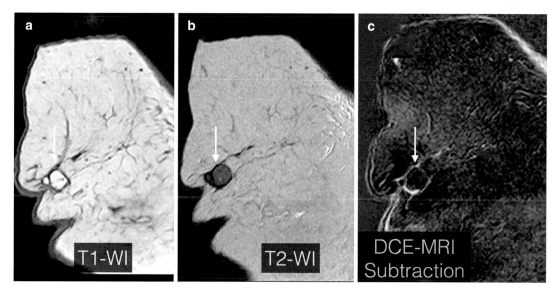

Fig. 5 Chronic hematoma: (**a**) hyperintense appearance on unenhanced T1-weighted images, (**b**) hypointense on T2-weighted images, and (**c**) dynamic contrast-enhanced T1-weighted images, where a subtle well-defined rim enhancement can be seen

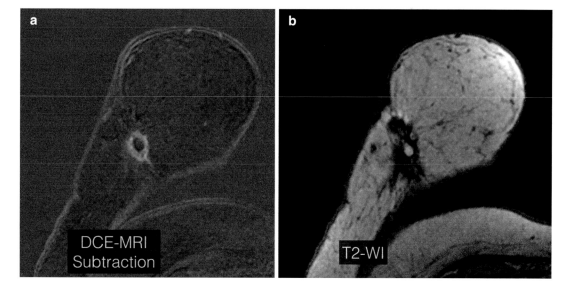

Fig. 6 Fat necrosis, inflammatory phase. (**a**) Dynamic contrast-enhanced T1-weighted images, where a peripheral rim enhancement can be seen. (**b**) T2-weighted image where the hypointense and partially enhancing (in T1-WI) fibrosis or scar tissue surrounds a hyperintense central area that corresponds with fat. If fat saturation methods are used, the central area would be hypointense, just like the rest of the fatty tissue

2.2 Timeline for Iatrogenic Changes in Breast

1. Edema and skin thickening are present in all patients and gradually resolve over time, being present only in 20% of the patients after 36 months.
2. Scarring and fibrosis are present in all patients after 36 months and remain stable thereafter.

3. Fluid collections are present only in 40% of the patients and start to disappear after 6–12 months, being very rare after 36 months.
4. Calcifications are rare during the first 12 months but will be present in 60% of the patients after 36 months (Fig. 1).

Granulation tissue starts forming 2–3 weeks after surgery. In case of performing MRI for residual disease, it should be performed during the first week after surgery, or we will encounter enhancement secondary to granulation tissue formation that can lead us to false-positive findings (Fig. 7).

It is also important to know that radiation therapy changes show enhancement up to 18 months after the end of the treatment. Any enhancement seen after 18–20 months should be viewed with suspicion, and recurrence should be ruled out.

2.3 Mastectomy

Mastectomy is the complete excision of the breast tissue. The state of the art recommends the excision of the nipple-areolar complex (NAC), the skin overlying, and the pectoral fascia. Despite that, residual tissue sometimes exists and then the recurrence is possible. That is why it is important to determine if there is residual tissue after a mastectomy since that will change the patient's follow-up protocol (Neal et al. 2014).

2.3.1 Radiological Tests and Findings
1. Mammography is not routinely performed in mastectomy patients, but it should be performed in order to determine the presence of residual breast tissue whenever it is feasible. In those cases, a fatty breast or breast with scattered fibroglandular tissue can be seen, difficult to differentiate sometimes from scar tissue (Fig. 8).
2. Ultrasound is the technique of choice for examining the mastectomy bed. Subcutaneous fat, pectoral muscle, and fibrosis can be seen as well as possible complications as seromas or hematomas. Nodular lesions suggest recur-

rence. Distortions or acoustic posterior shadowing can be a postsurgical finding or a recurrence (Lee et al. 2013).
3. MRI is the best technique for evaluating the type of surgery and the anatomical structures, showing the pectoral muscle when present, the axillary region, and the internal mammary chain. It is the choice technique for differentiating scar from recurrence, especially in those doubtful cases on ultrasound. In addition, in those patients without a mammography after the surgery for evaluating breast residual tissue, one MRI should be performed, and patients with residual tissue should be followed up with MRI every year or every 2 years (Fig. 8).

2.3.2 Recurrence and Follow-Up
Although mastectomy is supposed to entail a complete resection of the breast tissue, histologic exams have shown that some glandular breast tissue remains after the surgery, so recurrence is possible, and surveillance is still needed.

About 10–15% of patients will develop a locoregional recurrence, and nearly one-third will present with synchronous metastases at diagnosis (Kim et al. 2010). The most common form of recurrence is local (50–70%), which tends to be symptomatic (Fig. 9). Single or multiple masses, skin or chest wall involvement (Fig. 10), and presence of suspicious calcifications can be seen (Yilmaz et al. 2007). Those findings should be differentiated from dystrophic calcifications or fat necrosis. The other form of presentation is with regional or distant lymph node involvement (30–40%), which is usually asymptomatic. Some locations such as supraclavicular, axillar, and internal mammary regions can cause pain, brachial plexopathy, or arm lymphedema (Fig. 11). A recurrence should be ruled out with any new-onset lymphedema after treatment (Perez et al. 2017).

There is no consensus about the follow-up of these patients, but at least one MRI or mammography examination after the surgery should be performed to evaluate the presence of residual fibroglandular tissue (Fig. 12). Ultrasound and MRI are the techniques of choice for follow-up,

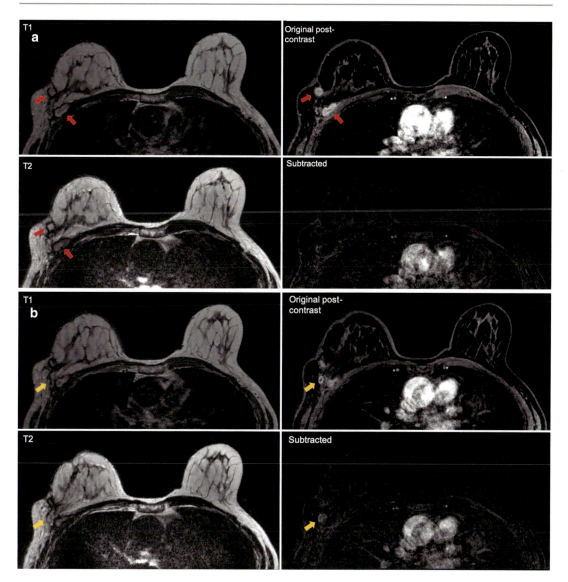

Fig. 7 Patient treated of hormonal receptor-positive IDC in UOQ of right breast. Axillary lymph node dissection was also performed showing one lymph node involved with IDC grade III with a different morphologic pattern being HER2+. Then, a second tumor in breast was suspected. MRI was performed 2 weeks after surgery. (**a**) Postsurgical changes were noted in the lumpectomy area with some collections related to evolved hematomas, hyperintense on T1 and T2 sequences (red arrow), but without enhancement in subtracted sequence. (**b**) Close to the postsurgical changes, there was an oval lesion (yellow arrow) with a rim enhancement in the subtracted images that corresponded to a second primary breast cancer

but the screening should be adapted to the patient risk. If the patient has an increased risk of breast cancer (>20%) or the breast cancer diagnosis was at an age younger than 50 years or premenopausal, annual MRI is recommended in addition to the screening ultrasound.

2.4 Breast-Conserving Treatment

Breast-conserving surgery is considered the first choice of treatment. It includes a surgical procedure in which only a portion of breast is removed (lumpectomy, segmentectomy, or quadrantec-

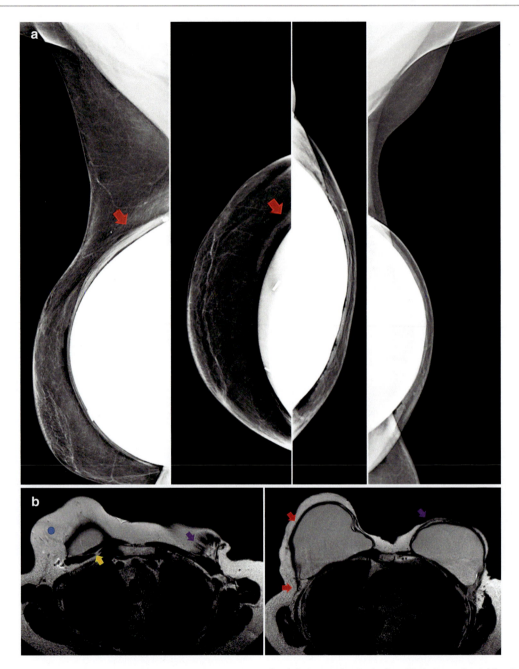

Fig. 8 Patient with a personal history of DCIS in right breast and posteriorly bilateral IDC. Patient underwent bilateral mastectomy and mixed reconstruction with latissimus dorsi and silicone implant in right breast and with a heterologous reconstruction with silicone implant in left breast. Fat-free injection (lipofilling) was performed in both breasts. (**a**) Bilateral mammography with CC and MLO views was performed to determine the presence of residual fibroglandular tissue. There was an absence of residual tissue in left breast, but there were doubts about the right breast due to the fat of latissimus dorsi. The density of latissimus dorsi can be seen (red arrow) on the right breast. (**b**, **c**) Axial and sagittal planes on T2-WI confirmed the presence of residual tissue on the right breast (blue circles). In the right breast, the implant is located between the latissimus dorsi, which comes from the back (red arrow), and the pectoral muscle (yellow arrow). In the left breast, the implant has a retro-pectoral location behind the pectoral muscle (purple arrow)

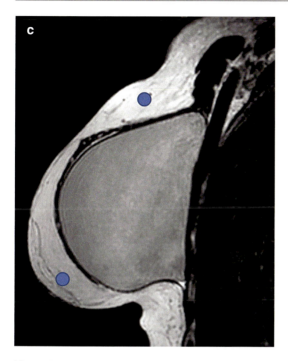

Fig. 8 (continued)

tomy) and adjuvant RT. The breast surgeon usually leaves metallic clips in the cavity edges to mark the outline of the surgical resection (Neal et al. 2014; Chansakul et al. 2012a).

2.4.1 Radiological Tests and Findings

Normal radiological findings after a conservative treatment can be misinterpreted as a recurrence, mainly because of the presence of fibrous and scar tissue and because of fat necrosis (Tayyab et al. 2018). It is essential to be familiar with the chronological changes that will occur (Mendelson 1992) (Fig. 1). These benign changes should decrease or remain stable over time at least 2–3 years after the radiation treatment (RT).

1. Mammography is routinely performed after conservative treatment. The most common findings are skin thickening, increased breast density, seroma, architectural distortion, scarring, dystrophic calcifications, and asymmetries (Neal et al. 2014; Ramani et al. 2017).
    (a) Edema and skin thickening will present the highest expression at 6 months after RT, and later they usually regress. It may be focal in the surgical area because of postsurgical changes or diffuse because of post-RT changes (Fig. 13). If there is an increase in edema, a differential diagnosis has to be established with obstruction of venous drainage, congestive heart failure (Fig. 14), infection, or lymph vessel involvement (Mertz et al. 1998; Libshitz et al. 1978).
    (b) Seroma or hematoma can be seen on the initial mammography following surgery. It appears as a round and oval mass or well-defined density due to the fluid-filled cavity. Sometimes, the mass or density may be partially obscured by the surrounding breast edema. Most of them will be replaced by connective tissue and fibrosis during the following months and disappear within 12–18 months after surgery, but sometimes they remain stable over time.
    (c) Architectural distortion appears as a spiculated or irregular density, poorly defined, associated with skin retraction. The presence of a central radiolucency, thick spiculations, and different imaging appearances with different mammographic views suggest more likely a postsurgical origin (Fig. 15). In addition, it should reach its highest expression at 2 years and later, be stable, or decrease in size and density. Other techniques like tomosynthesis, magnified and spot compressed views, are very useful. Comparison with previous studies and correlation with unchanged mammograms can lead to a correct interpretation. In case of doubt, an MRI or biopsy can be performed.
    (d) Asymmetries in size and density can be noted after postsurgical changes. Sometimes, they may be the only radiological finding of a previous surgery especially when the metallic clips are not present.
    (e) Calcifications usually appear as typically benign, as large (>5 mm), lucent-centered, eggshell, or rim-like calcifications.

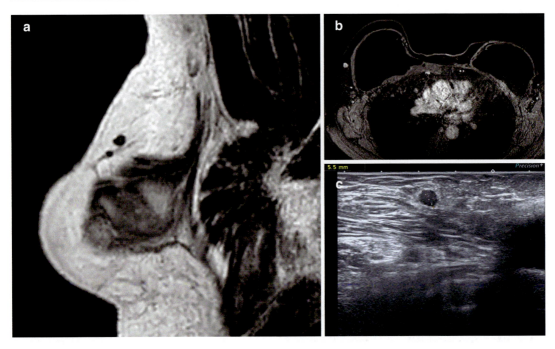

Fig. 9 Same patient as in Fig. 8. The surveillance was annually performed with right mammogram (due to the autologous flap) and MRI (due to the high risk of cancer). One routinely performed MRI showed a nodular lesion in UOQ of the right breast that resembled an intramammary lymph node. (**a**) In T2 sagittal plane, a fatty center seemed to be seen. (**b**) Axial first dynamic sequence showed rim enhancement. (**c**) Second-look ultrasound showed a nodular lesion without fatty center. Then, core needle biopsy was performed with an IDC recurrence. Note that in this case, the recurrence was asymptomatic and only detected by MRI

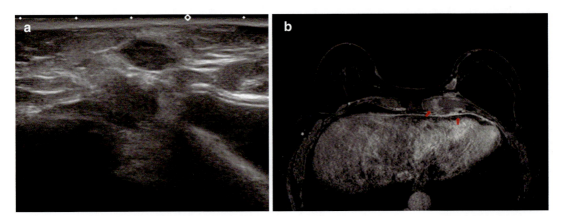

Fig. 10 Patient with a personal history of left-breast carcinoma, mastectomy, and implant-based reconstruction. (**a**) Ultrasound was performed due to a palpable lump in LIQ showing a nodular hypoechoic and well-circumscribed lesion. (**b**) Axial first post-contrast sequence at MRI showed a nodular and circumscribed lesion with rim enhancement. Additionally, enhancement of the area of mammary internal chain and a pericardiac enhancement (red arrows) were observed suggesting malignancy. These findings were only seen at MRI. Core true cut was performed with IDC result, and PET/CT was also performed detecting pericardiac involvement

Post-therapy Evaluation (Including Breast Implants) 387

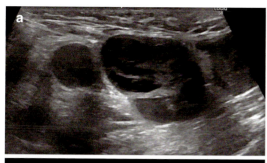
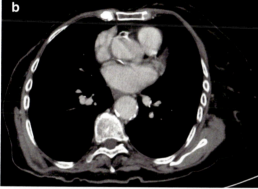
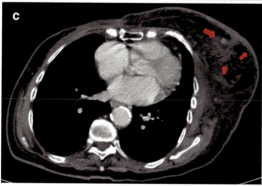

Fig. 11 Patient with a personal history of right-breast carcinoma and mastectomy without reconstruction. Patient developed a left-arm lymphedema and inflammatory changes of left breast (contralateral to the breast carcinoma). (**a**) Axillary ultrasound showed multiple pathological lymph nodes. (**b**) Thoracic CT performed before the onset of lymphedema, in the year 2017, was normal. (**c**) Thoracic CT performed after the onset of lymphedema, in the year 2018, showed marked skin thickening, subcutaneous edema, and some nodular lesions (red arrows). The patient underwent surgery with the result of contralateral sarcoma metastasis. Then, any new-onset lymphedema after treatment should rule out a recurrence or new tumor

Commonly, dystrophic and suture calcifications due to fat necrosis or calcium over the suture material can be seen (Fig. 13). Linear, branching, and pleomorphic calcifications should be considered suspicious and warrant a stereotactic biopsy or MRI to distinguish from scarring and fat necrosis.

2. Ultrasound may be complementary to mammography in order to distinguish recurrence from postsurgical changes. Some of the benign findings that can be observed are architectural distortion or a mass.
   (a) Skin thickening, trabecular thickening in the subcutaneous fat, and edema can be produced because of postsurgical and post-RT changes. Some fluid collections can be seen interspersed with the fatty tissue (Fig. 13).
   (b) Posterior acoustic shadowing related to postsurgical scarring is usually seen. Sometimes, the posterior aspect of a lesion is obscured. A practical tip for the differential diagnosis with recurrence is to change the orientation of the probe (Fig. 16). If the image is present in both views, an MRI or biopsy may be required.
   (c) A poorly marginated soft-tissue mass can be noted as a part of the evolutionary process towards a scar, but it usually contains radiolucent areas centrally and decreases in size and density over time.
   (d) Postoperative seroma or hematoma can have variable appearances on ultrasound (Boostrom et al. 2009). An anechoic or hypoechoic, round or oval, and well-defined mass is usually seen, but sometimes a complex (solid-cystic) mass which usually decreases over time can appear (Fig. 17). In some cases, these lesions remain unchanged over time and become chronic. In this case, the differential diagnosis with a recurrent or suspicious mass may warrant a biopsy if previous studies are not available.

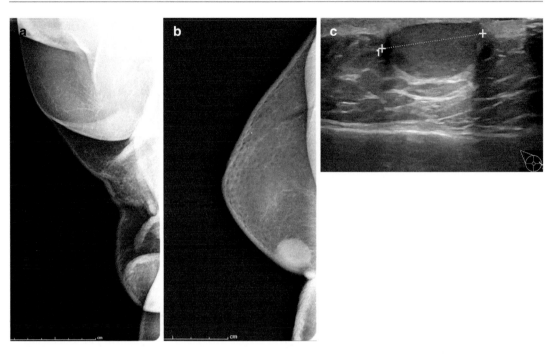

Fig. 12 Patient with a personal history of right-breast carcinoma without reconstruction. Bilateral mammography was performed 1 year after surgery, including the right breast, to evaluate the presence of residual parenchyma. (**a**) Although right MLO view did not show evidence of residual fibroglandular tissue, CC view (**b**) showed a benign nodule in inner quadrants. (**c**) Ultrasound confirmed the presence of that nodule

3. MRI is the technique of choice for differentiation of scar from recurrence due to its high negative predictive value (Chansakul et al. 2012b; Gigli et al. 2017; Soderstrom et al. 1997). Benign findings as skin thickening, trabecular thickening, breast edema related to post-RT changes, and fluid-filled cavities related to seromas are common (Fig. 7). An artifact due to surgical sutures or clips can be observed, especially in gradient-echo sequences, and sometimes is the only radiological finding of a previous surgery. The presence of a complex cystic and solid lesion can be seen when a hematoma or seroma becomes chronic. The most specific signs are the absence of enhancement in the dynamic sequences or the presence of a thin and smooth rim enhancement around the seroma. However, the presence of a nodular or an irregular enhancement should require a second-look ultrasound and a biopsy.

2.4.2 Recurrence and Follow-Up

The risk of recurrence is about 1–2% per year. There are two types of recurrences, early or late. Early recurrence usually occurs at the site of the original tumor, within the two first years after surgery, and represents a failure of treatment over the primary tumor (Fig. 18) (Gigli et al. 2017; Dershaw et al. 1990). Late recurrence can occur at a distance from the treated area; it is most common after 10 years of treatment completion and usually represents a new primary tumor. Early detection is crucial because it is associated to improved survival (Colleoni et al. 2016).

Follow-up of these patients can be overwhelming, but knowledge of the previous history, comparison with previous studies, and evolution are essential for differentiating benign from recurrence since stability is usually achieved 2–3 years after treatment (Gunhan-Bilgen and Oktay 2007). After this period of time, any new density, mass, or suspicious calcifications should be biopsied to rule out recurrence (Fig. 19).

In cases of primary tumors with calcifications, a baseline mammogram just before RT could be performed in order to ensure their complete excision. A baseline mammography should be performed 6–8 months after finishing treatment.

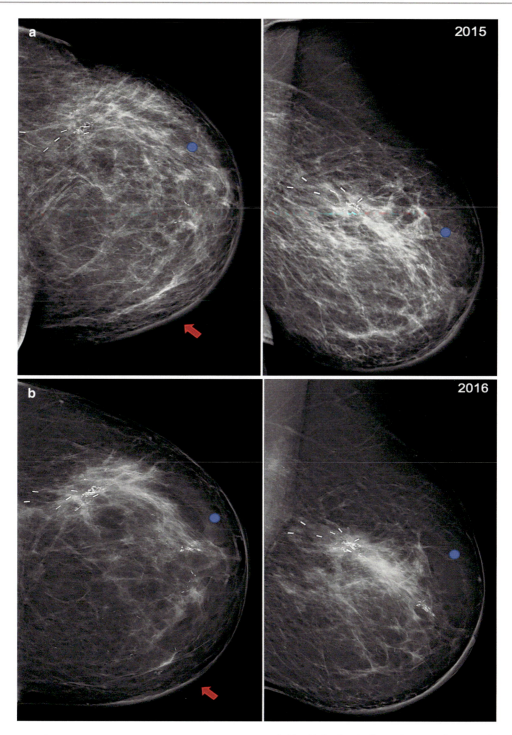

Fig. 13 Patient with a previous history of breast carcinoma in UOQ of left breast with conservative surgery and radiotherapy. (**a**) CC and MLO views of left mammography 1 year later showed diffuse edema (blue dot) and skin thickening (red arrow). (**b**) Follow-up mammography performed next year showed decrease of the edema (blue dot) and skin thickening (red arrow), suggesting normal evolution. (**c**) Magnified view showed multiple benign calcifications, dystrophic (yellow arrow) and suture calcifications (red arrows). (**d**) Ultrasound performed some months after the surgery showed edema and trabecular thickening in the subcutaneous fat

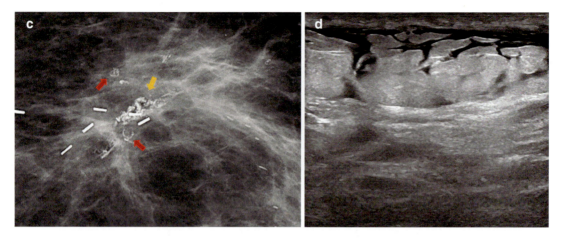

Fig. 13 (continued)

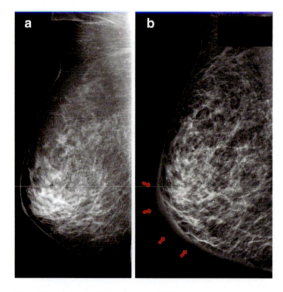

Fig. 14 Patient with a personal history of breast cancer. The surveillance was performed with mammography every year. (**a**) MLO view of right breast with benign findings. (**b**) MLO view of right breast performed the next year showed diffuse skin thickening (red arrow) and marked edema compared to previous mammography. A carcinoma was ruled out being those findings related to a congestive heart failure

After that, an annual mammography performed 2 years after RT is recommended, since thereafter the posttreatment changes should remain unchanged or decrease. An annual complementary ultrasound is optional (Berg et al. 2008). MRI is the most useful imaging technique during the follow-up period due to its high negative predictive value, but the cost and the availability can be a problem in some hospitals (Chansakul et al. 2012b; Swinnen et al. 2018; Lam et al. 2017; Spronk et al. 2018; Cho et al. 2017; Shah et al. 2016).

3 Heterologous and Implant-Based Breast Reconstruction (IBR)

Heterologous reconstruction is the most common type of breast reconstruction following cancer treatment. After mastectomy or conservative treatment, exogenous materials like implants or free injection of different substances as hyaluronic acid are used to compensate for the tissue defect to remodel the breast (Leibman and Misra 2011; Lui et al. 2008; Khedher et al. 2011; Teo and Wang 2008). The hyaluronic acid has been withdrawn for this purpose due to safety concerns because of the possibility of migration to other parts of the body, because of promoting the development of breast cancer, and because sometimes it produces radiological findings that can be difficult to differentiate from malignancy (Wong et al. 2016; Margolis et al. 2014).

Implant-based reconstruction or IBR is the heterologous reconstruction most commonly per-

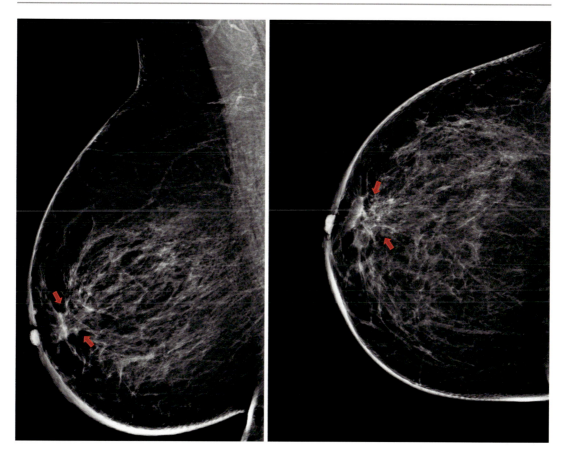

Fig. 15 Forty-two-year-old patient with a previous history of IDC in UQ of right breast in periareolar region, undergoing conserving surgery and RT. Follow-up mammography with CC and MLO views was performed 1 year and 3 months after surgery showing a distortion with thick spiculations and a central radiolucency corresponding to postsurgical changes (red arrows). In this case, there were no metallic clips. Note the presence of skin thickening

formed, and, in some cases, it can involve a biological mesh or acellular dermal matrix (ADM) additionally to the implant (Dellacroce and Wolfe 2013). Some of the advantages of the IBR over the autologous breast reconstruction (ABR) are lower morbidity rates since there is no donor site and it is a simpler procedure, shorter surgical and recovery times, no additional scars, and similar aesthetic aspect in color and texture to the adjacent tissue. However, there are also some disadvantages which include often necessary long-term adjustment, worse natural-looking breast, RT results in 40–50% capsular contractures, and implant-related complications (Gerber et al. 2015).

3.1 Breast Implants

Since the introduction of breast augmentation in the 1960s, many women have undergone these procedures for aesthetic reasons as well as reconstructive surgery following breast cancer. Their use has increased in the last decades. Therefore, the American College of Radiology (ACR) has included implant evaluation in the latest edition of the BI-RADS lexicon.

Breast implants are devices composed of silicone gel, saline (Fig. 20), or a combination of both, surrounded by an elastomer silicone shell. The immune system recognizes them as a foreign body and reacts forming a fibrous or external cap-

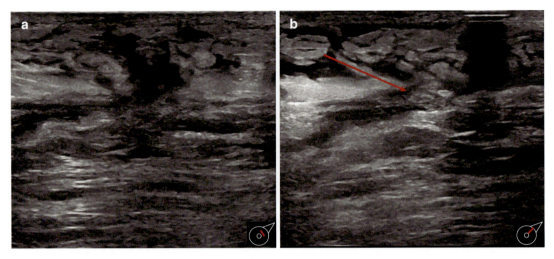

Fig. 16 Patient with a previous history of breast-conserving surgery. (**a**) Ultrasound showed a poorly circumscribed lesion, hypoechoic with posterior shadowing. (**b**) Ultrasound changing the orientation of the probe showed changes in the lesion appearance, adopting a linear morphology (red arrow) which allowed to do the differential diagnosis with a recurrence

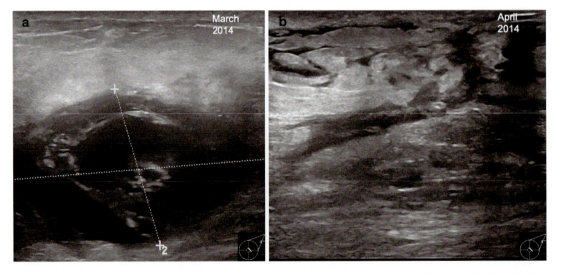

Fig. 17 Patient with a previous history of breast-conservative surgery and RT. Some months after the surgery, the patient consulted for pain, redness, and lump in that area. (**a**) Ultrasound showed a complex fluid collection related to an evolving hematoma that shortly after decreased. (**b**) Ultrasound 1 month later, the collection had decreased significantly

sule. They are placed in retro-glandular (Figs. 21 and 23) or retro-pectoral location (Figs. 22 and 23). There are various types regarding the number of lumen and their content, but the most common are unicameral (Figs. 20 and 23) (single lumen with saline or silicone-gel filled) and bicameral (or double lumen, usually with saline inner lumen and silicone outer lumen but being able to be the opposite). Both single- and double-lumen implants can have a permanent or temporary purpose. After mastectomy, if the skin and pectoral muscle could not cover an implant of the required

Post-therapy Evaluation (Including Breast Implants)

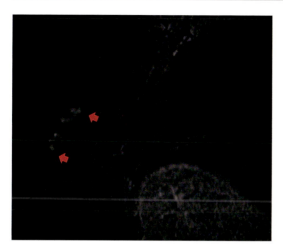

Fig. 18 Patient with a personal history of breast-conserving surgery in UOQ of the right breast. Follow-up was performed with bilateral mammography and breast MRI. Sagittal reconstruction of the axial first subtracted image showed some non-mass enhancements in that quadrant, with a linear distribution. Two MRI-guided biopsies of both ends were performed (red arrows) with a positive result for malignancy

size, a temporary implant or expander with at least one saline lumen is placed and the surgeon goes filling it over time until reaching the desirable volume. The unicameral expander (Fig. 24) has a metallic fill-in valve in its anterior margin. The bicameral expander (Fig. 25) has a connector or tube (lying posteriorly) that extends from the inner lumen to the titanium fill-in valve, which is separated and located, as a subcutaneous port, lateral to the implant. Posteriorly, the expander can be placed indefinitely or be replaced by a definitive and common silicone-gel implant.

3.1.1 Radiological Tests

Clinical examination is limited in implant evaluation and has low sensitivity for detecting ruptures. Therefore, imaging tests are necessary (Glynn and Litherland 2008; Berg et al. 1993; Shah and Jankharia 2016; Juanpere et al. 2011; Gorczyca et al. 2007; Brenner 2013; Pinel-Giroux et al. 2013).

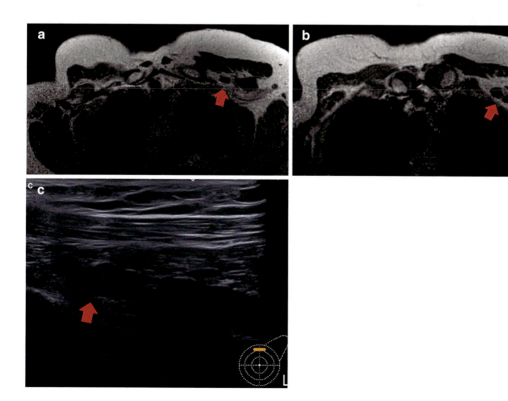

Fig. 19 Patient with a personal history of breast-conserving surgery in UOQ of the right breast 11 years ago. Follow-up was performed with bilateral mammography and breast MRI. (**a, b**) Axial T1-WI sequences showed the presence of some pathological contralateral axillary lymph nodes at the second and third levels. (**c**) Ultrasound was performed and showed those enlarged lymph nodes of left axilla without fatty hilum. A core needle biopsy was performed with the result of malignancy

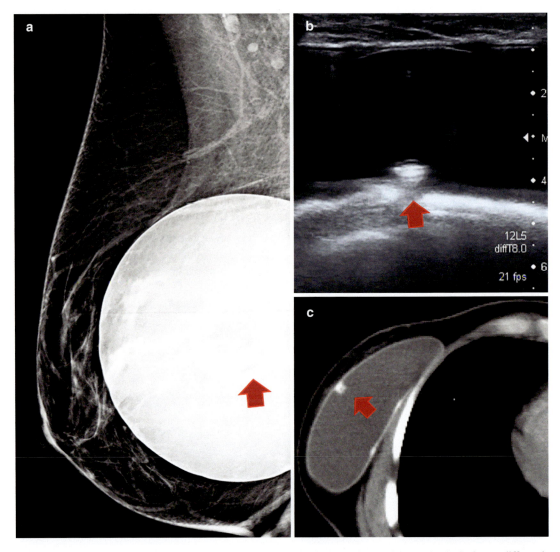

Fig. 20 Patient with a personal history of breast-conserving surgery in UOQ of the left breast and bilateral heterologous reconstruction with saline implants. (**a**) MLO view of the right breast shows lower density of the implant than that of a silicone implant. (**b**) Ultrasound shows anechoic appearance, identical to that of a silicone implant. Note that the filling valve is the key to differentiate a silicone implant. (**c**) CT is also showing the filling valve and the water density of the implant. (**d**) MRI axial T2-WI shows identical intensity to fluid. The filling valve is pointed with a red arrow in all the images

Mammography has limited sensitivity to evaluate implant integrity, being useful only to show evident deformities, capsular contractures, capsular calcifications (Fig. 26), extracapsular ruptures, and silicone migration through the glandular parenchyma, a very specific sign (Miglioretti et al. 2004).

Ultrasound is a safe and noninvasive test for evaluation of the integrity of the implant, as well as intracapsular and extracapsular rupture. Overall sensitivity and specificity rates range between 59–85% and 55–79%, respectively. It is the technique of choice in guiding interventional procedures without damaging the implant because it provides a direct view of the breast and implant in real time. However, it is an operator-dependent technique, and it is limited in evaluating the posterior aspect of the implant and to

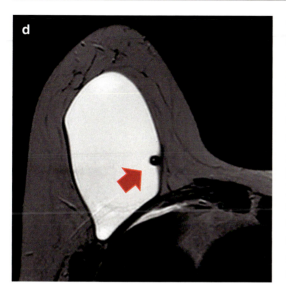

Fig. 20 (continued)

distinguish silicone and saline material (both are anechoic) (Lake et al. 2013).

MRI is the most reliable technique to assess implant integrity. It has high sensitivity (80–90%) and specificity (90–70%) for implant rupture. It has the ability to differentiate silicone from saline and single from double lumen, as well as the expanders. Therefore, it is very useful to detect intracapsular and extracapsular rupture and also silicone migration to axillary and internal mammary lymph nodes as well as to soft tissues. Cost, availability, motion, and artifacts are some of its disadvantages (Belli et al. 2002; Middleton 1998). In order to obtain high-quality images, specific examination protocols are necessary. It is recommended to obtain implant images at least in two perpendicular planes (axial and coronal or axial and sagittal). The sequences used to assess the implant integrity are variable, but at least a white silicone sequence (where fat and water are suppressed, and silicone is white) is necessary. Other complementary sequences are axial T1W, axial T2W, and black silicone (axial STIR with silicone suppression) (Fig. 27). This protocol makes no sense in saline single-lumen implant evaluation since saline will look exactly like liquid in all sequences (Fig. 28), and then if there is a rupture, the patient will know it because the implant volume will decrease. In a similar way, the use of MRI to evaluate saline single-lumen expander with anterior fill valve also makes no sense, since the metallic valve will produce an artifact that will prevent the assessment of that hemithorax. However, MRI is still useful to evaluate the contralateral breast (Fig. 24). The possibility of small movement of the metallic valve because of the magnetic field is not a problem, since the surgeon can locate the valve with the help of a magnet. Therefore, the only obstacle to MRI could be a burning sensation on the skin of the patient which is uncommon. The use of contrast is not necessary if MRI is only intended to evaluate the implant, but in the setting of IBR after breast cancer it is recommended (Wong et al. 2016).

3.1.2 Normal Findings

Implants are seen as well-defined oval masses. The presence of radial or subcapsular folds, a small amount of periprosthetic fluid, rippling, and fibrous bands are considered normal (Perez et al. 2017; Juanpere et al. 2011; Gorczyca et al. 2007).

1. Mammography will show the implant as a hyperdense mass. The oblique view will reveal the implant location with respect to the pectoral muscle. Silicone appears denser than saline (especially if the window is narrowed), and it is possible to distinguish both type of implants when they are unicameral or both chambers when they are bicameral (Figs. 20a and 21a, b).
2. At ultrasound, the implant shows the intact shell as a thin and continuous echogenic line at the parenchyma tissue-implant interface. Both silicone and saline materials have an anechoic appearance (Fig. 25c). Therefore, it is not possible to distinguish both components when there is a bicameral implant or to identify a saline unicameral implant if the clinical history is unknown and the patient also ignores it. Sometimes, the filling valve in saline unicameral implants may be seen in the posterior aspect of it (Fig. 20c). Some normal findings that can be seen are the following:

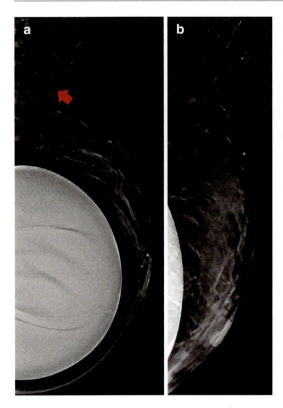

Fig. 21 Patient with a personal history of bilateral breast implants for aesthetic reasons. Screening mammography was performed. (**a**) MLO view showed a unicameral silicone implant and part of the fibroglandular tissue. The pectoral muscle (red arrow) is seen behind the implant which indicates a retro-glandular position. (**b**) Implant-displaced views were performed to be able to view all the fibroglandular tissue avoiding the implant interposition

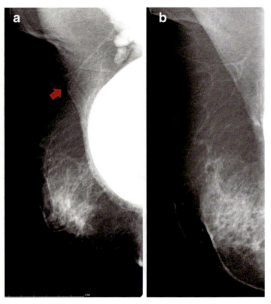

Fig. 22 Patient with a personal history of bilateral unicameral silicone breast implants for aesthetic reasons. Screening mammography was performed. (**a**) MLO view showed silicone implant without abnormalities and the retro-pectoral location with the pectoral muscle (red arrow) above the implant. Part of the fibroglandular tissue is also seen. (**b**) Implant-displaced views (Eklund views) were performed to be able to view all the fibroglandular tissue avoiding the implant interposition

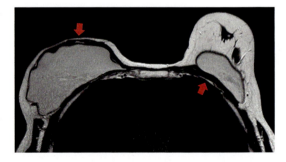

Fig. 23 Patient with a personal history of right-breast carcinoma treated with mastectomy. A reconstruction with a unicameral silicone implant with retro-pectoral location in right breast and with a left mastopexy and unicameral silicone implant with retro-glandular location. Axial T2-WI showing the pectoral muscle pointed with a red arrow going above the implant in the right breast and behind the implant in the left breast

(a) Reverberation artifacts are noted along the anterior aspect of the implant (Fig. 28b).
(b) Subcapsular and radial folds due to in-folding of the implant elastomer can be seen as echogenic lines extending from the periphery to the center of the implant (Fig. 29).
(c) Small amounts of peri-implant fluid (Fig. 29). One must be careful with any new onset of peri-implant fluid time after surgery due to a possible breast implant-associated anaplastic large-cell lymphoma (ALCL) (Adrada et al. 2014; O'Neill et al. 2017; Leberfinger et al. 2017). A FNA will be necessary to do the differential diagnosis with infection, hematoma, and inflammation (Fig. 30).

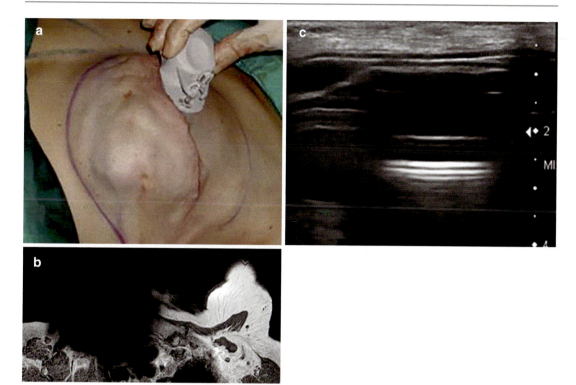

Fig. 24 Patient with a personal history of right mastectomy and temporary reconstruction with a single-lumen expander, which has the filling valve in the front of the implant with a metallic part that the surgeon identifies with a magnet (**a**). (**b**) Axial T1-WI sequence where the right breast is not valuable. However, the contralateral breast can be examined without any problem. (**c**) Ultrasound image can show an inner hyperechoic line below the elastomer that could be misinterpreted as an intracapsular rupture. (**c**) The key is to identify the metallic valve

(d) Some pitfalls can be seen. In patients with bicameral implants (but unknown to us and to the patient), the elastomer of the inner lumen can be misinterpreted as a subcapsular line of a unicameral implant, leading to an incorrect diagnosis of intracapsular rupture (Fig. 25c). Radial and intracapsular folds can also be misinterpreted as an intracapsular rupture, although the radial folds are usually smooth lines presenting as a prolongation of the elastomer. The presence of peri-implant calcifications in old implants with capsular contracture can appear as an irregular or discontinuous line that can be misinterpreted as a shell rupture, especially when there is no previous mammogram or CT (Fig. 26).

3. MRI allows for correct identification of the number of lumens and type of implant. Silicone material will be hypointense in T1 and STIR-weighted images, hyperintense in T2-weighted images, white in white silicone sequences, and black in black silicone sequences. It will show the relationship of the implant to the pectoral muscle. In cases of bicameral expanders, the connector route and valve location can be observed, but it is important to widen the field of view and review the gradient-echo sequences where both components are more evident (Figs. 20, 21, 22, 23, 24, and 25).

   (a) Radial folds are often seen as a normal feature, although, when complex, it can occasionally be difficult to differentiate from an intracapsular rupture. The presence of fluid outside of the elastomer is the key to make the differential diagnosis (Fig. 29).

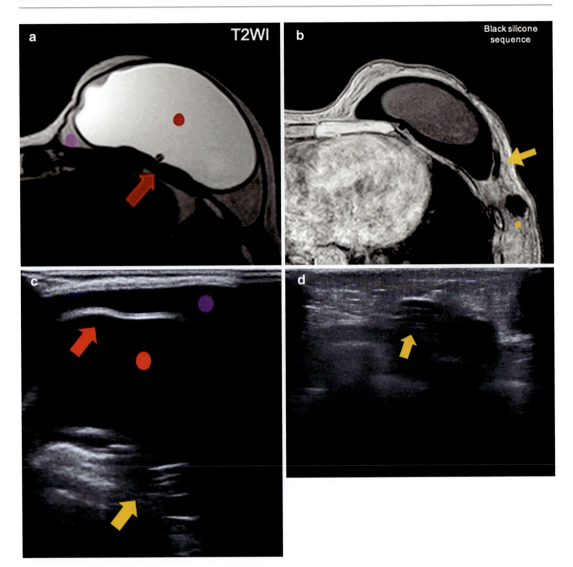

Fig. 25 Patient with a personal history of left-breast cancer treated with a mastectomy. Reconstruction was performed with a double-lumen expander with saline inner lumen and silicone outer lumen. Saline inner lumen is filled over time through a tube that is connected with a titanium fill-in valve located, as a subcutaneous port, lateral to the implant. (**a**) Axial plane T2-WI. Saline inner lumen is hyperintense (red dot), and silicone outer lumen is isointense (purple dot). The tube is lying posteriorly and extends from the inner lumen to the fill-in valve (red arrow). (**b**) Axial plane black-silicone sequence. Silicone outer lumen is hypointense. The tube (yellow arrow) is connecting the inner lumen, going lateral to the implant to the titanium fill-in valve (yellow dot). (**c**) At ultrasound, a line can be seen separating both chambers (red arrow), the inner lumen with saline (red dot) and outer lumen with silicone (purple dot). The ultrasonographic appearance is then the same for both (anechoic), so it is impossible to distinguish them if you do not know the type of implant. (**d**) The connector tube can be seen lying posteriorly and can be continued going towards the fill-in valve. The appearance is like a train track (yellow arrow)

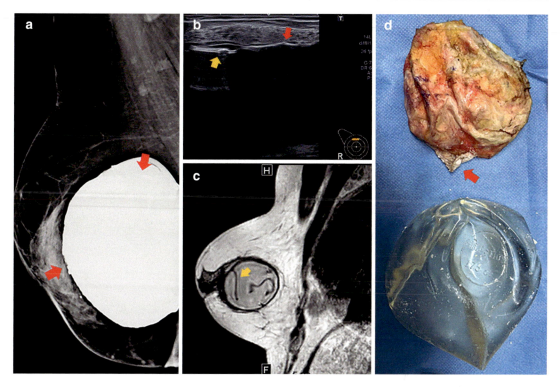

Fig. 26 Patient with augmented mammoplasty with silicone unicameral implants. Patient suffered a trauma, and the right implant changed the shape. Clinical capsulitis was present in both implants. (**a**) MLO-view mammography is showing some irregularities in the implant surface that corresponded to some calcifications (red arrows). The shape was not normal, but it was not possible to rule out a rupture. (**b**) Ultrasound showed also the irregularities of the implant surface (red arrow) and double line in the surface (yellow arrow). Then, MRI was recommended. (**c**) Sagittal T2-WI showed some hypointense lines inside the implant (yellow arrow) but was difficult to define if they corresponded to prominent radial folds or intracapsular rupture because neither silicone nor fluid was seen on the outside of the fold. An extracapsular rupture was not seen. (**d**) Surgical picture showed the capsule with grade IV capsulitis and calcifications (red arrow) and the implant without intracapsular rupture. (Pictures provided by the Dr. Martina Marin-Gutzke (Plastic surgeon MD. San Rafael Hospital. Madrid. Spain))

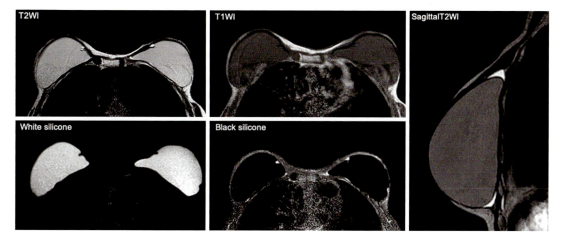

Fig. 27 Patient with bilateral mastectomy with heterologous reconstruction with silicone unicameral implants for evaluating implant complications. The protocol should include axial images on T2-WI (silicone is hyperintense), on T1-WI (silicone is hypointense), on white silicone sequence (silicone and only silicone is completely white), and on black silicone sequence (silicone is dark). Sagittal image acquisition is also recommended

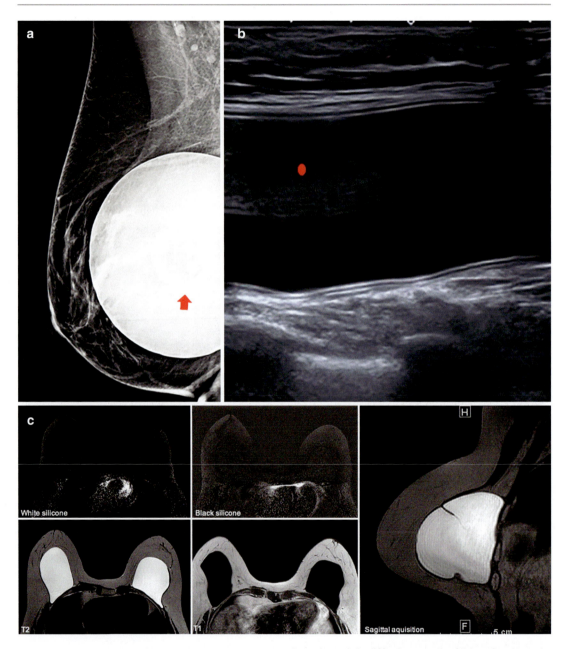

Fig. 28 Patient with a personal history of left-breast carcinoma with bilateral reconstruction with saline implants. (**a**) Mammography MLO view shows a hyperdense and oval implant, but the density is lower than that of silicone implants, and in fact the fill-in valve can be seen (red arrow). (**b**) Ultrasound shows an oval and well-defined implant with anechoic content, identical to that of silicone. The red dot is pointing to the reverberation artifact. Sometimes, it is difficult to see the fill-in valve due to its location. (**c**) At MRI, the implant shows fluid appearance in all the sequences. If the technician ignores the type of implant and uses white silicone and black silicone sequences, the images will appear all dark gray in both cases, and then a failure in the fat and water suppression might be misinterpreted

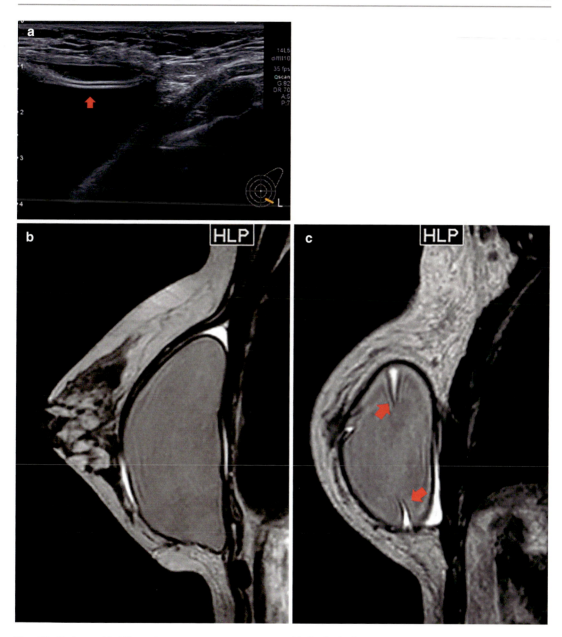

Fig. 29 Patient with bilateral mammoplasty with unicameral silicone implants. (**a**) Ultrasound shows hyperechoic line inside the implant that corresponds to a subcapsular fold (red arrow). (**b**) Sagittal plane on T2-WI shows a small and normal amount of peri-implant fluid. (**c**) Sagittal plane on T2-WI shows a radial fold going through the inside of the silicone (red arrow). Fluid is seen on one side of the fold, while silicone is seen on the other, which differentiates it from an intracapsular rupture

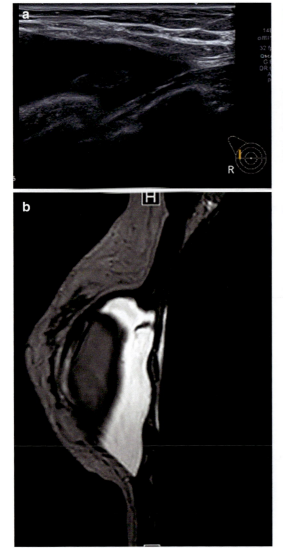

Fig. 30 Patient with a personal history of bilateral mammoplasty with silicone implant came for pain and increase of volume to right breast. (**a**) Ultrasound revealed the presence of new onset of peri-implant fluid with some septa inside. (**b**) Axial plane in T2-WI showed the same findings. A breast implant-associated anaplastic large lymphoma should be ruled out, so a FNA was performed to do the differential diagnosis with infection, hematoma, or inflammation. This patient had a streptococcus infection

(b) Thickening of the fibrous capsule with or without calcifications that can be associated to a certain degree of capsular contracture.

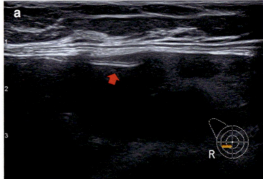

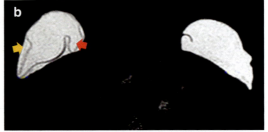

Fig. 31 Patient with a personal history of bilateral mammoplasty with silicone implant came for a follow-up with mammography and ultrasound. (**a**) Ultrasound revealed the presence of the elastomer floating in the silicone gel, which is called "*stepladder sign*." Additionally, there was a hyperechoic content inside the implant. (**b**) Axial plane in white silicone sequence showed the signs of "*keyhole*" (red arrow) and "*subcapsular line*" (yellow arrow) suggesting an intracapsular rupture with minimal collapse

(c) Small amount of peri-implant fluid: It is important to note that T2-weighted images should have a high TR value in order to obtain the hyperintensity of the fluid and be able to differentiate it from the fatty tissue.

3.1.3 Intracapsular Rupture

The diagnosis is usually made with ultrasound or MRI (Perez et al. 2017; Berg et al. 1993; Juanperc et al. 2011; Gorczyca et al. 2007; Scaranelo et al. 2004; Hillard et al. 2017):

1. At ultrasound, subcapsular and irregular lines or hyperechoic content inside the implant can be indirect signs, but the most reliable finding is the "*stepladder sign*," which corresponds to the ruptured elastomer floating in the silicone gel and is seen as hyperechoic lines extending

beyond the interior of the implant resembling a ladder or railway (Fig. 31a).

2. At MRI, silicone outside the elastomer can be seen but still contained by the fibrous and external capsule. There can be different grades of rupture:

   (a) Without collapse: "*keyhole*," "*teardrop*," "*inverted loop*," or "*noose*" signs. The silicone has spread more over the elastomer in a focal area being the extravasation confined to the fibrous capsule and with adhesions at their ends. Therefore, the appearance is similar to a radial fold but with silicone on both sides of elastomer. None of these signs is a reliable sign of rupture on its own but combined with other imaging features may suggest intracapsular rupture. In fact, these signs can also be seen as a result of "*gel bleed*," which occurs when silicone passes through an apparently intact elastomer (Fig. 31b).

   (b) With minimal collapse: "*Subcapsular line*" is a parallel and hypointense line to the fibrous capsule, also with silicone on both sides and with a wider and circumferential extension. It represents an evolution of the previous stage, with a greater extravasation and wider base of the invagination of the elastomer than without collapse (Fig. 31b).

   (c) With partial or total collapse: "*Linguine*" or "*wavy line*" signs. There is free-floating elastomer within the implant. Some curved and hypointense lines are seen inside the shell. It represents a complete rupture of the elastomer with the presence of free silicone between it and the fibrous capsule. It is the most reliable sign of intracapsular rupture (sensitivity and specificity of 96 and 76–97%, respectively) (Fig. 32).

   (d) The "*salad oil*" or "*droplet*" sign is the presence of one or multiple pockets of fluid inside the silicone, and it is not a necessary sign of intracapsular rupture. It can be seen in addition to other signs of rupture (Fig. 33).

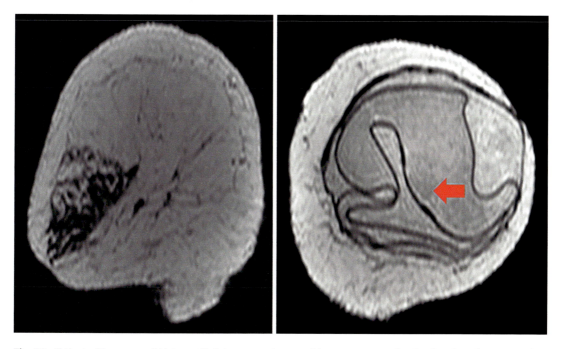

Fig. 32 Patient with a personal history of left-breast carcinoma with mastectomy and an implant-based reconstruction. On coronal T2 sequence MRI, a linguine sign can be observed regarding a collapsed intracapsular rupture

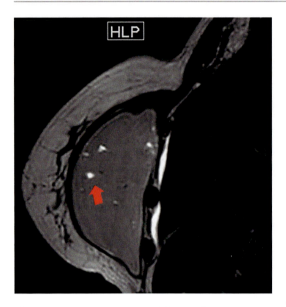

Fig. 33 Patient with a personal history of bilateral mammoplasty with silicone implants. On sagittal T2 sequence MRI, some fluid signal drops can be observed inside the silicone of the right implant but without any other sign of rupture

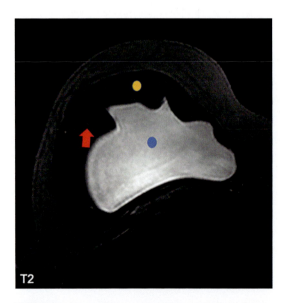

Fig. 34 Patient with a personal history of bilateral mastectomy with double-lumen implants. Axial T2 sequence MRI shows the implant with the inner lumen with saline content (blue dot) and outer lumen with silicone content (yellow dot). The red arrow is pointing to the elastomer floating inside the silicone of the outer lumen

The most common double-lumen implants are filled with saline in the inner lumen and with silicone in the outer lumen. An intracapsular rupture is possible in both lumens. The inner lumen rupture results in a disruption of the normal internal architecture of the implant (Fig. 34). The outer lumen rupture results in radiological finding similar to that in a silicone one-lumen implant rupture. Sometimes and during the expansion process, the inner lumen might not be fully inflated and thus may appear to have multiple folds or wrinkles in the surface for example on CT evaluation. This should not be interpreted as a rupture (Glynn and Litherland 2008).

3.1.4 Extracapsular Rupture

It is less common than intracapsular rupture, especially since new cohesive materials have developed. There is a rupture of both implant elastomer and fibrous capsule. Macroscopic silicone is thus seen beyond fibrous capsule, in peri-implant regions like the breast parenchyma, and a siliconoma may be seen when the body reacts against a foreign material like silicone. Silicone can also migrate to axillary or internal mammary lymph nodes, soft tissues, or other lymphatic regions (Perez et al. 2017; Berg et al. 1993; Juanpere et al. 2011; Gorczyca et al. 2007; Scaranelo et al. 2004; Hillard et al. 2017; Caskey et al. 1999). The presence of free silicone outside the fibrous capsule without an evidence of an extracapsular rupture can be explained by the presence of a previous implant ruptured and posterior replacement or by a gel bleeding or leakage of silicone that is picked up by the lymphatic vessels and carried to the lymph nodes (Fig. 35). In the latter, the lymph nodes can show a snowstorm sign or be enlarged due to reactive lymphadenitis.

1. At mammography, a well- or ill-defined hyperdense mass outside the implant is the most common finding. Change of the contour of the implant or enlarged and hyperdense axillary lymph nodes due to silicone migration can be noted (Fig. 35a).

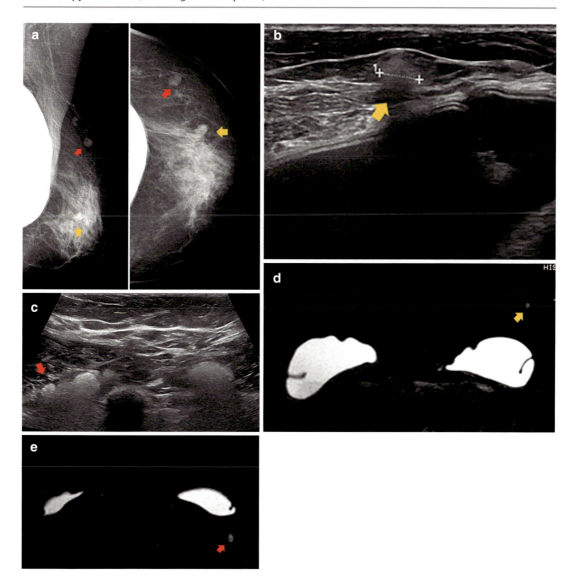

Fig. 35 Patient with bilateral mammoplasty with unicameral silicone implants. The patient had a previous extracapsular rupture some years ago and changed the implants. (**a**) Left mammogram shows dense, oval, and circumscribed nodules in breast tail (red arrow) and in outer quadrant (yellow quadrant). (**b**) Ultrasound shows the mammographic nodules corresponding to a hyperechoic nodule with snowstorm sign in breast parenchyma (yellow arrow) and in axillary tail (**c**) regarding an infiltrated lymph node (red arrow). (**d, e**) Axial plane on white silicone sequence shows silicone inside both nodules in breast parenchyma (yellow arrow) and in axillary lymph nodes (red arrow) related to the previous extracapsular rupture

2. At ultrasound, hypoechoic nodular lesions related to granulomatous reaction to foreign body or a loss of normal implant-parenchymal interface might be seen. However, the most specific sign is the "*snowstorm*" sign that appears as a diffusely increased echogenicity with posterior enhancement (Fig. 35b, c).

3. MRI is the most sensitive technique for detecting small foci of migration. Extracapsular silicone can be seen in the parenchyma, lymph nodes, or soft tissues. Free silicone will show the same signal intensity than intracapsular silicone in all sequences and no enhancement in recent ruptures. Over time, with granulomatous reac-

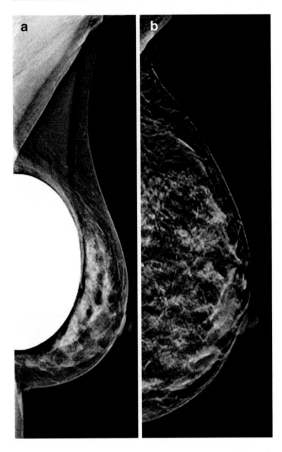

Fig. 36 Patient with bilateral mammoplasty with unicameral silicone implants. (**a**) Left mammogram with OML view with the implant visible, decreasing the breast tissue visualization. (**b**) Eklund technique where the implant is pushed towards the chest wall to increase the parenchymal visibility

parenchymal visibility) (Fig. 36b) and ultrasound in addition to the routine projection mammograms should be performed. MRI is the most sensitive and specific technique for evaluating implant integrity (about 72–94% and 85–100%, respectively). In addition, the risk of rupture increases with the longevity of the implant. Both aspects have led the FDA to recommend MRI every 2 years from 3 after implant placement. However, due to the cost and availability, MRI has been recommended only for cases with suspicion of rupture after mammography and ultrasound or in cases of normal findings on conventional techniques but clinical suspicion for rupture.

In patients with IBR due to a previous history of breast cancer, screening should be adapted to the type of surgery (see recurrence and follow-up of mastectomy and conservative treatment; Sects. 2.3.2 and 2.4.2) and to the patient's risk.

3.2 Complementary Meshes

Meshes are used preferentially for immediate reconstruction when skin or pectoral muscle cannot cover the implant. They make a one-stop reconstruction with reduced muscle defects and placement of a definitive implant instead of a temporary expander followed by a second surgery for the definitive implant possible. They provide an improved aesthetic outcome with natural shape (Gerber et al. 2015; Jacobs and Salzberg 2015; Reitsamer and Peintinger 2015).

However, the radiologist should be aware of the radiological findings. Mammography is not commonly performed in those patients who have undergone mastectomy or extensive surgeries. Ultrasound can show irregular masses (Fig. 37a), sometimes with posterior shadowing, adjacent to the implant that corresponds to folds of the mesh and might be interpreted as suspicious findings, leading to biopsy and possible damage of the mesh. MRI will show absence of uptake of these images (Fig. 37b) that usually are bilateral and symmetrical.

tion, the signal intensity may change and present some enhancement after intravenous contrast administration (Fig. 35d, e).

3.1.5 Recurrence and Follow-Up

The risk of breast cancer in women with or without breast implants is the same (Brett et al. 2018). Thus, there is no consensus on the follow-up of women with implants for aesthetic purposes. However, implants may interfere with early detection of cancer since breast tissue visualization decreases by 30–50% (Fig. 36a). Therefore, the Eklund technique (where the implant is pushed towards the chest wall to increase the

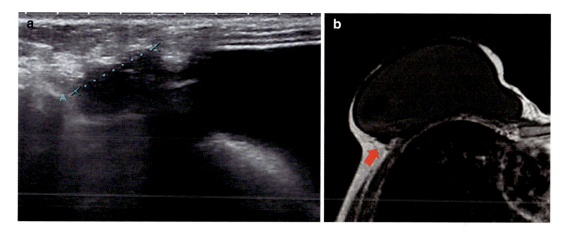

Fig. 37 Patient with bilateral mastectomy with the first follow-up 1 year after the surgery. US shows a hypoechoic, ill-defined mass adjacent to the implant (**a**) that corresponds to a fold of the mesh that did not show enhancement after the IVC administration (**b**)

4 Autologous Breast Reconstruction (ABR)

It involves the use of endogenous material from the patient's own body to reshape the breast. It can include autologous tissue flaps or free-fat injection. Sometimes, immediate autologous and heterologous reconstructions are supplementary rather than opposing each other, as for example the latissimus dorsi flap or the free-fat injection when combined with implant reconstruction (Margolis et al. 2014; Pinel-Giroux et al. 2013).

4.1 Autologous Flaps

They involve the use of skin, fatty tissue, and sometimes muscle from the patient's own body to reshape the breast. Advances in oncoplastic surgery over the past years have led to an increasing number of women requesting autologous flap reconstruction. Pedicle flaps, mainly from the abdomen, are the standard procedure (Neal et al. 2014). The most common free-flap surgery is the deep inferior epigastric perforator (DIEP) flap. The choice of procedure depends on the habitus, patient's wishes and ideas, risk factors (smoking, diabetes mellitus, obesity, previous surgeries, radiation, history of thrombosis, cardiovascular disease, etc.), possible postmastectomy radiotherapy (PMRT), and skills of the surgeon. Some of the advantages of the ABR over the IBR are no implant needed, natural appearance and aesthetic outcome, better long-term outcomes with natural aging process, suitable for irradiated tissue, shorter surgical and recovery times, no additional scars, and similar aesthetic aspect in color and texture to the adjacent tissue. However, there are also some disadvantages which include higher complexity, higher morbidity with higher rate of complications of the donor site, longer surgery, need of highly experienced surgeons, and higher cost, although autologous reconstruction can even become more cost effective than implant-based reconstruction in the long term (Perez et al. 2017; Gerber et al. 2015; Dialani et al. 2012).

4.1.1 Classification

There are different types of autologous flaps, depending on the following (Table 1):

1. Donor site: abdominal, dorsal, gluteal, inner thigh, or other regions.
2. Composition: myocutaneous flap (with skin, fat, muscle, and vascular pedicle) or muscle-sparing free flap (with skin, fat, and vascular supply; then the muscle is not transferred).
3. Connection between the vasculature and the donor site: pedicle (connected with the donor site over a vascular pedicle; there is no micro-

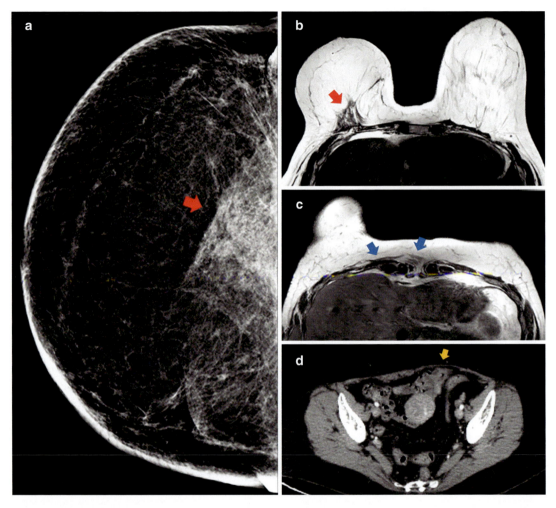

Fig. 38 Patient with a personal history of right-breast carcinoma with autologous reconstruction with pedicle TRAM flap. (**a**) Mammography CC view shows a radiolucent breast with a dense and triangular shape corresponding to the abdominis rectus muscle above the pectoral muscle (red arrow). (**b**) T1-WI at MRI shows the rectus muscle with hyperintense lines inside corresponding to fatty degeneration (red arrow). (**c**) Same sequence but in an inferior slice shows the rectus muscle crossing the midline going to the abdomen (blue arrows). (**d**) Abdominal CT shows the absence of the left rectus muscle (yellow arrow)

surgery of vessels) or free flap (there is no connection between the donor site and the flap; microsurgery is needed between a pedicle transferred and new vessels).

Taking into account the aforementioned factors, autologous flaps can be classified as follows (Dellacroce and Wolfe 2013; Dialani et al. 2012; Pinel-Giroux et al. 2013; Granzow et al. 2006):

1. Pedicle transverse rectus abdominis muscle (TRAM) flap: It is a myocutaneous flap. The abdominis rectus muscle is transferred with its corresponding vascular supply (superior epigastric artery) (Devon et al. 2004) (Fig. 38).
2. Free TRAM flap: It is a myocutaneous flap, but only a portion of the abdominis rectus muscle is transferred. Therefore, the abdominal wall morbidity is less than that in pedicle TRAM. The vascularization depends on perforating branches of the deep epigastric artery, which comes from the inferior epigastric artery. Microsurgery with the mammary internal vessels is required (Chen et al. 2007).

3. Deep inferior epigastric perforator (DIEP) flap: It is a muscle-sparing free flap. The donor site is the abdomen, where only a portion of the skin and fat is transferred. Unlike the TRAM flap, the abdominis rectus muscle is preserved. The vascularization also depends on perforating branches of the deep epigastric artery and then microsurgery is needed (Fig. 39).

4. Superficial inferior epigastric artery (SIEA) flap: It is a muscle-sparing free flap of abdominal origin. It is similar to DIEP (the muscle is preserved), but the vascular supply depends on the superficial epigastric artery.

5. Latissimus dorsi (LD) flap: It is a myocutaneous flap. The muscle transferred is the latissimus dorsi with its corresponding vascular supply (thoracodorsal artery). It is usually combined with an implant to increase the volume of the muscle (Monticciolo et al. 1996; Rainsbury 2002; Taglialatela Scafati et al. 2017; Demiri et al. 2018) (Fig. 40).

6. Thoracodorsal artery perforator (TDAP) flap: It is a muscle-sparing free flap originated in the back. The vascular supply depends on perforator branches of thoracodorsal artery. Unlike the LD flap, the latissimus dorsi muscle is preserved. Microsurgery is not required.

7. Originated in other regions, as for example the transverse upper gracilis (TUG) flap from the inner thigh or SGAP or IGAP (superior or inferior gluteal artery perforator) flaps (Lotempio and Allen 2010).

4.1.2   Radiological Tests

The main and common characteristic of all autologous flaps is the transfer of skin and fat for modeling a new breast. Therefore, fatty tissue is seen with all imaging techniques (Dialani et al. 2012).

Mammography will be essentially fatty tissue and so radiolucent (Figs. 38a, 39a, and 40a). If there is a myocutaneous flap, variable density due to the muscle component or postoperative scarring can be seen. Therefore, the presence of microcalcifications or new densities will be of higher contrast and easier detected (Mele et al. 2017).

Ultrasound is less productive in these patients than in patients who have undergone mastectomy with other types of reconstruction because of low contrast between lesions and surrounding fat. Frequent scars and fat necrosis can produce hard palpable lumps that make the interpretation of the findings difficult.

MRI will show the fatty flap as well as if there is residual breast tissue. It is very useful in differentiating scar or fat necrosis from recurrence, since it can demonstrate the presence of fat inside the lesion (Fig. 39a, c) or the absence of enhancement after IVC administration. Additionally, it is the only technique that can show with precision the vascular supply of the flap and the region of the internal mammary chain.

4.1.3   Normal Findings

Radiologists have to be familiar with the normal and abnormal appearance of the different types of autologous flaps. All techniques will show a fatty breast. The presence of a muscle will reveal a myocutaneous flap (Figs. 39 and 40) although over time the muscle will suffer atrophic changes and its appearance will become fattier. The presence of vascular anastomosis will reveal a muscle-sparing free flap (Fig. 39). The anastomosis is usually performed with the internal mammary vessels located in the first or second intercostal space, so these findings can be the only sign of a previous failed autologous reconstruction. Besides, it is important to assess the viability of the flap, especially at MRI.

1. At mammography, a radiolucent breast is seen (Figs. 38a, 39a, and 40a). Thin radiopaque line in the periphery corresponding to the dermal tissue of the flaps is observed. A higher density above the pectoral muscle, which decreases over time due to fatty infiltration, can be seen in myocutaneous flaps. When the donor site is the abdomen, the muscle transferred is usually seen as a triangular shape above the pectoral muscle (Fig. 38) unlike the back origin where the muscle is usually seen in a parallel distribution (Fig. 40). The microsurgery cannot be seen due to the location (Mele et al. 2017).

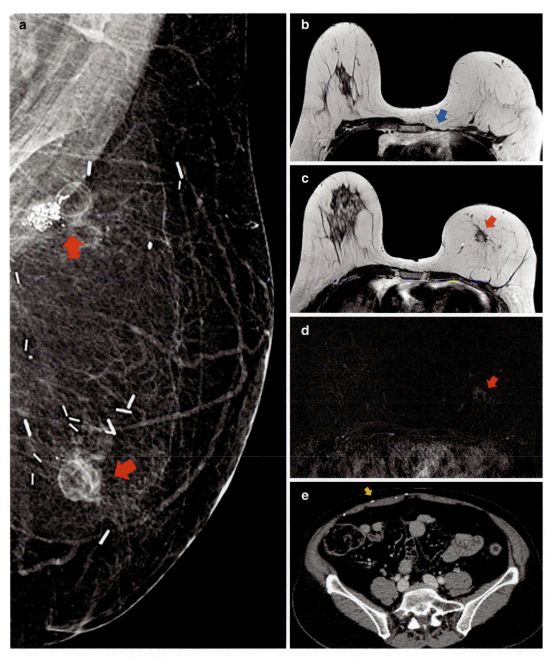

Fig. 39 Patient with a personal history of left-breast carcinoma with autologous reconstruction with DIEP flap. (**a**) Mammography OML view shows a radiolucent breast. Two nodular and calcified images (red arrows) are seen in correlation with fat necrosis. (**b**) T1-WI at MRI shows postsurgical changes in the first intercostal space (blue arrow) due to the vascular anastomosis. (**c, d**) T1-WI and subtracted images in the same slice show fat inside the fat necrosis despite the presence of peripheral enhancement (red arrows). (**e**) Abdominal CT shows postsurgical clips in the abdominal wall but with the rectus muscle preserved

2. At ultrasound, a hypoechoic breast is seen. A thin hyperechoic band in the periphery can be noted under the skin. The muscle transferred can be identified and can be followed if the technique of the flap is known. With the Doppler technique, the intravas-

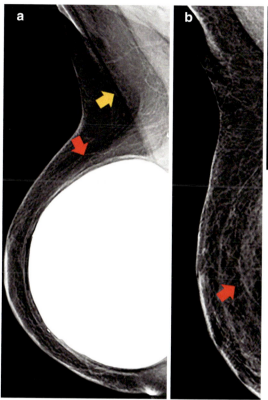
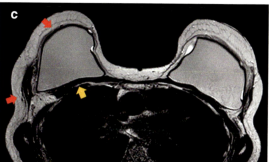

Fig. 40 Patient with a personal history of bilateral mastectomy with autologous reconstruction with latissimus dorsi flap combined with a silicone implant. (**a**) Mammography OML view shows a radiolucent breast with the latissimus dorsi muscle above the implant in a parallel distribution (red arrow) and the pectoral muscle shadow behind the implant. (**b**) Eklund technique shows the latissimus dorsi muscle (red arrow) and absence of residual fibroglandular tissue. (**c**) T2-WI at MRI shows the pectoral muscle behind the implant (yellow arrow) and the latissimus dorsi coming from the back (red arrow)

cular flow in the anastomosis can be assessed.
3. At MRI, the type of flap can be perfectly distinguished. The muscle is seen in myocutaneous flaps (Figs. 38 and 40), and if one follows it, one can see the origin. In the same way, one can examine the first intercostal spaces (Fig. 39b) to detect an anastomosis with the internal mammary chain or the lateral chest wall to detect vessels or muscle towards the back (Fig. 40c). It is important to review the T1 and T2W images to see the muscles despite the atrophic changes and also to use a wide field of view (FOV) to see the lateral chest wall. MRI is also the best technique to assess a good vascularization of the flap.
4. At abdominal CT, we can see the rectus abdominis area and distinguish the type of flap when the origin is abdominal. The pedicle TRAM shows absence of one rectus abdominis muscle (Fig. 38d). The free TRAM flap shows a partial defect of the muscle. The DIEP flap shows postsurgical clips surrounding the muscle, but the latter will be preserved (Fig. 39e). The SIEA flap shows an intact muscle, and postsurgical clips are seen at the origin of the superficial epigastric artery.

4.1.4 Complications

Fat necrosis is one of the most common complications, especially in abdominal flaps (Devon et al. 2004; Tayyab et al. 2018) (Fig. 39). It is clinically suspected when a new hard and palpable lump appears close to scarring areas. Differential diagnosis with a recurrence should be established, and radiological tests are needed.

Vascular complications such as venous congestion or arterial failure can be seen, especially when a microsurgery with anastomosis is required. Inflammatory changes are seen in cases of venous congestion with skin thickening, edema, and enhancement. A failure of the flap occurs when there is an arterial failure, and then a new anastomosis or new reconstruction is required.

Fluid collections as seromas, hematomas, or abscesses (Keidan et al. 1990) can be seen in some cases.

4.1.5 Recurrence and Follow Up

No statistically significant differences in recurrence rates of reconstructed and non-reconstructed patients have been demonstrated. The recurrences in these patients can be located predominantly in two areas. One of them is the superficial region, in the transition line between the flap and the subcutaneous fat of the native breast, which may be clinically detected. The other one is the deep portion of the flap, anteriorly to the pectoral muscle, which is rarely detected clinically.

Clinical examination is less sensitive than in surgeries without reconstruction or with heterologous reconstruction. Therefore, radiological tests are needed, and as previously stated, screening should be adapted to the type of surgery (see recurrence and follow-up of mastectomy and conservative treatment; Sects. 2.3.2 and 2.4.2) and to the patient's risk (Zakhireh et al. 2010). However, and unlike mastectomy without reconstruction, an annual mammogram has been recommended due to the presence of calcifications, fat necrosis, and possible recurrences in the deep portion of the flap. Ultrasound is less sensitive due to less contrast between the fat of the flap and possible recurrences (both with hypoechoic appearance). MRI is the most sensitive and specific test with a high negative predictive value (NPV) in these types of reconstruction. It is very useful showing the fat inside the lesion when it is fat necrosis and also showing other types of complications and differentiating recurrence from scarring (Brett et al. 2018) (Fig. 41).

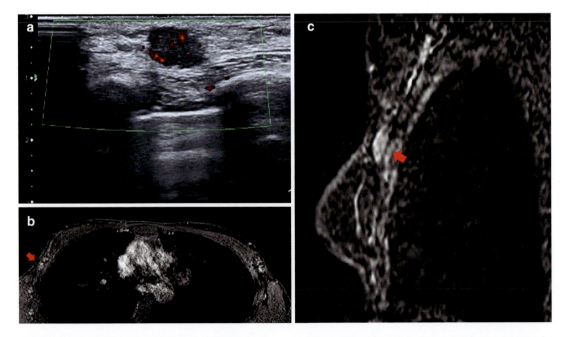

Fig. 41 Patient with a personal history of right mastectomy with DIEP. (**a**) US shows an irregular and new nodule in the breast tail. (**b**) MRI dynamic shows an ill-defined nodule, with enhancement after IVC administration, in the transition area between the flap and the subcutaneous fat of the native breast. In axial plane, it seems to be a small nodule but in sagittal reconstruction it has 2 cm (**c**)

4.2 Lipofilling, Lipomodeling, or Free-Fat Injection

Since the beginning of the use of IBR and ABR, other techniques like free injection of different substances have been developed. One of these substances is the fatty tissue of the patient. The fat derives from the liposuction of other parts of the body, and it is injected inside the breast, either in the surface, in the middle, or in the deep part of it (Ogawa et al. 2008). It is a very versatile technique as a complement of conservative surgery without reconstruction, of IBR and ABR, and also of surgery with aesthetic purpose only. It has shown to be secure for the patient, not increasing the risk of cancer.

4.2.1 Radiological Tests

As the substance injected is free fat, it is supposed that no radiological findings are observed. Then, no specific test should be used to study these patients because free fat would have the same appearance than breast fat, making the breast fattier. Then, the sensibility of mammography would be higher due to higher contrast between calcifications and lesions and fat of the breast (Wang et al. 2011). However, it has been shown that free fat can evolve to fat necrosis, and in those cases, MRI has shown the highest specificity and NPV.

4.2.2 Radiological Findings

This technique can show a wide spectrum of radiological findings, ranging from benign to suspicious findings. It is important to be familiar with these findings (Carvajal and Patino 2008; Pulagam et al. 2006).

1. BI-RADS® 1: Identical to normal breast. The injected fat is mixed with the fat of the breast with no specific radiological findings. If the patient does not refer the lipofilling and the previous history is unknown for the radiologist, those findings are not identified.
2. BI-RADS® 2: Benign findings. It is the most common finding when there are radiological abnormalities. The oil cyst is the most common manifestation in this group, with radiolucent aspect on mammogram, simulating a simple cyst appearance on ultrasound but showing a fatty appearance on T1W and fat-suppressed images on MRI (Fig. 42).
3. BI-RADS® 3: Probably benign findings. New onset of round or oval, circumscribed, and well defined solid lesions, without enhancement or with type 1 enhancement curve.
4. BI-RADS® 4: Suspicious findings. Fat necrosis in the inflammatory phase is the most common cause. Solid lesions which do not meet all the benign criteria on mammogram or ultrasound or with type 2 or 3 enhancement curves on MRI may be seen. On mammogram, suspicious calcifications may also be seen (Upadhyaya et al. 2018; De Decker et al. 2016; Mineda et al. 2014) (Fig. 43).

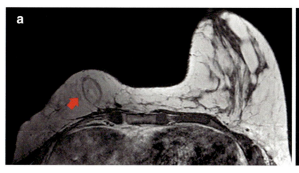
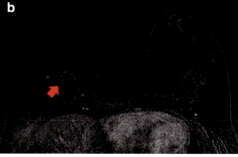
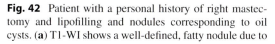

Fig. 42 Patient with a personal history of right mastectomy and lipofilling and nodules corresponding to oil cysts. (**a**) T1-WI shows a well-defined, fatty nodule due to lipofilling (red arrow). (**b**) Dynamic sequences do not show enhancement

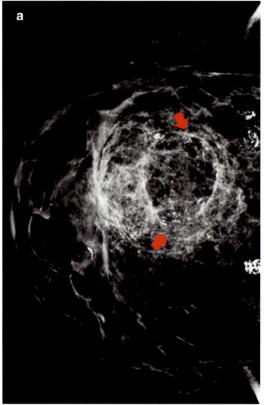

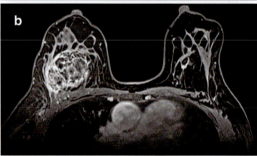

Fig. 43 Patient with a personal history of lipofilling in the outer quadrant of right breast. (**a**) Mammogram with CC view shows an ill-defined mass that apparently presents fat inside. However, multiple and pleomorphic microcalcifications were new (red arrows). (**b**) Dynamic sequence at MRI shows an irregular mass with heterogeneous enhancement. Stereotactic guided VABB was performed with fat necrosis result. Courtesy of Dr. Jaime Marcano

4.2.3 Recurrence and Follow-Up

The rate of recurrence is the same as in patients without lipofilling (Kaoutzanis et al. 2016; Groen et al. 2016; Brett et al. 2018; Kanchwala et al. 2009; Krastev et al. 2018). However, the differential diagnosis of recurrence when there is a fat necrosis is required. Additionally, fat necrosis usually appears after the procedure as a new-onset palpable and stiff mass; then, conventional test may not be enough to make the diagnosis (Pinell-White et al. 2015). In this case, an MRI should be performed, and if it shows fat inside the lesion, the biopsy is not needed. If MRI also reveals a suspicious finding, biopsy will be required. Screening should be adapted to the type of surgery and reconstruction complementary to the lipofilling when it is present (see recurrence and follow-up of mastectomy, conservative treatment, IBR, and ABR) (Sects. 2.3.2, 2.4.2, 3.1.5, and 4.1.5), and also to the patient's risk (Kaoutzanis et al. 2016). However, mammography is recommended in case of autologous reconstruction with lipofilling to rule out calcifications and MRI in almost all cases since it can show the fat necrosis and other possible complications in implants or flaps.

References

Adrada BE, Miranda RN, Rauch GM, Arribas E, Kanagal-Shamanna R, Clemens MW, Fanale M, Haideri N, Mustafa E, Larrinaga J, Reisman NR, Jaso J, You MJ, Young KH, Medeiros LJ, Yang W (2014) Breast implant-associated anaplastic large cell lymphoma: sensitivity, specificity, and findings of imaging studies in 44 patients. Breast Cancer Res Treat 147:1–14

Belli P, Romani M, Magistrelli A, Masetti R, Pastore G, Costantini M (2002) Diagnostic imaging of breast implants: role of MRI. Rays 27:259–277

Berg WA, Caskey CI, Hamper UM, Anderson ND, Chang BW, Sheth S, Zerhouni EA, Kuhlman JE (1993) Diagnosing breast implant rupture with MR imaging, US, and mammography. Radiographics 13:1323–1336

Berg WA, Blume JD, Cormack JB, Mendelson EB, Lehrer D, Bohm-Velez M, Pisano ED, Jong RA, Evans WP, Morton MJ, Mahoney MC, Larsen LH, Barr RG, Farria DM, Marques HS, Boparai K, ACRIN 6666 Investigators (2008) Combined screening with ultrasound and mammography vs mammography alone in women at elevated risk of breast cancer. JAMA 299:2151–2163

Boostrom SY, Throckmorton AD, Boughey JC, Holifield AC, Zakaria S, Hoskin TL, Degnim AC (2009) Incidence of clinically significant seroma after breast and axillary surgery. J Am Coll Surg 208:148–150

Brenner RJ (2013) Evaluation of breast silicone implants. Magn Reson Imaging Clin N Am 21:547–560

Brett EA, Aitzetmuller MM, Sauter MA, Huemer GM, Machens HG, Duscher D (2018) Breast cancer recurrence after reconstruction: know thine enemy. Oncotarget 9:27895–27906

Carvajal J, Patino JH (2008) Mammographic findings after breast augmentation with autologous fat injection. Aesthet Surg J 28:153–162

Caskey CI, Berg WA, Hamper UM, Sheth S, Chang BW, Anderson ND (1999) Imaging spectrum of extracapsular silicone: correlation of US, MR imaging, mammographic, and histopathologic findings. Radiographics 19 Spec No:S39–S51; Quiz S261–S262

Chansakul T, Lai KC, Slanetz PJ (2012a) The postconservation breast: Part 1, Expected imaging findings. AJR Am J Roentgenol 198:321–330

Chansakul T, Lai KC, Slanetz PJ (2012b) The postconservation breast: Part 2, Imaging findings of tumor recurrence and other long-term sequelae. AJR Am J Roentgenol 198:331–343

Chen CM, Halvorson EG, Disa JJ, Mccarthy C, Hu QY, Pusic AL, Cordeiro PG, Mehrara BJ (2007) Immediate postoperative complications in DIEP versus free/muscle-sparing TRAM flaps. Plast Reconstr Surg 120:1477–1482

Cho N, Han W, Han BK, Bae MS, Ko ES, Nam SJ, Chae EY, Lee JW, Kim SH, Kang BJ, Song BJ, Kim EK, Moon HJ, Kim SI, Kim SM, Kang E, Choi Y, Kim HH, Moon WK (2017) Breast cancer screening with mammography plus ultrasonography or magnetic resonance imaging in women 50 years or younger at diagnosis and treated with breast conservation therapy. JAMA Oncol 3:1495–1502

Colleoni M, Sun Z, Price KN, Karlsson P, Forbes JF, Thurlimann B, Gianni L, Castiglione M, Gelber RD, Coates AS, Goldhirsch A (2016) Annual hazard rates of recurrence for breast cancer during 24 years of follow-up: results from the International Breast Cancer Study Group Trials I to V. J Clin Oncol 34:927–935

De Decker M, De Schrijver L, Thiessen F, Tondu T, Van Goethem M, Tjalma WA (2016) Breast cancer and fat grafting: efficacy, safety and complications-a systematic review. Eur J Obstet Gynecol Reprod Biol 207:100–108

Dellacroce FJ, Wolfe ET (2013) Breast reconstruction. Surg Clin North Am 93:445–454

Demiri EC, Dionyssiou DD, Tsimponis A, Goula CO, Pavlidis LC, Spyropoulou GA (2018) Outcomes of fat-augmented latissimus dorsi (FALD) flap versus implant-based latissimus dorsi flap for delayed post-radiation breast reconstruction. Aesthetic Plast Surg 42:692–701

Dershaw DD, Mccormick B, Cox L, Osborne MP (1990) Differentiation of benign and malignant local tumor recurrence after lumpectomy. AJR Am J Roentgenol 155:35–38

Devon RK, Rosen MA, Mies C, Orel SG (2004) Breast reconstruction with a transverse rectus abdominis myocutaneous flap: spectrum of normal and abnormal MR imaging findings. Radiographics 24:1287–1299

Dialani V, Lai KC, Slanetz PJ (2012) MR imaging of the reconstructed breast: what the radiologist needs to know. Insights Imaging 3:201–213

Ganau S, Tortajada L, Escribano F, Andreu X, Sentis M (2009) The great mimicker: fat necrosis of the breast—magnetic resonance mammography approach. Curr Probl Diagn Radiol 38:189–197

Gerber B, Marx M, Untch M, Faridi A (2015) Breast reconstruction following cancer treatment. Dtsch Arztebl Int 112:593–600

Gigli S, Amabile MI, Di Pastena F, Manganaro L, David E, Monti M, D'Orazi V, Catalano C, Ballesio L (2017) Magnetic resonance imaging after breast oncoplastic surgery: an update. Breast Care (Basel) 12:260–265

Glynn C, Litherland J (2008) Imaging breast augmentation and reconstruction. Br J Radiol 81:587–595

Gorczyca DP, Gorczyca SM, Gorczyca KL (2007) The diagnosis of silicone breast implant rupture. Plast Reconstr Surg 120:49s–61s

Granzow JW, Levine JL, Chiu ES, Allen RJ (2006) Breast reconstruction using perforator flaps. J Surg Oncol 94:441–454

Groen JW, Negenborn VL, Twisk D, Rizopoulos D, Ket JCF, Smit JM, Mullender MG (2016) Autologous fat grafting in onco-plastic breast reconstruction: a systematic review on oncological and radiological safety, complications, volume retention and patient/surgeon satisfaction. J Plast Reconstr Aesthet Surg 69:742–764

Gunhan-Bilgen I, Oktay A (2007) Mammographic features of local recurrence after conservative surgery and radiation therapy: comparison with that of the primary tumor. Acta Radiol 48:390–397

Hillard C, Fowler JD, Barta R, Cunningham B (2017) Silicone breast implant rupture: a review. Gland Surg 6:163–168

Jacobs JM, Salzberg CA (2015) Implant-based breast reconstruction with meshes and matrices: biological vs synthetic. Br J Hosp Med (Lond) 76:211–216

Juanpere S, Perez E, Huc O, Motos N, Pont J, Pedraza S (2011) Imaging of breast implants-a pictorial review. Insights Imaging 2:653–670

Kanchwala SK, Glatt BS, Conant EF, Bucky LP (2009) Autologous fat grafting to the reconstructed breast: the management of acquired contour deformities. Plast Reconstr Surg 124:409–418

Kaoutzanis C, Xin M, Ballard TN, Welch KB, Momoh AO, Kozlow JH, Brown DL, Cederna PS, Wilkins EG (2016) Autologous fat grafting after breast reconstruction in postmastectomy patients: complications, biopsy rates, and locoregional cancer recurrence rates. Ann Plast Surg 76:270–275

Keidan RD, Hoffman JP, Weese JL, Hanks GE, Solin LJ, Eisenberg BL, Ottery FD, Boraas M (1990) Delayed breast abscesses after lumpectomy and radiation therapy. Am Surg 56:440–444

Khedher NB, David J, Trop I, Drouin S, Peloquin L, Lalonde L (2011) Imaging findings of breast augmentation with injected hydrophilic polyacrylamide gel: patient reports and literature review. Eur J Radiol 78:104–111

Kim HJ, Kwak JY, Choi JW, Bae JH, Shin KM, Lee HJ, Kim GC, Jung JH, Park JY (2010) Impact of US surveillance on detection of clinically occult locoregional recurrence after mastectomy for breast cancer. Ann Surg Oncol 17:2670–2676

Krastev TK, Schop SJ, Hommes J, Piatkowski AA, Heuts EM, Van Der Hulst R (2018) Meta-analysis of the oncological safety of autologous fat transfer after breast cancer. Br J Surg 105:1082–1097

Lake E, Ahmad S, Dobrashian R (2013) The sonographic appearances of breast implant rupture. Clin Radiol 68:851–858

Lam DL, Houssami N, Lee JM (2017) Imaging surveillance after primary breast cancer treatment. AJR Am J Roentgenol 208:676–686

Leberfinger AN, Behar BJ, Williams NC, Rakszawski KL, Potochny JD, Mackay DR, Ravnic DJ (2017) Breast implant-associated anaplastic large cell lymphoma: a systematic review. JAMA Surg 152:1161–1168

Lee JH, Kim EK, Oh JY, Kwon HC, Kim SH, Kim DC, Lee M, Cho SH, Nam KJ (2013) US screening for detection of nonpalpable locoregional recurrence after mastectomy. Eur J Radiol 82:485–489

Leibman AJ, Misra M (2011) Spectrum of imaging findings in the silicone-injected breast. Plast Reconstr Surg 128:28e–29e

Libshitz HI, Montague ED, Paulus DD Jr (1978) Skin thickness in the therapeutically irradiated breast. AJR Am J Roentgenol 130:345–347

Lotempio MM, Allen RJ (2010) Breast reconstruction with SGAP and IGAP flaps. Plast Reconstr Surg 126:393–401

Lui CY, Ho CM, Iu PP, Cheung WY, Lam HS, Cheng MS, Liu HL (2008) Evaluation of MRI findings after polyacrylamide gel injection for breast augmentation. AJR Am J Roentgenol 191:677–688

Margolis NE, Morley C, Lotfi P, Shaylor SD, Palestrant S, Moy L, Melsaether AN (2014) Update on imaging of the postsurgical breast. Radiographics 34:642–660

Mele S, Wright D, Paramanathan N, Laws S, Peiris L, Rainsbury R (2017) Long-term effect of oncoplastic breast-conserving surgery using latissimus dorsi miniflaps on mammographic surveillance and the detection of local recurrence. J Plast Reconstr Aesthet Surg 70:1203–1209

Mendelson EB (1989) Imaging the post-surgical breast. Semin Ultrasound CT MR 10:154–170

Mendelson EB (1992) Evaluation of the postoperative breast. Radiol Clin North Am 30:107–138

Mertz KR, Baddour LM, Bell JL, Gwin JL (1998) Breast cellulitis following breast conservation therapy: a novel complication of medical progress. Clin Infect Dis 26:481–486

Middleton MS (1998) Magnetic resonance evaluation of breast implants and soft-tissue silicone. Top Magn Reson Imaging 9:92–137

Miglioretti DL, Rutter CM, Geller BM, Cutter G, Barlow WE, Rosenberg R, Weaver DL, Taplin SH, Ballard-Barbash R, Carney PA, Yankaskas BC, Kerlikowske K (2004) Effect of breast augmentation on the accuracy of mammography and cancer characteristics. JAMA 291:442–450

Mineda K, Kuno S, Kato H, Kinoshita K, Doi K, Hashimoto I, Nakanishi H, Yoshimura K (2014) Chronic inflammation and progressive calcification as a result of fat necrosis: the worst outcome in fat grafting. Plast Reconstr Surg 133:1064–1072

Monticciolo DL, Ross D, Bostwick J III, Eaves F, Styblo T (1996) Autologous breast reconstruction with endoscopic latissimus dorsi musculosubcutaneous flaps in patients choosing breast-conserving therapy: mammographic appearance. AJR Am J Roentgenol 167:385–389

Neal CH, Yilmaz ZN, Noroozian M, Klein KA, Sundaram B, Kazerooni EA, Stojanovska J (2014) Imaging of breast cancer-related changes after surgical therapy. AJR Am J Roentgenol 202:262–272

O'Neill AC, Zhong T, Hofer SOP (2017) Implications of breast implant-associated anaplastic large cell lymphoma (BIA-ALCL) for breast cancer reconstruction: an update for surgical oncologists. Ann Surg Oncol 24:3174–3179

Ogawa R, Hyakusoku H, Ishii N, Ono S (2008) Fat grafting to the breast. Plast Reconstr Surg 121:341–342

Perez RS, Morris EA (2017) Breast Cancer. Innov Res Manag 277–315. https://doi.org/10.1007/978-3-319-48848-6_21

Pinel-Giroux FM, El Khoury MM, Trop I, Bernier C, David J, Lalonde L (2013) Breast reconstruction: review of surgical methods and spectrum of imaging findings. Radiographics 33:435–453

Pinell-White XA, Etra J, Newell M, Tuscano D, Shin K, Losken A (2015) Radiographic implications of fat grafting to the reconstructed breast. Breast J 21:520–525

Pulagam SR, Poulton T, Mamounas EP (2006) Long-term clinical and radiologic results with autologous fat transplantation for breast augmentation: case reports and review of the literature. Breast J 12:63–65

Rainsbury RM (2002) Breast-sparing reconstruction with latissimus dorsi miniflaps. Eur J Surg Oncol 28:891–895

Ramani SK, Rastogi A, Mahajan A, Nair N, Shet T, Thakur MH (2017) Imaging of the treated breast post breast conservation surgery/oncoplasty: pictorial review. World J Radiol 9:321–329

Reitsamer R, Peintinger F (2015) Prepectoral implant placement and complete coverage with porcine acellular dermal matrix: a new technique for direct-to-implant breast reconstruction after nipple-sparing mastectomy. J Plast Reconstr Aesthet Surg 68:162–167

Scaranelo AM, Marques AF, Smialowski EB, Lederman HM (2004) Evaluation of the rupture of silicone breast implants by mammography, ultrasonography and magnetic resonance imaging in asymptomatic patients: correlation with surgical findings. Sao Paulo Med J 122:41–47

Shah AT, Jankharia BB (2016) Imaging of common breast implants and implant-related complications: a pictorial essay. Indian J Radiol Imaging 26:216–225

Shah C, Ahlawat S, Khan A, Tendulkar RD, Wazer DE, Shah SS, Vicini F (2016) The role of MRI in the follow-up of women undergoing breast-conserving therapy. Am J Clin Oncol 39:314–319

Siegel RL, Miller KD, Jemal A (2016) Cancer statistics, 2016. CA Cancer J Clin 66:7–30

Soderstrom CE, Harms SE, Farrell RS Jr, Pruneda JM, Flamig DP (1997) Detection with MR imaging of residual tumor in the breast soon after surgery. AJR Am J Roentgenol 168:485–488

Spronk I, Schellevis FG, Burgers JS, De Bock GH, Korevaar JC (2018) Incidence of isolated local breast cancer recurrence and contralateral breast cancer: a systematic review. Breast 39:70–79

Swinnen J, Keupers M, Soens J, Lavens M, Postema S, Van Ongeval C (2018) Breast imaging surveillance after curative treatment for primary non-metastasised breast cancer in non-high-risk women: a systematic review. Insights Imaging 9:961–970

Taglialatela Scafati S, Cavaliere A, Aceto B, Somma F, Cremone L (2017) Combining autologous and prosthetic techniques: the breast reconstruction scale principle. Plast Reconstr Surg Glob Open 5:E1602

Tayyab SJ, Adrada BE, Rauch GM, Yang WT (2018) A pictorial review: multimodality imaging of benign and suspicious features of fat necrosis in the breast. Br J Radiol 91:20180213

Teo SY, Wang SC (2008) Radiologic features of poly-acrylamide gel mammoplasty. AJR Am J Roentgenol 191:W89–W95

Upadhyaya SN, Bernard SL, Grobmyer SR, Yanda C, Tu C, Valente SA (2018) Outcomes of autologous fat grafting in mastectomy patients following breast reconstruction. Ann Surg Oncol 25:3052–3056

Wang CF, Zhou Z, Yan YJ, Zhao DM, Chen F, Qiao Q (2011) Clinical analyses of clustered microcalcifications after autologous fat injection for breast augmentation. Plast Reconstr Surg 127:1669–1673

Wong T, Lo LW, Fung PY, Lai HY, She HL, Ng WK, Kwok KM, Lee CM (2016) Magnetic resonance imaging of breast augmentation: a pictorial review. Insights Imaging 7:399–410

Yilmaz MH, Esen G, Ayarcan Y, Aydogan F, Ozguroglu M, Demir G, Bese N, Mandel NM (2007) The role of US and MR imaging in detecting local chest wall tumor recurrence after mastectomy. Diagn Interv Radiol 13:13–18

Zakhireh J, Fowble B, Esserman LJ (2010) Application of screening principles to the reconstructed breast. J Clin Oncol 28:173–180

Impact and Assessment of Breast Density

Georg J. Wengert, Katja Pinker, and Thomas Helbich

Contents

1   **Introduction** 420

2   **Breast Density and the Risk for Breast Cancer** 420
     2.1   Masking Effect 420
     2.2   Independent Risk Factor 421

3   **Assessment Methods** 423
     3.1   Mammography 423
     3.2   Ultrasound 425
     3.3   Magnetic Resonance Imaging 426

4   **New Avenues for Risk-Adapted Screening** 428

5   **Summary** 430

   References 430

Abstract

Breast density, or the amount of fibroglandular tissue in the breast, is a recognized and independent marker for breast cancer risk. In addition, breast density reduces the sensitivity of mammography due to a masking effect. Public awareness of the importance of breast density has resulted in legislation for reporting breast density for risk stratification purposes. To date, breast density assessment is performed with mammography and to some extent with magnetic resonance imaging. Data indicate that computerized, quantitative techniques in comparison with subjective, visual estimations are characterized by higher reproducibility and

---

G. J. Wengert · T. Helbich (✉)
Division of Molecular and Gender Imaging, Department of Biomedical Imaging and Image-Guided Therapy, Medical University of Vienna, Vienna, Austria
e-mail: georg.wengert@meduniwien.ac.at; thomas.helbich@meduniwien.ac.at

K. Pinker
Division of Molecular and Gender Imaging, Department of Biomedical Imaging and Image-Guided Therapy, Medical University of Vienna, Vienna, Austria

Breast Imaging Service, Department of Radiology, Memorial Sloan Kettering Cancer Center, New York, NY, USA
e-mail: katja.pinker@meduniwien.ac.at; pinkerdk@mskcc.org

© Springer Nature Switzerland AG 2022
M. Fuchsjäger et al. (eds.), *Breast Imaging*, Medical Radiology Diagnostic Imaging,
https://doi.org/10.1007/978-3-030-94918-1_19

robustness. Standardized breast density assessment using automated volumetric quantitative methods has the potential to be useful for risk prediction, stratification, and determining the best screening plan for each woman. This chapter provides a comprehensive overview of the currently available imaging modalities for qualitative and quantitative breast density assessment and the current evidence on breast density and breast cancer risk assessment.

1 Introduction

Breast density is defined as the amount of fibroglandular breast components relative to fatty components within the breast. Fibroglandular breast components are composed of a mixture of connective, stromal, and parenchymal tissue (Boyd et al. 1992; Ghosh et al. 2008) and appear radiopaque on mammography; on the other hand, fatty components appear radiolucent. Large variations of breast tissue composition exist between women; breast composition also changes over the course of time and during the menstrual cycle, as influenced by endogenous and exogenous factors (Table 1) (Boyd et al. 2006; Byrne et al. 2017; Sterns and Zee 2000; van Duijnhoven et al. 2007). According to the American College of Radiology (ACR), 50% of women in the USA have high breast density, with 40% being categorized as having heterogeneously dense breasts (ACR category c) and 10% as having extremely dense breasts (ACR category d) (D'Orsi et al. 2013).

Based on a large twin study, Nguyen et al. reported that breast density is significantly influenced by the number of childbirths and by body mass index (BMI). Increased childbirths were found to be associated with a decrease of mammographic breast density as well as a corresponding breast cancer risk reduction of up to 4% per live birth (Nguyen et al. 2013). In studies on postmenopausal women, women with the greatest increase in weight and BMI experienced the greatest reduction in breast density (Wanders et al. 2015); however, higher BMI is also associated with higher breast cancer risk in this population (Keum et al. 2015; Huo et al. 2014). Using data from a longitudinal cohort, Hopper and colleagues reported a negative association between adolescent BMI at the age of 7–15 years and breast density at the age of 47–50 years, concluding that adolescent BMI is negatively associated with breast cancer risk (Hopper et al. 2016), in line with other publications in the literature (Harris et al. 2011; Andersen et al. 2014). Several studies have reported that lower BMI or a moderate reduction of body weight during adulthood, before or after menopause, has resulted in the reduction of postmenopausal breast cancer risk of up to 50% (Eliassen et al. 2006; Harvie et al. 2005). A recent study reported that breast density is associated with parity and BMI regardless of age (Krishnan et al. 2017).

Table 1 Summary of endogenous and exogenous factors influencing breast tissue composition to increased breast density (does not claim completeness)

Endogenous factors	Exogenous factors
Older age/ postmenopause	Smoking
High parity/nulliparity	Alcohol
High body mass index	HRT
Circulating estrogens/ IGF-1	Oral contraceptive
African-American	Obesity
Early age at menarche (≤12a)	Sedentary time
Age threshold at first live birth	Physical inactivity
CYP1A2 status	Tamoxifen/Vit C, D/folate/ NSAID

2 Breast Density and the Risk for Breast Cancer

2.1 Masking Effect

Breast composition impacts the risk for breast cancer in different ways. Mammographic sensitivity for detecting breast cancer decreases as breast density increases (Kerlikowske et al. 2007; Boyd et al. 2007; McCormack and dos Santos 2006). Breast density is known for producing tissue overlap that leads to a masking effect. Two-dimensional imaging modalities including mammography are particularly susceptible to the masking effect. While the masking effect is a source of false-negative readings and correspondingly a low efficiency of screening examinations (Bailey et al. 2010), an increased density also leads to increased false positives and recall rates (Ballard-Barbash et al. 1997; Carney et al. 2003). High breast density leads to overlapping normal breast tissue, resulting in coalescent areas of breast parenchyma and obliteration of tissues with underlying tumors on imaging (D'Orsi et al. 2013; Rhodes et al. 2015). As a result, women with higher breast density are more often diagnosed with larger breast tumors and advanced stages with lymphatic involvement at initial diagnosis (Ghosh et al. 2008; Aiello et al. 2005; Roubidoux et al. 2004). Interval cancers also increase 6- to 17-fold in women with higher density breasts (Boyd et al. 2007; McCormack and dos Santos 2006).

Most of the evidence on the reduced sensitivity of mammography in dense breasts is from studies employing screen-film mammography (SFM) (D'Orsi et al. 2013; Price et al. 2013). With the introduction of full-field digital mammography (FFDM), the masking effect of dense breasts on cancer detection has been greatly reduced (Carney et al. 2003; Pisano et al. 2005). Kerlikowske et al. (2011) also showed that FFDM improves the detection of hormone receptor-negative breast cancers compared with SFM (FFDM 78.5% vs. SFM 65.8%, sensitivity $p = 0.016$, in women aged 40–79 years; 95.2% vs. 54.9%, sensitivity, $p = 0.007$, in women aged 40–49 years). As hormone receptor-negative breast cancers usually present with a higher grade, carry a poorer prognosis, and often manifest as interval cancers, they presumably constitute some proportion of the cancers masked at SFM screening in women with higher density categories. Recently, digital breast tomosynthesis (DBT), a three-dimensional imaging modality, has also been introduced. Several large-scale studies worldwide have investigated DBT in the screening setting, demonstrating an increase in cancer detection as well as a significant reduction

in recall rates compared with FFDM, which is most likely attributable to a decreased masking effect (Destounis et al. 2015; Friedewald et al. 2014; McDonald et al. 2016). However, the value of DBT for breast cancer detection as related to breast density has not been fully elucidated. Ciatto et al. evaluated DBT in combination with FFDM in the STORM-1 trial, showing an improved cancer detection rate from 5.3 cancers to 8.1 cancers per 1000 screening examinations and a reduction of recalls by 17.2% (Ciatto et al. 2013). Bernardi et al. demonstrated similar results in the STORM-2 trial, showing cancer detection rates of up to 8.5 cancers per 1000 screening examinations when FFDM is combined with DBT, and up to 8.8 cancers per 1000 screening examinations when a synthesized two-dimensional mammographic image is reconstructed and combined with DBT. However, false-positive readings also increased when using DBT: 3.97% FFDM plus DBT and 4.45% synthetic FFDM plus DBT, respectively, compared with 3.42% for FFDM only (Bernardi et al. 2016).

2.2 Independent Risk Factor

Although the masking effect as related to breast density is an important issue to be considered, it must be noted that the association between breast density and risk for breast cancer is not merely a masking bias and cannot be explained by the reduced sensitivity of mammography alone. Conclusive data have shown that increased breast density is a strong and independent imaging biomarker for increased risk of breast cancer (McCormack and dos Santos 2006; Checka et al. 2012; Vachon et al. 2007; Boyd et al. 2010). Epithelial and glandular structures in the breast are the site of origin for most breast cancers; consequently, higher dense breast parenchyma is associated with an increased chance of future breast cancer development (Freer 2015). In a meta-analysis by McCormack et al. that investigated breast density as an independent risk factor for breast cancer, the relative risk associated with dense breasts was 2.92 for breasts that were

50–74% dense and 4.64 for breasts that were 75% or more dense (McCormack and dos Santos 2006). Boyd et al. summarized studies evaluating breast cancer risk with respect to quantitatively measured tissue density, and the odds ratio of the risk for breast cancer was found to range from 3.6 to 6.0 (Boyd et al. 2011).

Studies investigating breast density under screening conditions arrived at a similar conclusion regarding breast density as a strong predictor of breast cancer risk. Data from the TOMMY trial indicates that absolute measurements of fibroglandular tissue volume were significantly associated with increased breast cancer risk in higher density groups (Gilbert et al. 2015). After adjusting for age, a 2–3% increase of the odds of breast cancer was found per increase of 10 cm^3 dense tissue depending on the automated breast density measurement system. The relative risk for breast cancer can differ based on whether a quantitative or qualitative approach is used to determine breast density. However, in either approach, higher breast density is associated with an increased relative risk. In their review, Destounis et al. reported that the relative risk for breast cancer was higher when using semiquantitative percentage calculation methods (up to 4.64) than when using subjective qualitative assessments (up to 3.98) to determine mammographic breast density (Destounis et al. 2017). This is concordant with other studies comparing qualitative and quantitative methods of density measurement that demonstrated an increased risk when using quantitative approaches (Jeffers et al. 2017; Keller et al. 2015). It must be pointed out that most studies that have investigated the association between breast density and breast cancer risk did not use ACR Breast Imaging Reporting and Data System (BI-RADS) categories but instead used quantitative measures or a different classification such as the Wolfe classification. The use of the BI-RADS categories results in a similar but milder association of risk with breast density (Freer 2015).

Many studies focusing on the association between mammographic breast density and relative risk of breast cancer have also compared women with almost entirely fatty breasts and women with extremely dense breasts, finding that the relative risk for breast cancer is 4–6 in women with extremely dense breasts compared with women with almost entirely fatty breasts (Sickles 2010). However, as only approximately 10% of women have almost entirely fatty breasts and another 10% have extremely dense breasts, the results are potentially misleading (D'Orsi et al. 2013). Compared with the average women, the relative risk for breast cancer is approximately 1.2 in women with heterogeneously dense breasts and 2.1 in women with extremely dense breasts.

Although the relative risk of breast density as a risk factor is much smaller than age, family history, reproductive history, and genetic mutations, it is not negligible as mammographically dense breasts are relatively common (approximately 50% of the screening population). Therefore, breast density contributes significantly more to cancer risk in the population than other much stronger but less common risk factors, such as a BRCA 1 or 2 mutation carrier or high-risk status (McCormack and dos Santos 2006; Freer 2015; Boyd et al. 2011). The consistent association between increased breast density and cancer risk emphasizes its potential for risk prediction and risk stratification; thus, it might become a valuable tool in determining the best individualized screening plan for each woman.

In the past decade, breast density notification laws have been passed with the intent of informing women about their own breast density and possible benefits from supplemental screening methods such as breast ultrasound (Hooley 2017). Currently, there are 38 states of the USA with a legal obligation to provide a patient and her primary care physician with her breast density status and the risk posed by breast density. In addition, breast density notification legislation laws are in progress in other states and will be issued shortly. Breast density legislation provides a unique opportunity to strengthen patient-provider relationships by encouraging physicians to engage women in a conversation about the limitations, risks, and benefits of screening, as well as to provide women with greater autonomy; however, ineffective transfer of information may cause anxiety and patient confusion, which emphasizes the need for innovative information tools creating a better understanding for risk and health-care management (Miles et al. 2019; Slanetz et al. 2015; Are You Dense? 2018).

3 Assessment Methods

3.1 Mammography

3.1.1 Subjective Qualitative Assessment

The assessment of breast density is usually performed based on the appearance of the amount of fibroglandular tissue relative to fatty tissue on mammography. To date, there are no recommendations or criteria for standardized assessment of breast density (Winkler et al. 2015; Colin et al. 2014). Methods range from the initial classification systems of Wolfe (1976) and Tabár (He et al. 2015) to the recent BI-RADS classification of the ACR, which is currently the most commonly used classification system. The differences of these classification systems are summarized in Table 2 (D'Orsi et al. 2013). The BI-RADS lexicon classification of breast density is mainly performed based on the subjective visual estimation. According to the current revised fifth edition of

the BI-RADS atlas, published in 2013, breast density can be classified into ACR-MG-a, wherein the breasts are almost entirely fatty; ACR-MG-b, in which there are scattered areas of fibroglandular density; ACR-MG-c, wherein the breasts are heterogeneously dense, which may obscure small masses; and ACR-MG-d, in which the breasts are extremely dense, which lowers the sensitivity of mammography (D'Orsi et al. 2013). Women classified as either ACR-MG-a or -b are considered as having non-dense breasts, whereas women classified as either ACR-MG-c or -d are considered as having dense breasts. The revised fifth edition replaced a percentage categorization of total breast density with descriptive categories and identification of coalescent areas on the mammogram, acknowledging the possible masking of underlying breast masses, Fig. 1, and the potential benefit of supplemental screening (van der Waal et al. 2017).

Several studies have shown that subjective visual estimation of mammographic breast density is prone to error, with great inter- and intra-observer variability (Ciatto et al. 2012; Lee et al. 2015; Morrish et al. 2015; Wengert et al. 2016a). While training and experience can improve reader variability (Wengert et al. 2016a; Gao et al. 2008; Raza et al. 2016), subjective qualita-

Table 2 Summary of different available classification systems to describe parenchymal patterns of mammographic density in breast imaging, with the recommended current gold standard and ubiquitously used BI-RADS classification system from the American College of Radiology

Wolfe		Tabár		BI-RADS	
N1 (Normal)	The breast consists mainly of fat	I	Balanced distribution with slightly fibrous predominance	ACR-a	Almost entirely fatty breast
P1	Fatty breast with no more than 25% of linear densities	II	Predominance of fatty tissue	ACR-b	Scattered areas of fibroglandular tissue
P2	Linear densities more than 25% of the breast	III	Predominance of fatty tissue with retroareolar fibrous	ACR-c	Heterogeneously dense, small masses may obscure
Dy (dysplasia)	Dense, radiopaque breast	IV	Predominantly nodular densities	ACR-d	Extremely dense breast, lowering the sensitivity of mammography
Qdy (quasi-dysplasia)	Dense breast with spongy texture due to fatty infiltration	V	Dense breast, predominantly fibrous tissue		
	Low risk (N1 and P1) High risk (P2 and Dy)		Low risk (I, II, and III) High risk (IV and V)		Low risk (ACR-a und -b) High risk (ACR-c and -d)

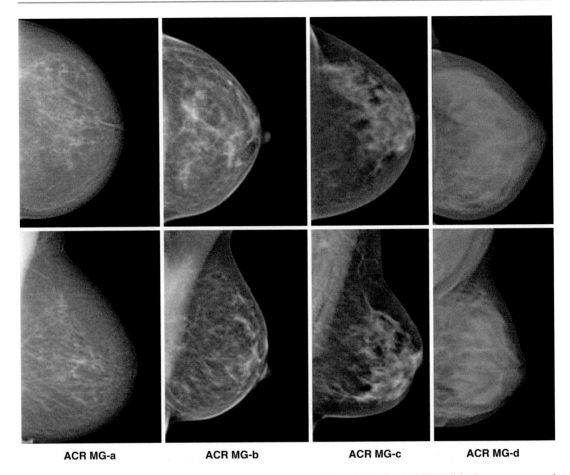

Fig. 1 Example images of the four breast density/composition categories defined by the fifth edition of the BI-RADS mammography atlas with descriptive categories indicating coalescent breast tissue with possible masking of underlying masses. ACR MG-a, the breasts are almost entirely fatty; ACR MG-b, there are scattered areas of fibroglandular density; ACR MG-c, the breasts are heterogeneously dense, which may obscure small masses; and ACR MG-d, the breasts are extremely dense, which lowers the sensitivity of mammography

tive breast density assessment is not equipped to provide a reliable and reproducible objective assessment of breast density as a risk factor.

3.1.2 Objective Automated Quantitative Assessment

To overcome the limitations of subjective visual assessments, attempts have been made to develop automated quantitative technologies for breast density measurement. There are computer-aided semiautomated and fully automated measurement approaches available that allow either a two- or three-dimensional assessment of breast tissue structures. Cumulus™, the so-called gold standard of breast density assessment on mammography that has been validated by epidemiological studies, allows the estimation of the percentage area of dense breast tissue from mammographic images (Byng et al. 1994), yielding a higher reproducibility compared with BI-RADS visual assessment (Boyd et al. 2011). The limitation of Cumulus™ is that breast density measurements are derived from two-dimensional images and thus requires some user interaction, which renders it prone to bias. Recently, other three-dimensional mammography-based breast density measurement techniques have become available. Highnam (Highnam et al. 2007) and van Engeland (van Engeland et al. 2006) introduced fully automated approaches, Quantra (Morrish et al. 2015;

Brandt et al. 2015; Wang et al. 2013) and Volpara (Lee et al. 2015; Morrish et al. 2015; Brandt et al. 2015; Wang et al. 2013), which allow mammography-based, volumetric, quantitative breast density measurements. Recently, yet another fully automated volumetric breast density measurement system "insight breast density," which is integrated into the new MAMMOMAT Revelation (Siemens Healthineers, Erlangen, Germany) unit for three-dimensional mammography, has become available (Fig. 2).

Although the above approaches are fully automated, breast density calculation based on mammography may vary due to differences in tissue compression and breast positioning (Kopans 2008). All these approaches have in common a positive association between breast density and breast cancer risk. However, a paper from Gastounioti et al. (2016) discussed how the differences in quantitative breast density measurements are influenced by processed or raw mammographic images, as well as specific features of image acquisition, physical properties, and vendors.

3.2 Ultrasound

Ultrasound (US) of the breast is a ubiquitous, cost-effective, and reliable imaging modality, which is easily performed without the need for intravenous contrast application or ionizing radiation. To date, breast US cannot be reliably used for either a qualitative or quantitative breast density assessment. However, the latest version of the US BI-RADS atlas recommends an assessment of breast tissue composition with US using three descriptive categories: ACR-US-a, homogeneous background echotexture—fat; ACR-US-b, homogeneous background echotexture—fibroglandular; and ACR-US-c, heterogeneous background echotexture, Fig. 3 (D'Orsi et al. 2013). To over-

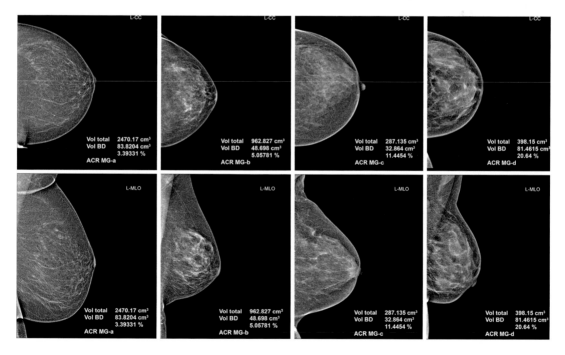

Fig. 2 Examples of increasing mammographic breast densities from left to right. Left craniocaudal (L-CC) and left mediolateral-oblique (L-MLO) were acquired with a Siemens MAMMOMAT Revelation (Siemens Healthcare GmbH, Erlangen, Germany). Density was assessed using the integrated insight breast density application, which calculates the total breast volume (Vol total, cm^3) and the breast density volume (Vol BD, cm^3 and %). Fully automated volumetric breast density measurements are displayed quantitatively and as the corresponding ACR BI-RADS category, A to D

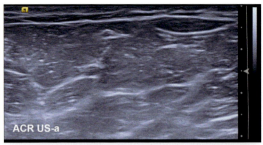
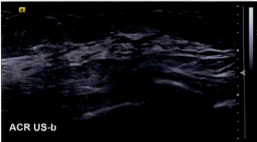
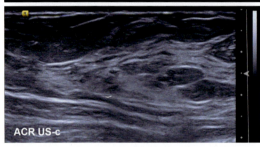

Fig. 3 Example images of the three breast density/tissue composition categories defined by the fifth edition of the BI-RADS ultrasound atlas for screening-only purposes. ACR US-a, homogeneous background echotexture—fat; ACR US-b, homogeneous background echotexture—fibroglandular; and ACR US-c, heterogenous background echotexture

come the drawback of handheld US, automated 3D whole-breast US (ABUS) has been introduced (Chae et al. 2013) and attempts have also been made to assess breast density with 3D ABUS using semiautomated techniques (Chen et al. 2016; Moon et al. 2011). Initial results suggest that ABUS might provide 3D volumetric imaging and accurate breast density measurement (Chen et al. 2016; Moon et al. 2011). US of the breast may be a valuable supplemental imaging modality to mammography in asymptomatic women with dense breast tissue to enable the detection of additional breast cancers invisible on mammography (Houssami and Ciatto 2011).

3.3 Magnetic Resonance Imaging

To address the problems of 2D mammography-based breast density assessment, promising approaches of volumetric, quantitative assessment of the amount of fibroglandular tissue on magnetic resonance imaging (MRI) have been developed and investigated.

In contrast to mammography, MRI allows radiation- and compression-free 3D imaging, which allows a standardized assessment of breast areas near the chest wall and axilla. MRI provides images related to the fat and water composition of the breast. Since the water composition is highly correlated with the prevalence of fibroglandular tissue, these images can be used for slice-by-slice segmentation of fibroglandular and fatty components and thereby allow quantitative breast density assessment (O'Flynn et al. 2015).

Many of the currently available approaches rely on the use of T1-weighted sequences, which provide grayscale images and therefore not enough tissue contrast to allow an objective assessment of breast parenchyma. In addition, most of these approaches require user interaction for breast area segmentation or threshold adjustments (van Engeland et al. 2006; Klifa et al. 2004, 2010; Lee et al. 1997; Thompson et al. 2009; Nie et al. 2008, 2010). Allowing accurate segmentation is one of the most important steps to precisely define breast and tissue borders. The boundaries for the segmentation are usually the anterior border of the major pectoral muscle and the anterior chest wall. The inferior border of the manubrium sterni and the submammary fold is the cranial and caudal boundaries. In addition, preferentially the variable subcutaneous fatty tissue of the cleavage should also be excluded from the segmentation. To overcome these, atlas- (Gubern-Merida et al. 2015; Wu et al. 2013) or template-aided (Wengert et al. 2015) semiautomated approaches with predefined breast models and automated adaption in real time have been investigated for an individual breast segmentation with high accuracy and robustness.

Meanwhile, there are already fully automated, volumetric measurement approaches for MRI-based measurements of the amount of fibroglandular breast tissue. Gubern-Mérida et al. (2014) used an expectation-maximization algorithm based on fuzzy C-means clustering, and Wu et al. (2013) developed a fully automated segmentation approach based on two-dimensional C-means clustering. Wengert et al. introduced an iterative segmentation for the separation of the bivariate signal intensity values on Dixon sequences, Fig. 4 (Wengert et al. 2015). The use of Dixon sequences for MRI-based measurements of the amount of fibroglandular tissue has been suggested previously (Graham et al. 1995) and tested with promising results (Wengert et al. 2015; Tagliafico et al. 2013, 2014), Fig. 5. Dixon sequences allow for improved reproducibility and accuracy of breast density measurements compared with conventional sequences (Wengert et al. 2016b, 2017). The integration of Dixon sequences into standard clinical dynamic contrast-enhanced MRI protocols, as well as for fibroglandular tissue quantification, is easily executed (Wengert et al. 2016b; Kuhl et al. 2014). Therefore, objective fibroglandular tissue segmentation derived from high-resolution Dixon sequences as the MRI-based reference standard for the assessment of the amount of FGT is a practical recommendation (Wengert et al. 2016b; Kuhl et al. 2014; Clauser et al. 2014; Mann et al. 2014).

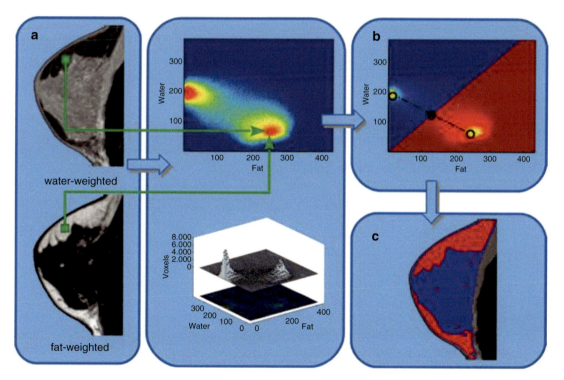

Fig. 4 Diagram of the process of fibroglandular tissue segmentation. For each individual breast and water/fat-based sequence, the program automatically segments an individual breast model, representing the identical 3D breast volume, with exclusion of the skin and the pectoralis muscle. (A) The signal intensity (SI) values of fat- and water-weighted pixel intensities were recorded and collected into a 2D histogram (top image). On the bottom, there is the 3D illustration of the histogram. (B) Thresholds for the corresponding fat and water SI values were automatically calculated by dividing the histogram into two regions half the distance between the two cluster peaks of the bimodal distribution of measured SI values. (C) Graphical illustration of the assignment for each voxel to be either fat tissue (red) or dense tissue (blue) into the 3D breast model. (Reprinted with permission from: Wengert GJ, Helbich TH, Vogl WD, et al. Introduction of an automated user independent quantitative volumetric magnetic resonance imaging breast density measurement system using the Dixon sequence: comparison with mammographic breast density assessment. Investigative Radiology. 2015;50(2):73–80. https://doi.org/10.1097/RLI.0000000000000102)

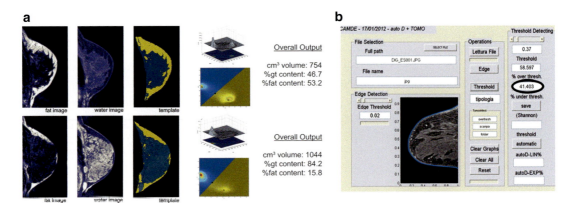

Fig. 5 Examples of MRI-based breast density calculation; (**a**) fully automated measurements of fibroglandular (%gt) breast tissue based on the fat and water high-resolution Dixon images of a moderate (top row) and extremely dense breast (bottom row); with the corresponding threshold segmentation (template) and scatterplots, breast compartments are represented by the total segmented volume (cm^3 volume), percentage of fibroglandular tissue (%gt), and percentage of fat tissue (%fat) (published in Wengert et al. 2015); (**b**) extract of the graphical computer interface illustrating the selection and thresholding process of the semiautomated assessment of fibroglandular breast tissue, with the output of the percentage of breast density (black circle). (Reprinted under a Creative Commons Attribution 4.0 International (CC BY 4.0) from Tagliafico A, Bignotti B, Tagliafigo G, et al. "Breast density assessment using a 3T MRI system: comparison among different sequences." PLoS One. 2014;9(6):e99027. https://doi.org/10.1371/journal.pone.0099027)

A drawback of fully automated, volumetric MRI-based measurements is that the output of percentage values of breast density is not included in the current fifth edition of the ACR BI-RADS lexicon. The MRI BI-RADS lexicon currently contains the recommendation to assess the amount of fibroglandular tissue with MRI similar to mammography on a four-grade scale, Fig. 6: ACR-MRI-a, almost entirely fat; ACR-MRI-b, scattered fibroglandular tissue; ACR-MRI-c, heterogeneous fibroglandular tissue; and ACR-MRI-d, extreme fibroglandular tissue (D'Orsi et al. 2013). Recent studies have shown that subjective visual estimation of breast density on mammography and the amount of FGT on MRI are both prone to error with great inter- and intra-observer variability (Wengert et al. 2016a; Gao et al. 2008; Raza et al. 2016). While subjective visual estimation can be improved by reader training, similar to mammography, this seems a suboptimal solution compared with the objective quantitative MRI-based assessment of breast density as a risk factor (Lee et al. 2015; Morrish et al. 2015; Wengert et al. 2016a; Wang et al. 2013; Ciatto et al. 2005).

4 New Avenues for Risk-Adapted Screening

While population-based screening programs using mammography with the aim of detecting breast cancer at an early stage have reduced cancer mortality by up to 49% (Broeders et al. 2012; Nickson et al. 2012), to date, there are no recommendations for risk-adapted screening.

Breast cancer risk estimation tools like the Gail and Tyrer-Cuzick models have been introduced with the purpose of identifying women who are at risk of developing breast cancer (Gail et al. 1989; Smith et al. 2014; Tyrer et al. 2004). The Gail model from the National Cancer Institute based on the general population is an eight-question tool using age, hormonal factors, benign disease, and number of fist-degree relatives who have already been diagnosed with breast cancer to estimate the relative risk of developing invasive breast cancer (Costantino et al. 1999). The Tyrer-Cuzick model uses similar risk factors from the Gail approach in conjunction with personal and genetic factors including the BRCA 1/2 genes for risk assessment of inva-

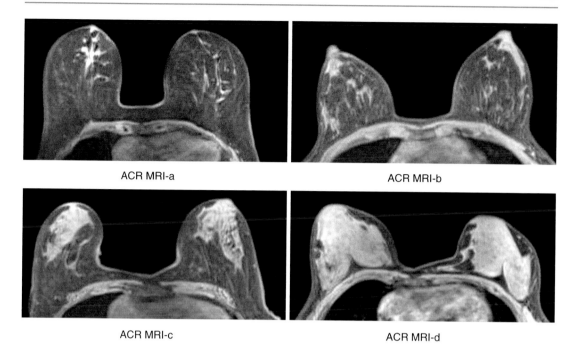

Fig. 6 Example of T1-weighted high-resolution Dixon images of the four breast density/composition categories defined by the fifth edition of the BI-RADS MRI atlas with four categories similar to mammography. ACR MRI-a, almost entirely fat; ACR MRI-b, scattered fibroglandular tissue; ACR MRI-c, heterogeneous fibroglandular tissue, which may obscure small masses; and ACR MRI-d, extreme fibroglandular tissue. (Reprinted under a Creative Commons Attribution 4.0 International License from: Wengert GJ, Helbich, TH, Leithner D, et al. Multimodality Imaging of Breast Parenchymal Density and Correlation with Risk Assessment. Curr Breast Cancer Rep. 2019;11:23–33. https://doi.org/10.1007/s12609-019-0302-6)

sive breast cancer (Tyrer et al. 2004). However, it has been demonstrated that mammographic density is a stronger risk factor than any of the risk factors used in the Gail and Tyrer-Cuzick models; the combination of breast density with either the Gail or the Tyrer-Cuzick model resulted in a better breast cancer risk assessment (Brentnall et al. 2015). The Gail model, which is based on demographic and clinical data for breast cancer risk stratification, can be assessed online: https://www.mdcalc.com/gail-model-breast-cancer-risk. The Tyrer-Cuzick model providing a personal risk and risk of mutation carrier assessment can be found at http://ibis.ikonopedia.com/.

Moreover, the process of screening for breast cancer remains controversial with different recommendations between national breast cancer screening programs concerning the start points and the intervals for screening. A potential model for risk-adapted screening could include an initial risk stratification incorporating family and personal history, breast density assessed with mammography, and, potentially, lifestyle risk factors such as obesity (Mahoney et al. 2008) and alcohol (Zhang et al. 2007). Based on this model, women could be classified into different risk categories, e.g., low, intermediate, and high, and would undergo screening tailored to their individual risk.

Other avenues that can be explored for a more refined breast cancer risk stratification include the use of radiomics analyses and machine-learning techniques, such as deep learning.

Based on such refined risk stratification, women could then be offered risk-adapted screening with different imaging modalities. Low-risk women could continue to be screened with FFDM or, when available, DBT with synthesized mammography annually, biannually, or triennially based on national recommendations. Intermediate-risk women could undergo additional supplemental screening with US or

MRI. High-risk women, who constitute a minority, could be offered MRI and mammography only in whom benefit has been demonstrated (e.g., BRCA 2 mutation carrier) (Phi et al. 2016). In this context, the Dutch DENSE trial investigates the effectiveness and cost-effectiveness of screening with mammography and MRI compared with those of screening with mammography alone in women with extremely dense breasts (Emaus et al. 2015). Recently published results showed that supplemental MRI screening of women with extremely dense breasts resulted in significantly fewer interval cancers compared to mammography as the sole screening methodology (2.5/1000 vs. 5.0/1000). The authors reported furthermore a cancer detection rate of 16.5/1000 women screened with MRI for breast cancer with a false-positive rate of 8.0% (Bakker et al. 2019). In addition, about 60% of the total screening population accepted the invitation of supplemental MRI screening. The most frequently stated reasons for not participating in this trial were MRI-related inconveniences, self-reported contraindications, and anxiety regarding the screening outcome (de Lange et al. 2018). Further results to better understand the role of MRI in this patient population are expected in the coming years after two rounds of screening are completed.

5   Summary

Breast density has recently become one of the hottest topics in breast imaging: firstly as it is an independent risk factor for breast cancer and secondly because high breast density reduces mammographic sensitivity due to a masking effect. Although the exact extent to which breast density is an independent risk factor remains controversial, there is consensus that the increased breast cancer risk is not solely attributable to the masking effect. This emphasizes the potential of breast density for cancer risk prediction and stratification, potentially becoming a valuable tool in determining the best screening plan for each woman and guiding supplemental screening methods. However, to be used in this context, breast density assessment must be reliable, reproducible, and accurate. Breast density has been predominantly assessed with mammography using qualitatively subjective visual inspection and the ACR BI-RADS classification. Due to substantial intra/inter-reader variability, semi/automated volumetric breast density measurement approaches with both mammography and MRI have been developed with excellent results. Initial attempts for automated volumetric breast density measurements with ABUS are promising. It is expected that these advances in breast density assessment will further define its role in breast cancer risk assessment and help tailoring breast cancer screening strategies to an individual woman's risk, values, and preferences while also accounting for cost, potential harms, and important patient outcomes.

Acknowledgements Funding was provided in part by the European Union's Horizon 2020 Research and Innovation Programme under grant agreement Nr. 688188.

References

Aiello EJ, Buist DS, White E, Porter PL (2005) Association between mammographic breast density and breast cancer tumor characteristics. Cancer Epidemiol Biomarkers Prev 14(3):662–668

Andersen ZJ, Baker JL, Bihrmann K, Vejborg I, Sorensen TI, Lynge E (2014) Birth weight, childhood body mass index, and height in relation to mammographic density and breast cancer: a register-based cohort study. Breast Cancer Res 16(1):R4

Are You Dense? 2008 (2018) https://www.areyoudenseadvocacy.org/dense

Bailey SL, Sigal BM, Plevritis SK (2010) A simulation model investigating the impact of tumor volume doubling time and mammographic tumor detectability on screening outcomes in women aged 40–49 years. J Natl Cancer Inst 102(16):1263–1271

Bakker MF, de Lange SV, Pijnappel RM, Mann RM, Peeters PHM, Monninkhof EM et al (2019) Supplemental MRI screening for women with extremely dense breast tissue. N Engl J Med 381(22):2091–2102

Ballard-Barbash R, Taplin SH, Yankaskas BC, Ernster VL, Rosenberg RD, Carney PA et al (1997) Breast Cancer Surveillance Consortium: a national mammography screening and outcomes database. AJR Am J Roentgenol 169(4):1001–1008

Bernardi D, Macaskill P, Pellegrini M, Valentini M, Fanto C, Ostillio L et al (2016) Breast cancer screening with tomosynthesis (3D mammography) with acquired or synthetic 2D mammography compared with 2D mammography alone (STORM-2): a population-based prospective study. Lancet Oncol 17(8):1105–1113

Boyd NF, Jensen HM, Cooke G, Han HL (1992) Relationship between mammographic and histological risk factors for breast cancer. J Natl Cancer Inst 84(15):1170–1179

Boyd NF, Martin LJ, Yaffe MJ, Minkin S (2006) Mammographic density: a hormonally responsive risk factor for breast cancer. J Br Menopause Soc 12(4):186–193

Boyd NF, Guo H, Martin LJ, Sun L, Stone J, Fishell E et al (2007) Mammographic density and the risk and detection of breast cancer. N Engl J Med 356(3):227–236

Boyd NF, Martin LJ, Bronskill M, Yaffe MJ, Duric N, Minkin S (2010) Breast tissue composition and susceptibility to breast cancer. J Natl Cancer Inst 102(16):1224–1237

Boyd NF, Martin LJ, Yaffe MJ, Minkin S (2011) Mammographic density and breast cancer risk: current understanding and future prospects. Breast Cancer Res 13(6):223

Brandt KR, Scott CG, Ma L, Mahmoudzadeh AP, Jensen MR, Whaley DH et al (2015) Comparison of clinical and automated breast density measurements: implications for risk prediction and supplemental screening. Radiology 2015:151261

Brentnall AR, Harkness EF, Astley SM, Donnelly LS, Stavrinos P, Sampson S et al (2015) Mammographic density adds accuracy to both the Tyrer-Cuzick and Gail breast cancer risk models in a prospective UK screening cohort. Breast Cancer Res 17(1):147

Broeders M, Moss S, Nystrom L, Njor S, Jonsson H, Paap E et al (2012) The impact of mammographic screening on breast cancer mortality in Europe: a review of observational studies. J Med Screen 19(Suppl 1):14–25

Byng JW, Boyd NF, Fishell E, Jong RA, Yaffe MJ (1994) The quantitative analysis of mammographic densities. Phys Med Biol 39(10):1629–1638

Byrne C, Ursin G, Martin CF, Peck JD, Cole EB, Zeng D et al (2017) Mammographic density change with estrogen and progestin therapy and breast cancer risk. J Natl Cancer Inst 109(9):djx001

Carney PA, Miglioretti DL, Yankaskas BC, Kerlikowske K, Rosenberg R, Rutter CM et al (2003) Individual and combined effects of age, breast density, and hormone replacement therapy use on the accuracy of screening mammography. Ann Intern Med 138(3):168–175

Chae EY, Shin HJ, Kim HJ, Yoo H, Baek S, Cha JH et al (2013) Diagnostic performance of automated breast ultrasound as a replacement for a hand-held second-look ultrasound for breast lesions detected initially on magnetic resonance imaging. Ultrasound Med Biol 39(12):2246–2254

Checka CM, Chun JE, Schnabel FR, Lee J, Toth H (2012) The relationship of mammographic density and age: implications for breast cancer screening. AJR Am J Roentgenol 198(3):W292–W295

Chen JH, Lee YW, Chan SW, Yeh DC, Chang RF (2016) Breast density analysis with automated whole-breast ultrasound: comparison with 3-D magnetic resonance imaging. Ultrasound Med Biol 42(5):1211–1220

Ciatto S, Houssami N, Apruzzese A, Bassetti E, Brancato B, Carozzi F et al (2005) Categorizing breast mammographic density: intra- and interobserver reproducibility of BI-RADS density categories. Breast 14(4):269–275

Ciatto S, Bernardi D, Calabrese M, Durando M, Gentilini MA, Mariscotti G et al (2012) A first evaluation of breast radiological density assessment by QUANTRA software as compared to visual classification. Breast 21(4):503–506

Ciatto S, Houssami N, Bernardi D, Caumo F, Pellegrini M, Brunelli S et al (2013) Integration of 3D digital mammography with tomosynthesis for population breast-cancer screening (STORM): a prospective comparison study. Lancet Oncol 14(7):583–589

Clauser P, Pinker K, Helbich TH, Kapetas P, Bernathova M, Baltzer PA (2014) Fat saturation in dynamic breast MRI at 3 Tesla: is the Dixon technique superior to spectral fat saturation? A visual grading characteristics study. Eur Radiol 24(9):2213–2219

Colin C, Schott AM, Valette PJ (2014) Mammographic density is not a worthwhile examination to distinguish high cancer risk women in screening. Eur Radiol 24(10):2412–2416

Costantino JP, Gail MH, Pee D, Anderson S, Redmond CK, Benichou J et al (1999) Validation studies for models projecting the risk of invasive and total breast cancer incidence. J Natl Cancer Inst 91(18):1541–1548

D'Orsi CJ, Sickles EA, Mendelson EB, Morris EA (2013) ACR BI-RADS® Atlas, Breast Imaging Reporting and Data System. American College of Radiology, Reston, VA

de Lange SV, Bakker MF, Monninkhof EM, Peeters PHM, de Koekkoek-Doll PK, Mann RM et al (2018) Reasons for (non)participation in supplemental population-based MRI breast screening for women with extremely dense breasts. Clin Radiol 73(8):759.e1–759.e9

Destounis SV, Morgan R, Arieno A (2015) Screening for dense breasts: digital breast tomosynthesis. AJR Am J Roentgenol 204(2):261–264

Destounis S, Arieno A, Morgan R, Roberts C, Chan A (2017) Qualitative versus quantitative mammographic breast density assessment: applications for the US and abroad. Diagnostics (Basel) 7(2):30

Eliassen AH, Colditz GA, Rosner B, Willett WC, Hankinson SE (2006) Adult weight change and risk of postmenopausal breast cancer. JAMA 296(2):193–201

Emaus MJ, Bakker MF, Peeters PH, Loo CE, Mann RM, de Jong MD et al (2015) MR imaging as an additional screening modality for the detection of breast cancer in women aged 50–75 years with extremely dense breasts: The DENSE Trial Study Design. Radiology 277(2):527–537

Freer PE (2015) Mammographic breast density: impact on breast cancer risk and implications for screening. Radiographics 35(2):302–315

Friedewald SM, Rafferty EA, Rose SL, Durand MA, Plecha DM, Greenberg JS et al (2014) Breast cancer screening using tomosynthesis in combination with digital mammography. JAMA 311(24):2499–2507

Gail MH, Brinton LA, Byar DP, Corle DK, Green SB, Schairer C et al (1989) Projecting individualized probabilities of developing breast cancer for white females who are being examined annually. J Natl Cancer Inst 81(24):1879–1886

Gao J, Warren R, Warren-Forward H, Forbes JF (2008) Reproducibility of visual assessment on mammographic density. Breast Cancer Res Treat 108(1):121–127

Gastounioti A, Oustimov A, Keller BM, Pantalone L, Hsich MK, Conant EF et al (2016) Breast parenchymal patterns in processed versus raw digital mammograms: a large population study toward assessing differences in quantitative measures across image representations. Med Phys 43(11):5862

Ghosh K, Brandt KR, Sellers TA, Reynolds C, Scott CG, Maloney SD et al (2008) Association of mammographic density with the pathology of subsequent breast cancer among postmenopausal women. Cancer Epidemiol Biomarkers Prev 17(4):872–879

Gilbert FJ, Tucker L, Gillan MG, Willsher P, Cooke J, Duncan KA et al (2015) The TOMMY trial: a comparison of TOMosynthesis with digital MammographY in the UK NHS Breast Screening Programme—a multicentre retrospective reading study comparing the diagnostic performance of digital breast tomosynthesis and digital mammography with digital mammography alone. Health Technol Assess 19(4):i–xxv, 1–136

Graham SJ, Stanchev PL, Lloyd-Smith JO, Bronskill MJ, Plewes DB (1995) Changes in fibroglandular volume and water content of breast tissue during the menstrual cycle observed by MR imaging at 1.5 T. J Magn Reson Imaging 5(6):695–701

Gubern-Merida A, Kallenberg M, Platel B, Mann RM, Marti R, Karssemeijer N (2014) Volumetric breast density estimation from full-field digital mammograms: a validation study. PLoS One 9(1):e85952

Gubern-Merida A, Kallenberg M, Mann RM, Marti R, Karssemeijer N (2015) Breast segmentation and density estimation in breast MRI: a fully automatic framework. IEEE J Biomed Health Inform 19(1):349–357

Harris HR, Tamimi RM, Willett WC, Hankinson SE, Michels KB (2011) Body size across the life course, mammographic density, and risk of breast cancer. Am J Epidemiol 174(8):909–918

Harvie M, Howell A, Vierkant RA, Kumar N, Cerhan JR, Kelemen LE et al (2005) Association of gain and loss of weight before and after menopause with risk of postmenopausal breast cancer in the Iowa women's health study. Cancer Epidemiol Biomarkers Prev 14(3):656–661

He W, Hogg P, Juette A, Denton ER, Zwiggelaar R (2015) Breast image pre-processing for mammographic tissue segmentation. Comput Biol Med 67:61–73

Highnam R, Jeffreys M, McCormack V, Warren R, Davey Smith G, Brady M (2007) Comparing measurements of breast density. Phys Med Biol 52(19):5881–5895

Hooley RJ (2017) Breast density legislation and clinical evidence. Radiol Clin North Am 55(3):513–526

Hopper JL, Nguyen TL, Stone J, Aujard K, Matheson MC, Abramson MJ et al (2016) Childhood body mass index and adult mammographic density measures that predict breast cancer risk. Breast Cancer Res Treat 156(1):163–170

Houssami N, Ciatto S (2011) The evolving role of new imaging methods in breast screening. Prev Med 53(3):123–126

Huo CW, Chew GL, Britt KL, Ingman WV, Henderson MA, Hopper JL et al (2014) Mammographic density-a review on the current understanding of its association with breast cancer. Breast Cancer Res Treat 144(3):479–502

Jeffers AM, Sieh W, Lipson JA, Rothstein JH, McGuire V, Whittemore AS et al (2017) Breast cancer risk and mammographic density assessed with semi-automated and fully automated methods and BI-RADS. Radiology 282(2):348–355

Keller BM, Chen J, Daye D, Conant EF, Kontos D (2015) Preliminary evaluation of the publicly available Laboratory for Breast Radiodensity Assessment (LIBRA) software tool: comparison of fully automated area and volumetric density measures in a case-control study with digital mammography. Breast Cancer Res 17:117

Kerlikowske K, Ichikawa L, Miglioretti DL, Buist DS, Vacek PM, Smith-Bindman R et al (2007) Longitudinal measurement of clinical mammographic breast density to improve estimation of breast cancer risk. J Natl Cancer Inst 99(5):386–395

Kerlikowske K, Hubbard RA, Miglioretti DL, Geller BM, Yankaskas BC, Lehman CD et al (2011) Comparative effectiveness of digital versus film-screen mammography in community practice in the United States: a cohort study. Ann Intern Med 155(8):493–502

Keum N, Greenwood DC, Lee DH, Kim R, Aune D, Ju W et al (2015) Adult weight gain and adiposity-related cancers: a dose-response meta-analysis of prospective observational studies. J Natl Cancer Inst 107(3):djv088

Klifa C, Carballido-Gamio J, Wilmes L, Laprie A, Lobo C, Demicco E et al (2004) Quantification of breast tissue index from MR data using fuzzy clustering. Conf Proc IEEE Eng Med Biol Soc 3:1667–1670

Klifa C, Carballido-Gamio J, Wilmes L, Laprie A, Shepherd J, Gibbs J et al (2010) Magnetic resonance imaging for secondary assessment of breast density in a high-risk cohort. Magn Reson Imaging 28(1):8–15

Kopans DB (2008) Basic physics and doubts about relationship between mammographically determined tissue density and breast cancer risk. Radiology 246(2):348–353

Krishnan K, Baglietto L, Stone J, Simpson JA, Severi G, Evans CF et al (2017) Longitudinal study of mammographic density measures that predict breast cancer risk. Cancer Epidemiol Biomarkers Prev 26(4):651–660

Kuhl CK, Schrading S, Strobel K, Schild HH, Hilgers RD, Bieling HB (2014) Abbreviated breast magnetic resonance imaging (MRI): first postcontrast subtracted images and maximum-intensity projection-a novel approach to breast cancer screening with MRI. J Clin Oncol 32(22):2304–2310

Lee NA, Rusinek H, Weinreb J, Chandra R, Toth H, Singer C et al (1997) Fatty and fibroglandular tissue volumes in the breasts of women 20–83 years old: comparison of X-ray mammography and computer-assisted MR imaging. AJR Am J Roentgenol 168(2):501–506

Lee HN, Sohn YM, Han KH (2015) Comparison of mammographic density estimation by Volpara software with radiologists' visual assessment: analysis of clinical-radiologic factors affecting discrepancy between them. Acta Radiol 56(9):1061–1068

Mahoney MC, Bevers T, Linos E, Willett WC (2008) Opportunities and strategies for breast cancer prevention through risk reduction. CA Cancer J Clin 58(6):347–371

Mann RM, Mus RD, van Zelst J, Geppert C, Karssemeijer N, Platel B (2014) A novel approach to contrast-enhanced breast magnetic resonance imaging for screening: high-resolution ultrafast dynamic imaging. Invest Radiol 49(9):579–585

McCormack VA, dos Santos SI (2006) Breast density and parenchymal patterns as markers of breast cancer risk: a meta-analysis. Cancer Epidemiol Biomarkers Prev 15(6):1159–1169

McDonald ES, Oustimov A, Weinstein SP, Synnestvedt MB, Schnall M, Conant EF (2016) Effectiveness of digital breast tomosynthesis compared with digital mammography: outcomes analysis from 3 years of breast cancer screening. JAMA Oncol 2(6):737–743

Miles RC, Lehman C, Warner E, Tuttle A, Saksena M (2019) Patient-reported breast density awareness and knowledge after breast density legislation passage. Acad Radiol 26(6):726–731

Moon WK, Shen YW, Huang CS, Luo SC, Kuzucan A, Chen JH et al (2011) Comparative study of density analysis using automated whole breast ultrasound and MRI. Med Phys 38(1):382–389

Morrish OW, Tucker L, Black R, Willsher P, Duffy SW, Gilbert FJ (2015) Mammographic breast density: comparison of methods for quantitative evaluation. Radiology 2015:141508

Nguyen TL, Schmidt DF, Makalic E, Dite GS, Stone J, Apicella C et al (2013) Explaining variance in the cumulus mammographic measures that predict breast cancer risk: a twins and sisters study. Cancer Epidemiol Biomarkers Prev 22(12):2395–2403

Nickson C, Mason KE, English DR, Kavanagh AM (2012) Mammographic screening and breast cancer mortality: a case-control study and meta-analysis. Cancer Epidemiol Biomarkers Prev 21(9):1479–1488

Nie K, Chen JH, Chan S, Chau MK, Yu HJ, Bahri S et al (2008) Development of a quantitative method for analysis of breast density based on three-dimensional breast MRI. Med Phys 35(12):5253–5262

Nie K, Chang D, Chen JH, Hsu CC, Nalcioglu O, Su MY (2010) Quantitative analysis of breast parenchymal patterns using 3D fibroglandular tissues segmented based on MRI. Med Phys 37(1):217–226

O'Flynn EA, Ledger AE, deSouza NM (2015) Alternative screening for dense breasts: MRI. AJR Am J Roentgenol 204(2):W141–W149

Phi XA, Saadatmand S, De Bock GH, Warner E, Sardanelli F, Leach MO et al (2016) Contribution of mammography to MRI screening in BRCA mutation carriers by BRCA status and age: individual patient data meta-analysis. Br J Cancer 114(6):631–637

Pisano ED, Gatsonis CA, Yaffe MJ, Hendrick RE, Tosteson AN, Fryback DG et al (2005) American College of Radiology Imaging Network digital mammographic imaging screening trial: objectives and methodology. Radiology 236(2):404–412

Price ER, Hargreaves J, Lipson JA, Sickles EA, Brenner RJ, Lindfors KK et al (2013) The California breast density information group: a collaborative response to the issues of breast density, breast cancer risk, and breast density notification legislation. Radiology 269(3):887–892

Raza S, Mackesy MM, Winkler NS, Hurwitz S, Birdwell RL (2016) Effect of training on qualitative mammographic density assessment. J Am Coll Radiol 13(3):310–315

Rhodes DJ, Radecki Breitkopf C, Ziegenfuss JY, Jenkins SM, Vachon CM (2015) Awareness of breast density and its impact on breast cancer detection and risk. J Clin Oncol 33(10):1143–1150

Roubidoux MA, Bailey JE, Wray LA, Helvie MA (2004) Invasive cancers detected after breast cancer screening yielded a negative result: relationship of mammographic density to tumor prognostic factors. Radiology 230(1):42–48

Sickles EA (2010) The use of breast imaging to screen women at high risk for cancer. Radiol Clin North Am 48(5):859–878

Slanetz PJ, Freer PE, Birdwell RL (2015) Breast-density legislation—practical considerations. N Engl J Med 372(7):593–595

Smith RA, Manassaram-Baptiste D, Brooks D, Cokkinides V, Doroshenk M, Saslow D et al (2014) Cancer screening in the United States, 2014: a review of current American Cancer Society guidelines and current issues in cancer screening. CA Cancer J Clin 64(1):30–51

Sterns EE, Zee B (2000) Mammographic density changes in perimenopausal and postmenopausal women: is effect of hormone replacement therapy predictable? Breast Cancer Res Treat 59(2):125–132

Tagliafico A, Tagliafico G, Astengo D, Airaldi S, Calabrese M, Houssami N (2013) Comparative estimation of percentage breast tissue density for digital mammography, digital breast tomosynthesis, and magnetic resonance imaging. Breast Cancer Res Treat 138(1):311–317

Tagliafico A, Bignotti B, Tagliafico G, Astengo D, Martino L, Airaldi S et al (2014) Breast density assessment using a 3T MRI system: comparison among different sequences. PLoS One 9(6):e99027

Thompson DJ, Leach MO, Kwan-Lim G, Gayther SA, Ramus SJ, Warsi I et al (2009) Assessing the usefulness of a novel MRI-based breast density estimation algorithm in a cohort of women at high genetic risk of breast cancer: the UK MARIBS study. Breast Cancer Res 11(6):R80

Tyrer J, Duffy SW, Cuzick J (2004) A breast cancer prediction model incorporating familial and personal risk factors. Stat Med 23(7):1111–1130

Vachon CM, Pankratz VS, Scott CG, Maloney SD, Ghosh K, Brandt KR et al (2007) Longitudinal trends in mammographic percent density and breast cancer risk. Cancer Epidemiol Biomarkers Prev 16(5):921–928

van der Waal D, Ripping TM, Verbeek AL, Broeders MJ (2017) Breast cancer screening effect across breast density strata: a case-control study. Int J Cancer 140(1):41–49

van Duijnhoven FJ, Peeters PH, Warren RM, Bingham SA, van Noord PA, Monninkhof EM et al (2007) Postmenopausal hormone therapy and changes in mammographic density. J Clin Oncol 25(11):1323–1328

van Engeland S, Snoeren PR, Huisman H, Boetes C, Karssemeijer N (2006) Volumetric breast density estimation from full-field digital mammograms. IEEE Trans Med Imaging 25(3):273–282

Wanders JO, Bakker MF, Veldhuis WB, Peeters PH, van Gils CH (2015) The effect of weight change on changes in breast density measures over menopause in a breast cancer screening cohort. Breast Cancer Res 17:74

Wang J, Azziz A, Fan B, Malkov S, Klifa C, Newitt D et al (2013) Agreement of mammographic measures of volumetric breast density to MRI. PLoS One 8(12):e81653

Wengert GJ, Helbich TH, Vogl WD, Baltzer P, Langs G, Weber M et al (2015) Introduction of an automated user-independent quantitative volumetric magnetic resonance imaging breast density measurement system using the Dixon sequence: comparison with mammographic breast density assessment. Invest Radiol 50(2):73–80

Wengert GJ, Helbich TH, Woitek R, Kapetas P, Clauser P, Baltzer PA et al (2016a) Inter- and intra-observer agreement of BI-RADS-based subjective visual estimation of amount of fibroglandular breast tissue with magnetic resonance imaging: comparison to automated quantitative assessment. Eur Radiol 26(11):3917–3922

Wengert GJ, Pinker-Domenig K, Helbich TH, Vogl WD, Clauser P, Bickel H et al (2016b) Influence of fat-water separation and spatial resolution on automated volumetric MRI measurements of fibroglandular breast tissue. NMR Biomed 29(6):702–708

Wengert GJ, Pinker K, Helbich TH, Vogl WD, Spijker SM, Bickel H et al (2017) Accuracy of fully automated, quantitative, volumetric measurement of the amount of fibroglandular breast tissue using MRI: correlation with anthropomorphic breast phantoms. NMR Biomed. https://doi.org/10.1002/nbm.3705

Winkler NS, Raza S, Mackesy M, Birdwell RL (2015) Breast density: clinical implications and assessment methods. Radiographics 35(2):316–324

Wolfe JN (1976) Breast patterns as an index of risk for developing breast cancer. AJR Am J Roentgenol 126(6):1130–1137

Wu S, Weinstein SP, Conant EF, Kontos D (2013) Automated fibroglandular tissue segmentation and volumetric density estimation in breast MRI using an atlas-aided fuzzy C-means method. Med Phys 40(12):122302

Zhang SM, Lee IM, Manson JE, Cook NR, Willett WC, Buring JE (2007) Alcohol consumption and breast cancer risk in the Women's Health Study. Am J Epidemiol 165(6):667–676

Artificial Intelligence in Breast Imaging

Xin Wang, Nikita Moriakov, Yuan Gao,
Tianyu Zhang, Luyi Han, and Ritse M. Mann

Contents

1 Introduction 436

2 A Brief Overview: From Conventional CAD to Deep Learning Based—A More Comprehensive Range of Applications 436

3 AI Systems in Various Clinical Applications 437
    3.1 Breast Cancer Risk Assessment for Screening: Mainly in Mammography 437
    3.2 Lesion Detection and Classification for Diagnosis 438
    3.3 Therapy Selection and Outcome Prediction for Interventions 445

4 Challenges and Future Directions 447

References 449

Abstract

The development and implementation of artificial intelligence (AI) for breast imaging have been ongoing for several decades and have played an important role in clinical practice. With the emergence and maturity of deep learning (DL) algorithms, the application of AI technology in medical imaging has gradually moved to a higher level and broader range. It may break the performance bottleneck of traditional computer-aided detection/diagnosis (CAD) systems. This chapter reviews the three domains of clinical use cases for AI techniques in breast imaging, including risk assessment for screening, breast cancer detection and classification for diagnosis, and therapy selection and outcome prediction for interventions. As for future directions, it is necessary to improve the AI-based system's interpretability and performance in a clinical application and maximize its clinical impact.

X. Wang · Y. Gao · T. Zhang
GROW School for Oncology and Development
Biology, Maastricht University,
Maastricht, The Netherlands

Department of Radiology, The Netherlands Cancer
Institute, Amsterdam, The Netherlands

N. Moriakov · L. Han · R. M. Mann (✉)
Department of Radiology, The Netherlands Cancer
Institute, Amsterdam, The Netherlands

Department of Medical Imaging, Radboud University
Medical Center, Nijmegen, The Netherlands
e-mail: Ritse.Mann@radboudumc.nl

© Springer Nature Switzerland AG 2022
M. Fuchsjäger et al. (eds.), *Breast Imaging*, Medical Radiology,
https://doi.org/10.1007/978-3-030-94918-1_20

1 Introduction

Breast cancer is one of the most common cancers in the world and is the cause of a large fraction of cancer-related mortality among women (Sun et al. 2017). Many studies have shown that widely used regular screening mammography can prevent the spread of the disease, reduce breast cancer mortality substantially, improve the quality of life of breast cancer patients, and reduce treatment costs (Boulehmi et al. 2016; Tabar et al. 2019). Precise and efficient imaging screening can diagnose breast diseases early and can effectively be used to tailor intervention. Recent advances in artificial intelligence (AI) have impacted many scientific fields including breast imaging (Geras et al. 2019; Mann et al. 2020). The rapid development in the field of AI for breast imaging has the potential to affect clinical screening, diagnosis, and prognosis of breast cancer (Meyer-Base et al. 2020), by enhancing, for example, risk prediction, detection, classification, therapy selection, and outcome prediction. Implementation of AI into clinical breast imaging is currently still limited but may largely change current practice.

In clinical screening and diagnosis of breast cancer, challenges remain in the accurate detection and characterization of breast lesions. Interpretation of breast images varies with radiologists' experience (Elmore et al. 2009) and is subjective (Miglioretti et al. 2007). False positives can lead to patient anxiety (Tosteson et al. 2014), unnecessary follow-up, and invasive diagnostic procedures. Cancers missed at screening may not be identified until they are more advanced and less amenable to treatment (Houssami and Hunter 2017). However, AI may be uniquely poised to help with this challenge (McKinney et al. 2020). Previous studies indicated that the use of machine learning (ML)-based computer-aided detection/diagnosis (CAD) systems for mammography significantly increased the radiologist's sensitivity with specificity at the same level (Brem et al. 2003; Nishikawa 2007), but did not eventually lead to better screening performance (Fenton et al. 2007; Lehman et al. 2016). In recent years, with the emergence and maturity of deep learning (DL) algorithms, the application of AI technology in medical imaging has gradually moved to a higher level and has improved the stand-alone performance of DL-based AI applications for mammography.

On the other hand, in clinical practice, treatment of breast cancer also faces many challenges. Just as for early detection, many breast cancer patients will miss optimal treatment opportunities due to inappropriate therapy selection or incomplete monitoring of the tumor response to treatment, leading to disease progression and higher mortality rates (Bejnordi et al. 2017). However, AI technology adequately using follow-up images allows to improve tracking radiographic changes of tumors over time for smarter personalized prognosis and therapy selection and outcome prediction (Huynh et al. 2017). Specifically, AI systems may predict the most beneficial specific treatments for breast cancer patients, avoiding unnecessary surgery and other treatments, thus improving patient care (El Adoui et al. 2020).

In this chapter, we review the developments of AI systems for breast imaging, discussing the various clinical use cases for AI techniques in breast imaging that have been developed. Moreover, an overview of the challenges and future directions of AI in breast imaging will be given.

2 A Brief Overview: From Conventional CAD to Deep Learning Based—A More Comprehensive Range of Applications

In breast radiology, the notion of utilizing computer technologies to aid radiologists is not novel. Computer-aided detection/diagnosis (CAD) system for breast imaging was first developed in the 1960s (Winsberg et al. 1967). CAD systems use a combination of computer, mathematics, statistics, image processing, and analysis methods to extract features from medical images, mark the location of suspicious lesions, and judge whether lesions are benign or malignant. Several investigators have attempted to detect breast abnormalities automatically (Winsberg et al. 1967; Kimme et al. 1977; Spiesberger 1979; Semmlow et al. 1980).

Systematic development of machine learning techniques for medical imaging began in the 1980s (Chan et al. 2020) with a more realistic goal to develop CAD systems as a second reader to assist radiologists in image interpretation rather than full automation. Several studies demonstrated the potential of machine learning-based CAD in improving the detection of breast cancer in an early stage (Chan et al. 1987, 1990), specifically significantly enhancing radiologists' performance in detecting microcalcifications (Chan et al. 1987). The US Food and Drug Administration (FDA) approved the first commercial CAD system to detect cancer for screening mammography in 1998 (R2 ImageChecker; Hologic, Marlborough, Massachusetts) (Roehrig et al. 1998). Since then, the use of AI for the evaluation of breast images has dramatically expanded (Huang et al. 2018; Dorrius et al. 2011; Thrall et al. 2018). However, the performance of conventional CAD systems is limited. Conventional techniques depend heavily on prior, low-level, handcrafted features to detect microcalcifications or classify masses as benign or malignant (Al-Antari et al. 2018). It is challenging to capture all the signs of breast cancer recognized by humans in handcrafted mathematical formulations. Therefore, hardly any of the conventional algorithms ever approached the performance of breast radiologists or could automatically perform diagnosis tasks (Al-Antari et al. 2018). Moreover, Fenton et al. (2007) indicated that the use of conventional CAD leads to higher false-positive rates, recall rates, and biopsy rates.

In recent years, with the enhancement of computing power and the maturity of deep learning, it has become possible to break the performance bottleneck of traditional machine learning-based CAD systems. Deep learning is a type of machine learning method but enables end-to-end training and extraction of relevant features automatically from input data. This is achieved by transforming the input information into multiple layers of abstraction in a deep neural network architecture (LeCun et al. 2015). This implies that deep learning-based CAD systems can even learn from features that are unseen or unknown by radiologists, making them independent from how a radiologist reads images (Ou et al. 2021). Several deep learning CAD systems for mammography have been presented and in general achieve better performance than conventional ones (Geras et al. 2019; Chan et al. 2020; Ou et al. 2021; Sechopoulos et al. 2020; Le et al. 2019).

In recent years, there has been a steadily growing interest in the use of deep learning for other goals in breast imaging. The developments of deep learning in computer vision have made these techniques relatively straightforward to apply to various types of breast imaging. Deep learning-based CAD systems may, for example, automatically analyze imaging information combined with other clinical data and can be developed to provide decision support for many applications in the patient care process. They are far more powerful than conventional CAD systems and have a wide range of potential clinical applications.

3 AI Systems in Various Clinical Applications

Applications of AI in three domains will be reviewed: risk assessment for screening, breast cancer detection and classification for diagnosis, and therapy selection and outcome prediction for interventions.

3.1 Breast Cancer Risk Assessment for Screening: Mainly in Mammography

The most important task of the breast cancer risk assessment (or prediction) so far is to stratify women into high-risk and low-risk populations for screening (Louro et al. 2019). With risk-based guidelines, we can offer more tailored screening examinations to women in different risk categories, achieving earlier detection while reducing unnecessary screening for the low-risk population to reduce costs and anxiety caused by the overtreatment and false-positive assessments (Louro et al. 2019). Previous researches explored questionnaires exploring lifestyle, hormonal, and genetic information. Others focused on mammographic density assessment or combined these aspects (Brentnall et al. 2015). Although many mathematically defined image features have shown risk associations (Dembrower et al. 2020), human-specified features may not be able to capture all risk-relevant information in the image (Li et al. 2017), since, in fact, we do not know specifically what we are looking for.

Image-based deep learning models have recently focused on mammography for risk prediction. This could improve the accuracy of breast cancer prediction tools and improve their accuracy (Table 1) (Dembrower et al. 2020; Yala et al. 2019a, 2021; Liu et al. 2020; Ha et al. 2019a). A handful of recent breakthrough studies showed substantial improvements in long-term risk prediction using neural networks on large population-level cohorts, obtaining area under the curves (AUCs) up to 0.70 for assessing 5-year risk and advancing state of the art (Dembrower et al. 2020; Yala et al. 2019a). To further bring the image-based risk model to the clinic, Yala et al. (2021) developed MIRAI and validated its performance at scale across diverse populations and clinical settings with significantly higher 5-year ROC AUCs than the Tyrer-Cuzick model and prior methods (Fig. 1). Still several studies showed that it is also possible to select a similar subset of patients using a likelihood of malignancy threshold on the AI findings, which would contain a higher fraction of women with occult early breast cancer than a selection based on more classical risk prediction. These studies suggested also to exclude images with a very low likelihood of malignancy according to the AI system from human reading (referred to as preselection) to reduce the reading workload in mammography screening while not decreasing radiologists' detection performance (Rodriguez-Ruiz et al. 2019a; Yala et al. 2019b). In addition, women with the highest risks could be offered supplemental screening strategies to detect more cancer early (Dembrower et al. 2020).

Except for pushing better performance across different races and large population-level cohorts in clinical practice, the decision of the risk prediction model should also be explained in a form that humans can understand. However, only a few of these studies could visualize image cues that were used to obtain the risk score (Liu et al. 2020; Arefan et al. 2020), and none of these studies did find a biomarker in the medical images that could intuitively be used to predict the tumor area. Potentially, larger numbers of screening mammograms, as well as better ways to visualize AI outputs, may in the future alleviate this problem. In the context of the gradual application of other screening methods, breast cancer risk prediction models based on other different image modalities, such as ultrasound and MRI, are also needed. It is anticipated that such risk assessment models using other different image modalities, when trained on sufficiently large databases, will obtain at least a similar performance to that achieved with mammography.

3.2 Lesion Detection and Classification for Diagnosis

Lesion detection and classification on medical images have long been the only components of CAD systems in radiology. A large number of clinical studies, aimed at early lesion detection, have been conducted in different imaging modalities, including mammography, breast ultrasound, and MRI (Tables 2, 3, and 4). Currently, these AI systems are achieving remarkable results in object classification and detection tasks due to the incorporation of modern deep learning algorithms (Fathy and Ghoneim 2019), and for mammography their performance is now even on par with that of breast radiologists (McKinney et al. 2020). It is, therefore, widely believed that AI-based CAD systems will soon play a major role in screening to improve radiologists' efficiency and performance or act as an independent second reader. Even stand-alone use of such AI systems—for a subset of mammograms—is now widely discussed.

Artificial Intelligence in Breast Imaging

Table 1 AI in breast imaging for breast cancer risk prediction

Term	Reference	Image modality	Dataset	Outcome	Key findings
Short term and long term	Liu et al. (2020)	Mammography	Included 147,476 screening mammograms in 16,621 women	<1-year AUC = 0.72 >1-year AUC = 0.72 >2-year AUC = 0.62 >5-year AUC = 0.61	In particular, short-term risk (≤1 year) should rely on cancer sign models. Long-term risk models should be trained exclusively on images with no visible cancer signs or use other strategies to mitigate model conflation.
	Yala et al. (2021)	Mammography	Included 80,134 patients from 2009 to 2016 at MGH, 11,303 patients from 2008 to 2016 at Karolinska, and 15,178 patients from 2010 to 2011 at CGMH	1-year AUC = 0.84 2-year AUC = 0.80 3-year AUC = 0.78 4-year AUC = 0.76 5-year AUC = 0.76	Mirai demonstrated improved discriminatory capacity over the state-of-the-art clinically adopted Tyrer-Cuzick and prior deep learning approaches hybrid DL and image-only DL.
Long term	Yala et al. (2019a)	Mammography	Included 134,924 mammograms in 60,886 women between 1/2009 and 12/2012	AUC = 0.70	Deep learning models that use full-field mammograms yield substantially improved risk discrimination compared with the Tyrer-Cuzick (version 8) model.
	Ha et al. (2019a)	Mammography	Included 1474 mammograms in 737 women between 1/2011 and 1/2017	Accuracy = 0.72	Novel pixel-wise mammographic breast evaluation using a CNN architecture can stratify breast cancer risk, independent of the BD.
	Dembrower et al. (2020)	Mammography	More than 500,000 women, 1 million images, and approximately 10,000 breast cancer cases between 2008 and 2015	AUC = 0.66	Compared with density-based models, a deep neural network can more accurately predict which women are at risk for future breast cancer, with a lower false-negative rate for more aggressive cancers.

At present, in the task of breast cancer detection and classification, most AI-based CAD systems still focus on mammography (Bi et al. 2019), as the large number of available screening mammograms permits the leverage of big datasets. It is therefore easier to train the deep learning models (Geras et al. 2019). While initial studies aimed at the detection or classification of microcalcifications, masses, and lesions separately, modern AI programs integrate these approaches for early diagnosis of all types of lesions (Table 2) (McKinney et al. 2020; Rodriguez-Ruiz et al. 2019a, b; Yala et al. 2019b; Fathy and Ghoneim 2019; Samala et al. 2016, 2018; Wu et al. 2020; Conant et al. 2019; Al-Masni et al. 2018). Currently, these systems detect regular lesions that remain unobserved by human readers, even after double reading (Fig. 2) (McKinney et al. 2020; Rodriguez-Ruiz et al. 2019b; Wu et al. 2020).

Since digital breast tomosynthesis (DBT) is now gaining solid ground in breast cancer screening and diagnostic settings (Mann et al. 2020), it is important to develop state-of-the-art AI applications for DBT too. Due to the similarity between mammography and DBT, mammo-

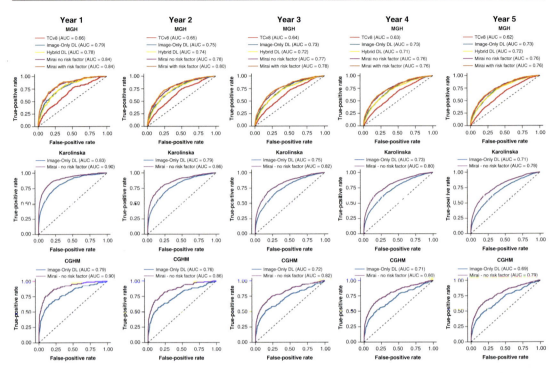

Fig. 1 Receiver operating characteristic (ROC) curves for model predictions on MGH, Karolinska, and CGMH test sets. To further bring the image-based risk model to the clinic, Yala et al. (2021) developed Mirai and validated its performance at scale across diverse populations and clinical settings with significantly higher ROC AUCs than the Tyrer-Cuzick model and prior methods. Results are shown in the top, middle, and bottom rows, respectively. The curves are arranged left to right from 1- to 5-year outcomes. *TCv8* Tyrer-Cuzick version 8, *DL* deep learning, *hybrid DL* DL model that uses both imaging and the traditional risk factors in risk factor logistic regression. (Quoted from Yala A, et al. Toward robust mammography-based models for breast cancer risk. Science Translational Medicine, 2021)

graphic images can be used to improve the performance of DBT-based systems by using transfer learning methods to make up for the currently still present lack of data (Samala et al. 2016, 2018). Therefore, DBT studies already report similar performance (Conant et al. 2019; Lee and Elmore 2019).

Ultrasound is often used for supplemental screening in dense breasts and for diagnostic workup of symptomatic or otherwise detected breast lesions. Unfortunately, ultrasound has been associated with high false-positive rates, as commonly only cysts are classified as certainly benign, which may lead to a large amount of unnecessary biopsy procedures. An increasing number of AI applications in breast ultrasound have been described. The majority of these are related to breast mass detection and classification (Table 3) (Yap et al. 2017; Ciritsis et al. 2019; Fujioka et al. 2019; Cho et al. 2018; van Zelst et al. 2018; Xu et al. 2018). In recent years, several studies reported that AI achieves humanlike performance (Ciritsis et al. 2019; Fujioka et al. 2019) and may support radiologists to improve specificity and reduce in false-positive assessments (Barinov et al. 2019). This has even been used commercially (Fig. 3) (Cho et al. 2018; van Zelst et al. 2018; Xu et al. 2018). Especially for the use of US as supplemental screening modality, image acquisition is more dependent on the operator's experience compared to mammography and MRI, which accordingly limits the maximum potential of AI for ultrasound (Mann et al. 2020). Automated breast ultrasound, which makes use of a wide transducer and a standardized acquisition protocol, may improve this situ-

Artificial Intelligence in Breast Imaging

Table 2 AI for breast cancer detection and classification in mammography

Image modality	Reference	Task	Dataset	Performance	Key findings
Mammography	McKinney et al. (2020)	Breast cancer classification	Included 25,856 women from the UK and 3097 women from the USA	AUC = 0.96	The AI system outperforms radiologists in breast cancer identification.
	Fathy and Ghoneim (2019)	Breast mass detection and classification	Included 2620 cases (695 normal, 141 benign without callback, 870 benign, and 914 malignant)	Classification: AUC = 0.96; sensitivity = 0.998; specificity = 0.821 Detection: sensitivity = 0.9367	The pre-trained CNN was able to automatically learn the most discriminative features in mammograms and achieve excellent results in breast cancer classification (normal or mass).
	Rodríguez-Ruiz et al. (2019b)	Breast cancer detection	Included 240 women (100 cancers, 40 false-positive recalls, 100 normal)	AUC = 0.89 (with AI) AUC = 0.87 (without AI)	Radiologists improved their cancer detection at mammography when using an artificial intelligence system for support.
	Wu et al. (2020)	Breast cancer classification	Included 1,001,093 images from 141,473 patients	AUC = 0.895	Averaging the probability of malignancy predicted by radiologists and proposed deep learning modal is more accurate than either of the two separately.
	Al-Masni et al. (2018)	Breast mass detection and classification	Included 600 mammograms	Detection: Accuracy = 0.997 Classification: Accuracy = 0.97; AUC = 0.9645	The proposed system even works on some challenging breast cancer cases where the masses exist over the pectoral muscles or dense regions.
	Rodriguez-Ruiz et al. (2019a)	Normal mammography classification	Included 2652 exams (653 cancer)	Reduce workload by 47%	It is possible to automatically preselect exams using AI to significantly reduce the breast cancer screening reading workload.
	Yala et al. (2019b)	Normal mammography classification	Included 223,109 mammograms from 66,661 women	Sensitivity = 0.906; specificity = 0.935 (without AI) Sensitivity = 0.901; specificity = 0.942 (with AI)	This deep learning model has the potential to reduce radiologist workload and significantly improve specificity without harming sensitivity.

(continued)

Table 2 (continued)

Image modality	Reference	Task	Dataset	Performance	Key findings
MammographyDBT	Samala et al. (2018)	Mass classification	Included 4039 unique ROIs (1797 malignant and 2242 benign)	AUC = 0.85 (single-stage transfer learning) AUC = 0.91 (multistage transfer learning)	When the training sample size from the target domain is limited, an additional stage of transfer-learning using data from a similar auxiliary domain is advantageous.
	Samala et al. (2016)	Breast mass detection	Included 2282 mammograms and 324 DBT volumes	AUC = 0.81 (before transfer learning) AUC = 0.90 (after transfer learning)	Large datasets collected from mammography are useful for developing new CAD systems for DBT, alleviating the problem and effort of collecting entirely new large datasets for the new modality.
DBT	Conant et al. (2019)	Suspicious soft-tissue and calcified lesion detection	Included 260 DBT examinations (65 cancer cases)	AUC = 0.795 (without AI) AUC = 0.852 (with AI)	The concurrent use of an accurate DBT AI system was found to improve cancer detection efficacy with increases in AUC, sensitivity, and specificity and a reduction in recall rate and reading time.

ation and could create reproducible breast evaluations. AI programs for the automated assessment of automated breast ultrasound acquisitions are under development, albeit they are currently not as advanced as other applications.

Breast MRI has the advantage of being a standardized technique, just like mammography. However, due to the fact that scanner types and acquisition protocols vary, the image characteristics are not uniform; therefore, the datasets available for training are actually limited (Jackson et al. 2007). Breast MRI is commonly used as a (supplemental) screening technology for women at high risk, and several preliminary studies have been conducted on AI-based automatic detection (Dalmış et al. 2018; Herent et al. 2019; Zhou et al. 2020) and automated lesion classification, differentiating between benign and malignant breast lesions to enhance specificity and improve accuracy (Truhn et al. 2019; Dalmis et al. 2019) (Table 4). Unsurprisingly, the performance is still below human standards, and currently, in clinical applications, it is limited to prevent false-positive recalls (Mann et al. 2020; Reig et al. 2020). Only, once images from various vendors can be standardized using image synthesis-based deep learning models, AI algorithms may arrive at or even move beyond humanlike performance for breast lesion detection and classification in MRI screening.

Most of the above CAD methods generally consider one modality, while different modalities may be complementary. Due to the limitation of processing-related information from heterogeneous sources, there are currently only some related studies using small datasets (Wang et al. 2020; Habib et al. 2020; Cong et al. 2017). Habib et al. (2020) propose a deep learning method for the classification of breast lesions that combine mammography and ultrasound images showing the potential of multimodal classification in clinical application. Likewise, He et al. (2019) propose a multimodal risk assessment model by combining mammography and ultrasound images

Table 3 AI for breast cancer detection and classification in ultrasound

Image modality	Reference	Task	Dataset	Performance	Key findings
Ultrasound (US)	Yap et al. (2017)	Breast lesion detection	Dataset A comprises 306 images (60 malignant and 246 benign) Dataset B comprises 163 images (53 malignant and 110 benign)	True positive fraction (TPF) = 0.99 (Dataset A) TPF = 0.93 (Dataset B)	The study investigated the use of different deep learning approaches and presents a comprehensive evaluation of the most representative lesion detection methodologies.
	Ciritsis et al. (2019)	Breast mass classification	Included 1090 images from 582 patients	Accuracy = 0.871 (BI-RADS 2 versus BI-RADS 3–5) Accuracy = 0.931 (BI-RADS 2–3 versus BI-RADS 4–5) AUC = 0.838	Deep learning may be used to mimic human decision-making in the evaluation of single US images of breast lesions according to the BI-RADS catalog.
	Fujioka et al. (2019)	Breast mass classification	Included 947 images of 235 patients	Sensitivity = 0.958 Specificity = 0.925 Accuracy = 0.925 AUC = 0.913	Deep learning shows high diagnostic performance to discriminate between benign and malignant breast masses on ultrasound.
	Cho et al. (2018)	Breast cancer detection	Included 119 breast masses (54 malignant and 65 benign) from 116 women	Specificity = 0.908 (S-Detect) Specificity = 0.492 (Radiologist 1) Specificity = 0.554 (Radiologist 2)	S-Detect is a clinically feasible diagnostic tool that can be used to improve the specificity and accuracy of breast US, with a moderate degree of agreement in final assessments, regardless of the experience of the radiologist.

(continued)

Table 3 (continued)

Image modality	Reference	Task	Dataset	Performance	Key findings
Automated breast ultrasound (ABUS)	van Zelst et al. (2018)	Breast cancer detection	Included 120 women (30 malignant, 30 benign, and 60 normal cases)	Average reading time (RT) = 133.4 s/case (with CAD-ABUS) Average RT = 158.3 s/case (without CAD-ABUS)	CAD software for ABUS may decrease the time needed to screen for breast cancer without compromising the screening performance of radiologists.
	Xu et al. (2018)	Breast cancer detection	Included 1000 cases (206 malignant, 486 benign, and 308 normal cases)	AUC = 0.784 (with CADe) AUC = 0.747 (without CADe)	The CADe improves radiologist performance with respect to both accuracy and reading time for the detection of breast cancer using the automated breast volume scanner (ABVS) images.

Table 4 AI for breast cancer detection and classification in MRI

Image modality	Reference	Task	Dataset	Performance	Key findings
DCE-MRI	Dalmış et al. (2018)	Breast cancer detection	Included 385 MRI scans (161 malignant lesions)	Sensitivity = 0.6429	The developed CADe system is able to exploit the spatial information obtained from the early-phase scans and can be used in screening programs where abbreviated MRI protocols are used.
	Herent et al. (2019)	Breast lesion classification	Included 335 MR images from 335 patients	AUC = 0.816	The study shows good performance of a supervised attention model with deep learning for breast MRI.
	Truhn et al. (2019)	Breast lesion classification	Included 447 patients with 1294 enhancing lesions (787 malignant, 507 benign)	AUC = 0.88 Deep learning AUC = 0.81 Radiomic analysis AUC = 0.98 Radiologist	Deep learning and radiomic analysis approaches were inferior to radiologists' performance for the classification of enhancing lesions as benign or malignant at multiparametric breast MRI.
	Zhou et al. (2020)	Breast lesion classification	Included 227 patients (139 malignant and 88 benign lesions)	AUC = 0.97	Using the smallest bounding box containing proximal peritumor tissue as input had higher accuracy compared to using tumor alone or larger boxes.
	Dalmis et al. (2019)	Breast lesion classification	Included 576 lesions imaged with MRI (368 malignant and 149 benign lesions)	AUC = 0.852	The developed AI system for interpretation of multiparametric ultrafast breast MRI may improve specificity.

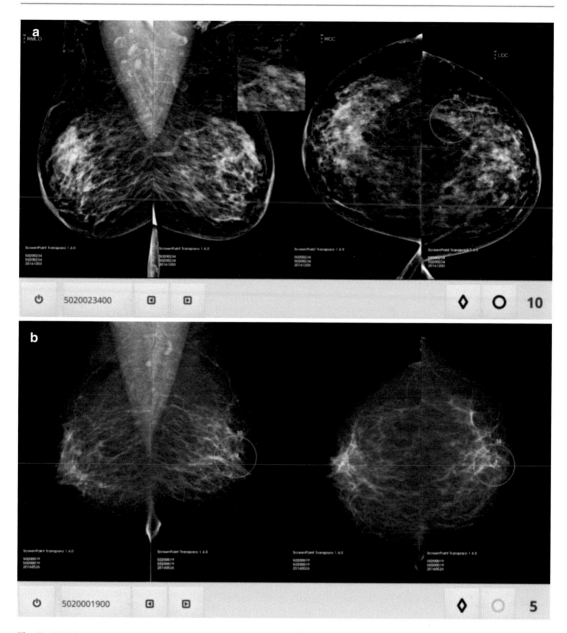

Fig. 2 (**a**) Mammograms of a patient with invasive ductal carcinoma (outlined and with the level of suspicion score assigned by AI system). (**b**) Mammograms of a normal woman with a low level of suspicion score assigned by the AI system. (Quoted from Rodríguez-Ruiz A, et al. Detection of Breast Cancer with Mammography: Effect of an Artificial Intelligence Support System. Radiology, 2019)

from BI-RADS 4 patients to facilitate biopsy decision. It should be realized that most studies on AI and breast imaging are retrospective. To further improve the generalizability of CAD systems in clinical applications, prospective studies in different ethnicities and larger populations are necessary.

3.3 Therapy Selection and Outcome Prediction for Interventions

In women with breast cancer, choosing the right therapy is the first, and in many ways most essential, "intervention" (Schaffter et al. 2020). Apart

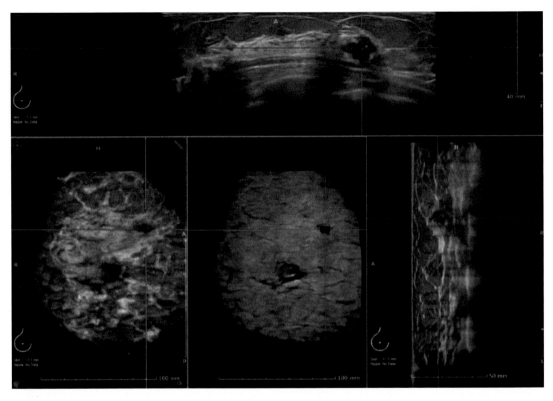

Fig. 3 CAD-based minimum-intensity projection (MinIP) integrated in a multiplanar hanging protocol for ABUS that shows the conventional ABUS planes. The top plane shows the transverse acquisitions, the lower left plane the coronal reconstructions, and the lower right plane the sagittal reconstruction. The MinIP (bottom row in the middle) is a 2D image where lower intensity regions in the 3D ABUS volume are enhanced as dark spots. By clicking on the dark spot, the 3D multiplanar hanging automatically snaps to the corresponding 3D location. The CAD marks (colored square) are displayed on the MinIP. (Quoted from van Zelst, et al. Dedicated computer-aided detection software for automated 3D breast ultrasound; an efficient tool for the radiologist in supplemental screening of women with dense breasts. European Radiology, 2018)

from surgery, there are many other therapeutic options that may be considered, including different forms of radiotherapy, and systemic therapy (e.g., partial breast irradiation, intraoperative radiotherapy, various forms of chemotherapy, targeted therapy, immunotherapy, and endocrine therapy). Treatment for high-risk and/or locally advanced breast cancer patients often aims to reduce the volume of cancer and clinical stage before surgery is performed (Faneyte et al. 2003; Schott and Hayes 2012; Thompson and Moulder-Thompson 2012; Kaufmann et al. 2006). This not only offers the potential to convert mastectomy to breast-conserving therapy, but also enables preservation of the axillary lymph nodes in women with initial stage IIb disease. Consequently, neoadjuvant systemic therapy (NST), the administration of chemotherapy and other agents prior to surgery, constitutes the first avenue of treatment for an expanding portion of breast cancer patients (Braman et al. 2020). However, it is not clear which patients are sensitive or not sensitive to initial treatment with a specific therapy. This may cause some patients to miss optimal opportunities for treatment due to initial inappropriate therapy selection.

Therefore, AI systems based on different modalities of breast imaging are gradually being applied in intervention studies to alleviate this plight (Table 5) (Huynh et al. 2017; El Adoui et al. 2020; Braman et al. 2020; Qu et al. 2020; Ha et al. 2019b; Choi et al. 2020; Ravichandran et al.

2018; Rabinovici-Cohen et al. 2020). AI systems are being trained to predict to which specific treatments breast cancer patients will likely respond or not respond. Moreover, even for responding patients, it might be useful to determine beforehand whether there is a high likelihood that they will not achieve a pathological complete response (pCR). It is also possible to produce probability heatmaps that visualize tumor regions that are most likely to respond well, and those that are unlikely to respond, to obtain relevant prognostic information in breast cancer patients prior to therapy (Ravichandran et al. 2018). Then likely non-responders will probably be delivered to alternative therapeutic approaches or immediate surgery, thus improving patient care. This would both expedite the delivery of effective treatment and eliminate therapies that are potentially toxic and ineffective. These are all potential directions for deep learning AI-based CAD systems that could aid in the choice of therapy for breast cancer patients (Ravichandran et al. 2018; Pang et al. 2020; Chen and Guestrin 2016).

Recently, some studies showed the potential effectiveness of deep learning in AI for prediction and discrimination of chemotherapy response, mainly focusing on MRI (Table 5) (Huynh et al. 2017; El Adoui et al. 2020; Braman et al. 2020; Qu et al. 2020; Ha et al. 2019b; Choi et al. 2020; Ravichandran et al. 2018; Rabinovici-Cohen et al. 2020). For instance, Braman et al. (2020) evaluated the ability of deep learning to predict response to human epidermal receptor 2-negative (HER2−) targeted neoadjuvant chemotherapy (NAC) from pretreatment dynamic contrast-enhanced (DCE) MRI acquired prior to treatment and achieved an impressive response prediction within the validation set (AUC = 0.93). Other researchers focused on multi-time points of MRI, comparing the different DCE-MRI contrast time points with regard to how well their extracted features predict response to NAC within a deep convolutional neural network. Typically, they found that the classifier trained on features from the pre-contrast time point only performed best with an AUC of 0.85 (Huynh et al. 2017). A study from Rabinovici-Cohen et al. (2020) explored multimodal clinical and radiomics metrics, including quantitative features from mammography, to assess in advance complete response to chemotherapy. Their model could correctly predict in advance which women would not achieve pCR. As for AI-associated multimodal breast imaging studies, Choi et al. investigated the predictive efficacy of PET/CT and MRI for the pathological response of advanced breast cancer to NAC (Choi et al. 2020), showing that a PET/MRI-based deep learning model might predict pathological responses to NAC in patients with advanced breast cancer. Studies based on other multimodality combinations have not yet been published.

However, there are limitations to current research. The major limitation of the present studies is the small, retrospective single-institution nature. Deep learning models can evaluate high-dimensional features of images, but a substantial amount of data is necessary to obtain good results (Tajbakhsh et al. 2016). In the future, prospective and multicenter studies may help to construct a more generalizable prediction model that is appropriate for different clinical situations. Additionally, the current research datasets usually contain a mix of histological and molecular breast cancer subtypes, which are known to possess distinct imaging phenotypes and disparate rates of therapeutic response (Carey et al. 2006; Nguyen et al. 2008). Ideally, a deep learning-based approach to response prediction would either consist of distinct CNNs trained to recognize responses within individual subtypes or leverage enough training examples of each subtype for a single network to learn their individual nuances. Furthermore, integration of the radiological characteristics with histopathological data from biopsy specimen, genetic information, and general patient characteristics should be pursued to enhance the classification robustness and performance.

4 Challenges and Future Directions

The development and implementation of artificial intelligence (AI) for breast imaging have been ongoing for several decades, and AI is

Table 5 AI in breast imaging for therapy selection and outcome prediction

Image modality	Reference	Collected term	Dataset	Outcome	Key findings
DCE-MRI	Ha et al. (2019b)	Pre-NAC	Included 141 patients (46 pCR, 57 partial response, 38 non-pCR)	AUC = 0.98 (three-class prediction) Accuracy = 0.88	It is feasible for current deep learning architectures to be trained to predict NAC treatment response using a breast MRI dataset obtained prior to initiation of chemotherapy.
	Ravichandran et al. (2018)	Pre-NAC	Included 166 patients (49 pCR, 117 non-pCR)	AUC = 0.77	The proposed deep learning model was able to predict therapy response and produce probability heatmaps that visualized tumor regions that most strongly predicted therapeutic response.
	Huynh et al. (2017)	Pre-NAC	Included 64 patients (39 pCR, 25 non-pCR)	AUC = 0.85	The pre-contrast time point seems to be the most effective at predicting response to therapy.
	Braman et al. (2020)	Pre-NAC	Included 157 patients: 85 patients (50 pCR, 50 non-pCR) External test 1: 28 patients (16 pCR, 13 non-pCR) External test 2: 29 patients (10 pCR, 19 non-pCR)	AUC = 0.93 (internal date) AUC = 0.85 (external test 1) AUC = 0.77 (external test 2)	A multi-input deep learning model leveraging both pre-contrast and late post-contrast DCE-MRI acquisitions was identified to achieve optimal response prediction within the validation set.
	Qu et al. (2020)	Pre-NAC and post-NAC	Included 302 patients (132 pCR, 170 non-pCR)	AUC = 0.553 (pre-NAC) AUC = 0.968 (post-NAC) AUC = 0.970 (combined)	The ensemble model performed better than using pre-NAC data only and also performed better than using post-NAC data only.
	El Adoui et al. (2020)	Pre-NAC and post-NAC	Included 42 patients (14 pCR, 28 non-pCR) External test:14 cases (6 responders and 8 nonresponders)	AUC = 0.91	The proposed and developed deep learning model using DCE-MR images acquired before and after the first chemotherapy was able to classify pCR and non-pCR patients with substantial accuracy.
PET/MRI	Choi et al. (2020)	Pre-NAC and post-NAC	Included 56 patients (6 pCR, 50 non-pCR)	AUC = 0.805	The deep learning model could predict pathologic responses to NAC in patients with advanced breast cancer.
Mammography	Rabinovici-Cohen et al. (2020)	Pre-NAC	Included 528 patients (140 pCR, 388 non-pCR)	AUC = 0.708	Deep learning model with texture extractions is used on mammograms for NACT prediction.

poised to play a more critical role in breast cancer screening, diagnosis, and therapy selection. Still, there are large challenges to these novel AI applications.

Interpretability is the first challenge of AI systems. To effectively apply the AI systems to the clinic, their findings must be comprehensible for humans (Geras et al. 2019; Chan et al. 2020). Some researchers have developed visualization methods that use a heatmap or feature map to display the corresponding regions on the input image that can influence the prediction made by AI systems (Zeiler and Fergus 2014; Yosinski et al. 2015; Zhou et al. 2016). However, these visualization methods are only preliminary and cannot be used clinically. This problem must therefore be further addressed and, beyond improving the understanding of the AI system's predictions, indicates which suspicious areas in breast images could be used to plan and analyze subsequent examinations.

The second challenge regards to the datasets. For the purpose of improving the performance of the AI-based system in a specific clinical application, it is necessary to collect large datasets with appropriate labeling from trained professionals (Chan et al. 2020; Thrall et al. 2018; Bi et al. 2019). Because the training sample size is an important factor that impacts the robustness of the trained model, specifically, only a sufficiently large and accurately labeled dataset can enable the deep learning model to learn various types and subtleties from cancer images (Chan et al. 2020). Certain techniques can be used in limited datasets, such as transfer learning, but these methods do not obviate the need for adequate representation of the disease of interest in the training dataset (Chan et al. 2020; Chartrand et al. 2017; Do et al. 2020; Litjens et al. 2017; Bahl 2020). Prior to widespread deployment, AI systems require thorough tests with true independent sets and evaluation in a clinical setting with large and heterogeneous populations. This urgently requires collaborative efforts from multiple institutions to compile big patient datasets across vendors.

Finally, the ultimate target is to implement the advances in AI in such a way that their clinical impact is maximized. For this target, national and international collaborations between radiologists, computer scientists, academia, and industry are necessary to regulate the integration of AI systems rapidly, safely, and effectively (Le et al. 2019). In addition, physicians will require training to understand the appropriate use and limitations of AI systems (Chan et al. 2020; Bahl 2020) that could be used in various clinical scenarios.

Overall, even with these challenges, it is expected that AI will play a major role in various clinical applications of breast imaging, albeit the level of autonomy is likely dependent on the use case for which it is employed.

References

Al-Antari MA, Al-Masni MA, Choi MT, Han SM, Kim TS (2018) A fully integrated computer-aided diagnosis system for digital X-ray mammograms via deep learning detection, segmentation, and classification. Int J Med Inform 117:44–54

Al-Masni MA, Al-Antari MA, Park J-M, Gi G, Kim T-Y, Rivera P et al (2018) Simultaneous detection and classification of breast masses in digital mammograms via a deep learning YOLO-based CAD system. Comput Methods Programs Biomed 157:85–94

Arefan D, Mohamed AA, Berg WA, Zuley ML, Sumkin JH, Wu S (2020) Deep learning modeling using normal mammograms for predicting breast cancer risk. Med Phys 47(1):110–118

Bahl M (2020) Artificial intelligence: a primer for breast imaging radiologists. J Breast Imaging 2(4):304–314

Barinov L, Jairaj A, Becker M, Seymour S, Lee E, Schram A et al (2019) Impact of data presentation on physician performance utilizing artificial intelligence-based computer-aided diagnosis and decision support systems. J Digit Imaging 32(3):408–416

Bejnordi BE, Veta M, Van Diest PJ, Van Ginneken B, Karssemeijer N, Litjens G et al (2017) Diagnostic assessment of deep learning algorithms for detection of lymph node metastases in women with breast cancer. JAMA 318(22):2199–2210

Bi WL, Hosny A, Schabath MB, Giger ML, Birkbak NJ, Mehrtash A et al (2019) Artificial intelligence in cancer imaging: clinical challenges and applications. CA Cancer J Clin 69(2):127–157

Boulehmi H, Mahersia H, Hamrouni K (2016) A new CAD system for breast microcalcifications diagnosis. Int J Adv Comput Sci Appl 7(4):133–143

Braman N, Adoui ME, Vulchi M, Turk P, Etesami M, Fu P et al (2020) Deep learning-based prediction of response to HER2-targeted neoadjuvant chemotherapy from pre-treatment dynamic breast MRI: a multi-institutional validation study. arXiv preprint arXiv:08570

Brem RF, Baum J, Lechner M, Kaplan S, Souders S, Naul LG et al (2003) Improvement in sensitivity of screening mammography with computer-aided detection: a multiinstitutional trial. AJR Am J Roentgenol 181(3):687–693

Brentnall AR, Harkness EF, Astley SM, Donnelly LS, Stavrinos P, Sampson S et al (2015) Mammographic density adds accuracy to both the Tyrer-Cuzick and Gail breast cancer risk models in a prospective UK screening cohort. Breast Cancer Res 17(1):1–10

Carey LA, Perou CM, Livasy CA, Dressler LG, Cowan D, Conway K et al (2006) Race, breast cancer subtypes, and survival in the Carolina Breast Cancer Study. JAMA 295(21):2492–2502

Chan HP, Doi K, Galhotra S, Vyborny CJ, MacMahon H, Jokich PM (1987) Image feature analysis and computer-aided diagnosis in digital radiography. I. Automated detection of microcalcifications in mammography. Med Phys 14(4):538–548

Chan HP, Doi K, Vyborny CJ, Schmidt RA, Metz CE, Lam KL et al (1990) Improvement in radiologists' detection of clustered microcalcifications on mammograms. The potential of computer-aided diagnosis. Invest Radiol 25(10):1102–1110

Chan HP, Samala RK, Hadjiiski LM (2020) CAD and AI for breast cancer-recent development and challenges. Br J Radiol 93(1108):20190580

Chartrand G, Cheng PM, Vorontsov E, Drozdzal M, Turcotte S, Pal CJ et al (2017) Deep learning: a primer for radiologists. Radiographics 37(7):2113–2131

Chen T, Guestrin C (2016) Xgboost: a scalable tree boosting system. In: Proceedings of the 22nd ACM SIGKDD international conference on knowledge discovery and data mining

Cho E, Kim EK, Song MK, Yoon JH (2018) Application of computer-aided diagnosis on breast ultrasonography: evaluation of diagnostic performances and agreement of radiologists according to different levels of experience. J Ultrasound Med 37(1):209–216

Choi JH, Kim H-A, Kim W, Lim I, Lee I, Byun BH et al (2020) Early prediction of neoadjuvant chemotherapy response for advanced breast cancer using PET/MRI image deep learning. Sci Rep 10(1):1–11

Ciritsis A, Rossi C, Eberhard M, Marcon M, Becker AS, Boss A (2019) Automatic classification of ultrasound breast lesions using a deep convolutional neural network mimicking human decision-making. Eur Radiol 29(10):5458–5468

Conant EF, Toledano AY, Periaswamy S, Fotin SV, Go J, Boatsman JE et al (2019) Improving accuracy and efficiency with concurrent use of artificial intelligence for digital breast tomosynthesis. Radiol Artif Intell 1(4):e180096

Cong J, Wei B, He Y, Yin Y, Zheng Y (2017) A selective ensemble classification method combining mammography images with ultrasound images for breast cancer diagnosis. Comput Math Methods Med 2017:4896386

Dalmış MU, Vreemann S, Kooi T, Mann RM, Karssemeijer N, Gubern-Mérida A (2018) Fully automated detection of breast cancer in screening MRI using convolutional neural networks. J Med Imaging 5(1):014502

Dalmis MU, Gubern-Merida A, Vreemann S, Bult P, Karssemeijer N, Mann R et al (2019) Artificial intelligence-based classification of breast lesions imaged with a multiparametric breast MRI protocol with ultrafast DCE-MRI, T2, and DWI. Invest Radiol 54(6):325–332

Dembrower K, Liu Y, Azizpour H, Eklund M, Smith K, Lindholm P et al (2020) Comparison of a deep learning risk score and standard mammographic density score for breast cancer risk prediction. Radiology 294(2):265–272

Do S, Song KD, Chung JW (2020) Basics of deep learning: a radiologist's guide to understanding published radiology articles on deep learning. Korean J Radiol 21(1):33–41

Dorrius MD, Jansen-van der Weide MC, van Ooijen PM, Pijnappel RM, Oudkerk M (2011) Computer-aided detection in breast MRI: a systematic review and meta-analysis. Eur Radiol 21(8):1600–1608

El Adoui M, Drisis S, Benjelloun M (2020) Multi-input deep learning architecture for predicting breast tumor response to chemotherapy using quantitative MR images. Int J Comput Assist Radiol Surg 15(9):1491–1500

Elmore JG, Jackson SL, Abraham L, Miglioretti DL, Carney PA, Geller BM et al (2009) Variability in interpretive performance at screening mammography and radiologists' characteristics associated with accuracy. Radiology 253(3):641–651

Faneyte IF, Schrama JG, Peterse JL, Remijnse PL, Rodenhuis S, van de Vijver MJ (2003) Breast cancer response to neoadjuvant chemotherapy: predictive markers and relation with outcome. Br J Cancer 88(3):406–412

Fathy WE, Ghoneim AS (2019) A deep learning approach for breast cancer mass detection. Int J Adv Comput Sci Appl 10(1). https://doi.org/10.14569/IJACSA.2019.0100123

Fenton JJ, Taplin SH, Carney PA, Abraham L, Sickles EA, D'Orsi C et al (2007) Influence of computer-aided detection on performance of screening mammography. N Engl J Med 356(14):1399–1409

Fujioka T, Kubota K, Mori M, Kikuchi Y, Katsuta L, Kasahara M et al (2019) Distinction between benign and malignant breast masses at breast ultrasound using deep learning method with convolutional neural network. Jpn J Radiol 37(6):466–472

Geras KJ, Mann RM, Moy L (2019) Artificial intelligence for mammography and digital breast tomosynthesis: current concepts and future perspectives. Radiology 293(2):246–259

Ha R, Chang P, Karcich J, Mutasa S, Van Sant EP, Liu MZ et al (2019a) Convolutional neural network based breast cancer risk stratification using a mammographic dataset. Acad Radiol 26(4):544–549

Ha R, Chin C, Karcich J, Liu MZ, Chang P, Mutasa S et al (2019b) Prior to initiation of chemotherapy, can we predict breast tumor response? Deep learning convolutional neural networks approach using a breast MRI tumor dataset. J Digit Imaging 32(5):693–701

Habib G, Kiryati N, Sklair-Levy M, Shalmon A, Neiman OH, Weidenfeld RF et al (2020) Automatic breast lesion classification by joint neural analysis of mammography and ultrasound. Multimodal learning for clinical decision support and clinical image-based procedures. Springer, New York, pp 125–135

He T, Puppala M, Ezeana CF, Huang YS, Chou PH, Yu X et al (2019) A deep learning-based decision support tool for precision risk assessment of breast cancer. JCO Clin Cancer Inform 3:1–12

Herent P, Schmauch B, Jehanno P, Dehaene O, Saillard C, Balleyguier C et al (2019) Detection and characterization of MRI breast lesions using deep learning. Diagn Interv Imaging 100(4):219–225

Houssami N, Hunter K (2017) The epidemiology, radiology and biological characteristics of interval breast cancers in population mammography screening. NPJ Breast Cancer 3(1):12

Huang Q, Zhang F, Li X (2018) Machine learning in ultrasound computer-aided diagnostic systems: a survey. Biomed Res Int 2018:5137904

Huynh BQ, Antropova N, Giger ML (2017) Comparison of breast DCE-MRI contrast time points for predicting response to neoadjuvant chemotherapy using deep convolutional neural network features with transfer learning. In: Medical imaging 2017: computer-aided diagnosis. International Society for Optics and Photonics, Bellingham, WA

Jackson A, O'Connor JP, Parker GJ, Jayson GC (2007) Imaging tumor vascular heterogeneity and angiogenesis using dynamic contrast-enhanced magnetic resonance imaging. Clin Cancer Res 13(12):3449–3459

Kaufmann M, Hortobagyi GN, Goldhirsch A, Scholl S, Makris A, Valagussa P et al (2006) Recommendations from an international expert panel on the use of neoadjuvant (primary) systemic treatment of operable breast cancer: an update. J Clin Oncol 24(12):1940–1949

Kimme C, O'Loughlin BJ, Sklansky J (1977) Automatic detection of suspicious abnormalities in breast radiographs. In: Data structures, computer graphics, and pattern recognition. Elsevier, Amsterdam, pp 427–447

Le EPV, Wang Y, Huang Y, Hickman S, Gilbert FJ (2019) Artificial intelligence in breast imaging. Clin Radiol 74(5):357–366

LeCun Y, Bengio Y, Hinton G (2015) Deep learning. Nature 521(7553):436–444

Lee CI, Elmore JG (2019) Artificial intelligence for breast cancer imaging: the new frontier? Oxford University Press, Oxford

Lehman CD, Lee JM, DeMartini WB, Hippe DS, Rendi MH, Kalish G et al (2016) Screening MRI in women with a personal history of breast cancer. J Natl Cancer Inst 108(3):djv349

Li H, Giger ML, Huynh BQ, Antropova NO (2017) Deep learning in breast cancer risk assessment: evaluation of convolutional neural networks on a clinical dataset of full-field digital mammograms. J Med Imaging (Bellingham) 4(4):041304

Litjens G, Kooi T, Bejnordi BE, Setio AAA, Ciompi F, Ghafoorian M et al (2017) A survey on deep learning in medical image analysis. Med Image Anal 42:60–88

Liu Y, Azizpour H, Strand F, Smith K (eds) (2020) Decoupling inherent risk and early cancer signs in image-based breast cancer risk models. International conference on medical image computing and computer-assisted intervention. Springer, New York

Louro J, Posso M, Hilton Boon M, Roman M, Domingo L, Castells X et al (2019) A systematic review and quality assessment of individualised breast cancer risk prediction models. Br J Cancer 121(1):76–85

Mann RM, Hooley R, Barr RG, Moy L (2020) Novel approaches to screening for breast cancer. Radiology 297(2):266–285

McKinney SM, Sieniek M, Godbole V, Godwin J, Antropova N, Ashrafian H et al (2020) International evaluation of an AI system for breast cancer screening. Nature 577(7788):89–94

Meyer-Base A, Morra L, Meyer-Base U, Pinker K (2020) Current status and future perspectives of artificial intelligence in magnetic resonance breast imaging. Contrast Media Mol Imaging 2020:6805710

Miglioretti DL, Smith-Bindman R, Abraham L, Brenner RJ, Carney PA, Bowles EJ et al (2007) Radiologist characteristics associated with interpretive performance of diagnostic mammography. J Natl Cancer Inst 99(24):1854–1863

Nguyen PL, Taghian AG, Katz MS, Niemierko A, Abi Raad RF, Boon WL et al (2008) Breast cancer subtype approximated by estrogen receptor, progesterone receptor, and HER-2 is associated with local and distant recurrence after breast-conserving therapy. J Clin Oncol 26(14):2373–2378

Nishikawa RM (2007) Current status and future directions of computer-aided diagnosis in mammography. Comput Med Imaging Graph 31(4–5):224–235

Ou WC, Polat D, Dogan BE (2021) Deep learning in breast radiology: current progress and future directions. Eur Radiol 31(7):4872–4885

Pang T, Wong JHD, Ng WL, Chan CS (2020) Deep learning radiomics in breast cancer with different modalities: overview and future. Expert Syst Appl 2020:113501

Qu YH, Zhu HT, Cao K, Li XT, Ye M, Sun YS (2020) Prediction of pathological complete response to neoadjuvant chemotherapy in breast cancer using a deep learning (DL) method. Thorac Cancer 11(3):651–658

Rabinovici-Cohen S, Tlusty T, Abutbul A, Antila K, Fernandez X, Rejo BG et al (2020) Radiomics for predicting response to neoadjuvant chemotherapy treatment in breast cancer. In: Medical imaging 2020: imaging informatics for healthcare, research, and applications. International Society for Optics and Photonics, Bellingham, WA

Ravichandran K, Braman N, Janowczyk A, Madabhushi A (2018) A deep learning classifier for prediction of pathological complete response to neoadjuvant chemotherapy from baseline breast DCE-MRI. In: Medical imaging 2018: computer-aided diagnosis. International Society for Optics and Photonics, Bellingham, WA

Reig B, Heacock L, Geras KJ, Moy L (2020) Machine learning in breast MRI. J Magn Reson Imaging 52(4):998–1018

Rodriguez-Ruiz A, Lång K, Gubern-Merida A, Teuwen J, Broeders M, Gennaro G et al (2019a) Can we reduce the workload of mammographic screening by automatic identification of normal exams with artificial intelligence? A feasibility study. Eur Radiol 29(9):4825–4832

Rodriguez-Ruiz A, Krupinski E, Mordang JJ, Schilling K, Heywang-Kobrunner SH, Sechopoulos I et al (2019b) Detection of breast cancer with mammography: effect of an artificial intelligence support system. Radiology 290(2):305–314

Roehrig J, Doi T, Hasegawa A, Hunt B, Marshall J, Romsdahl H et al (1998) Clinical results with R2 imagechecker system. In: Digital mammography. Springer, New York, pp 395–400

Samala RK, Chan HP, Hadjiiski L, Helvie MA, Wei J, Cha K (2016) Mass detection in digital breast tomosynthesis: deep convolutional neural network with transfer learning from mammography. Med Phys 43(12):6654

Samala RK, Chan H-P, Hadjiiski L, Helvie MA, Richter CD, Cha KH (2018) Breast cancer diagnosis in digital breast tomosynthesis: effects of training sample size on multi-stage transfer learning using deep neural nets. IEEE Trans Med Imaging 38(3):686–696

Schaffter T, Buist DSM, Lee CI, Nikulin Y, Ribli D, Guan Y et al (2020) Evaluation of combined artificial intelligence and radiologist assessment to interpret screening mammograms. JAMA Netw Open 3(3):e200265

Schott AF, Hayes DF (2012) Defining the benefits of neoadjuvant chemotherapy for breast cancer. J Clin Oncol 30(15):1747–1749

Sechopoulos I, Teuwen J, Mann R (eds) (2020) Artificial intelligence for breast cancer detection in mammography and digital breast tomosynthesis: state of the art, Seminars in cancer biology. Elsevier, Amsterdam

Semmlow JL, Shadagopappan A, Ackerman LV, Hand W, Alcorn FS (1980) A fully automated system for screening xeromammograms. Comput Biomed Res 13(4):350–362

Spiesberger W (1979) Mammogram inspection by computer. IEEE Trans Biomed Eng 26(4):213–219

Sun YS, Zhao Z, Yang ZN, Xu F, Lu HJ, Zhu ZY et al (2017) Risk factors and preventions of breast cancer. Int J Biol Sci 13(11):1387–1397

Tabar L, Dean PB, Chen TH, Yen AM, Chen SL, Fann JC et al (2019) The incidence of fatal breast cancer measures the increased effectiveness of therapy in women participating in mammography screening. Cancer 125(4):515–523

Tajbakhsh N, Shin JY, Gurudu SR, Hurst RT, Kendall CB, Gotway MB et al (2016) Convolutional neural networks for medical image analysis: full training or fine tuning? IEEE Trans Med Imaging 35(5):1299–1312

Thompson AM, Moulder-Thompson SL (2012) Neoadjuvant treatment of breast cancer. Ann Oncol 23(Suppl 10):x231–x236

Thrall JH, Li X, Li Q, Cruz C, Do S, Dreyer K et al (2018) Artificial intelligence and machine learning in radiology: opportunities, challenges, pitfalls, and criteria for success. J Am Coll Radiol 15(3 Pt B):504–508

Tosteson AN, Fryback DG, Hammond CS, Hanna LG, Grove MR, Brown M et al (2014) Consequences of false-positive screening mammograms. JAMA Intern Med 174(6):954–961

Truhn D, Schrading S, Haarburger C, Schneider H, Merhof D, Kuhl C (2019) Radiomic versus convolutional neural networks analysis for classification of contrast-enhancing lesions at multiparametric breast MRI. Radiology 290(2):290–297

van Zelst JCM, Tan T, Clauser P, Domingo A, Dorrius MD, Drieling D et al (2018) Dedicated computer-aided detection software for automated 3D breast ultrasound; an efficient tool for the radiologist in supplemental screening of women with dense breasts. Eur Radiol 28(7):2996–3006

Wang J, Miao J, Yang X, Li R, Zhou G, Huang Y et al (eds) (2020) Auto-weighting for breast cancer classification in multimodal ultrasound. International conference on medical image computing and computer-assisted intervention. Springer, New York

Winsberg F, Elkin M, Macy J Jr, Bordaz V, Weymouth W (1967) Detection of radiographic abnormalities in mammograms by means of optical scanning and computer analysis. Radiology 89(2):211–215

Wu N, Phang J, Park J, Shen Y, Huang Z, Zorin M et al (2020) Deep neural networks improve radiologists' performance in breast cancer screening. IEEE Trans Med Imaging 39(4):1184–1194

Xu X, Bao L, Tan Y, Zhu L, Kong F, Wang W (2018) 1000-Case reader study of radiologists' performance in interpretation of automated breast volume scanner images with a computer-aided detection system. Ultrasound Med Biol 44(8):1694–1702

Yala A, Lehman C, Schuster T, Portnoi T, Barzilay R (2019a) A deep learning mammography-based model for improved breast cancer risk prediction. Radiology 292(1):60–66

Yala A, Schuster T, Miles R, Barzilay R, Lehman C (2019b) A deep learning model to triage screening mammograms: a simulation study. Radiology 293(1):38–46

Yala A, Mikhael PG, Strand F, Lin G, Smith K, Wan YL et al (2021) Toward robust mammography-based models for breast cancer risk. Sci Transl Med 13(578):eaba4373

Yap MH, Pons G, Marti J, Ganau S, Sentis M, Zwiggelaar R et al (2017) Automated breast ultrasound lesions detection using convolutional neural networks. IEEE J Biomed Health Inform 22(4):1218–1226

Yosinski J, Clune J, Nguyen A, Fuchs T, Lipson H (2015) Understanding neural networks through deep visualization. arXiv preprint arXiv:06579

Zeiler MD, Fergus R (2014) Visualizing and understanding convolutional networks. European conference on computer vision. Springer, New York

Zhou B, Khosla A, Lapedriza A, Oliva A, Torralba A, editors. Learning deep features for discriminative localization. Proceedings of the IEEE conference on computer vision and pattern recognition; 2016

Zhou J, Zhang Y, Chang KT, Lee KE, Wang O, Li J et al (2020) Diagnosis of benign and malignant breast lesions on DCE-MRI by using radiomics and deep learning with consideration of peritumor tissue. J Magn Reson Imaging 51(3):798–809